Drug	Use	Dosage	Route	Side effects	Other medical issues
Antihypertensives					
ACE inhibitors	Antihypertensive	—	PO, IV	Nephrotic syndrome	Works via inhibition of renin-angiotensin conversion
α-Blockers (Minipress)	Antihypertensive, treatment to control sympathetic dystrophy	—	PO, IV	Syncope, sedation, headache, urinary retention	Acts as a vasodilator via peripheral vasodilation or central inhibitors
β-Blockers	Antihypertensive	—	PO, IV	CHF, bradycardia, hypotension, PVD	Decreases cardiac contractility and inotropy
Calcium-channel blockers	Antihypertensive	—	PO, IV	Dizziness, headache, hypotension	Acts as a vasodilator via a calcium channel blockade
Direct vasodilators	Antihypertensive	—	PO, IV	Tachycardia, hypotension, headache	—
Diuretics	Antihypertensive	—	PO, IV	Metabolic or electrolyte imbalance, cramps, hypotension, renal failure	Decreases volume in vascular spaces
Postganglionic neuron inhibitors	Antihypertensive	—	PO, IV	Diarrhea, hypotension, depression	Acts as a vasodilator via inhibition of postganglionic sympathetic neurons
Antidepressants					
Fluoxetine (Prozac)	Antidepressant	20-80 mg qd-bid	PO	Anxiety, tremor, insomnia, nausea, diarrhea	—
MAO inhibitors	Antidepressant	—	PO	Dizziness, vertigo, headache, constipation, HTN	Should avoid concurrent use of tyramine/tryptophan
Sertraline (Zoloft)	Antidepressant	50-200 mg qd-bid	PO	Anxiety, tremor, insomnia, nausea, diarrhea	—
Tricyclics, e.g., amitriptyline, nortriptyline, desipramine	Antidepressant, treatment to control pain, adjuvant	—	PO	MI, hypotension, seizures, confusion, leukopenia, parasthesias, nausea and vomiting, coma, constipation, hepatitis	Is best for treating continuous neuropathic pain
Steroids					
Androgenic steroids	Treatment for testicular insufficiency, antineoplastic	25-50 mg monthly	IM	Muscle wasting, weakness	Only used for hormonal replacement
Betamethasone (Celestone)	Treatment for inflammation and pain	1-9 mg injection per treatment	IM, intra-articular	Mental status changes, osteoporosis, peptic ulcer, glaucoma, DM, HTN	—
Cortisone	Treatment for Addison's disease and conditions such as inflammation, swelling, rashes, asthma, and arthritis	35-70 mg qd	PO	Mental status changes, osteoporosis, peptic ulcer, glaucoma, DM, HTN	—
Dexamethasone (Decadron)	Treatment for acute spinal cord injury, inflammation, and swelling	0.75-10 mg up to 1 g per treatment	PO, IV	Mental status changes, osteoporosis, peptic ulcer, glaucoma, DM, HTN	1 mg = 20 mg cortisone
Hydrocortisone	Treatment for conditions such as inflammation, swelling, rashes, asthma, and arthritis	Depends on route	IV, PO, IM, topical	Mental status changes, osteoporosis, peptic ulcer, glaucoma, DM, HTN	1 mg = 1 mg cortisone
Prednisone (Deltasone)	Treatment for conditions such as inflammation, swelling, asthma, and arthritis	5-60 mg qd	PO	Mental status changes, osteoporosis, peptic ulcer, glaucoma, DM, HTN	1 mg = 5 mg cortisone

Continued on back inside cover

Stroke Rehabilitation

A Function-Based Approach

Stroke Rehabilitation

A Function-Based Approach

Stroke Rehabilitation

A Function-Based Approach

GLEN GILLEN, MPA, OTR/L, BCN

Supervisor, Inpatient Rehabilitation
Occupational Therapy, Department of Rehabilitation Medicine,
Columbia-Presbyterian Medical Center;
Clinical Instructor, Program in Occupational Therapy,
College of Physicians and Surgeons, Columbia University,
New York, New York

ANN BURKHARDT, MA, OTR/L, BCN

Assistant Director,
Occupational Therapy, Department of Rehabilitation Medicine,
Columbia-Presbyterian Medical Center;
Clinical Instructor, Program in Occupational Therapy,
College of Physicians and Surgeons, Columbia University,
New York, New York

with 29 contributors
with 458 illustrations

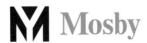 Mosby

St. Louis Baltimore Boston Carlsbad Chicago Minneapolis New York Philadelphia Portland
London Milan Sydney Tokyo Toronto

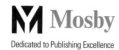
Mosby
Dedicated to Publishing Excellence

Vice President and Publisher Don Ladig
Executive Editor Martha Sasser
Developmental Editor Amy Christopher
Editorial Assistant Laura MacAdam
Project Manager Linda McKinley
Senior Production Editor Catherine Comer
Designer Elizabeth Young
Illustrations by Jeanne Robertson

Composition by Top Graphics
Printing/binding by Maple-Vail

Mosby, Inc.
11830 Westline Industrial Drive
St. Louis, MO 63146

International Standard Book Number: 0-8151-3460-6

98 99 00 01 02 / 9 8 7 6 5 4 3 2

Contributors

Lorraine Aloisio, OTR
Private Practitioner,
Pediatric Therapy Unlimited;
Consultant,
Long Island School Districts,
Long Island, New York

Guðrún Árnadóttir, MA, BOT
Private Practitioner,
Reykjavík, Iceland

Beverly K. Bain, EdD, OTR, FAOTA
Coordinator of RSA Technology
   Grant,
Occupational Therapy
   Department,
New York University,
New York, New York

Matthew N. Bartels, MD, MPH
Assistant Attending,
Department of Rehabilitation
   Medicine,
Columbia-Presbyterian Medical
   Center;
Assistant Professor of Clinical
   Rehabilitation Medicine,
College of Physicians and
   Surgeons,
Columbia University,
New York, New York

Karen A. Buckley, MA, OTR/L
Clinical Assistant Professor,
Department of Occupational
   Therapy,
New York University,
New York, New York

Ann Burkhardt, MA, OTR/L, BCN
Assistant Director,
Occupational Therapy,
Department of Rehabilitation
   Medicine,
Columbia-Presbyterian Medical
   Center;
Clinical Instructor,
Program in Occupational Therapy,
College of Physicians and
   Surgeons,
Columbia University,
New York, New York

Salvatore DiMauro, MD
Lucy G. Moses Professor of
   Neurology,
Department of Neurology,
College of Physicians and
   Surgeons,
Columbia University,
New York, New York

Susan M. Donato, BS, OT
Director of Occupational Therapy,
Occupational Therapy
   Department,
Greenery of North Andover,
Rehab Works,
North Andover, MA

Jessica Farman, MS, OTR/L
Occupational Therapist,
Department of Rehabilitation,
VNA of Boston,
Boston, Massachusetts

Carol G. Fraley, MA, OTR
Director, Occupational Therapy,
Department of Rehabilitation
   Medicine,
Columbia Presbyterian Medical
   Center,
Associate in Clinical Occupational
   Therapy,
Columbia University,
New York, New York

Judith Dicker Friedman, MA, OTR/L
Adjunct Faculty,
Occupational Therapy
   Department,
New York University,
New York, New York

Glen Gillen, MPA, OTR/L, BCN
Supervisor,
Inpatient Rehabilitation,
Occupational Therapy,
Department of Rehabilitation
   Medicine,
Columbia-Presbyterian Medical
   Center;
Clinical Instructor,
Program in Occupational Therapy,
College of Physicians and
   Surgeons,
Columbia University,
New York, New York

Sheila M. Hayes, BS, RN, MS, PT
Advanced Clinician in
   Rehabilitation,
Physical Therapy Department,
Columbia-Presbyterian Medical
   Center,
New York, New York

Lauren Joachim-Grizzaffi, MA, OTR/L
Supervisor,
Acute Care Occupational Therapy Department,
Columbia-Presbyterian Medical Center;
Clinical Instructor,
Occupational Therapy Department,
New York University,
New York, New York

Christine M. Johann, OTR
Seating and Positioning Consultant,
Private Practitioner,
Long Island, New York;
Adjunct Professor;
Clinical Instructor,
Occupational Therapy Department,
School of Health Technology,
State University of New York at Stony Brook,
Stony Brook, New York

Leslie A. Kane, OTR/L
Clinical Program Advisor,
Brain Injury Unit,
Mount Sinai Medical Center,
New York, New York

Stephanie Milazzo, MA, OTR
Department of Hand and Occupational Therapy,
HealthSouth—Somers,
Somers, New York

Steve Park, MS, OTR/L
Assistant Professor,
School of Occupational Therapy,
Pacific University,
Forest Grove, Oregon

Terry A. Pavlou, COTA
Occupational Therapy,
Department of Rehabilitation Medicine,
Columbia-Presbyterian Medical Center,
New York, New York

Susan L. Pierce, BS, OTR, CDRS
President,
Adaptive Mobility Services, Inc.,
Orlando, Florida

Karen Halliday Pulaski, MS, OTR/L
Supervisor,
Occupational Therapy Inpatient Rehabilitation,
Rehabilitation Services Department,
Moses Cone Memorial Hospital,
Greensboro, North Carolina

Kerry Brockmann Rubio, MHS, OTR/L, BCN
Staff Occupational Therapist,
Rehab Management, Inc,
Raleigh, North Carolina

Patricia A. Ryan, MA, OTR/L
Senior Occupational Therapist,
Department of Occupational Therapy,
Columbia-Presbyterian Medical Center;
Lecturer,
Programs in Occupational Therapy,
Columbia University,
New York, New York

Joyce Shapero Sabari, PhD, OTR, BCN
Associate Professor,
Department of Occupational Therapy,
New York University,
New York, New York

Catherine A. Salerno, OTR/L, BCN
Advanced Clinician,
Occupational Therapy Department,
Columbia-Presbyterian Medical Center;
Lecturer,
Program in Occupational Therapy,
Columbia University,
New York, New York

Roberta Ann Schroeder-Lopez, MS, OTR
Supervisor of Occupational Therapy,
The Allen Pavillion,
Columbia-Presbyterian Medical Center,
New York, New York

Anne Marie Skvarla, MA, CCC-SLP
Director,
Speech Pathology,
Department of Rehabilitation Medicine,
Columbia-Presbyterian Medical Center;
Clinical Instructor,
Columbia University,
College of Physicians and Surgeons;
Adjunct Assistant Professor,
Speech and Language Pathology Department,
New York University,
New York, New York

Jennie W. Sullivan, MA, OTR/L
Private Practitioner,
New York, New York

Denise A. Supon, MA, OTR/L
Senior Occupational Therapist,
Outpatient Occupational Therapy Department,
Rusk Institute of Rehabilitation Medicine,
New York University Medical Center,
New York, New York

Jeffrey L. Tomlinson, OTR, CSW
Senior Occupational Therapist,
N.Y.S. Psychiatric Institute,
New York, New York

Nancy C. Whyte, OTR/L
Clinical Supervisor,
Occupational Therapy Department,
Rusk Institute,
New York University Medical Center,
New York, New York

To the patients who have challenged us and taught us to value and appreciate each day of life, without whom we would not have meaning or purpose in our professional lives.

To the talented professionals with whom we have worked and by whom we have been trained. You have challenged our minds and given us inspiration to share our experiences and to contribute to the development of theory in functionally based rehabilitation. We hope our contribution will challenge currently practicing therapists to think and question treatment approaches so that there is ongoing development of theory and practice in neuro-rehabilitation in the future.

Glen Gillen and Ann Burkhardt

To Gary, who taught me how to fish.

Glen Gillen

To Ken, Betty, Hattie, and Elva, who always told me I could.

Ann Burkhardt

Foreword

In an era of scientific breakthroughs the reality that 550,000 men and women are affected by strokes each year serves as a strong motivator to search for the most effective ways of providing services to this special population. Equally, the fact that a majority of employed occupational therapists treat stroke patients gives rise to the imperative underlying the publication of *Stroke Rehabilitation: A Function-Based Approach*, the first comprehensive text on stroke written primarily by and for occupational therapists and other neurorehabilitation specialists. This book is long overdue—a text that provides professionals an exhaustive resource in a single volume. Editors Glen Gillen and Ann Burkhardt are to be commended for taking on the immense task of conceptualizing and organizing the book. Both have considerable experience as clinicians and educators and know the needs of learners at all levels. They have succeeded in selecting a group of authors with extensive knowledge in particular aspects of stroke rehabilitation.

The overall plan for the book reflects the global nature of a full rehabilitation program that takes the patient from acute care through all aspects of therapy to reentry into community living. The 27 chapters cover direct intervention with patients, approaches that address environmental changes for facilitating function, and approaches that focus on aspects of the total system in which the rehabilitation takes place. This structure allows for presentation of issues such as psychosocial aspects of coping with stroke; working with families; the partnership between the occupational therapist and the certified occupational therapy assistant; total quality assurance; and topics such as sexuality, leisure, and driving that are particularly relevant for patients nearing the end of their rehabilitation.

Each author introduces new information through a thorough review of literature on the chapter topic. The writing also keeps the focus on function in its broadest sense. The content is directed toward remediation, as well as attaining function through adaptation.

This function-based approach to stroke rehabilitation not only acknowledges the complexity of patient needs, but also the economic realities of providing health care in an environment of managed care and reimbursement restrictions. The sound, practical focus of the book's content provides a solid foundation for students who are learning about stroke rehabilitation for the first time, as well as for occupational therapy practitioners who need to enrich their clinical base with new knowledge. Each chapter provides useful learning tools such as objectives, key terms, and review questions to develop the reasoning skills of the learners. The case studies that accompany the chapters furnish readers with helpful examples of ways to apply theoretical information. An extensive list of references on each topic directs the reader to additional resources. The numerous illustrations throughout the text and the detailed information regarding several standardized assessment tools are particularly valuable.

Stroke Rehabilitation: A Function-Based Approach fills a vital need for current clinical information and will be a valuable addition to rehabilitation literature.

Barbara E. Neuhaus, EdD, OTR, FAOTA
Adjunct Associate Professor,
Programs in Occupational Therapy,
Columbia University,
New York, New York

Preface

The original idea for this text came about after teaching a class on motor control to occupational therapy students. We began discussing our frustration that there was not a single text available that was a comprehensive reference on stroke rehabilitation. As advanced-level neurorehabilitation practitioners, we also felt there was not a single resource available to us to complement the knowledge base we had attained and to use as an easy yet comprehensive reference in the clinical setting.

We were concerned that many therapists we knew were using splinter skills and nonfunctionally based approaches to evaluation and treatment—approaches that had little relationship or meaning to life beyond the clinical setting. Occupational therapy practitioners were being challenged to demonstrate functional outcomes and cost effectiveness. We challenged ourselves to develop a text that occupational therapy practitioners as well as students would use and value—one that would cover multiple areas of intervention including mobility, self-care, and limb function, as well as specific skill areas such as driving and gait.

We thought that this text would have to combine aspects of background medical information; a critical review; and samples of functionally based evaluations, treatment techniques, and interventions. It would also have to contain the most up-to-date research on stroke rehabilitation from a variety of rehabilitation settings and professions without losing its holistic perspective on the overall care of the people whose lives we touch.

We were frustrated by the standard yet not standardized evaluations commonly used by therapists. It was highly questionable whether these evaluation tools and the treatments based on them were meaningful to patients and affected their overall quality of life after stroke. We began reading and hearing about new standardized tests developed both in the United States (e.g., the Assessment of Motor and Process Skills [AMPS]) and abroad (e.g., the Árnadóttir Occupational Therapy Neurobehavioral Evaluation [A-ONE], the Canadian Occupational Performance Measure [COPM]) that embraced occupational therapy principles and the philosophy we hoped to emulate.

In addition, treatment philosophies often seemed ambiguous and were often not based on research or current understanding of impairments resulting from stroke. Popular treatment philosophies seemed to focus on and emphasize the impairments after stroke rather than the disability and handicaps caused by the impairments. Cost effectiveness and treatment outcomes demanded a change in practice and the current way we conducted business.

Our goal in writing this book was to frame and compile evaluation and treatment approaches for a specialized population in one comprehensive text. Although this book is written for and by occupational therapy practitioners, it is an appropriate reference for a variety of rehabilitation professionals including physiatrists, physical therapists, speech and language pathologists, rehabilitation nurses, social workers, vocational counselors, and therapeutic recreation specialists. We have grown to value the multidisciplinary team approach to the treatment of individuals with neurologic diagnoses. This text may also be beneficial to therapists who practice virtually alone in the community or as a case manager because its research on the specific topic of stroke rehabilitation is comprehensive. Throughout this text, we have used the term *occupational therapy practitioner* to refer both to registered occupational therapists (OTRs) and certified occupational therapy assistants (COTAs). Although we use the term *patient* for consistency, we recognize that stroke rehabilitation can take place in multiple settings other than the hospital.

Educators and students can use this text in the classroom setting. Key terms, chapter objectives, and review questions have been provided as learning tools, as well as COTA considerations and case studies. A text that can appeal to the basic learner and the specialist alike, this book is a good investment for any occupational therapy practitioner who plans to work with neurologically impaired persons—adults who have had a stroke. This text spans the continuum of care—from acute care to long-term management—in a variety of roles and settings.

The opening chapters of the book provide the necessary medical (Chapter 1) and therapeutic foundations that should be the basis of any treatment plan. The information in Chapter 2 (Application of Learning and Environmental Strategies to Activity-Based Treatment) as well as in Chapter 3 (Psychological Aspects of Stroke Rehabilitation) should be implicit in any therapeutic interaction with members of this population.

This text contains chapters on specific functional aspects of living after a stroke, such as driving, sexuality, leisure, instrumental ADL, mobility and gait, and self-care. In addition, the book highlights function-based approaches to working with patients who have balance dysfunction, upper extremity impairments, and neurobehavioral defi-

cits. Specific interventions highlighted include splinting and casting, edema control, entrapment neuropathies, dysphagia management, home adaptation, wheeled mobility and seating prescription, and the integration of assistive technology for the stroke population.

The standardized evaluations in this text were selected because they focus on disability and handicaps associated with stroke instead of impairments. The evaluations are based on skilled observations of functional tasks and embrace the principles of occupational therapy. The treatments are based on functional tasks and active participation of the person receiving treatment. Adaptations are highlighted to compensate for deficits after stroke.

It is our hope that this text will challenge practicing clinicians to consider their present approaches to stroke rehabilitation and serve as a foundation on which students can build their philosophies for intervention with the stroke population.

Glen Gillen
Ann Burkhardt

Acknowledgments

We are grateful to all of the professionals from our own community, across the country, and internationally for their contributions to this book. They have contributed not only to this text but to the profession of occupational therapy as a whole. They accepted our challenge to put their knowledge and skill base into words. Their dedication to this project will inspire future generations of clinicians.

We appreciate the dedication and persistence of the staff at Mosby, specifically Amy Christopher, Martha Sasser, Laura MacAdam, and Cathy Comer. Their open-mindedness when we contacted them initially about the possibility of this book, their encouragement, and their support throughout this project has been admirable. We would also like to acknowledge the support of Carol Fraley, the director of our department, who not only contributed to the text but encouraged us and added direction and perspective at all times. The support staff in our department, in particular Bobbi Sussman, Gracie Wright, and Somari Colon, were ever-willing to assist us throughout this project.

The practitioners who have "paved the road" for us by developing theory and being creative challenged us to use and expand on their knowledge base. We view this text as a continuation of this development of acceptable theory and standards of care. As health care professionals, we all need to continue to study, learn, challenge, and change throughout our careers.

Contents

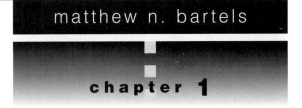

matthew n. bartels

chapter 1

Pathophysiology and Medical Management of Stroke

key terms

stroke prevention	stroke diagnosis	ischemic stroke
stroke management	stroke complications	hemorrhagic stroke

chapter objectives

After completing this chapter, the reader will be able to accomplish the following:

1. Describe the pathophysiology of stroke.
2. Explain the diagnostic workup of stroke survivors.
3. Understand the medical management of various stroke syndromes.
4. Describe interventions to prevent the recurrence of stroke and its complications.

PREVALENCE AND IMPACT OF STROKE

Stroke is the third leading cause of mortality in the United States after cardiovascular disease and cancer, accounting for 10% to 12% of all deaths.[8] There are an estimated 550,000 strokes each year resulting in 150,000 deaths and more than 300,000 individuals with significant disability.[86] There are an estimated 3 million stroke survivors in the United States today, which is double the number of survivors 25 years ago.[37] The economic impact of stroke in 1993 was estimated at $30 billion, of which $17 billion are direct medical costs and $13 billion are indirect costs from lost productivity.[86] Fortunately there are signs that modern medical interventions (mostly risk factor modifications) have decreased stroke mortality by approximately 7% per year in industrialized nations since 1970.[8]

EPIDEMIOLOGY OF STROKE

Stroke is essentially a preventable disease with known, manageable risk factors.[7] The established risk factors for stroke include hypertension, cigarette smoking, obesity, elevated serum fibrinogen levels, diabetes, a sedentary lifestyle, and the use of contraceptives with high doses of estrogen.[71] The most important and easily treated of these risk factors is systolic hypertension. In the multiple risk factor intervention trial (MRFIT), 40% of strokes were attributed to systolic blood pressures greater than 140 mm Hg.[93] Stroke incidence also increases exponentially with aging, with an increase in stroke from 3 in 100,000 individuals per year in the third and fourth decades of age to 300 in 100,000 individuals per year in the eighth and ninth decades of life.[7] Eighty-eight percent of stroke deaths occur among people aged 65 or older.[8] (Modifiable and non-modifiable risks are outlined in Table 1-1.)

Stroke prevention interventions have reduced mortality in industrialized nations primarily through treating hypertension in the elderly. Another cause of decreased mortality has been the establishment of dedicated stroke units that can prevent acute death and later development of life-threatening complications.

PATHOGENESIS AND PATHOLOGY OF STROKE

Definition and Description of Stroke Syndromes

Stroke

Stroke is essentially a disease of the cerebral vasculature in which a failure to supply oxygen to brain cells, which are the most susceptible to ischemic damage, leads to their death. The syndromes that lead to stroke comprise two broad categories, ischemic and hemorrhagic stroke. Ischemic strokes account for approximately 80% of strokes, whereas hemorrhagic strokes account for the remaining 20%.[91]

Transient Ischemic Attack

Symptoms of a transient ischemic attack (TIA) include the focal deficits of an ischemic stroke and a clearly vascular distribution, but TIAs are reversible defects because no cerebral infarction ensues. The causes of TIAs can be both thrombotic and embolic in nature and could also be a result of a cerebral vasospasm. By definition the effects of TIAs must resolve in less than 24 hours. A patient who has had a TIA should have a complete evaluation for cere-

brovascular disease and sources of embolism as 35% of patients who have had TIAs have a stroke within 5 years.[120] The treatment of TIAs depends on the source of the emboli or thrombi and can include anticoagulation therapy and/or surgery.

Ischemic Stroke

An ischemic stroke is the most common form of stroke, and its etiology varies. The one common factor among all the different subtypes of ischemic strokes is that the cause of injury is tissue anoxia caused by cessation of cerebral blood flow.

Embolic Stroke

Cerebral embolic strokes are the most common ischemic stroke subtype.[57] Embolic strokes are usually characterized by an abrupt onset, although they can also be associated with stuttering symptoms. There usually are no heralding events such as TIAs or previous small strokes evolving into larger strokes.[57] Microemboli that cause smaller events are uncommon, and the usual clue to a possible embolic source is a completed stroke.[91] The source of approximately 40% of embolic strokes is unknown, even after the common sources have been extensively evaluated. Most embolic strokes of known cause are secondary to emboli that are cardiac in origin.[16] The second most common sources of emboli are atherothrombotic lesions that result in artery-to-artery embolisms. These lesions can be in the aorta, the carotid and vertebrobasilar systems, and less frequently smaller arteries.

Sources of Emboli

Cardiac

Cardiac emboli can develop from numerous areas in the heart. Cardiac arrhythmias, structural anomalies, and acute infarctions all can be sources of emboli. Classically, the most common source is the left atrium in patients with atrial fibrillation. Atrial fibrillation causes thrombi through clot formation in the left atrial appendage, which then breaks off and embolizes through the arterial system. Patients older than age 60 are particularly prone to this type of embolization.

The most common cardiac structural cause of a cerebral embolism is a result of a myocardial infarction.[57] In patients with left ventricular infarcts, particularly anterior wall and apical infarctions, the endocardial damage associated with a subendocardial or transmural infarction is an excellent nidus (a focal point where bacteria or other infectious agents thrive) for thrombus formation. The emboli most often develop during the first several weeks after the infarction, although the risk for developing them can persist for much longer.

Valvular heart disease can also result in thrombi, but they more frequently develop after valve replacement rather than resulting directly from the native valve. More

Table 1-1

Modifiable and Nonmodifiable Risks	
TYPE OF RISK	**RELATIVE RISK (per 1000 people)**
Modifiable risks	
Hypertension	4-5
Cardiac disease	2-4
Atrial fibrillation	5.6-17.6
Diabetes mellitus	1.5-3
Cigarette smoking	1.5-2.9
Alcohol abuse	1-4
Hyperlipidemia	1-2
Nonmodifiable risks	
Age	1-2 at ages 45-54; 20 at ages 75-84
Gender	1.2-2.1
Race (Black or Hispanic)	2
Heredity	1-2

commonly the native valvular heart disease causes the patient to be in atrial fibrillation and then develop an embolus. Mechanical heart valves (e.g. St. Jude valves) are much more likely to cause emboli than porcine valves, so patients with the mechanical type always continue to receive anticoagulation therapy.

Much less common sources of cardiac emboli are the vegetations resulting from bacterial endocarditis. These emboli cause small septic infarcts called *mycotic aneurysms*, which are at high risk of conversion to hemorrhagic infarcts. Other rare causes of cardiac emboli are atrial myxomas, which are tumors of the heart endocardium. In addition, embolic infarctions may also result from cardiac and thoracic surgery.[57]

Cardiac emboli usually (80% of the time) occlude the middle cerebral artery, 10% of cardiac emboli occlude the posterior cerebral artery, and the remainder occlude the vertebral artery or its branches.[57] Anterior cerebral artery embolization from the heart is rare. The severity of the clinical syndrome is related to the size of the embolus. An embolus of 3 to 4 mm can cause a large stroke by occluding the larger brain arteries. Blood clots undergo lysis over a period of a few days with the establishment of recanalization through the clot. Because clots naturally lyse, a stroke can convert from ischemic to hemorrhagic when reperfusion distal to the occlusion is present because the blood vessels in the ischemic distribution may no longer be intact. This can lead to leakage from these damaged arteries, arterioles, and capillaries, leading to a phenomenon called *hemorrhagic conversion*. The possibility of hemorrhagic conversion contraindicates the use of anticoagulation therapy as initial treatment for large embolic strokes.

Vascular

Strokes that are vascular in origin are far less common than cardiac strokes but are still one major type of embolic stroke. The sources of vascular emboli are usually atheromatous plaques in the walls of the aorta, carotid arteries, or smaller vessels in the cerebral circulation. Platelet activation and the formation of a fibrin clot can occur rapidly. The most common areas affected by the emboli of the vascular system are the same as those affected by cardiac sources of emboli. The most common areas for ulcerated plaques in the cerebral blood supply are the aorta and the proximal internal carotid artery. The plaques in the carotid artery can be visualized by Doppler sonography of the carotid artery system.[91]

Paradoxical

Congenital atrial septal defects can create the opportunity for emboli to cross from the right-sided (venous) circulation to the left-sided (arterial) circulation—a relatively rare source of cerebral emboli. A common source of paradoxical embolic material is deep venous thrombosis (DVT). The modern techniques of transesophageal echocardiography with a "bubble study" help identify patients at risk for this condition. A bubble study is performed by injecting a small bolus of air into the venous circulation while the echocardiographer observes the heart. If the air bolus, which is easily seen, has no portion cross over to the left-sided circulation, then no shunt is present. If the bubbles cross into the left-sided circulation, then a shunt is possible. One of the most common atrial shunting abnormalities is a patent foramen ovale. In young patients or patients who have had TIAs or strokes, the treatment of choice is surgical repair of the lesion.

Unknown Source

Thrombi of unknown source are often seen in patients with known hypercoagulability syndromes. These can be a result of acquired diseases (e.g., lupus anticoagulant, metastatic tumors) or inborn errors of the coagulation system (e.g., protein S and C deficiencies). Iatrogenic causes of hypercoagulable states can be induced by surgery or medication therapies such as estrogen replacement. Even when the patient is known to be in a hypercoagulable state, the source of the emboli may remain unknown. In many patients the entire workup is unrevealing.

Thrombotic Stroke

A thrombotic stroke can be a result of a variety of causes, but most are related to the development of abnormalities in the arterial vessel wall. Atherosclerosis, arteritis, dissections, and external compression of the vessels are all causes. In addition, some patients with hematologic disorders develop thrombosis. The spectrum of disease includes stroke and TIA, and often the difference between a thrombotic and an embolic stroke may be difficult to determine. Thrombosis and embolism are often both present, especially in patients with atherosclerotic disease. The exact mechanism of infarction from thrombosis is still being debated, but atherosclerosis does play a significant role. Hypertension with associated microtrauma of the arterial intima is thought to play a role, as is hypercholesterolemia.[73,91] TIAs may be a result of both the formation of microthrombi and their embolization. Large vessel thrombosis can also occur in extracranial vessels, such as the vertebral and carotid arteries, leading to devastating strokes.[84]

Pathophysiology

Atherosclerotic plaque formation is greatest at the branching points of major vessels and also forms in areas of turbulent flow. Chronic hypertension is a common precursor, and damage to the intimal wall may be followed by lymphocyte infiltration. Foam cells then develop, and the first stage of atherosclerosis is formed. This is followed by calcification and narrowing with resultant turbulent flow. In this setting of turbulent flow, plaque ulceration can become a site for thrombus formation. If the thrombus forms and is rapidly degraded, a transient ischemic phenomenon can occur, which is the setting of a TIA. Classically the symptoms of internal carotid disease include amaurosis fugax and monocular blindness. If the clot does not break up or lyse, a cerebral infarction can occur. The size and severity of the infarction depends on available collateral circulation and the size of the occluded vessel. In patients with extensive atherosclerotic disease, however, a limited amount of collateral circulation is available, and the sparing from collateral circulation may be limited.

Atherothrombotic Disease

The most common site for the development of atherosclerosis and the subsequent development of atherothrombosis that leads to TIAs and stroke in the anterior circulation is the origin of the carotid artery and in the posterior circulation is the top of the basilar artery. Other sites of atherosclerosis include the carotid siphon and the stems (bases) of the middle cerebral artery (MCA), anterior cerebral artery (ACA), and origin of the basilar artery.[36] The atheromatous plaques are sources of emboli that can cause distal symptoms in a TIA or stroke. These embolic events are similar events from other embolic sources. (Table 1-2 lists common stroke syndromes and Figures 1-1, 1-2, and 1-3 explain the anatomy of these strokes.) Atherosclerotic disease is most readily screened by carotid Doppler ultrasonography and transcranial Doppler imaging. Magnetic resonance angiography (MRA) and carotid and cerebral

Table 1-2

Common Stroke Syndromes

ANATOMIC DISTRIBUTION	STROKE SYNDROMES
Common carotid artery	Often resembles MCA but can be asymptomatic if circle of Willis is competent
Internal carotid artery	Often resembles MCA but can be asymptomatic if circle of Willis is competent
Middle cerebral artery (MCA)	
Main stem	Contralateral hemiplegia
	Contralateral hemianopia
	Contralateral hemianesthesia
	Head/eye turning toward lesion
	Dysphagia
	Uninhibited neurogenic bladder
	Dominant hemisphere
	Global aphasia
	Apraxia
	Nondominant hemisphere
	Aprosody and affective agnosia
	Visuospatial deficit
	Neglect syndrome
Upper division	Contralateral hemiplegia, leg more spared
	Contralateral hemianopia
	Contralateral hemianesthesia
	Head/eye turning toward lesion
	Dysphagia
	Uninhibited neurogenic bladder
	Dominant hemisphere
	Broca (motor) aphasia
	Apraxia
	Nondominant hemisphere
	Aprosody and affective agnosia
	Visuospatial deficit
	Neglect syndrome
Lower division	Contralateral hemianopia
	Dominant hemisphere
	Wernicke aphasia
	Nondominant hemisphere
	Affective agnosia

Table 1-2

Common Stroke Syndromes—cont'd

ANATOMIC DISTRIBUTION	STROKE SYNDROMES
Anterior cerebral artery (ACA)	
Proximal (precommunal) segment (A1)	Can be asymptomatic if circle of Willis is competent, but if both ACA arise from the same stem:
	Profound abulia (akinetic mutism)
	Bilateral pyramidal signs
	Paraplegia
Postcommunal segment (A2)	Contralateral hemiplegia, arm more spared
	Contralateral hemianesthesia
	Head/eye turning toward lesion
	Grasp reflex, sucking reflex, gegenhalten
	Disconnection apraxia
	Abulia
	Gait apraxia
	Urinary incontinence
Anterior choroidal artery	Contralateral hemiplegia
	Hemianesthesia
	Homonymous hemianopsia
Posterior cerebral artery (PCA)	
Proximal (precommunal) segment (P1)	Thalamic syndrome:
	Choreoathetosis
	Spontaneous pain and dysesthesias
	Sensory loss (all modalities)
	Intention tremor
	Mild hemiparesis
	Thalamoperforate syndrome:
	Crossed cerebellar ataxia
	Ipsilateral third nerve palsy
	Weber's syndrome:
	Contralateral hemiplegia
	Ipsilateral third nerve palsy
	Contralateral hemiplegia
	Paralysis of vertical eye movement
	Contralateral action tremor
Postcommunal segment (P2)	Homonymous hemianopsia
	Cortical blindness
	Visual agnosia
	Prosopagnosia
	Dyschromatopsia
	Alexia without agraphia
	Memory deficits
	Complex hallucinations
Vertebrobasilar syndromes	
Superior cerebellar artery	Ipsilateral cerebellar ataxia
	Nausea/vomiting
	Dysarthria
	Contralateral loss of pain and temperature sensation
	Partial deafness
	Horner's syndrome
	Ipsilateral ataxic tremor

Continued

Table 1-2

Common Stroke Syndromes—cont'd

ANATOMIC DISTRIBUTION	STROKE SYNDROMES
Vertebrobasilar syndromes—cont'd	
Anterior inferior cerebellar artery	Ipsilateral deafness
	Ipsilateral facial weakness
	Nausea/vomiting
	Vertigo
	Nystagmus
	Tinnitus
	Cerebellar ataxia
	Paresis of conjugate lateral gaze
	Contralateral loss of pain and temperature sensation
Medial basal midbrain (Weber's)	Contralateral hemiplegia
	Ipsilateral third nerve palsy
Tegmentum of midbrain (Benedict's)	Ipsilateral third nerve palsy
	Contralateral loss of pain and temperature sensation
	Contralateral loss of joint position sensation
	Contralateral ataxia
	Contralateral chorea
Bilateral basal pons (locked in)	Bilateral hemiplegia
	Bilateral cranial nerve palsy (upward gaze spared)
Lateral pons (Millard-Gubler)	Ipsilateral sixth nerve palsy
	Ipsilateral facial weakness
	Contralateral hemiplegia
Lateral medulla (Wallenberg's)	Ipsilateral hemiataxia
	Ipsilateral loss of facial pain and sensation
	Contralateral loss of body pain and temperature sensation
	Nystagmus
	Ipsilateral Horner's syndrome
	Dysphagia and dysphonia

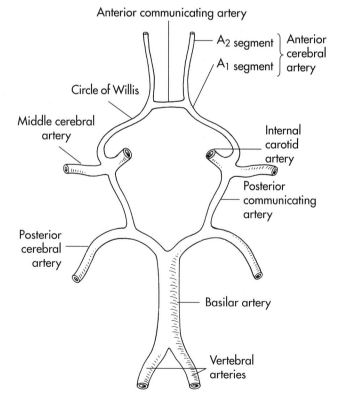

Figure 1-1 Circle of Willis and cerebral circulation.

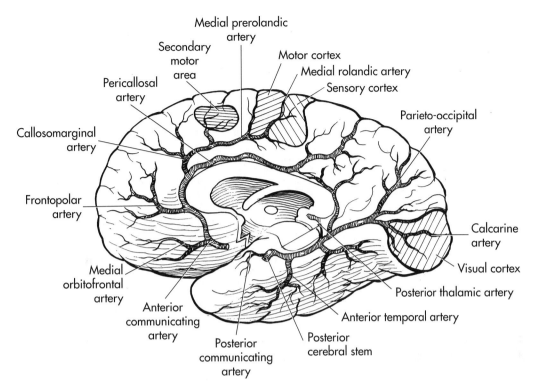

Figure 1-2 Medial view of brain with anterior and posterior cerebral artery circulation and areas of cortical function.

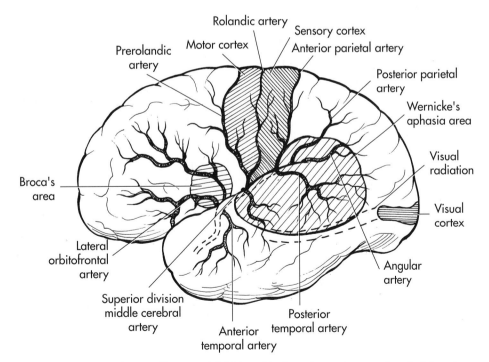

Figure 1-3 Lateral view of brain with MCA and its branches and areas of cortical function.

angiography can further elucidate lesions, which can be treated surgically or medically.

Lacunar Syndrome

A lacunar stroke is a stroke in one of the perforating branches of the circle of Willis, the middle cerebral artery stem, or the vertebral or basilar arteries. The occlusion of these vessels is a result of the atherothrombotic or lipohyalinotic blockage of one of these arteries. The development of disease in these arteries is closely correlated with the presence of chronic hypertension and diabetic microvascular disease.[77,91] These are small vessels, 100 to 300 μm in diameter, that branch off the main artery and penetrate into the deep gray or white matter of the cerebrum.[77] The resulting infarcts are from 2 mm to 3 cm in size and account for roughly 20% of all strokes. These types of strokes usually evolve over a few hours and can sometimes be heralded by transient symptoms in lacunar TIAs. Lacunar strokes can cause recognizable syndromes (Table 1-3). The basic lacunar syndromes are (1) pure motor hemiparesis from an infarct in the posterior limb of the interior capsule or pons, (2) pure sensory stroke from an infarct in the ventrolateral thalamus, (3) ataxic hemiparesis from an infarct in the base of the pons or the genu of the internal capsule, and (4) pure motor hemiparesis with motor apraxia resulting from an infarct in the genu of the anterior

Table 1-3

Lacunar Stroke Syndromes and Their Anatomic Sites

LACUNAR SYNDROME	ANATOMIC SITES
Pure motor	Posterior limb of internal capsule
	Basis pontis
	Pyramids
Pure sensory	Ventrolateral thalamus
	Thalamocortical projections
Ataxic hemiparesis	Pons
	Genu of internal capsule
	Corona radiata
	Cerebellum
Motor hemiparesis with apraxia	Genu of the anterior limb of the internal capsule
	Corona radiata
Hemibalismus	Head of caudate
	Thalamus
	Subthalamic nucleus
Dysarthria/clumsy hand	Base of pons
	Genu of anterior limb of the internal capsule
Sensorimotor	Junction of the internal capsule and thalamus
Anarthric psuedobulbar	Bilateral internal capsule

limb of the internal capsule and the adjacent white matter in the corona radiata. Recovery from a lacunar stroke can often be dramatic and in some individuals, near complete or complete resolution of deficits can occur in several weeks or months. In patients who have had multiple lacunar infarcts a syndrome characterized by emotional instability, slow abulia (impairment in or loss of volition), and bilateral pyramidal signs known as *pseudobulbar palsy* will develop. This diagnosis is made on the basis of the symptoms and the use of computerized tomography (CT) or magnetic resonance imaging (MRI). MRI is especially useful in this situation for the detection of small lesions in the deep brain structures or brain stem; the ability of CT to clearly see lesions in these areas is limited.[17]

Hemorrhagic Conversion

As a sequela of an embolic or ischemic infarction, a purely ischemic infarct may convert into a hemorrhagic lesion. Thrombi can migrate, lyse, and reperfuse into an ischemic area, leading to small hemorrhages (petechial hemorrhages) because the damaged capillaries and small blood vessels no longer maintain their integrity. These damaged areas can then coalesce (combine) and form a hemorrhage into ischemia.[57] These conversions are more common in large infarcts, such as an occluded MCA, or in a large infarction in the distribution of a lenticulostrate artery. In patients who have large infarcts with possibility of hemorrhage, anticoagulation therapy is not used because of the risk of hemorrhagic conversion. These types of hemorrhages have characteristics in common with hemorrhagic strokes.

Hemorrhagic Stroke

Hemorrhagic strokes have numerous causes. The four most common types are deep hypertensive intracerebral hemorrhages, ruptured saccular aneurysms, bleeding from an arteriovenous malformation (AVM), and spontaneous lobar hemorrhages.[57]

Hypertensive Bleed

Hypertensive cerebral hemorrhages usually occur in four sites: the putamen and internal capsule, the pons, the thalamus, and the cerebellum. Usually these hemorrhages develop from small penetrating arteries in the deep brain that have had damage from hypertension. The pathologic features of hypertension include lipohyalinosis (fat infiltration of pathologically degenerated tissue) and Charcot-Bouchard aneurysms.[34] The usual hypertensive intracerebral hemorrhage (ICH) develops over the span of a few minutes but can occasionally take as long as 60 minutes. Unlike ischemic infarcts, hemorrhagic bleeds do not follow the anatomic distribution of blood vessels but dissect through tissue planes spherically. This commonly leads to severe damage and complications such as hydrocephalus and mass shift (movement of brain tissues to one side to accommodate the volume of the hemorrhage).[57,91] Within 48 hours of the hemorrhage, macrophages begin to phagocytize the hemorrhage at its outer margins. Patients with a cerebral hemorrhage often experience a rapid recovery within the first 2 to 3 months after the hemorrhage. ICHs usually occur while patients are awake and often while they are under emotional stress. Vomiting and headache are commonly associated with ICH and are unique features that differentiate ICHs from ischemic strokes. (The four major hypertensive ICH syndromes are outlined in Table 1-4.)

Lobar Intracerebral Bleed

Lobar hemorrhages are ICHs that occur outside the basal ganglia and thalamus in the white matter of the cerebral cortex. These types of hemorrhages and hypertension are not clearly correlated; the most common underlying condition in patients with this type of ICH is the presence of AVMs.[57] Other associated conditions include bleeding diatheses, tumors (such as melanoma or glioma), aneurysms in the circle of Willis, and a large number of idiopathic cases.[35] The lobar ICH patients are initially seen with acute onset of symptoms, and most lobar ICHs are small enough to cause discrete clinical syndromes that may resemble focal ischemic events. Because lobar bleeds occur far from the thalamus and the brain stem, coma and

stupor are much less common than they are in patients with hypertensive ICHs. Headaches are also common and can help differentiate lobar bleeds from ischemic strokes, which they can so closely resemble.[90] Detecting a hemorrhage on a CT scan or MRI is the best way to distinguish these two entities.

Saccular Aneurysm and Subarachnoid Bleed

A saccular aneurysm rupture is the most common cause of a subarachnoid hemorrhage (SAH).[109] Saccular aneurysms occur at the bifurcation (branching) points of the large arteries in the brain and most commonly found in the anterior portion of the circle of Willis.[57] An estimated 0.5% to 1% of normal individuals harbor saccular aneurysms.[114] Despite the high number, bleeding from them is quite rare (6 to 16 per 100,000). Unlike other stroke syndromes, however, the incidence of SAH has not declined since 1970.[72] The rupture risk is best correlated with the size of the aneurysm. Aneurysms smaller than 3 mm have little chance of hemorrhage, whereas aneurysms 10 mm or larger have the greatest chance of rupture.[67] SAH is usually characterized by acute, abrupt onset of a severe headache of atypical quality.[72] These headaches are often the most severe that patients have ever experienced. A brief loss of consciousness, nausea and vomiting, focal

Table 1-4

The Four Major Hypertension ICH Syndromes

TYPE OF ICH	STRUCTURES INVOLVED	CLINICAL SYNDROME	COMMENTS
Putamenal	Internal capsule Basal ganglia	Contralateral hemiplegia Coma in large infarcts Deviation of eyes away from lesion Stupor/coma with brain stem compression Decerebrate rigidity	Most common
Thalamic	Thalamus Internal capsule	Contralateral hemiplegia Prominent contralateral sensory deficit for all modalities Aphasia if dominant (left) thalamus involved Homonymous visual field defect Gaze palsies Horner's syndrome Downward eye deviation	—
Pontine	Pons Brain stem Midbrain	Coma Quadriparesis Decerebrate rigidity Severe acute hypertension Death	Can lead to a "locked in" syndrome
Cerebellar	Cerebellum	Nausea and vomiting Ataxia Vertigo/dizziness Occipital headache Gaze toward the lesion Occasional dysarthria and dysphagia	Relatively rarely, can have nystagmus and limb ataxia

neurologic deficits, and a stiff neck at the onset of symptoms may also occur. The diagnosis is based on clinical suspicion, subarachnoid blood found on the CT scan, or blood found in the cerebrospinal fluid (CSF) from a spinal tap. The definitive location of the aneurysm is determined by cerebral angiography.

The development of further delayed neurologic deficits result from three major events: rerupture, hydrocephalus, and cerebral vasospasm. Rerupture occurs in 20% to 30% of cases within 1 month if there is no aggressive treatment, and rebleeding has an associated mortality rate of up to 70%.[72] Hydrocephalus occurs in up to 20% of cases, and aggressive management is often required. Chronic hydrocephalus is also common and often requires permanent CSF drainage (shunting). Vasospasm also is a common problem after SAHs, occurring in approximately 30% of cases.[72] The normal time course for vasospasm is an onset in 3 to 5 days, peak narrowing in 5 to 14 days, and resolution in 2 to 4 weeks. In one half of cases the vasospasm is severe enough to cause a cerebral infarction with resulting stroke or death. Even with modern management, 15% to 20% of patients who develop vasospasms still suffer strokes or die.[68] A permanent ischemic deficit develops in approximately 50% of patients with symptomatic vasospasms after SAHs.[46] Vasospasm must therefore be treated rapidly and aggressively as possible to prevent permanent ischemic damage.

Arteriovenous Malformation

AVMs are found throughout the body and can occur in any part of the brain. They are usually congenital and consist of an abnormal tangle of blood vessels between the arterial and venous systems. They range from a few millimeters in size to large masses that can increase cardiac output because of the size of their blood flow. The larger AVMs in the brain tend to be found in the posterior portions of the cerebral hemispheres.[34] AVMs occur more frequently in men and if found in one family member, they have a tendency to be found in other members. AVMs are present from birth, but bleeding most often occurs in the second and third decades of life. Headaches and seizures are common symptoms, as is hemiplegia. Half of AVMs are initially seen as intracerebral hemorrhages. Although rebleeding in the first month is rare, it is common in larger lesions as more time passes. Contrast CT, MRA, and MRI are useful noninvasive tests, whereas cerebral angiography is the best test for delineating the nature of the lesion. The management of these lesions is best accomplished by a team approach; a combination of surgical treatment and interventional angiography is used for definitive management. Treatment of hydrocephalus and increased intracranial pressure is the same as treatment for SAH and ICH.

Posttraumatic

A traumatic brain injury (TBI) commonly results in hemorrhagic damage to the brain in addition to ischemic and other injuries. The four major types of injury caused by TBI include SAH and ICH, diffuse axonal injury, contusions, and anoxic injury from hypoperfusion (decreased flow in the vessels) and hypoxemia (decreased oxygen level). This combination of injuries leads to a complex constellation of findings that mixes the features of a number of individual ischemic and hemorrhagic injuries.

Other Causes of Stroke and Strokelike Syndromes

Arterial and Medical Disease

Numerous medical conditions can result in arterial system diseases and lead to thrombosis and thromboembolism. Some conditions may cause disease in the cerebral vasculature (Table 1-5).

Strokelike Syndromes

There are a number of conditions in addition to TIAs and cerebral infarctions that can cause transient paralysis. These conditions all generally resolve spontaneously with no long-term sequelae. The most common cause of transient hemiparesis is Todd's paralysis, which develops postictally (after a seizure). This is a result of neurotransmitter depletion and neuronal fatigue in focal areas of the brain caused by the extremely high neuronal firing rate during a seizure.[23] Patients usually regain function within 24 hours. Another common cause of focal neurologic deficits is migraine headaches. These are actually thought to be a result of cerebral vasospasms, but an actual ischemic infarct rarely if ever occurs. The deficits resolve with the resolution of the migraine and leave no permanent deficits.

Cerebral Neoplasm

Obviously, cerebral neoplasms (whether primary or metastatic) can lead to focal neurologic deficits that resemble a stroke. The treatment of the sequelae and the long-term management of the deficits are the same as they are in stroke patients. Treating the primary lesions is the focus of the acute care. Often the initial symptoms are seizures and ICHs.

STROKE DIAGNOSIS

The diagnosis of stroke and differentiation of stroke from strokelike syndromes is based on the clinical presentation and physical examination of the patient. The examiner needs to differentiate a true stroke from syndromes that can mimic a stroke, such as Todd's paralysis, seizures, multiple sclerosis, tumors, and metabolic syndromes. Most often, the patient's symptoms in the emergency room include an acute onset of weakness or other neurologic deficits. The patient history can help identify the risk factors for stroke and the nature of the lesion. The physical examination includes a general medical examination as well as a neurologic examination. Only after a diagnosis of stroke

Table 1-5

Medical Conditions That Cause Arterial System Disease

CONDITION	FEATURES	TREATMENT
Vasculitic/Inflammatory		
Systemic lupus erythematosis	Most commonly associated vasculitis with stroke Involves vasculitic, thrombotic, and embolic events Has over a 50% recurrence rate Possible antiphospholipid antibody participation	Treatment of lupus Anticoagulation with warfarin
Binswanger's disease	Is a rare condition Involves diffuse subcortical infarction Involves diffuse lipohyalinosis of small arteries	No clear treatment Anticoagulation
Scleroderma	Causes stroke in 6% of patients May have antiphospholipid antibody participation	No clear treatment Anticoagulation
Periarteritis nodosa	Can cause CNS vasculitis Can cause embolic stroke	Treatment of underlying condition
Temporal arteritis	Can cause CNS vasculitis Can cause embolic stroke	Treatment of underlying condition
Wegener's granulomatosis	Can cause CNS necrotizing vasculitis Can cause thrombotic stroke	Treatment of underlying condition
Takayasu's arteritis	Can cause embolic stroke	Treatment of underlying condition Anticoagulation
Isolated angiitis of the CNS	Is a rare primary CNS vasculitis Includes symptoms such as headache, multiinfarct dementia, lethargy	Treatment of underlying condition
Fibromuscular dysplasia	Occurs mostly in young women Is often asymptomatic Can be associated with TIA and stroke	Anticoagulation Surgical dilation of the carotid arteries if necessary
Moyamoya disease	Is a vasoocclusive disease of large intracranial arteries Is mainly in Asian population Causes of strokes in children and young adults	Role of anticoagulation controversial because of hemorrhage risk Role of surgery controversial
Hypercoagulable state		
Antiphospholipid antibodies	Associated with recurrent thrombosis Involves both embolic and thrombotic strokes	Anticoagulation with warfarin
Oral contraceptive agents	Increases relative risk to 4 times controls Is thought to result from hypercoagulability	Cessation of oral contraceptive use
Sickle cell disease	Causes microvascular occlusion because of sickled cells Is seen in 5% to 17% of patients with sickle cell disease	No good treatments
Polycythemia	Causes vascular occlusion resulting from increased viscosity and hypercoagulability	Treatment of underlying cause (if known)
Inherited thrombotic tendencies	Include many familial clotting abnormalities	Treatment of abnormality (if possible) Anticoagulation
Others		
Venous thrombosis	Seen in patients with meningitis or hypercoagulable states or after trauma Increases intracranial pressure, headache, seizures Causes focal neurologic signs, especially in legs (more than arms) Is diagnosed with angiography	Anticoagulation May need surgical decompression
Arterial dissection	Is more common in children and young adults May present with TIA Is often preceded by mild to severe trauma	Surgical treatment as needed Anticoagulation after acute state

based on the clinical history and examination can a further diagnostic evaluation be performed. Modern technology has improved the tools available for the accurate diagnosis of stroke and includes an armamentarium of imaging studies to diagnose the exact nature of the lesions that may cause neurologic deficits. Each imaging study available has benefits and limitations that are useful to know when assessing a patient who has had a stroke. The stroke evaluation should also include an evaluation for the cause of the stroke.

Cerebrovascular Imaging

The main tool used in stroke diagnostic evaluations is cerebral imaging, which historically included pneumoencephalography and other studies that are no longer performed. CT is probably the most common and the best known of the studies. MRI is becoming more common and has some advantages over CT, but availability and cost are still prohibitive. Positron emission tomography (PET) scans and single photon emission computerized tomography (SPECT) scans are just being introduced and may have a role in stroke diagnosis.

Computerized Axial Tomography

CT is a readily available and useful technique that has become the standard for the evaluation of a patient experiencing an acute onset of stroke. The most important functions of CT scanning in an acute patient are ruling out other conditions (such as tumor or abscess) and helping identify whether there is evidence of hemorrhage into the infarction. In the acute phase of stroke, most CT scans are actually negative with no clear evidence of abnormalities. A negative immediate CT scan with an acute neurologic deficit determined by physical examination can actually verify the impression of stroke because it rules out tumors, hemorrhages, and other brain lesions.[17] The few changes seen in an acute stroke by CT are subtle and can include loss of distinction between gray and white matter and sulcal effacement. Acute bleeding, however, is very visible on CT scanning, and can be present in as many as 39% to 43% of patients.[17] By definition, hemorrhagic infarction occurs within 24 hours of infarction, and hemorrhagic transformation (HT) occurs after 24 hours of infarction. The cause of the hemorrhagic change is thought to be a result of reperfusion into areas of damaged capillary endothelium. This is common in large infarcts with extensive injury. HT occurs equally in all distributions of infarcts[81] and is not necessarily associated with hypertension or older age.[16] HT can be detected in the acute phase by CT; in this case anticoagulants should not be used because they may increase in the severity of the cerebral hemorrhage.

In the subacute phase the findings from CT clearly show the development of cerebral edema within 3 days, which then fades over the next 2 to 3 weeks; there is then a decrease in the signal intensity over the infarction. This corresponds with the change from the positive mass effect (swelling) of the acute phase to the negative mass effect (shrinkage) of the chronic phase. The infarct may actually be difficult to see again in 2 to 3 weeks but can be clearly seen with the addition of contrast material. Long-term parenchymal enhancement develops, which is consistent with the scar formation that becomes the permanent CT finding. The loss of tissue volume (negative mass effect) and the permanent scar tissue are the characteristic features of a chronic infarct (Figures 1-4 through 1-8).

Magnetic Resonance Imaging

MRI is not as commonly used in acute patients as CT because of cost (which is nearly double) and limited availability. It is, however, popular in research settings, and functional MRIs may become one of the future key dynamic flow studies. MRI can also rule out other conditions as well as screen for acute bleeding. In addition, MRI can be more sensitive for detecting cerebral infarctions in acute patients. MRI images are created by mapping out the re-

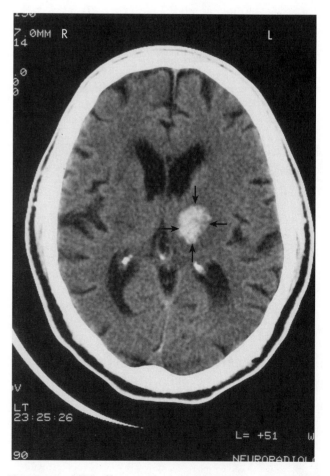

Figure 1-4   MRI of brain without gadolinium demonstrates an acute large left basal ganglia infarct. An acute infarct on MRI appears white and is indicated by arrows.

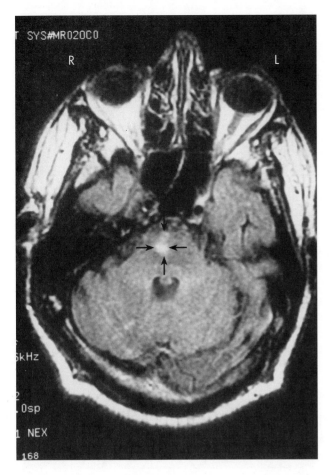

Figure 1-5 MRI of brain stem and cerebellum without gadolinium demonstrates an acute right pontine infarct. The infarct appears white and is indicated by arrows.

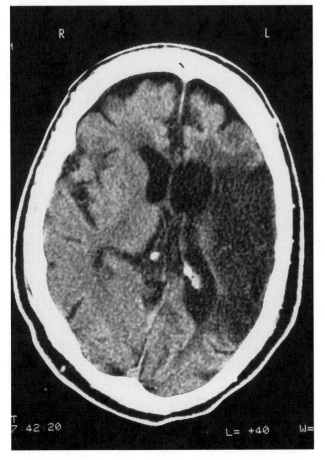

Figure 1-6 CT of the brain without contrast demonstrates a large, previous, left MCA distribution infarction. Note the loss of mass of brain tissue with dilated ventricles. There is no evidence of bleeding or acute infarction.

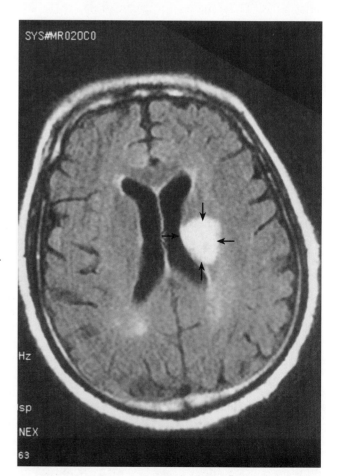

Figure 1-7 CT of the brain without contrast demonstrates a large subacute left MCA distribution infarction, indicated by the hollow arrows. Note there is no loss of brain tissue mass as compared to Figure 1-6. Evidence of acute bleeding is in the basal ganglia on the left, which is white on the scan and indicated with solid arrows.

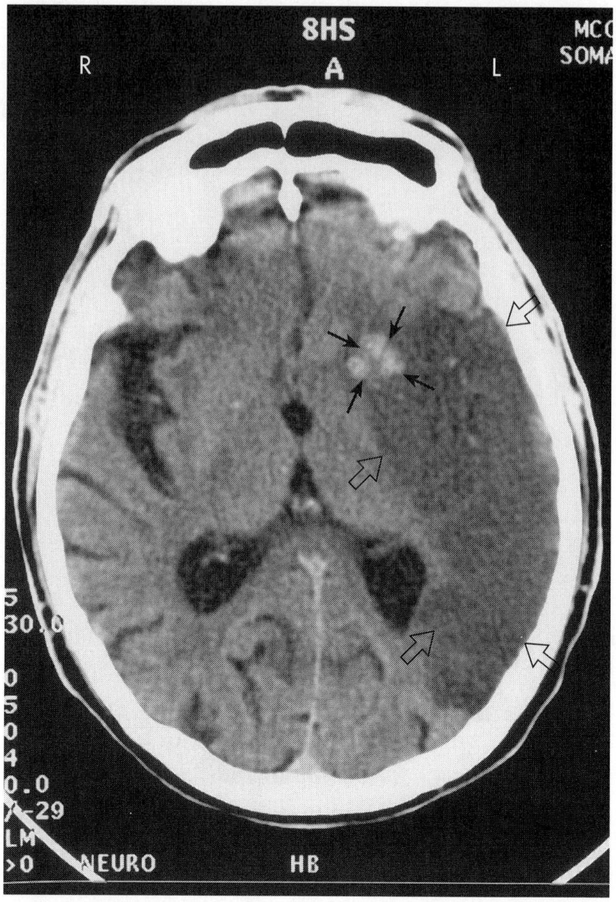

Figure 1-8 CT of the brain without contrast demonstrates a large, acute left thalamic hemorrhage. The acute bleeding in the thalamus on the left is white on the scan and indicated with arrows.

laxation of protons after the imposition of a strong magnetic field. These images are then taken in two ways—T1 and T2 weighted images. In T1 images, fat and tissues with similar proton densities are enhanced (bright). In T2 images, water and tissues that are rich in water are enhanced. As in CT scans, sulcal effacement can be seen, but there is also hyperintensity in affected areas on the T1 weighted images. MRI images, can show meningeal enhancement over the dura, which occurs in 35% of acute stroke cases.[30] Hemorrhage can also be detected by MRI in much the same way as it is by CT.

The subacute changes of edema and mass effect can be seen with MRI, and it may be necessary to use contrast to elucidate an infarct in the 2- to 3-week window. MRI has an advantage in determining a hemorrhage in a late stage because it can detect the degradation products of hemoglobin (*hemosiderin deposits)* and show hemorrhage areas well after CT can no longer detect a bleed. The MRI changes in a chronic infarction are similar to those on a CT scan.

PET and SPECT Scanning

PET and SPECT scanning are new techniques that are only available at selected centers. They have no clear role in the acute-stage evaluation of stroke.[1] In the subacute and chronic stages of stroke, they help to distinguish between infarcted and noninfarcted tissue and can help delineate areas of dysfunctional but potentially salvageable brain tissue. These studies can also be used to try to assess brain function in the chronic setting. However, because of cost, limited availability, and an unclear definition of their use, they are essentially only research tools and do not have a role in the routine management of stroke patients.

WORKUP FOR CAUSE OF STROKE

The workup for the diagnosis of stroke is aimed at answering three main questions:

1. Is the stroke thrombotic or embolic?
2. Is there an underlying cause that requires treatment?
3. Are there risk factors that require modification?

Transcranial and Carotid Doppler

These tests allow for noninvasive visualization of the cerebral vessels. The advantages are that they provide useful therapeutic information on the state of the cerebral vessels and the blood flow to the brain. Approximately one third of patients who have had ischemic strokes that are cardiac in origin have significant cerebrovascular disease.[15] Patients with symptoms or evidence of posterior circulation disease are best tested with a transcranial Doppler study including examination of the vertebrobasilar system. The cost is low compared to other tests such as MRA or cerebral angiography, which has significant associated mor-

bidity and mortality. The evidence of carotid disease can help shape the patient's treatment plan and encourage pursuit of definitive treatments such as carotid endarterectomy.

Electrocardiography

Electrocardiography is used to evaluate patients with stroke symptoms to detect arrhythmias (which may be a source of embolic material) or myocardial infarction or other acute cardiac events that may be related to an acute stroke.

Echocardiography

In patients with a history of cardiac disease and stroke, echocardiography is usually warranted. The types of cardiac disease that usually cause emboli and should be investigated with an echocardiograph include congestive heart failure (CHF), valvular heart disease, arrhythmias, and a recent myocardial infarction. In some individuals a patent foramen ovale (the fetal opening between the right and left sides of the heart) persists into adulthood and can be the source of a paradoxical embolus from the venous circulation that crosses from the right atrium into the left atrium. A transesophageal echocardiogram (TEE) can then be useful in combination with a bubble study to assess for a right-to-left shunt. This specialized study can also better visualize parts of the heart for emboli in areas such as the left atrial appendage when the standard transthoracic echocardiogram is inconclusive.

Blood Work

The standard acute evaluation of the stroke patient includes a complete screening set of blood analyses, including hematologic studies, serum electrolyte levels (ionizing substances such as sodium and potassium), and renal (e.g., serum creatinine) and hepatic chemical analyses (liver function tests). The typical hematologic evaluation has a complete blood count, platelet count, prothrombin time (PT), and partial thromboplastin time (PTT). These studies help to rule out other causes of strokelike symptoms, diagnose complications, and allow for a baseline analysis before the initiation of therapies such as anticoagulation. The blood chemistry analyses allow metabolic abnormalities to be ruled out, as do the renal and hepatic chemistry analyses. The latter part of the stroke evaluation can involve numerous specialized tests that are chosen according to the clinical symptoms and development of the differential diagnosis as the evaluation progresses (Figure 1-9). (Table 1-6 provides a sample of some of these studies and their associated conditions.)

MEDICAL STROKE MANAGEMENT

Principal Goals

As in the medical management of all patients, the care of stroke management requires good general patient care. All phases include caring for the conditions the patient may

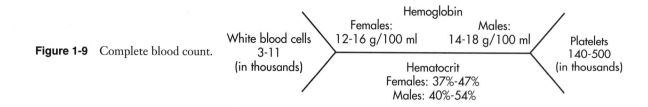

Figure 1-9 Complete blood count.

Table 1-6

Medical Studies Used to Clarify Differential Diagnoses in Stroke Evaluation

SPECIALIZED STUDIES IN STROKE EVALUATION	ASSOCIATED CONDITIONS
Protein S and C	Hypercoagulable state
Anticardiolipin antibodies (lupus anticoagulant)	Lupus erythematosis, hypercoagulable state
Erythrocyte sedimentation rate (ESR)	Collagen vascular disease
Rheumatoid factor	Lupus erythematosis, collagen vascular disease
Antinuclear antibody (ANA)	Lupus erythematosis, collagen vascular disease
Hemoglobin	Polycythemia
Sickle cell preparation	Sickle cell disease
Hemoglobin electrophoresis	Sickle cell disease
Blood/tissue cultures	Infectious emboli

have as well as preventing medical complications and anticipating needs that will arise as the patient progresses through the acute phase into the convalescent, rehabilitative, and long-term maintenance phases after stroke. Care for acute patients is best provided in a specialized stroke unit that commonly deals with the issues and concerns unique to these patients.[1a,72] Outcome studies have demonstrated the benefit of these units in the care of stroke patients.[62] Medical rehabilitation units have also been shown to be beneficial in the improvements of outcomes in the subacute and convalescent phases.

Acute Stroke Management

In management of acute stroke patients, basic medical needs have to be addressed and include such essentials as airway protection, maintenance of adequate circulation, and the treatment of fractures or other injuries and conditions that are present at the time of admission. The neurologic management of the acute stroke problems focus on identifying the cause of the stroke, preventing progression of the lesion, and treating acute neurologic complications. There are some specific approaches to treatment of each of the different types of stroke.

General Principles

The general principles of acute stroke management include attempting to stop progression of the lesion to limit deficits, reducing cerebral edema, decreasing the risk of hydrocephalus, treating seizures, and preventing complications such as DVT or aspiration that may lead to severe illness. See the previous sections for a discussion of the studies used in acute patients to diagnose stroke. Once the type of lesion has been defined, specific treatment can be instituted. Although numerous studies have been performed and are underway on the reduction of stroke mortality or disability,[98] no routine medical or surgical treatment has been shown to be effective. Currently, more aggressive methods such as angioplasty and thrombolysis are being studied, and it is hoped that the results of these trials will lead to treatments that will actually be able to improve the outcomes for individuals who have had strokes.

The basic principles in the approach to the treatment of acute stroke include an attempt to achieve improvement in cerebral perfusion by reestablishing blood flow, decreasing neuronal damage at the site of ischemia by modifying the pathophysiologic process, and decreasing edema in the area of damaged tissue (which can often lead to secondary damage to nonischemic brain tissue). Many pharmacologic and surgical treatments have been targeted toward at least one of these areas. Depending on the stroke mechanism, the agents and techniques of choice will be used.

Ischemic Stroke

In patients who have had ischemic strokes the restoration of blood flow and the control of neuronal damage at the area of ischemia are of the highest priority. In very large strokes, edema can play a very significant role, and mass shift can even lead to hydrocephalus. The pharmacologic therapies are divided broadly into antithrombotic, thrombolytic, neuroprotective, and antiedema therapies. The surgical therapies include endarterectomy, extracranial-intracranial bypass, and balloon angioplasty.

Pharmacologic Therapies
Antithrombotic Therapy (Antiplatelet and Anticoagulation)

The principal rationale behind the use of these agents is that rapid recanalization and reperfusion of occluded vessels reduces the infarction area. There is also the theoretical benefit of preventing clot propagation and recurring vascular thrombosis. The risks associated with the use of these treatments includes hemorrhagic conversion, hemorrhage, and increased cerebral edema, all of which are associated with worse outcomes.[63] Current research has not established a clear advantage to the use of aspirin or heparin in acute stroke patients, but these agents are still commonly used in the hope that they may decrease injury from acute stroke. Aspirin, an irreversible antiplatelet agent, is administered when symptoms appear. Heparin is administered intravenously in a continuous infusion.[49] Both of these agents are started only after determining by CT or MRI that there is no hemorrhage associated with the stroke. Ticlopidine, another antiplatelet agent, has been even less well studied, and its role if any in acute stroke treatment is unclear. A recent meta-analysis of the trials of heparin and oral anticoagulation in acute stroke treatment showed a marginal benefit from treatments with anticoagulation compared to no treatment at all.[97] There are currently numerous large, multicentric studies in the United States and Europe examining the best approach to the antithrombotic treatment of stroke that should provide better guidance as their results become known in the next few years.

Thrombolytic Therapy

Thrombolytic therapy is attractive as a therapy for acute stroke because it opens up occluded cerebral vessels and immediately restores blood flow to ischemic areas. However, a problem in using these agents in stroke treatment is that the treatment must start in 6 hours from onset of symptoms to be therapeutic. Most patients are symptomatic at a much later stage, and even if they have symptoms early enough a rapid workup to rule out a cerebral bleed must be performed prior to initiating therapy. The successful use of these agents—primarily urokinase, streptokinase, and tissue plasminogen activator (t-PA)—in the treatment of myocardial ischemia has aroused interest in similar use of these agents for acute stroke treatment. The agents' mechanism of action is to cause fibrin breakdown in the clots that have been formed and thus lead to lysis of the occlusions in the blood vessels. Reviews of thrombolytic therapy for stroke treatment have shown some reduction in mortality, but there is no definitive answer to date concerning efficacy.[116] As stated previously, these treatments can only be started in the absence of hemorrhage because the thrombolysis will result in massive hemorrhage and possibly death in patients with established intracerebral bleeding. In studies on cardiac thrombolytic therapy, there is a demonstrated increase in the risk of cerebral hemorrhage in acute myocardial infarction patients with hypertension and low body weight, who are using t-PA.[100] The definitive trials are now underway to elucidate the risks and possible utility of thrombolytic

therapies for stroke. Early data indicate a significant increase in early cerebral hemorrhage and death in some of the studies[63]; a final answer is expected in the next few years.

Other Treatments for Altering Cerebral Perfusion

A number of different treatments aimed at lowering blood viscosity or cerebral perfusion have been used, including hemodilution with agents such as dextran, albumin, and hetastarch. None of the 12 studies reviewed by Asplund demonstrated any clear benefit.[3] Similarly, studies of prostacyclins and several different types of cerebral vasodilators have also shown no clear evidence of increased survival rates or improvement in outcomes after treatment.[63] There continues to be active research in these areas, but so far none of these alternative treatments for increasing cerebral perfusion have yielded a favorable outcome.

Neuroprotective Agents

Neuroprotective agents are medications that can alter the course of metabolic events after the onset of ischemia and therefore have the potential to reduce stroke damage. There has not been any agent with clear benefits among this group of treatments. These agents include calcium-channel blockers, naloxone, gangliosides, glutamate antagonists, and free-radical scavengers. Each of these agents has had promise in the theoretical or laboratory realm, but none have proved to be clinically efficacious.

The use of naloxone, a narcotic antagonist, is based on the in vitro observation that naloxone has neuroprotective effects. Unfortunately, the clinical trials to date have not demonstrated any benefit.[20] The therapeutic rationale of using calcium-channel blockers is that they prevent injury to ischemic neurons by preventing calcium influx, which will decrease metabolic activity in the neuron.[63] Initial hope was that the treatment results for SAH, in which nimodipine decreases secondary ischemia, would be similar for stroke. Unfortunately, the results of several studies have not shown any clear benefits from treatment with these agents,[76] and none of them are currently used routinely for stroke treatment.

In animal experiments, glutamate antagonists decrease the size of infarction area in stroke.[63] However, the few studies done in humans have been inconclusive and there have been serious neuropsychiatric side effects.[20]

Gangliosides may reduce ischemic damage by counteracting toxic amino acids in ischemic tissue. Despite the many studies that have been performed, no clearly demonstrated benefits have resulted from use of these agents.[20]

The free-radical scavengers include 21-amino steroids (lazaroids), ascorbic acid (vitamin C), and tocopherol (vitamin E). They have not been well evaluated, and some studies to establish their clinical utility are being undertaken.[63] However, vitamin E has been clinically demonstrated to reduce the risk of heart disease, so secondarily its use may decrease the risk of stroke.

Agents for Cerebral Edema

Agents that reduce cerebral edema include corticosteroids, mannitol, glycerol, vinca alkaloids, and piracecam. All the studies done on persons receiving steroids[87] after an acute stroke demonstrated no clear benefits and there is a risk of diabetes and deep vein thrombosis with steroid use.[41] Use of the other agents also has no clear benefit in the treatment of acute stroke and are also not routinely used.

Surgical Therapies
Endarterectomy

A carotid endarterectomy is the surgical opening of the carotid arteries to remove plaque. This therapy has been shown to be extremely useful in the prevention of recurrent strokes or development of stroke in individuals with TIAs, but it has not been used to treat acute stroke. In theory the opening of the carotids could subject ischemic areas and their blood vessels to excessive pressure from restored blood flow and lead to hemorrhage.[26] Concerns about using major anesthesia in a patient with a new stroke makes this surgery too risky to treat acute stroke.

Extracranial-Intracranial Bypass

Despite the initial attraction of bringing extracranial blood flow into the intracranial vessels through the use of bypass procedures, the large trial done in the 1980s demonstrated no improvement in patient outcomes, and the procedure has been largely abandoned.[29]

Balloon Angioplasty

Despite its efficacy in opening blocked coronary arteries in patients with heart disease and its successful treatment of acute myocardial infarction, the use of balloon angioplasty in acute stroke has not been studied. There are clinical centers that are actively investigating its possible uses.

Hemorrhagic Stroke

In patients who have had a hemorrhagic stroke the size and location of the lesion determines the overall prognosis; supratentorial lesions greater than 5 cm have a poor prognosis, and brain stem lesions of 3 cm are usually fatal.[35] In these cases the control of edema is very important, and the techniques described previously can be used. In SAH patients the treatment regimen is usually more aggressive and focuses on several issues, which include the control of intracranial pressure, prevention of rebleeding, maintenance of cerebral perfusion, and control of vasospasm.

Prevention of Rebleeding

Before 1980, 6 weeks of bed rest were routinely prescribed for the care of acute SAH patients to prevent re-

bleeding. In 1981 a study demonstrated that bed rest was inferior to surgical treatment, lowering of blood pressure, and carotid ligation.[114] Antihypertensive medications for the prevention of rebleeding are still controversial, and there is no consensus as to their use.[72] Carotid ligation used to be popular, but more recent reevaluations of the benefits of the technique have not been as conclusive, and because of its surgical risks, direct repair of the aneurysm is a better choice.[72] Antifibrinolytic agents have been studied as well and have also been beneficial for low-risk patients in whom surgery must be delayed, but they seem to increase the risk of ischemic events. The placement of intraluminal coils, balloons, and polymers have shown some benefit in the short-term prevention of rebleeding, but the long-term efficacy is still unclear and the techniques still experimental.[72] Because the risk of rebleeding is also very high in post SAH seizures even though the incidence of seizure is low, it is recommended that patients receive antiseizure medications for prophylaxis.

Control of Vasospasm

The treatment of vasospasm is important for the reasons previously outlined. The current treatments include the use of oral nimodipine, a calcium-channel blocker that has been shown to improve outcomes of patients who have had an SAH with vasospasm. The results of using other calcium-channel antagonists are unclear.[72] The use of hypertension/hypervolemia/hemodilution (HHH) has been recommended by some studies. Creating more volume than normal results in hypertension. The stretch caused by the volume stimulates the smooth muscle pressure receptors that line the vessels. These receptors inhibit muscle action by a protective response and the blood vessel dilates to accommodate the increased volume. HHH is most effective in preventing vasospasm after surgically clipping the aneurysm. There are significant cardiac and hemodynamic risks associated with this therapy, so intensive care unit monitoring is required.[72]

PREVENTION OF STROKE RECURRENCE
Ischemic Stroke

In general, the strategies to prevent recurrence of ischemic stroke can be divided into two areas: risk factor modification (which also applies to primary prevention) and secondary prevention to treat the underlying cause of stroke in individuals with a history of stroke. Following is a discussion of the secondary interventions that can be used to prevent recurrence of stroke.

Hypertension

Although the treatment of hypertension is an important primary preventive measure in the management of stroke, whether blood pressure reduction after stroke is beneficial has not been definitively proven. The transient rise in blood pressure after stroke will usually settle without intervention.[118] Because of the uncertainty about whether overaggressive treatment of acute elevated blood pressure is harmful, definitive antihypertensive therapy should probably be delayed for 2 weeks.[63] At that time, the usual recommendations regarding adequate control of hypertension should be followed because there is some evidence that it is beneficial. This seems especially appropriate in patients who have had a lacunar stroke because the development of multiple lacunae is related to uncontrolled blood pressure.

Antiplatelet Medications

In patients who have had a TIA or stroke, long-term use of aspirin has been shown to decrease the incidence of death, myocardial infarction, and recurrent events by up to 23%.[2] The doses of aspirin in numerous studies have ranged from 30 mg to 600 mg; all doses resulted in a 14% to 18% reduction in recurrent cerebral events, but gastrointestinal complications increased with the higher doses.[33,111,112] In general, a standard dosage of one regular adult aspirin (325 mg a day) is the usual treatment for recurrent ischemic stroke. There are studies underway comparing the efficacy of warfarin versus aspirin in treating ischemic stroke; the results of these studies are not yet available. Ticlopidine is another antiplatelet medication that has been effective in reducing the incidence of recurrent stroke.[56] Ticlopidine is most efficacious in women, patients who are not helped by aspirin therapy, and patients with vertebrobasilar symptoms, hypertension, diabetes, and no severe carotid disease.[41]

Anticoagulation

The incidence of recurrent stroke and TIA in patients with atrial fibrillation is approximately 7% per year. For patients who have atrial fibrillation with cardiac sources of emboli, warfarin is the clear treatment of choice; this is true both for primary and secondary prevention.[63] Although aspirin has some preventive effects it is not *as* efficacious and in the presence of structural cardiac disease or atrial fibrillation should only be used to treat patients in whom warfarin anticoagulation is contraindicated.[63]

The odds ratio for recurrence is approximately 0.36 in those treated with warfarin versus control and 0.84 for those treated with aspirin versus control.[31] However, there are problems with warfarin anticoagulation in the elderly. Cognitive and compliance difficulties can lead to an increase in complications. Unclear issues in anticoagulation use include when to start anticoagulants after stroke, the safety of anticoagulants in clinical practice, and the optimum anticoagulant blood level. There are several studies currently examining these questions.

Treatment of Arrhythmias or Underlying Disease

Obviously, both primary and secondary prevention should treat the underlying cause of the ischemic stroke.

This can include cardioversion to normal sinus rhythm and treatment with antiarrhythmic medications as well as treatment of underlying medical conditions if they can be found. Unfortunately, only a small proportion of patients who have had TIAs and strokes can benefit from these specific treatments.

Carotid Endarterectomy

The surgical treatment of carotid artery stenosis has been shown to be beneficial in recent studies of stroke recurrence in patients with severely (>70%) stenosed carotid arteries.[32,79] The data on the intermediate group of patients (stenosis from 30% to 70%) are being collected. For patients with high-grade stenosis, carotid endarterectomy reduces the range of stroke risk from 22% to 26% down to 8% to 12%.

Hemorrhagic Stroke

The mainstay of ICH prevention is controlling systolic and diastolic hypertension. There is no clear benefit of one group of treatment agents versus another as long as adequate hypertension control is maintained. In patients in whom the ICH was secondary to vasculitis or the use of anticoagulants, the treatment for preventing recurrence includes treating the vasculitis or terminating anticoagulant use.[91]

The secondary prevention of recurrent stroke and SAH of AVMs and/or aneurysms includes surgical management of the lesions (the treatment of choice). Clipping or microsurgical dissection of the lesions is performed whenever possible and as soon as the patient is able to safely undergo the procedure.[72,108] In surgically unresectable lesions, alternatives include sclerotherapy, coating, trapping, and proximal arterial occlusion.[72]

PREVENTION OF COMPLICATIONS AND LONG-TERM SEQUELAE

General Principles

To prevent complications and long-term sequelae after a stroke, it is important to maximize function, decrease morbidity, and prevent rehospitalization from a complication. Prevention of these complications begins on the day the patient arrives at the hospital with symptoms of acute stroke. Many complications are associated with bed rest in general, but some are specific to stroke.

Musculoskeletal Complications

Contractures

Contractures are periarticular motion impairments that are a result of elasticity loss in the periarticular tissues, which include muscle, tendons, and ligaments. Contractures can occur in any immobilized joint but are particularly prevalent in the paretic limbs after a stroke. In fact, only 10% of stroke patients recover limb strength and mobility rapidly enough to avoid developing contractures.[42] Shoulder pain, contractures, and muscle pain occur in 70% to 80% of patients who have had a hemiplegic stroke.[91] The management and related issues of the hemiplegic shoulder are addressed in Chapter 6. Contractures also occur in other areas and begin to be problematic within a few days of onset or several days after the stroke when symptoms of immobility and spasticity may begin to develop. Usually contractures occur in a pattern of flexion, adduction, and internal rotation; muscles that span two joints are more susceptible to contracture formation.[43] To prevent shortening of the connective tissue in muscles and joints, an active range of motion (ROM) program has to be initiated. Because certain muscles span two joints, joints must be positioned to allow full physiologic stretch of the muscles involved. Once a contracture is present, the mainstay of treatment is gradual prolonged stretch. The minimal treatment is a sustained stretch greater than 30 minutes.[58] Other treatments include serial casting and splinting, deep-heating modalities,[13] and possible surgical release for long-standing tight contractures.[43] (For a more detailed overview of these treatments, see Chapters 8 and 9.)

Osteoporosis

Bone is a metabolically active tissue that is normally in a state of equilibrium between active bone resorption and deposition. The ratio of bone formation to bone resorption is influenced by the stressors that the bone is subjected to—a relationship that is known as *Wolff's Law*.[13] The lack of weight bearing and normal stress on long bones on the hemiplegic side of a stroke patient leads to a predominance of bone resorption. This loss of bone mass can start as early as 30 hours after the beginning of immobility,[113] and with bed rest can be as high as 25% to 45% in 30 to 36 weeks.[25] In patients who have had a stroke, osteoporosis is often worse and the rate of hip fracture is far higher on the side of the hemiplegia.[44]

Osteoporosis prevention is best accomplished with measures that include active weight-bearing exercise and active muscle contraction. Medical therapies for individuals at risk for osteoporosis should be initiated. Therapies include calcium and vitamin D supplementation, hormone replacement, and other measures as needed. (Box 1-1

Box 1-1

Treatments for Osteoporosis

Estrogen replacement
Calcitonin
Calcium supplementation
Vitamin D supplementation
Fluoride supplementation
Weight-bearing exercises

shows some of the medical treatments available for osteoporosis.)

Heterotopic Ossification

Heterotopic ossification (HO) is the deposition of calcium in the form of mature bone in the soft tissues. It is not particularly common after stroke but is seen with increased incidence after TBI. The incidence ranges from 11% to 76% in various studies.[9] Spasticity is associated with the development of HO as are long-bone fractures and a prolonged coma. Symptoms of HO usually develop 1 to 3 months after injury with pain and limited ROM.[14] The diagnosis is based on clinical examination, elevated alkaline phosphatase levels in the serum, and a positive bone scan.

Treatment for HO includes active ROM; there are no studies to indicate that the condition is caused or worsened by active ROM exercises.[9] Pharmacologic treatment options include the use of etidronate disodium and nonsteroidal antiinflammatory drugs.[14] Other treatments include radiation therapy and, for refractory cases after the lesion has matured, surgical excision of the HO. It is particularly important that ROM exercises be performed after surgery. Low-dose radiation or etidronate disodium can also be used to prevent recurrence.[21]

Falls

Falls are of particular concern in survivors of stroke. These patients are at increased risk of hip fracture because of developed osteoporosis, and the acuity of their balance, visual perceptions, and spatial perceptions are decreased. The increased risk of falls has been documented in several studies and is greater in patients who have had a right hemispheric stroke.[22,75,85] Fall prevention should emphasize balance and cognitive training, removing environmental hazards, and using adaptive devices. (These measures are reviewed in Chapters 5, 11, 14, and 20.)

Neurologic Complications

Seizures

Seizures after strokes have been documented since the nineteenth century. The incidence of late-onset seizures (epilepsy) in the individuals who have had strokes ranges from 6% to 18%,[45,115] whereas the incidence of early seizures is approximately 10%, with reports ranging from 3% to 38%.[6,121] The risk for seizures is highest right after stroke; 57% of seizures occur in the first week, and 88% of all seizures after strokes occur in the first year.[6] Seizures are more common in patients who have had an SAH, and 85% of these seizures are early seizures.[107] The timing of seizures that occur after stroke varies according to the mechanism of injury. The timing of seizures after thrombotic and embolic strokes seems to be about equal. SAH patients have more seizures soon after the stroke, whereas ICH patients are more similar to ischemic stroke patients and may have more late-onset seizures.[121]

The treatment and management of seizures associated with stroke are usually straightforward, and monotherapy often produces adequate results. If the patient only has acute-onset seizures in the setting of their stroke, they often will not require long-term antiseizure medication. A single, brief seizure or a nongeneralizing local seizure can also often be managed conservatively. If seizures do require treatment, a single agent usually suffices and is beneficial because there are less drug interactions and is better compliance with monotherapy. Carbamazepine and phenytoin are the preferred agents for treating epilepsy after stroke.[121] Management of the medication requires close follow-up to ensure that the desired outcome is achieved—an asymptomatic, seizure-free patient. Excessive medication can lead to a number of symptoms (Box 1-2). Inadequate control of the condition will lead to additional seizures. For situations in which seizures become refractory to treatment, there are several factors to remember.[121] Intercurrent illness or metabolic disarray that lowers the seizure threshold may make the seizures more frequent and difficult to treat. Patient compliance may be a problem, especially if the stroke created cognitive and behavioral deficits. Progressive lesions or new infarcts are also causes of increasing seizure frequency. Finally a stroke that occurs in highly epileptogenic areas, such as the hippocampus, the parieto-occipital cortex surrounding the rolandic fissure, and calcarine cortex, may engender refractory epilepsy and require combination therapy. (The common seizure medications and their side effects are listed in Table 1-7.)

Hydrocephalus

Hydrocephalus can occur acutely, especially in SAH and ICH patients as discussed previously, or it can develop symptoms later insidiously. It is usually hearalded by the gradual onset of a triad of symptoms, including lethargy with decreased mental function, ataxia, and urinary incontinence. Once hydrocephalus is suspected, a CT scan should promptly be performed because the increasing size of the ventricles can be readily seen. Once diagnosed, a ventricular shunt should be surgically placed. This is a

Box 1-2

Signs of Excess Antiseizure Medication

Lethargy
Drowsiness
Depression
Nystagmus
Ataxia
Irritability
Distractibility
Poor cognition
Poor memory

well-tolerated procedure and can lead to resolution of all the symptoms of hydrocephalus if performed promptly. Patients with an occluded shunt have symptoms that mimic the initial symptoms of hydrocephalus.

Spasticity

Spasticity is defined as a motor disorder characterized by a velocity-dependent increase in tonic stretch reflexes with exaggerated tendon jerks. It results from hyperexcitability of the stretch reflex (which is one component of the upper motor neuron syndrome).[61] In a normal recovery after a flaccid stroke, there is an initial period with little resistance to passive motion of the muscles and joints. Approximately 48 hours after the stroke, tendon reflexes and muscle resistance to passive motion begin to return.[43] Spasticity is most pronounced in the flexor muscles and occurs throughout the hemiplegic side. The lower extremity later develops a component of extensor spasticity that can assist with function, whereas the upper extremity spasticity is usually in a flexor pattern.[4]

The management of spasticity includes encouraging voluntary movement, ROM exercises, and a functional rehabilitative approach.[43] The research data on the different neurorehabilitative treatment approaches do not clearly define which approach is most effective, so an individualized approach to treating each patient is the best course. Pharmacologic treatments for spasticity are numerous, and they need to be individually tailored to each patient to find the best balance of side effects and efficacy. The most commonly used agents are baclofen, dantrolene sodium, and diazepam. These medications and a representative sample of the other medications used to treat patients who have had a stroke are presented in table of medications and their side effects on the inside cover of the book. Other treatments for severe spasticity that are more invasive include phenol blocks and neurolysis, botulinum toxin (BOTOX) injections, and implantable baclofen pumps. BOTOX injections and baclofen pumps are still experimental approaches, and ongoing studies will elucidate their future roles.

Other Complications

Deconditioning

Physiologic deconditioning in patients after a stroke is a result of the acute medical illness and the associated bed rest and immobility that may result. (Some of the effects of deconditioning are listed in Box 1-3.) All of these factors can alter the ability of the patient to recover. It is therefore important for the patient to get out of bed and increase activity as early and aggressively as possible.

Psychologic

Stroke is a major life event and is associated with significant alterations in the individual's well-being and independence. Negative emotional reactions are common in pa-

Table 1-7

Medical Management of Seizures: Drug Therapy

MEDICATION	SIDE EFFECTS	PRINCIPAL USES OF ANTISEIZURE MEDICATIONS
Phenytoin	Ataxia Incoordination Confusion Rash Gum hyperplasia Hirsuitism Osteomalacia	Tonic-clonic (grand mal) Partial
Carbamazepine	Ataxia Dizziness Diplopia Vertigo Bone marrow suppression Hepatotoxicity	Tonic-clonic (grand mal) Partial
Phenobarbital	Sedation Ataxia Confusion Dizziness Depression Decreased libido Rash	Tonic-clonic (grand mal) Partial
Primidone	Same as phenobarbital	Tonic-clonic (grand mal) Partial
Valproic acid	Ataxia Sedation Tremor Bone marrow suppression Hepatotoxicity Weight gain Transient alopecia	Absence (petit mal) Atypical absence Myoclonic Tonic-clonic (grand mal)
Clonazepam	Ataxia Sedation Lethargy Anorexia	Absence (petit mal) Atypical absence Myoclonic
Ethosuximide	Ataxia Lethargy Rash Bone marrow suppression	Absence (petit mal)

tients following a stroke[110] and can have a significant effect on the patient's eventual outcome. After a stroke, patients may go through the four stages of bereavement described by Worden.[125] These include accepting the loss, experiencing the pain of the loss, adjusting to a new environment in which previous abilities are missing, and investing in new activities. Not all patients will become depressed, and this lack of depression does not necessarily mean the patient is in denial.[126] Denial is a normal defense mechanism and as long as it does not interfere with the rehabilitative process,

it is not a concern.[110] The indifference reaction, a persistent denial reaction, is more common in patients who have had a right-sided stroke than a left-sided stroke.[38]

Another common consequence of stroke is emotional lability, which is rapidly shifting from one extreme emotion to another. Approximately 20% of patients have emotional lability 6 months after a stroke, and up to 10% have lability for 1 year.[51] Emotional lability is more common in patients with pseudobulbar palsy and right hemispheric strokes, particularly if the patient is depressed.[51]

Box 1-3

Deconditioning Effects of Stroke

MUSCULOSKELETAL

Atrophy
Decreased strength in tendons, ligaments, bones, muscles

CARDIOVASCULAR

↓Stroke volume
↑Heart rate
↓Oxygen consumption VO_2 max
↑Respiratory rate
↓Lean body mass
↑Body fat
Orthostatic hypotension

NEUROLOGIC EMOTIONAL

Sensory deprivation
↓Balance
↓Coordination
Fatigue
Depression
Anxiety
Sleep disturbance

GENITOURINARY

Diuresis
Difficulty voiding

ENDOCRINE

Impaired glucose tolerance
Altered hormone regulation

BODY COMPOSITION AND METABOLISM

Nitrogen loss
Calcium loss
Potassium loss
Phosphorus loss
Sulfur loss

Anxiety is also common after stroke and is more frequent in patients with left hemispheric strokes[66] and cortical lesions.[105] There are many sources of anxiety, including financial affairs, family issues, and a fear of dying or recurrent stroke. Reassurance and constant positive feedback during rehabilitation can help and in severe cases, treatment with anxiolytics and psychologic support may be needed.

Fortunately, outbursts and aggressive behavior are rare after a stroke, but when they occur, they are more common in patients with left-sided infarcts who are more aware of their deficits.[110] The approach to management of these outbursts should not include restraints and threats but should be based on avoiding excessive frustration in the patient by removing emotional triggers and alternating easy and difficult tasks.[110]

Depression is common after stroke, developing in 20% to 50% of stroke survivors, with 30% being the most commonly accepted figure.[110] The depression can either be a reaction to the stroke or a neuropsychologic sequela of the stroke. The consequences of depression after stroke are numerous: hospital stays are longer,[27] cognitive impairment is greater,[89] and motivation decreases.[101] Depression is more common in patients with left cortical lesions[104] and lesions close to the frontal poles and is shorter in patients with subcortical and brain stem lesions. Depression after stroke is often best treated with antidepressant medications.[110] In patients unable to tolerate antidepressants, who are unresponsive to therapy, or who have active suicidal ideation, electroconvulsive therapy can be a last resort.[78] (See Chapter 3 for more information about the psychologic effects of stroke.)

Urinary Tract Dysfunction

Urinary incontinence is common after stroke, affecting 51% to 60% of patients,[11] and can cause difficulties with rehabilitation, influence eventual discharge location, and place stress on caregivers.[28] One month and 6 months after stroke, 29% and 14% of patients respectively will still have urinary incontinence.[5] The usual pathophysiology of incontinence is detrusor hyperreflexia, which is quite common in patients with cortical lesions. The incontinence assessment includes a thorough history of the urinary symptoms and can include urodynamic studies to help define the problem. Incontinence treatment includes timed voiding and use of pharmacologic agents and intermittent catheterization. If these treatments do not work, incontinence may need to be treated by indwelling catheterization. This is performed on patients who cannot independently self-catheterize and do not have caretakers who can provide this care or in patients who have physical barriers such as urethral strictures that prevent regular catheterizations. Unfortunately, indwelling catheters have a high incidence of associated urinary tract infections. External condom catheters may also be used by male patients and can provide socially acceptable continence when the individual is traveling or physically active. Patients with continuous dribbling also benefit from condom catheters. The goals of all of these therapies is to maintain continence and prevent urinary tract infections and other complications such as skin breakdown from skin maceration.

Skin Breakdown and Decubiti

Pressure ulcer formation is a serious health problem in debilitated and immobilized patients. After a stroke, patients are at particular risk for pressure ulcers because they have numerous factors contributing to skin breakdown. Abnormal sensation, contracture, malnutrition, immobility, muscle and soft tissue atrophy, and advanced age often develop. Prevention of pressure ulcers rather than treatment of developing ulcers, should be the focus of care.

Preventive measures include frequent repositioning, keeping skin clean and dry, maintaining an adequate level of nutrition, and in especially high-risk patients, using pressure-relief mattresses.[94] Once pressure ulcers have formed, in addition to strictly observing the preventive and pressure relieving measures previously noted, treatments include meticulous wound care with a variety of agents and possibly surgical reconstruction.

Dysphagia

Swallowing disorders are common after a stroke. Dysphagia is more common in the elderly, with an incidence of 25% to 45%.[39,40] Aspiration can lead to pneumonia, and a decreased eating ability can lead to dehydration and malnutrition. The details of the pathology of aspiration and the methods of its treatment are covered in Chapter 17.

Aspiration

Aspiration causes chemical pneumonitis that can be followed by a secondary bacterial infection. Because there are numerous anaerobic organisms in the mouth, aspiration pneumonia can develop into an anaerobic abscess.[65] This occurs less frequently in edentulous individuals because they have less oral flora; it can occur in up to a third of cases in hospitalized patients.[69] The treatment of choice is to reduce the risk of aspiration and administer antibiotics. Examining an X ray for evidence of abscess cavities and the sputum for organisms can help develop a specific medical treatment. Sputum culture growth often requires up to 3 or 4 days, so initial treatment is often empiric and should be administration of a wide-spectrum antibiotic that is effective against hospital-acquired organisms (which are often resistant to certain antibiotics) as well as anaerobic bacteria.[65] The usual course of antibiotics is 7 to 10 days but cavitary pneumonia may require far longer treatment for erradication of the organism.[64] Determining which specific antibacterial agents will be used depends on the resistance patterns in the institution where the aspiration takes place, and the decision about which antibiotics will be used should be determined by the infectious disease team at that institution.

Deep Venous Thrombosis

DVT is a common problem after stroke, and has an incidence of 23% to 75% depending on the severity of the stroke. Most of the morbidity and mortality associated with DVT results from venous thromboembolism (VTE). Pulmonary embolism after stroke has an incidence of 10% to 29% and a mortality rate of 10%.[10] The formation of DVT is caused by the triad of risk factors outlined by Virchow's postulates: altered blood flow, damage to the blood vessel wall, and altered blood coagulability. The common risk factors for DVT are listed in Box 1-4. Of the risk factors for DVT, stasis is one of the most important. After a stroke, DVT is 10 times more common in the paretic

Box 1-4

Risk Factors for Deep Venous Thrombosis
Immobilization
Postoperative state
Age > 40
Cardiac disease
Limb trauma
Coagulation disorders
Obesity
Advanced neoplasm
Pregnancy

leg.[117] DVT usually begins in the calf, and although the emboli from calf thrombi are not dangerous, these thrombi propagate in about 20% of cases, and about 50% of the proximal deep venous thrombi will embolize. About 20% of symptomatic pulmonary emboli will be fatal.[96] After a stroke, ambulation in itself is not preventive in the subacute setting—pulmonary embolism occurred in 57% of ambulatory patients in the rehabilitation setting.[106] Lower extremity and pelvic DVT are the most common, but proximal upper extremity DVT can also occur, although it is rare. All of the diagnostic and management issues discussed in the VTE section that follows applies to this condition as well.

The diagnosis of DVT in the clinical setting is unreliable,[10] and many patients with life-threatening embolism and thrombosis will have no clinical symptoms of DVT. Other patients with swelling and tenderness may not have DVT at all and may have any of a number of other diagnoses. The differential diagnosis of lower extremity pain and swelling includes trauma, fracture, gout, cellulitis, and superficial phlebitis. The usual clinical signs of DVT include pain and tenderness, swelling, the presence of Homan's sign, superficial venous distention, a palpable cord, and fever. Some of these signs, such as Homan's, are unreliable indicators. Homan's sign is present in less than one third of patients with DVT and is present in half of patients without DVT.[48] Objective testing for DVT has venography as the gold standard, but this procedure is associated with significant risks, including anaphylaxis and causing DVT.[52] More commonly used, risk-free procedures are impedance plethysmography (IPG), which is a noninvasive test that measures volume changes in the leg with circumferential calf electrodes,[52] and Doppler ultrasound, which is also a noninvasive test that uses a handheld probe to detect blood flow in deep leg veins.[119] Doppler ultrasound and IPG have similar sensitivities and specificities for DVT detection, but Doppler ultrasound is not as portable and has a higher cost than IPG.[10]

The clinical diagnosis of pulmonary embolism is also unreliable, and only 30% of patients with pulmonary embolism have clinical DVT, even though 70% have venographic evidence of DVT.[10] The symptoms of submassive pulmonary embolism overlap with the symptoms of many other pulmonary conditions, including tachypnea, tachycardia, rales, hemoptysis, pleuritic chest pain, pleural effusion, general malaise, bronchospasm, and fever.[106] In patients with massive pulmonary embolism with greater than 60% of the pulmonary circulation obstructed, patients are critically ill and develop heart failure, circulatory collapse, hypotension and coma and can die suddenly.[106] The gold standard for testing for pulmonary embolism is the pulmonary angiogram, but it is associated with significant morbidity and mortality. The preferred noninvasive test is the ventilation/perfusion (V/Q) scan.[74]

The best approach to VTE is to prevent DVT. The National Institutes of Health Consensus Conference on the Prevention of Venous Thrombosis and Pulmonary Embolism recommends using low doses of subcutaneous heparin in all stroke patients with no hemorrhagic components.[80] In all other patients, external pneumatic calf compression is recommended. More recently, low molecular weight heparin has been introduced and may actually be more effective than standard heparin for DVT prophylaxis.[47] Low doses of warfarin for DVT prophylaxis in stroke patients has not been well studied, but its use in other conditions has proven its effectiveness in DVT reduction. Dextran, aspirin, and static compression stockings are not effective for preventing DVT.[10] Physical treatments alone, such as ROM exercises, have not been studied. Ambulatory patients must be able to walk at least 50 feet to have a reduction in risk of DVT[12] but as previously stated, there is still a significant risk of pulmonary embolism in ambulatory patients.[106] The length of time prophylaxis should continue is still not definite, but evidence shows that continuing prophylaxis well into the subacute phase is warranted.[10]

The treatment of venous thromboembolism (DVT and pulmonary embolism) is based on preventing pulmonary embolism, which can be fatal. A patient who is identified with acute VTE is started on intravenous heparin as long as no contraindications to anticoagulation exist.[50] The effectiveness of the heparin is determined by monitoring the PTT, and the heparin is adjusted to a dose between 1.5 to 2.5 times control. In a patient with only DVT, warfarin can be started on the first day, and the heparin can be discontinued when the warfarin dose is therapeutic as measured by the increase in the PT or International Normalized Ration (INR). Targets are a PT of 1.25 to 1.5 times control or an INR of 2 to 3.[10] In patients with PE, warfarin may be started a few days later, and after management of the acute stage the patient keeps receiving it longer; patients with DVT receive warfarin for approximately 3 months and with PE, 6 months.[47] All patients who have recently been diagnosed with VTE are placed on bed rest initially and are usually allowed to become mobile 2 days after the PTT has become therapeutic.[53] The rehabilitation of patients with VTE who are beginning treatment should continue at the bedside, and in the case of patients with lower extremity DVT the rehabilitation program should include activity of daily living training, upper extremity programs, communication work, and dysphagia treatments.

FUTURE TRENDS IN MEDICAL STROKE MANAGEMENT

Improved Primary Stroke Prevention

Because the treatments for stroke are so limited and the deficits that can result are so devastating, the primary prevention of stroke has to be the essential strategy to decrease morbidity and mortality from stroke. With a good understanding of the risk factors for stroke, risk factor modification can be targeted at groups and individuals who are at risk. The preventable and nonpreventable risk factors for stroke are listed in Table 1-1. Fortunately, many of the risk factors for stroke are the same as those for myocardial infarction and vascular disease leading to death, so the modification of stroke risk factors also decreases the risk of cardiac-related morbidity and mortality. As a result of greater awareness and risk factor modification and largely through the treatment of blood pressure, there has been a decline of greater than 50% in the stroke mortality rate in the last 20 years.[122] Each of the modifiable risk factors will be considered separately.

Hypertension

Diastolic and systolic hypertension are each independently and strongly implicated in causing stroke. Hypertension increases the risk of stroke in all age groups of men and women.[122] In fact, there is no threshold level of blood pressure below which the risk curve plateaus.[70] For every 7.5 mm Hg increase in diastolic pressure there is a 46% increase in stroke incidence and a 29% increase in coronary heart disease (CHD). Reducing blood pressure in hypertensive patients has been shown to decrease the risk of stroke significantly, with an average reduction of 5.8 mm Hg leading to a reduction in stroke incidence of 42% but only a 14% reduction in CHD incidence.[19] Because these trials only spanned 2 to 5 years, the reduction in stroke incidence is a direct result of decreased blood pressure and not an alteration in atherogenesis (production of plaque in the arteries), which would take longer to develop.[122] Systolic blood pressure is also a factor; the treatment of isolated systolic hypertension (>160 mm Hg) has been shown to reduce the incidence of stroke by 36% and CHD by 27% over 4.5 years.[99] It is therefore essential to treat all forms of hypertension in the older age groups because they are at increased risk for stroke, and most strokes occur in this age group. Screening for hypertension and aggressively treating both systolic and diastolic hypertension should be the cornerstone of any primary prevention program for stroke.

Cigarette Smoking

The results of both the Framingham Study and the Nurses' Health Study demonstrate that the cessation of cigarette smoking should lead to a prompt reduction in stroke mortality.[18,123] Risk of CHD decreases by 50% in 1 year and reaches the level of a nonsmoker's risk in 5 years. Smoking increases stroke risk by 40% in men and 60% in women (with no other risk factors being considered), and it seems to follow that smoking cessation leads to a reduction in stroke risk that is similar to the reduction in CHD incidence.

Cardiac Arrhythmia and Myocardial Infarction

CHD, atrial fibrillation, and CHF all lead to an increased incidence of stroke.[122] Preventing these conditions by modifying their associated risk factors leads to a reduction in incidence of stroke. In addition, treating patients who have established arrhythmias and CHF with anticoagulants such as warfarin will decrease the incidence of stroke (as explained previously).

Blood Lipids

The development of carotid artery atherosclerotic disease has been shown to be related to the levels of serum lipids.[95] However, it has been difficult to clearly relate accelerated atherosclerosis to an increase in the incidence of stroke, because other pathologies related to serum lipids have been observed. Levels of total serum cholesterol below 160 mg/dl seem to be associated with ICH and SAH, whereas higher levels of serum cholesterol are associated with atherothrombosis. There has been no relationship demonstrated between cholesterol and lacunar strokes.[122] This unusual relationship of low serum lipids and higher hemorrhagic infarct has been demonstrated in Japan and also recently in the United States in the group of patients studied in the MRFIT.[54,88] Because of the ambiguity of these data, it is difficult to clearly state guidelines for the management of cholesterol to reduce incidence.

Diabetes

The rate of atherosclerosis development in coronary, femoral, and cerebral vessels is increased in diabetics. Stroke is increased 2.5 to 4 times in diabetics compared to nondiabetics.[60] In the Framingham Study, glucose intolerance (a blood sugar greater than 150 mg/ml) is only a significant, independent contributor to stroke in older women and is greater for women than men at any age.[55] Because of the associated risk of stroke, it is prudent to carefully manage diabetes in addition to all other risk factors.

Oral Contraceptives

In female patients over the age of 35 who have other stroke risk factors, oral contraceptive (OC) use is associated with increased incidence of stroke.[102] The relative risk for OC users is approximately 5 times greater if they are already in the high-risk group. With the use of lower estrogen formulation OCs, the risk has substantially decreased in recent years.[103] It is noteworthy that the incidence of fatal SAH was increased in OC-using women with concomitant smoking; it is 4 times higher in the group over age 35.[92] It is therefore recommended that women over the age of 35 avoid using OCs, and younger women who smoke should be advised of the increased risks associated with concurrent OC use.

Alcohol

Heavy alcohol consumption is related to an increase in stroke and stroke deaths, whereas light to moderate alcohol consumption is associated with a reduced incidence of CHD.[24,59] Alcohol is clearly related to hemorrhagic stroke events, but there is not a definite association with thromboembolic events. Regardless, patients at risk for stroke should avoid heavy alcohol consumption.

Physical Activity

Despite the clear benefits of physical activity in the reduction of CHD morbidity and mortality, there has been no clear association between physical activity and the incidence of stroke.[82,83]

Public Education

The primary goal of primary and secondary prevention programs should be to educate individuals about risk factors and then teach them the way to modify their risks. During routine visits a physician should be able to identify at-risk patients through a combination of a history and physical. Routine blood pressure screening should be included in all evaluations, and patients who have hypertension should be treated. A stroke-risk profile has been assembled from the Framingham Study data and can be used by physicians[124] (e.g., to help a physician decide which borderline hypertensive patients to treat). Education can start in the physician's office and be continued by all the other health professionals with whom the patient comes into contact. If the community at large is educated about the risk factors of stroke, those individuals who are at highest risk can seek out the attention they require. This model has been implemented and supported through research such as The Agency for Health Care Policy and Research *Smoking Cessation Clinical Practice Guidelines.*[1b]

■

CASE STUDY

Ischemic stroke: management of acute case and complications with workup

GH is a 76-year-old woman who has a history of hypertension and diabetes mellitus and had a myocardial infarction 2 years ago. She arrives at her local emergency room 4 hours after an acute onset of weakness in her left arm and leg. She fell at home after trying to get up, and it was only after her neighbors heard her calls for help that the emergency services rescue team came to her aid. On admission to the emergency room, she has an elevated blood pressure of 200/100 and is alert and oriented. Her initial physical exam reveals left-sided weakness and sensory loss that is greater in her arm than her leg. The emergency room team has the impression that she has an acute stroke in evolution, so an emergency CT scan is ordered. The initial blood work and electrocardiogram are unremarkable. While she is in the CT scanner, the on call resident is paged and asked to come see her because the radiology technician notes that she has become unable to move while in the machine. She now has a dense left hemiplegia. Because of fear of stroke progression, she is admitted to the ICU.

Review of the CT scan shows some mild effacement of the sulci on the right side of the brain and no other clear abnormalities. The neurologic consultant advises the GH's treatment that night be conservative and supportive and recommends that GH be given an enteric-coated aspirin each day. By the next morning, she has had no further progression of her symptoms but has flaccid left hemiplegia and hemineglect. She remains medically stable during the next several days but is unable to achieve adequate oral intake and has to have a nasogastric tube placed for enteral feeding. A physiatric consultation is obtained, and physical and occupational therapy is started at the bedside in the ICU.

Another CT scan is performed on the third hospital day, which reveals a clear, acute infarct in the right temporoparietal area with associated edema and no mass effect or hemorrhage, so the neurologist recommends an extended workup. Carotid Doppler images are normal and the electrocardiogram indicates stability, but the echocardiogram reveals that GH has a decreased ejection fraction of 25% with a visible apical thrombus in the area of her previous myocardial infarction. The neurologist and cardiologist concur on anticoagulation with heparin followed by conversion to warfarin. Anticoagulant therapy is initiated, and the aspirin is no longer administered.

On the sixth hospital day, GH is successfully started on warfarin, her hemiparesis has improved, and she is able to move her leg against gravity and with gravity eliminated. However, she is still unable to swallow safely and still has a nasogastric tube. GH is accepted for inpatient rehabilitation and is transferred to the rehabilitation service on the eighth hospital day.

GH's rehabilitation course is notable because of swelling and pain in her left leg, which is by duplex Doppler scanning found to be the result of a DVT. Because she developed the thrombosis while receiving adequate anticoagulation medication, she has an umbrella filter placed in her inferior vena cava to prevent development of a pulmonary embolus. GH becomes severely depressed and after consultation with the psychiatry service begins receiving antidepressant medication, which has good results. GH progresses in therapy, but her left shoulder becomes painful because of a shoulder-hand syndrome, which responds well to aggressive therapeutic intervention. She also develops a progressive increase in skeletal muscle activity, particularly in her left hand, which only can be kept under control with aggressive ROM exercises. At the time of her discharge,

she is able to move short distances with a hemiwalker and needs assistance with dressing her lower extremities and setting up for her basic activities of daily living.

GH's 1-year follow-up is notable for the continuing intractable painful spasticity in her left arm, so treatment with BOTOX is instituted and results in adequate pain relief. She remains stable until 5 years after her stroke, when she suffers a fall with a subsequent hip fracture. Evaluation of bone density shows accelerated osteoporosis in the left hip. She needs left hip hemiarthroplasty but is unable to regain her previous level of function despite aggressive therapy and finally has to be admitted to a nursing home when discharged from the hospital.

Hemorrhagic stroke: management of acute case with workup

CC is a 25-year-old man who works as a sales manager in a local retail store. While dismissing a store clerk whom he caught stealing from the store safe, he suddenly complains of a severe headache, sinks to the chair in his office, and slumps over to the right. Within a few minutes he is unconscious, and the staff calls the ambulance. CC is admitted to the emergency room within 20 minutes accompanied by the fired clerk who is loudly proclaiming that she has done nothing to him. In the emergency room, CC is in a deep coma, breathing deeply, and has dilated pupils and absent reflexes. He is immediately intubated for airway protection and taken for an emergency CT scan. The study is not completed because CC has a seizure while in the CT scanner, but the partially completed study shows a great deal of blood in the ventricles. CC is diagnosed with a presumed SAH and treatment is started. Hyperventilation and treatment with mannitol begin. An intracranial pressure monitor is inserted, and is given phenytoin and nimodipine. CC is managed closely in the ICU and after 3 days comes out of the coma. He remains intubated and has an MRI/MRA performed that shows a probable berry aneurysm on the anterior communicating artery. A cerebral angiogram is performed, and a 2 cm aneurysm is clearly seen. CC has a good response to the treatment and is extubated on the sixth hospital day. His neurologic exam reveals mild disorientation, dysarthria, and tetraparesis that is more pronounced on the right than the left.

The neurologic and neurosurgical team, patient, and family have a discussion and decide that surgical clipping of the aneurysm is the best approach to treating the lesion. CC is scheduled for operative intervention the next day. However, in the middle of the night, he suddenly loses consciousness and stops breathing. He has a cardiac arrest but is successfully resuscitated. An emergency CT scan reveals a large recurrent hemorrhage that extends into the cerebral cortex and a herniated brain stem. Aggressive treatments are instituted, but despite all measures the herniation progresses, and CC lapses into an irreversible coma. One week later CC is declared brain dead, and according to his family's wishes his organs are donated for transplantation.

REVIEW QUESTIONS

1. Which stroke risk factors are considered modifiable?
2. Which procedures are utilized to diagnose a stroke?
3. Which clinical signs indicate a patient is receiving excessive seizure medication?
4. What are the risk factors and recommended treatments for DVTs?
5. Other than neurologic, what are the common complications that follow a stroke?

■ COTA Considerations ■

- A TIA is a reversible precursor to stroke.
- Strokes can occur from emboli, thrombi, or vasospasm, all of which cause an ischemic event (interruption of oxygenated blood flow to the brain).
- CT scans are the most common scans used to detect stroke.
- Once a stroke has been detected, it is important to diagnose and medically treat the underlying cause (e.g., cardiac, hemorrhagic, abnormally increased platelet levels, carotid plaques, infections, neoplasms).
- Treatment can be surgical (e.g., angioplasty, endarterectomy, extracranial-intracranial bypass, shunt placement for hydrocephalus) or medical (e.g., antithrombotic therapy, thrombolytic therapy, anti-edema therapy).
- Common long-term complications following stroke can include contractures, osteoporosis, heterotopic ossification, falling, seizures, hydrocephalus, and abnormal changes in muscle tone and length.
- Less common long-term effects of stroke include deconditioning, psychologic disorders, urinary tract dysfunction, skin breakdown, dysphagia, aspiration, and deep venous thrombosis.
- Modification of risk factors, such as control of hypertension, smoking cessation, antiarrythmic drug therapy or pacemaker insertion, control of blood lipid level (cholesterol/triglicerides) control of diabetes, elimination of use of oral contraceptives in persons with other risks, limited alcohol use, increased physical activity, and public education can prevent strokes.

REFERENCES

1a. Adams HP et al: Guidelines for the management of patients with acute ischemic stroke: a statement for healthcare professionals from a special writing group of the Stroke Council, American Heart Association, *Circulation* 90:1588, 1994.
1b. The Agency for Health Care Policy and Research: Smoking cessation clinical practice guidelines, *JAMA* 276:448, 1996.
2. Antiplatelet Trialists' Collaboration: Collaborative overview of randomized trials of antiplatelet therapy—I: prevention of death, myocardial infarction, and stroke by prolonged antiplatelet therapy in various categories of patients, *Br Med J*: 308:81, 1994.
3. Asplund K: Hemodilution in acute stroke, *Cerebrovasc Dis* 1(suppl):129, 1991.
4. Bah-y-rita P: Process of recovery from stroke. In Brandstser ME, Basmajian JV, editors: *Stroke rehabilitation*, Baltimore, Md, 1987, Williams & Wilkins.
5. Barer DH: Continence after stroke: useful predictor or goal of therapy? *Age Ageing* 18:183, 1989.
6. Black SE, Norris JW, Hachinski VC: Post stroke seizures, *Stroke* 14:134, 1983.
7. Bonita R, Beaglehole R, North JDK: Event, incidence and case fatality rates of cerebrovascular disease in Auckland, New Zealand, *Am J Epidemiol* 120:236, 1984.
8. Bonita R: Epidemiology of stroke, *Lancet* 339:342, 1992.
9. Bontke CF, Boake C: Principles of brain injury rehabilitation. In Braddom RL, editor: *Physical medicine and rehabilitation*, Philadelphia, 1996, WB Saunders.
10. Brandstater ME, Roth EJ, Siebens HC: Venous thromboembolism in stroke: literature review and implication for clinical practice, *Arch Phys Med Rehabl* 73(suppl):379, 1992.
11. Brockhurst JC et al: Incidence and correlates of incontinence in stroke patients, *J Am Geriatr Soc* 33:540, 1985.
12. Bromfield EB, Reding MJ: Relative risk of deep venous thrombosis or pulmonary embolism post-stroke based on ambulatory status, *J Neuro Rehab* 2:51, 1988.
13. Bushbacher RM: Deconditioning, conditioning, and the benefits of exercise. In Braddom RL, editor: *Physical medicine and rehabilitation*, Philadelphia, 1996, WB Saunders.
14. Bushbacher R: Heterotopic ossification: a review, *Crit Rev Phys Med Rehab* 4:199, 1992.
15. Caplan LR: Diagnosis and treatment of ischemic stroke, *JAMA* 266:2413, 1991.
16. Cerebral Embolism Study Group: Immediate anticoagulation of embolic stroke: Brain Hemorrhage and Cerebral Embolism Task Force: cardiogenic brain embolism: the second report of the cerebral embolism task force, *Arch Neurol* 46:727, 1989.
17. Cinnamon J et al: CT and MRI diagnosis of cerebrovascular disease: going beyond the pixels, *Sem CT MRI* 16:212, 1995.
18. Colditz GA et al: Cigarette smoking and risk for stroke in middle aged women, *N Engl J Med* 318:937, 1988.
19. Collins R et al: Blood pressure, stroke, and coronary heart disease: part II. Effects of short-term reductions in blood pressure and overview of the unconfounded randomized trials in an epidemiological context, *Lancet* 335:827, 1990.
20. Counsel C, Sandercock P: The management of patients with acute ischemic stroke, *Curr MedLit: Geriatr* 7:99, 1994.
21. Coventry MB, Scanlon PW: The use of radiation to discourage ectopic bone, *J Bone Joint Surg Am* 63:201, 1981.
22. DeVincenzo DK, Watkins S: Accidental falls in a rehabilitation setting, *Rehab Nurs* 12:248, 1987.
23. Dicter MA: In Isselbacher KJ et al, editors: *Harrison's principles of internal medicine*, New York, 1994, McGraw Hill.
24. Donahue RP et al: Alcohol and hemorrhagic stroke: the Honolulu Heart Program, *JAMA* 255:2311, 1986.
25. Donaldson CL et al: Effect of prolonged bed rest on bone mineral, *Metabolism* 19:1071, 1970.
26. Dyken ML: Trends in management and prognosis in stroke, *Ann Epidemiol* 3:535, 1993.
27. Ebrahim S: *Clinical epidemiology of stroke*, Oxford, Oxford University Press.
28. Ebrahim S, Nouri F: Caring for stroke patients at home, *Int Rehab Med* 8:171, 1987.
29. EC/IC Bypass Study Group: Failure of EC-IC arterial bypass to reduce the risk of ischemic stroke. Results of an international randomized trial, *N Engl J Med* 313:1191, 1985.
30. Elster AD, Moody DM: Early cerebral infarction: gadopentetate dimeblumine enhancement, *Radiology* 177:627, 1990.

31. European Atrial Fibrillation Trial Study Group: Secondary prevention in nonrheumatic atrial fibrillation after transient ischemic attack or minor stroke, *Lancet* 342:1255, 1993.

32. European Carotid Surgery Trial Collaborative Group: Medical research council carotid surgery trial: interim results for patients with severe (70% to 90%) or with mild (0% to 30%) carotid stenosis, *Lancet* 334:175, 1989.

33. Farrell B et al: The United Kingdom transient ischemic attack (UK-TIA) aspirin trial: final results, *J Neurol Neurosurg Psychiatry* 54:1044, 1991.

34. Fischer CM: Pathological observations in hypertensive cerebral hemorrhage, *J Neuropath Exp Neurol* 30:536, 1971.

35. Fisher CM: Clinical syndromes in cerebral thrombosis, hypertensive hemorrhage, and ruptured accular aneurysm, *Clin Neurosurg* 22:117, 1975.

36. Fisher CM et al: Atherosclerosis of the carotid and vertebral arteries: extracranial and intracranial, *J Neuropathol Exp Neurol* 24:455, 1965.

37. Garraway WM, Whisnant JP, Drury I: The changing pattern of survival after stroke, *Stroke* 14:699, 1983.

38. Gianotti G: Emotional behavior and hemispheric side of the lesion, *Cortex* 8:41, 1972.

39. Gordon C, Hewer RL, Wade DT: Dysphagia in acute stroke, *Br J Med* 295:411, 1987.

40. Groher ME, Bukatman R: The prevalence of swallowing disorders in two teaching hospitals, *Dysphagia* 1:3, 1986.

41. Grotta JC, Norris JW, Kamm B: Prevention of stroke with ticlopidine: who benefits most? *Neurology* 42:111, 1992.

42. Hachinski V, Norris JW: *The acute stroke*, Philadelphia, 1985, FA Davis.

43. Harburn KL, Potter PJ: Spasticity and contractures, *Phys Med Rehab: State Art Rev* 7:113, 1993.

44. Hassenfeld M: Increased incidence of hip fracture on the hemiplegic side of post stroke patients, Unpublished work presented at Columbia Presbyterian Medical Center, New York, May, 1993.

45. Hauser WA, Ramirez-Lassepas M, Rosenstein R: Risk for seizures and epilepsy following cerebrovascular insults, *Epilepsia* 25:666, 1984.

46. Heros RC, Zervas NT, Varsos V: Cerebral vasospasm after subarachnoid hemorrhage: an update, *Ann Neurol* 14:599, 1983.

47. Hirsh J, Genton E, Hull R: *Venous thromboembolism*, New York, 1981, Grune and Stratton.

48. Hirsh J, Hull R: Natural history and clinical features of venous thrombosis. In Coleman RW et al, editors: *Haemostasis and thrombosis: basic principles and clinical practice*, Philadelphia, 1982, JB Lippincott.

49. Hirsh J: From unfractionated heparins to low molecular weight heparins, *Acta Chir Scand Suppl* 556:42, 1990.

50. Hirsh J: Heparin, *N Engl J Med* 324:1565, 1991.

51. House A et al: Emotionalism after stroke, *BMJ* 298:991, 1989.

52. Hull R, Hirsh J: Diagnosis of venous thromboembolism. In Coleman RW et al, editors: *Haemostasis and thrombosis: basic principles and clinical practice*, Philadelphia, 1982, JB Lippincott.

53. Hull RD et al: Heparin for 5 days as compared with 10 days in the initial treatment of proximal venous thrombosis, *N Engl J Med* 322:1260, 1990.

54. Iso H, et al: Serum cholesterol levels and six year mortality from stroke in 350,977 men screened for the multiple risk factor intervention trial, *N Engl J Med* 320:904, 1989.

55. Kannel WB, McGee DL: Diabetes and cardiavascular disease: The Framingham Study, *JAMA* 241:2035, 1979.

56. Kanter MC, Sherman DG: Strategies for preventing stroke, *Curr Opin Neurol Neurosurg* 6:60, 1993.

57. Kistler JP, Ropper AH, Martin JB: Cerebrovascular disease. In Isselbacher KJ et al, editors: *Harrison's principles of internal medicine*, New York, 1994, McGraw Hill.

58. Kottke FJ, Pauley DL, Park RA: The rationale for prolonged stretching for correction of shortening of connective tissue, *Arch Phys Med Rehab* 47:345, 1966.

59. Kozarevic DJ et al: Frequency of alcohol consumption and morbidity and mortality: the Yugoslavia Cardiovascular Disease Study, *Lancet* 1:613, 1980.

60. Kuller LH, Dorman JS, Wolf PA: Cerebrovascular disease and diabetes. In *Diabetes in America: diabetes data compiled for 1984*, National Diabetes Data Group, Department of Health and Human Services, NIH Pub No 85-1468, August, 1985.

61. Lance JW: Pathophysiology of spasticity and clinical experience with baclofen. In Eldman RG, Young RR, Koella P, editors: *Spasticity—disordered motor control*, Chicago, 1980, Yearbook.

62. Langhorne P et al: Do stroke units save lives? *Lancet* 342:395, 1993.

63. Langhorne P, Stott DJ: Acute cerebral infarction: optimal management in older patients, *Drugs Aging* 6:445, 1995.

64. Levinson ME, Bush L: Pharmacodynamics of antimicrobial agents: bactericidal and postantibiotic effects, *Infect Dis Clin North Am* 3:415, 1989.

65. Levinson ME: Pneumonia, including necrotizing pulmonary infections (lung abscesses). In Isselbacher KJ et al, editors: *Harrison's principles of internal medicine*, New York, 1994, McGraw Hill.

66. Lezak MD: *Neuropsychological assessment*, ed 2, New York, 1983, Orford University Press.

67. Locksley HB: Natural history of subarachnoid hemorrhage, intracranial aneurysms, and arteriovenous malformations: based on 6368 cases in a cooperative study. In Sahs AL et al, editors: *Intracranial aneurysms and subarachnoid hemorrhage: a cooperative study*, Philadelphia, 1969, JB Lippincott.

68. Longstreth WT Jr, et al: Clinical course of spontaneous subarachnoid hemorrhage: a population based study in King County, Washington, *Neurology* 43:712, 1993.

69. Lorber B, Swenson RM: Bacteriology of aspiration pneumonia: a prospective study of community and hospital acquired cases, *Ann Intern Med* 81:329, 1974.

70. MacMahon S et al: Blood pressure, stroke, and coronary heart disease: part I. Effects of prolonged differences in blood pressure. Evidence from nine prospective observational studies corrected for regression dilution bias, *Lancet* 335:765, 1990.

71. Marmot MG, Poulter NR: Primary prevention of stroke, *Lancet* 339:344, 1992.

72. Mayerberg MR et al: Guidelines for the management of aneurysmal subarachnoid hemorrhage: a statement for healthcare professionals from a special writing group of the Stroke Council, American Heart Association, *Stroke* 25:2315, 1994.

73. McGill HC: The pathogenesis of atherosclerosis, *Clin Chem* 34:B34, 1988.

74. McNeil BJ, Bettman MA: The diagnosis of pulmonary embolism. In Coleman RW et al, editors: *Haemostasis and thrombosis: Basic principles and clinical practice*, Philadelphia, 1982, JB Lippincott.

75. Mion LC et al: Falls in the rehabilitation setting: incidence and characteristics, *Rehab Nurs* 14:17, 1989.

76. Mohr JP et al: Meta-analysis of nimodipine trials in acute ischemic stroke, *Cerebrovasc Dis* 4:197, 1994.

77. Mohr JP: Lacunes, *Stroke* 13:3-11, 1982.

78. Murray GB, Shea V, Conn DK: Electroconvulsive therapy for poststroke depression, *J Clin Psychiatry* 47:258, 1986.

79. NASCET Collaborators: Beneficial effect of carotid endarterectomy in symptomatic patients with high grade stenosis, *N Eng J Med* 325:445, 1991.

80. Office of Medical Applications of Research, NIH Consensus Conference: prevention of venous thrombosis and pulmonary embolism, *JAMA* 256:744, 1986.

81. Okada Y et al: Hemorrhagic transformation in cerebral embolism, *Stroke* 20:598, 1989.

82. Paffenbarger RS et al: Work activity of longshoremen as related to death from coronary heart disease and stroke, *N Engl J Med* 282:1109, 1970.

83. Paffenbarger RS, Wing AL, Hyde RT: Physical activity as an index of heart attack risk in college alumni, *Am J Epidemiol* 108:161, 1978.

84. Pessin MS et al: Clinical and angiographic features of carotid transient ischemic attacks, *N Engl J Med* 296:358, 1977.

85. Poplinger AR, Pillar T: Hip fracture in stroke patients: epidemiology and rehabilitation, *Acta Orthop Scand* 56:226, 1985.

86. PORT Study: Funded by the Agency for Health Care Policy and Research. Duke University Medical Center, Durham, NC, 1994.

87. Quizilbash N, Murphy M: Meta-analysis of trials of corticosteroids in acute stroke, *Age Ageing* 22(suppl):2, 1993.

88. Reed DM: The paradox of high risk of stroke in populations with low risk of coronary heart disease, *Am J Epidemiol* 131:579, 1990.

89. Robinson RG et al: Depression influenced intellectual impairment in stroke patients, *Br J Psychiatry* 148:541, 1986.

90. Ropper AH, Davis KR: Lobar cerebral hemorrhages: acute clinical syndromes in 26 patients, *Ann Neurol* 8:141, 1980.

91. Roth EJ, Harvey RL: Rehabilitation of stroke syndromes. In Braddom RL, editor: *Physical medicine and rehabilitation*, Philadelphia, 1996, WB Saunders.

92. Royal College of General Practitioners': Royal College of General Practitioners' Oral Contraceptive Study: further analyses of mortality in oral contraceptive users, *Lancet* 1:541, 1981.

93. Rutan GH et al: Mortality associated with diastolic hypertension and isolated systolic hypertension among men screened for the Multiple Risk Factor Intervention Trial, *Hypertension* 77:504, 1988.

94. Salcido R, Hart D, Smith AM: The prevention and management of pressure ulcers. In Braddom RL editor: *Physical medicine and rehabilitation*, Philadelphia, 1996, WB Saunders.

95. Salonen R et al: Prevalence of carotid atherosclerosis and serum cholesterol levels in eastern Finland, *Atherosclerosis* 8:788, 1988.

96. Salzman EW, Hirsh J: Prevention of venous thromboembolism. In Coleman RW et al, editors: *Haemostasis and thrombosis: basic principles and clinical practice*, Philadelphia, 1982, JB Lippincott.

97. Sandercock PAG et al: Antithrombotic therapy in acute ischemic stroke: an overview of the randomized trials, *J Neurol Neurosurg Psychiatry* 56:17, 1993.

98. Sandercock PAG, Williams H: Medical treatment of acute ischemic stroke, *Lancet* 339:537, 1992.

99. SHEP Cooperative Research Group: Prevention of stroke by antihypertensive drug treatment in older persons with isolated systolic hypertension: final results of the Systolic Hypertension in the Elderly Program (SHEP), *JAMA* 265:3255, 1991.

100. Simoons ML et al: Individaul risk assessment for intracranial hemorrhage during thrombolytic therapy, *Lancet* 342:1523, 1993.

101. Sinyor D et al: Post-stroke depression: relationships to functional impairment, coping strategies and rehabilitation outcome, *Stroke* 17:1102, 1986.

102. Stadel BV: Oral contraceptives and cardiovascular disease, *N Engl J Med* 288:672, 1981.

103. Stampfer MJ et al: A prospective study of the past use of oral contraceptive agents and the risk of cardiovascular diseases, *N Engl J Med* 319:1313, 1988.

104. Starkstein S, Robinson R, Price TR: Comparison of cortical and subcortical lesions in the production of post stroke mood disorders, *Brain* 110:1045, 1987.

105. Starkstein SE et al: Relationship between anxiety disorders and depressive disorders in patients with cerebrovascular injury, *Arch Gen Psychiatry* 47:246, 1990.

106. Subbarao J, Smith J: Pulmonary embolism during stroke rehabilitation, *Illinois Med J* 165:328, 1984.

107. Sundaram MBM, Chow F: Seizures associated with spontaneous subarachnoid hemorrhage, *Can J Neurol Sci* 13:229, 1986.

108. Sundt TM Jr et al: Results and complications of surgical management of 809 intracranial aneurysms in 722 cases: related and unrelated to grade of patient, type of aneurysm, and timing of surgery, *J Neurosurg* 56:753, 1982.

109. Sundt TM, Whisnant P: Subarachnoid hemorrhage from intracranial aneurysms, *N Engl J Med* 299:116, 1978.

110. Swartzman L, Teasell RW: Psychological consequences of stroke, *Phys Med Rehab: State Art Rev* 7:179, 1993.

111. The Dutch Transient Ischemic Attack Trial Study Group: A comparison of two doses of aspirin (30 mg versus 283 mg a day) in patients after a transient ischemic attack or minor ischemic stroke, *N Engl J Med* 325:1261, 1991.

112. The Swedish Aspirin Low-Dose Trial Collaborative Group: Swedish aspirin low-dose trial (SALT) of 75 mg aspirin as secondary prophylaxis after cerebrovascular ischemic events, *Lancet* 338:1345, 1991.

113. Thompson DD, Rodan GA: Indomethacin inhibition of tenotomy induced bone resorbtion in rats, *J Bone Miner Res* 3:409, 1988.

114. Torner JC, Nibbelink DW, Burmeister LF: Statistical comparisons of end results of a randomized treatment study. In Sahs AL, Nibbelink DW, Torner JC, editors: *Aneurysmal subarachnoid hemorrhage: report of the cooperative study*, Baltimore, 1981, Urban & Schwarzenberg.

115. Viitanen M, Eriksson S, Aspulund K: Risk of recurrent stroke, myocardial infarction and epilepsy during long-term follow-up after stroke, *Eur Neurol* 28:227, 1988.

116. Wardlaw JM, Warlow CP: Thrombolysis in acute ischemic stroke: does it work? *Stroke* 23:1826, 1992.

117. Warlow C, Ogston D, Douglas AS: Deep venous thrombosis of the legs after strokes. Part I. Incidence and predisposing factors. Part II. Natural history, *Br Med J* 1:1178, 1976.

118. Warlow C: Disorders of the cerebral circulation. In Walton J, editor: *Brain's disease of the nervous system*, ed 10, Oxford, 1993, Oxford University Press.

119. Wheeler HB, Anderson FA Jr: Diagnostic approaches for deep vein thrombosis, *Chest* 89(suppl):407, 1986.

120. Whisnant JP, Matsumotoa N, Elveback LR: The effect of anticoagulant therapy on the prognosis of patients with transient cerebral ischemic attacks in a community: Rochester, Minnesota 1955-1969, *Mayo Clinic Proc* 48:844, 1973.

121. Wiebe-Velasquez S, Blume WT: Seizures, *Phys Med Rehab: State Art Rev* 7:73, 1993.

122. Wolf PA, Belanger AJ, D'Agostino RB: Management of risk factors, *Neurol Clin* 10:177, 1992.

123. Wolf PA et al: Cigarette smoking as a risk factor for stroke: the Framingham Study, *JAMA* 259:1025, 1988.

124. Wolf PA et al: Probability of stroke: a risk profile from the Framingham Study, *Stroke* 22:312, 1991.

125. Worden JW: *Grief counseling and grief therapy*, New York, 1982, Springer.

126. Wortman CB, Silver RC: The myths of coping with loss, *J Consult Clin Psychol* 57:349, 1989.

joyce shapero sabari

chapter 2

Application of Learning and Environmental Strategies to Activity-Based Treatment

key terms

pathology	extrinsic feedback	closed tasks
impairment	concurrent feedback	variable motionless tasks
disability	terminal/summary feedback	consistent motion tasks
handicap/societal limitation	knowledge of performance (KP) feedback	open tasks
performance areas		purposeful activity
performance components	knowledge of results (KR) feedback	activity analysis
performance contexts		postural set
degrees of freedom	multicontext approach	postural adjustments
metacognition	practice conditions	disassociation between body segments
kinesiologic linkages	variable practice	
cognitive strategies	repetitive practice	compensatory strategies
task analysis	contextual interference	activity synthesis
generalization of learning	blocked practice	regulatory conditions
intrinsic feedback	random practice	occupational form

chapter objectives

After completing this chapter, the reader will be able to accomplish the following:

1. Identify the general goals and performance component goals of occupational therapy intervention for stroke survivors.
2. Describe which factors contribute to generalization of learning, and apply these concepts to occupational therapy intervention with stroke survivors.
3. Describe the way occupational therapists analyze, select, and synthesize activities during clinical intervention with stroke survivors.
4. Apply principles of activity analysis and synthesis when designing occupational therapy intervention for stroke survivors.

This chapter has been designed to serve as a foundation for the general understanding of occupational therapy intervention with stroke survivors. Although specific methods and goals may overlap with the contributions made by other professionals on the rehabilitation team, the totality of occupational therapy intervention is characterized by the following unique and distinguishable features:

1. Occupational therapists enable stroke survivors to be self-sufficient in tasks of daily life.
2. Occupational therapists enable stroke survivors to resume meaningful and productive life roles.
3. Occupational therapists implement strategies that will maximize generalization of learning from the clinical setting to nonclinical environments.
4. Occupational therapists use activity analysis, selection, and synthesis as interventions to assist stroke survivors in meeting their personal goals.

GENERAL GOALS OF OCCUPATIONAL THERAPY INTERVENTION FOR STROKE SURVIVORS

The World Health Organization's (WHO) International Classification of Impairment, Disability, and Handicap (ICIDH)[71] provides a useful framework for examining the effects of long-term disability and clarifies the roles of occupational therapy intervention in stroke rehabilitation (Figure 2-1).

Pathology refers to the direct anatomic and physiologic effects of a stroke (see Chapter 1). Impairments are the motor and cognitive residuals of the pathology. Primary impairments, such as paralysis or aphasia, are directly linked to the neuropathology associated with the cerebrovascular accident (CVA). Their severity varies greatly among stroke survivors, depending upon individual differences in stroke pathology. Secondary impairments are preventable dysfunctions, such as disruptions in postural alignment, joint deformities, or edema.

Disabilities are the difficulties a person has performing daily-life tasks such as self-care, work and leisure activities. Handicaps, or societal limitations, are limitations in social role performance.

Medical, pharmacologic, and surgical interventions play a critical role in preventing or minimizing the pathology associated with stroke. However, many stroke survivors must cope with life in spite of remaining pathology and impairments. Their quality of life after stroke depends on learning strategies to minimize their disabilities and societal limitations.

Occupational therapists play a major role in helping stroke survivors resume active, productive lives. The ultimate goal of occupational therapy is to enable individuals to perform the tasks that are essential for performing their unique roles. An occupational therapist assesses underlying motor, cognitive, perceptual, and interpersonal skills as well as task performance and valued roles. Depending on a person's current potential for recovery impairments, the occupational therapist facilitates task performance by improving relevant performance skills, developing and teaching compensatory strategies to overcome lost performance skills, or combining both of these strategies.

Occupational therapists implement activity-based intervention for the following reasons:

1. To maximize each individual's potential to improve primary impairments and prevent secondary impairments
2. To minimize disabilities by enabling each individual to perform relevant daily life tasks
3. To reduce handicaps/societal limitations by facilitating task performance and role achievement (Figure 2-2)

The American Occupational Therapy Association's (AOTA) framework for conceptualizing OT intervention[1,65] is quite consistent with WHO's ICIDH[71] (Table 2-1). A major difference is that the WHO framework uses negative terms to describe the sequelae of stroke, whereas

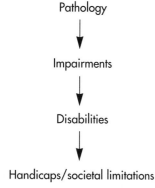

Figure 2-1 World Health Organization International Classification of Impairment, Disability, and Handicap.

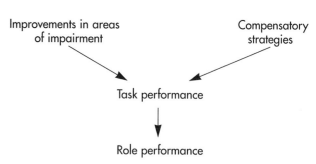

Figure 2-2 The occupational therapy process.

the occupational therapy framework uses positive terms to describe aspects of therapeutic intervention.

Performance areas "are broad categories of human activity that are typically part of daily life. They include activities of daily living, work, and leisure activities."[65] Intervention to improve function in performance areas corresponds directly to reducing disabilities in the WHO ICIDH classification.

Performance components "are fundamental human abilities that—to varying degrees and in differing combinations—are required for successful engagement in performance areas. These components are sensorimotor, cognitive, psychosocial, and psychological."[65] Performance component deficits are analogous to ICIDH impairments.

Performance contexts "are situations or factors that influence an individual's engagement in desired and/or required performance areas."[65] Societal limitations associated with an inability to resume meaningful roles after a stroke may be amenable to change by removing environmental barriers such as social, cultural, or physical constraints. For example, an occupational therapist may redesign a work site so that it is accessible to a stroke survivor who walks with a cane and has partial paralysis in the left arm. Social and cultural barriers, such as preconceived notions about what a person with a disability can achieve, may be more difficult to overcome than physical constraints. Occupational therapists educate stroke survivors, their families, and members of the community about the possibilities of performing role-related tasks in spite of residual impairments.

PERFORMANCE COMPONENT GOALS IN OCCUPATIONAL THERAPY INTERVENTION FOR STROKE SURVIVORS

Performance area and performance context goals are based on individual lifestyles, environments, interests, and needs. Performance component goals, however, are based on the impairments that are associated with a given diagnosis. Although stroke survivors can have a broad range of impairments that may vary in severity between individuals, it is still useful to understand which performance components are most likely to be impaired after a CVA. In addition, it is useful to determine which motor and cognitive impairments are amenable to positive change through rehabilitation.

Historically, prevailing theories about motor control have influenced therapeutic interventions for stroke survivors.[24,35] Previous rehabilitative efforts focused only on the limb paralysis associated with stroke. Therapists taught one-handed strategies for activity performance or attempted to improve muscle strength and range-of-motion (ROM) using treatments designed for individuals with orthopedic or peripheral nervous system disorders.

Beginning in the 1950s the ideas of Twitchell,[64] Brunnstrom,[8] and Bobath[7] focused attention on the positively associated symptoms associated with the neu-

ropathology of stroke. Therapy programs were designed to reduce spasticity and primitive reflexes so that they could facilitate limb movements. By the 1970s, Bobath[7] had expanded understanding of the motor residuals of CVAs. In addition to considering limb paralysis and abnormal muscle tone, therapists were encouraged to consider issues related to posture, balance, and motor control of the head, trunk, shoulder, and pelvic girdles.

Current theories about motor control, cognition, and learning have influenced recent strategies to improve functional performance after stroke. It is generally accepted that human performance requires complex interactions between perceptual, cognitive, and motor systems in relation to specific tasks and environments.[35,38,39,52] OT intervention strives to achieve the following five general performance component goals (Figure 2-3).

Preventing Secondary Impairments

Abnormal Muscle Shortening

Selected muscle weakness and loss of automatic control over complex postural adjustments are primary impairments that are related to stroke pathology. Abnormal muscle shortening develops when muscles do not have the opportunity to be lengthened by antagonist muscles or an

Table 2-1

Comparison Between ICIDH and AOTA Terminology

ICIDH	AOTA UNIFORM TERMINOLOGY
Pathology	—
Impairments	Performance components
Disabilities	Performance areas
Role limitations	Performance contexts

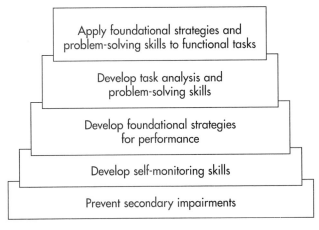

Figure 2-3 Occupational therapy performance component goals for stroke survivors.

external force. This loss of distensibility may lead to malalignments in posture that contribute to further muscle-length abnormalities. Selected muscle shortening also creates disturbances in the efficient mechanics of muscular function, resulting in additional problems in motor control. Furthermore, chronic muscle shortening eventually leads to shortening of ligaments and other articular structures, resulting in fixed limitations of joint motion and alignment.[11,12,16]

Prevention of abnormal muscle shortening is achieved by establishing appropriate postural alignment while lying down, sitting, and standing. In addition, shortly after a stroke, individuals are instructed to follow daily routines to maintain muscle length through the practice of a variety of motor tasks.[11,12,16,19] These strategies are discussed in Chapters 6, 10 and 19. Orthotic interventions to prevent abnormal muscle shortening are discussed in Chapters 8 and 9.

Fixation Patterns

When people feel unable to maintain their balance in posturally threatening situations, the natural response is to fixate selected body parts and thus decrease the number of motor elements (or degrees of freedom) the central nervous system must control.[5,68] An example of this strategy is a person's tendency to contract all the flexors and extensors of the trunk when attempting to ski or ice skate for the first time.[68] Individuals with postural adjustment deficits resulting from stroke feel insecure about their ability to maintain balance, even in routine sitting or standing positions. The strategy of fixating the pelvis on the lumbar spine or the scapula on the thorax has the short-term benefit of enhancing a person's sense of postural security. A negative consequence is that these fixation patterns lead to difficulty disassociating the scapula and pelvis from adjacent proximal structures. This lack of sufficient limb girdle mobility subsequently limits the normal kinematics of upper and lower extremity movement. Current therapeutic approaches[9,15,16,20,23] advocate the early introduction of techniques to enhance balance and postural control to prevent the development of abnormal fixation patterns. These techniques are discussed in Chapter 5.

Similarly, when people attempt to perform motor tasks that are too complex for them to control, they tend to "freeze degrees of freedom" by rigidly coupling their movements to two or more body segments.[68] An example is the novice tennis player's tendency to "simplify" the act of serving by limiting movements at the neck, trunk, and shoulder. Individuals with intact neuromuscular systems are often able to make a smooth transition from using these freezing strategies to developing a single motor program that allows smooth, coordinated control over multiple body segments. However, clinical observations indicate that neuropathology after a stroke limits individuals' ability to "unlearn" restricted motor strategies and progress to using more flexible and efficient patterns of movement.[7,9]

Some therapists* believe that the continual practice of fundamentally inappropriate compensatory strategies is a critical mechanism that limits recovery following brain damage. Therefore treatment efforts are geared toward ensuring that compensatory behaviors are not learned as a substitute for optimal performance. Therapists structure activities and environmental supports so that patients can accomplish motor tasks without using freezing or other inefficient compensatory strategies. Task demands are gradually increased as the individual's ability to control an increasing number of degrees of freedom increases.[45]

Other Secondary Impairments

Other secondary impairments related to stroke include psychosocial dysfunction, edema, pain, and shoulder subluxation. Prevention and management of these impairments are discussed in Chapters 3, 6, 7, 8, 9, and 19.

Developing Self-Monitoring Skills

Stroke survivors are faced with the challenge of resuming their lives in a body that is quite different from the one they inhabited before: sensory information may be difficult to interpret, muscles may no longer work in effortless synchrony, and postural preparation for movement may no longer be automatic.

Before stroke survivors can begin to learn effective strategies for movement and task performance, they need to become acutely aware of the way their bodies work, which movements are possible at different body segments, when their postures are optimally aligned, and when they are efficiently "set" to perform particular activities. These understandings are critical for redeveloping appropriate kinesiologic linkages that will serve as motor foundations for task performance.

Metacognition[57,58] is the knowledge and regulation of personal cognitive processes and capacities. It includes an awareness of personal strengths and limitations and the ability to evaluate task difficulty, plan ahead, choose appropriate strategies, and shift strategies in response to environmental cues. Toglia's multicontext approach to cognitive perceptual impairment[57,58] emphasizes developing insight about personal deficits (and strengths) as a first step toward developing strategies for functional performance after brain injury (see Chapter 14).

Understanding the concept of metacognition is important for understanding movement as well. Before individuals can generalize the way to use scapulohumeral rhythm in tasks requiring functional reach, they must first understand the amount of mobility their unaffected scapula has. Then they must acknowledge when their affected scapula is not moving freely so that they can develop internal feedback mechanisms that will enable them to correct their scapula movements when they are insufficient for accomplishing a given task. The ultimate goal is to use this per-

*References 6, 11, 12, 15, 16, 19.

sonal knowledge of movement to change the foundational strategy used for reaching tasks in a variety of contexts. "The individual's degree of effectiveness in the learning process (and thus in problem solving in general) will be limited by his or her ability for critical self-analysis and environmental analysis in light of the problems encountered and by his or her ability to generate and control the solutions to these problems."[25]

Redeveloping Appropriate Foundational Strategies for Task Performance

Appropriate Kinesiologic Linkages for Efficient Control of Balance, Gross Mobility, and Limb Movement

When the neuromuscular system is functioning optimally, a person can rely on automatic kinematic and kinetic linkages to serve as a foundation for functional movements. Although these linkages are described in a variety of ways,[5,49,50,52,55] motor control theorists and kinesiologists agree that they promote optimal mechanical interactions between muscles and body segments. Normal shoulder abduction is an example. Regardless of the task or the environment, kinematic linkages between the scapula and humerus result in the scapulohumeral rhythm that is required to achieve full ROM and force production[42] (Figure 2-4). In addition, the deltoid and rotator cuff muscles are kinetically linked to ensure that the deltoid fibers produce the desired rotary force on the humerus. Without this linkage an attempt to abduct the shoulder will instead result in a nonfunctional upward shrug of the shoulder[42] (Figure 2-5).

Stroke survivors have often lost the automatic kinesiologic linkages associated with efficient movement.[45] This may be a result of limited mobility of body segments, weakness of specific muscular components, or loss of the motor program that links muscles or joints during a given movement sequence. An occupational therapist determines which kinesiologic linkages are impaired and intervenes by assisting with reestablishing these general foundations for normal motor performance. Motion analysis studies of rolling,[44] getting out of bed,[36,37] standing up from a sitting position,[47] and moving the arms[30] provide useful information that can help an occupational therapist determine which components are essential in a variety of performance contexts.

Cognitive Strategies and Strategies That Compensate for Perceptual Impairments

Just as kinetic linkages serve as foundational strategies for efficient movement, cognitive processing strategies provide individuals with a framework for interpreting and acting on complex information in a variety of situations. These strategies are organized approaches that assist a person in selecting relevant cues from the environment and planning the most appropriate response.[58]

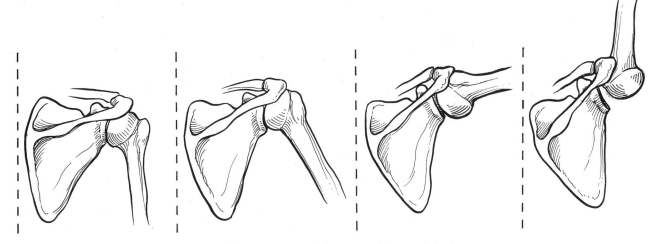

Figure 2-4   Kinematic linkage: scapulohumeral rhythm.

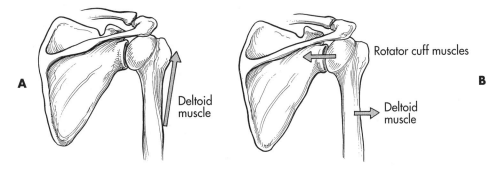

Figure 2-5   Kinetic linkage: relationship between deltoid and rotator cuff muscles. **A,** Deltoid muscle force acting alone. **B,** Deltoid and rotator cuff muscles working together.

Depending on the nature and location of the pathology associated with the CVA, a stroke survivor may demonstrate impairments in selecting and implementing appropriate cognitive strategies for accomplishing complex tasks. If these impairments are severe, they will limit performance of routine self-care tasks. However, the impairments usually become more apparent when the individual attempts to resume home management, work, or school activities. Toglia has been particularly influential in designing evaluation and treatment protocols to guide occupational therapists in this aspect of intervention.[57,58,59,60,61]

Occupational therapy intervention begins with helping patients develop insight about these deficits through a program that challenges them to estimate task difficulty, predict outcomes, and evaluate personal performance. Then the occupational therapist teaches general processing strategies that are practiced in a variety of contexts.

There are several examples of cognitive strategies. Prioritizing information before beginning a task is a strategy that can be applied to activities as varied as grocery shopping (using a list, coupons, and the weekly circular), doing a work-related task, or planning a family outing. Clustering related information together may be a useful strategy for a student who is attempting to master a difficult subject or for a person who is trying to remember what to purchase in the pharmacy. Blocking out irrelevant details is a foundational strategy that is necessary for reading a map as well as managing monthly bills. A left-to-right scanning strategy can be used to find a certain item in a bathroom cabinet as well as check typing for errors. Maintaining a daily notebook of things to do and remember is a strategy with wide applications in a range of situations. Additional strategies and their applications are discussed in Chapters 12, 13, 14, and 15. Each individual tests the strategies introduced by the therapist to determine whether they are effective and in which situations they can be successfully applied.

Developing Skills in Task Analysis and Problem Solving

Occupational therapists have always recognized that the therapist needs to be skillful at analyzing tasks. Task analysis enables an occupational therapist to establish treatment goals, synthesize treatment activities, and develop compensatory strategies.[27] Rehabilitation professionals are realizing more often that clients must also learn to analyze activities—or be perpetually dependent on their therapists for successful task achievement. A stroke survivor must learn to determine which motor, cognitive-perceptual, and psychologic challenges a task presents. Only then can effective strategies be chosen to "solve the problems"[5] inherent in the infinite variety of tasks encountered while actively engaging in meaningful life roles.

While reading subsequent chapters in this text, it should be remembered that occupational therapists strive to develop patients' insight and problem-solving skills, regardless of whether the intervention relates to balance, gross motor function, limb movement, visual skills, neurobehavioral performance, or daily living tasks.

Applying Foundational Strategies, Task Analysis, and Problem-Solving Skills to Functional Activity Performance

For many years, therapeutic outcomes were determined by assessing patients' abilities to perform isolated movements or through artificial tests of specific perceptual or cognitive functions. Research about motor control and learning has revealed that skilled performance is the ability to perform tasks in a number of different ways in accordance with variations in environmental demands.[25,35,45,55,70]

The ultimate goal of occupational therapy intervention is for stroke survivors to generalize their new skills to activities beyond the context of the treatment setting. Intervention is not complete until individuals are able to apply the strategies learned in therapy to performing activities that are personally relevant in their individual, daily lives. Successful achievement of this goal requires generalization of learning.

GENERALIZATION OF LEARNING

Learning is an internal phenomenon that cannot be observed directly. However, it can be assumed that learning has occurred if performance of a skill *improves* over time, the improvement in performance *persists* over time, and the improved performance remains *consistent* in a variety of situations.[33,52]

The following three stages of learning are important in the occupational therapy process:

1. The *acquisition phase* occurs during initial instruction on and practice of a skill (e.g., the initial treatment sessions in which a person learns to use the left arm for functional reach).
2. The *retention phase* occurs after the initial practice period as individuals are asked to demonstrate how well they perform the newly acquired skill; therapists often refer to this as *carry-over* (e.g., a patient's ability to perform previously learned reaching activities).
3. In the *transfer phase* the individual must use the skill in a new context (e.g., the patient's ability to perform the reaching strategy when getting dressed or preparing a meal). When a stroke survivor can generalize the strategies learned in the therapy setting and use them in real-life situations, learning has occurred.

Literature about skill acquisition presents several concepts that are helpful in guiding therapeutic intervention that promotes generalization of learning. These concepts can be categorized into three major groups: feedback, strategy development, and practice conditions (Figure 2-6).

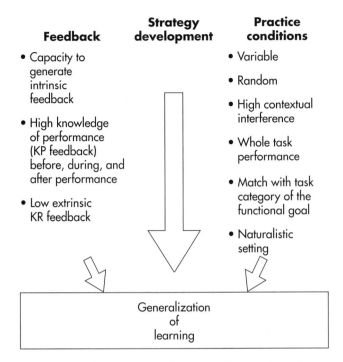

Feedback

- Capacity to generate intrinsic feedback
- High knowledge of performance (KP feedback) before, during, and after performance
- Low extrinsic KR feedback

Strategy development

Practice conditions

- Variable
- Random
- High contextual interference
- Whole task performance
- Match with task category of the functional goal
- Naturalistic setting

Generalization of learning

Figure 2-6 Factors promoting generalization of learning.

Feedback

Feedback, or information about a response, can be intrinsic or extrinsic, concurrent or terminal, and can provide knowledge of performance or results. Intrinsic feedback is a result of an individual's own proprioceptive, tactile, vestibular, visual, and auditory sensory systems. After a stroke the visual and somatosensory systems are often impaired, which limits the effectiveness of intrinsic feedback about motor performance. Extrinsic feedback from a therapist or feedback technology can provide useful supplementary information to facilitate early awareness and learning. Extrinsic feedback must be gradually decreased for generalization to occur, or the person may remain dependent on others for successful task performance.[52]

Concurrent feedback is provided during task performance. It includes intrinsic somatosensory feedback as well as ongoing verbal or manual guidance by a therapist. Terminal, or summary, feedback is given after task completion.[52] There are no published studies that compare the effectiveness of concurrent and terminal feedback.

Knowledge of Performance

Knowledge of performance (KP) feedback is information about the processes used during task performance, such as the way a person moves the pelvis or scapula or whether an appropriate cognitive strategy has been implemented. Individuals with intact proprioceptive systems receive concurrent, intrinsic KP feedback as they move. Stroke survivors, however, have often lost access to this continuous supply of information. Extrinsic KP can be provided before a task is initiated. For example, a therapist

can guide a person into assuming a postural set[6,19] that will facilitate motor performance or in planning a strategy that will enhance performance of a cognitively demanding task. KP can also be provided as concurrent or terminal feedback.

Knowledge of motor performance can relate to the kinetic or the kinematic aspects of movement. Varied kinetic information may be provided to stroke survivors through electromyography (EMG) biofeedback.[63] Although additional study is needed, biofeedback as a tool for increasing KP has been found to improve functional movement in the stroke population.[48] Kinematic feedback provides information about the direction and range of movement at selected body segments. Schmidt[51] cites a study by Lindahl[32] in which knowledge of kinematic performance was shown to be effective in industrial training. The researcher used measurements from highly skilled textile workers to determine the most effective pattern of foot motion for operating a cutting machine. He then used this pattern to provide feedback to new employees about their foot patterns. This kinematic feedback increased training efficiency significantly; new trainees achieved performance levels of skilled workers after only weeks of training. Physical and occupational therapists use a similar strategy when they use findings from kinematic studies of persons who move normally to guide the kinematic feedback provided to individuals who are regaining motor control after stroke.

Knowledge of Results

Knowledge of results (KR) is feedback about the outcome of an action in terms of accomplishing a goal. This information can serve as a basis for correcting errors for more effective performance on future trials. Extrinsic KR feedback has been more widely studied than KP feedback; however, most published research relates to normal subjects performing contrived tasks in laboratory settings.[52]

Results of laboratory research with normal subjects indicates that frequent, accurate, immediate KR tends to promote improved performance during the acquisition phase but poorer performance during the retention and transfer stages of learning.[46,69] Similarly, bandwidth KR, in which feedback is provided only when the performance response is outside a given range of acceptable performance, also leads to better generalization of learning.[69] Schmidt[51] provides the following theoretical explanation of these findings. When limited KR is provided during acquisition, individuals are forced to rely on relevant cues provided by intrinsic mechanisms to improve their performance on future trials. Thus they tend to develop less dependency on extrinsic feedback. Based on these findings, it is wise for therapists to limit the immediacy and frequency of KR feedback during stroke rehabilitation. Furthermore, therapists are advised to require that patients determine how effectively they performed therapeutic tasks. To generalize their knowledge for use in situations outside the treatment context, stroke survivors need to learn ways to assess their own performance of functional activities.

Strategy Development

Strategies are organized plans or sets of rules that guide action in a variety of situations. New knowledge is more likely to be generalized for use after the acquisition phase if the individual learns a foundational strategy that can be applied to performance of multiple tasks.[54]

Therapeutic approaches that advocate the importance of strategy formulation during task performance[11,57] rely heavily on KP feedback. A therapist teaches the individual to analyze personal performance in one or two selected domains and verifies the person's self-evaluation. To ensure generalization of the strategy the selected underlying skill is practiced repeatedly in a variety of contexts during a treatment session. For example, the therapist may decide to provide KP about pelvic mobility as a foundation for functional movement. Individuals will be instructed to be aware of the way their pelvis moves in the sagittal plane during different tasks. The session may begin with the therapist moving the patient's pelvis so that the person understands the kinematic model of action. The patient may then be asked to sit on a therapy ball, which is rocked forward and backward using anterior and posterior pelvic movement. After this, rising from sit to stand can direct focus to the required movement at the pelvis. The seemingly unrelated task of reaching for objects from the seated position will emphasize the appropriate pelvic movements to accompany trunk and arm trajectories.

Carr and Shepherd's motor relearning program for stroke[9,10,11,12] uses five major techniques to assist patients with developing motor strategies: (1) verbal instruction, (2) visual demonstration, (3) manual guidance, (4) accurate and timely feedback, and (5) consistency of practice. In addition, patients develop skill in providing themselves with intrinsic feedback about the kinematics of their motor performance. Two outcome studies[2,17] of individuals recovering from stroke provide support for this program's efficacy.

Toglia[57] has proposed a systematic approach to promoting generalization of cognitive strategies using KP feedback in a variety of settings. The therapist grades treatment by changing certain characteristics of a task but leaving the underlying strategy the same. To illustrate this approach the levels of transfer as they relate to treatment designed to facilitate learning and generalization of a strategy for categorizing information will be discussed.

The initial task is the first activity performed by the patient, such as sorting a deck of playing cards into a red group (hearts and diamonds) and a black group (spades and clubs).

Near transfer is an alternate form of the initial task. Using the previous example, the person might be instructed to sort the playing cards into four groups according to their suits or two groups of odd and even numbers.

Intermediate transfer has a moderate number of changes in task parameters but still has some similarities to the initial task. For example, the same person may be asked to create three categories for sorting a stack of photographs for eventual placement in a photo album.

Far transfer introduces an activity that is conceptually the same as but physically different from the initial task. Now the person may be asked to organize a collection of magazines into groups based on general interest areas (e.g., news, sports, fashion) for display in a clinic waiting room.

Very far transfer requires spontaneous use of the new strategy in daily functional activities. Before travelling to a neighborhood mall, the person may be asked to categorize items on a shopping list based on the type of store in which they can most likely be purchased.

In Toglia's multicontext approach, most of the KP feedback is intrinsic (provided by the individuals themselves rather than the therapist). Before attempting a new task, patients estimate their performance accuracy and efficiency and determine similarities and differences between the current task and previous activities. After completing a task, patients evaluate their performance and identify techniques that may be helpful in the future. The therapist's major roles are to structure the activity progression and guide patients in developing insights and strategies.

Practice Conditions

Concepts about practicing tasks to promote learning have changed significantly as a result of theoretical developments in cognitive psychology and motor control.[23,24,25,31,70] When performing isolated movements or testing specific perceptual impairments were the major goals of rehabilitation, practice was considered repetition of single movements or tasks. Currently, practice is considered an opportunity to develop and apply foundational strategies in a variety of contexts. Therefore, as discussed in the previous section, practice sessions in stroke rehabilitation settings are organized around a core group of strategies that are applied to performance of multiple tasks.

Several aspects of practice conditions have been studied under both laboratory and clinical conditions. Occupational therapists can use these findings to structure practice conditions in stroke rehabilitation programs. The key is to structure conditions during the acquisition phase that will produce optimal retention and transfer of the learned skills.[29]

Variable Versus Repetitive Practice

Subjects who participate in variable practice perform better on transfer tests than subjects who participate in repetitive practice.[13,50,51] Toglia[58] explains this finding by hypothesizing that variable practice facilitates generalization by preventing individuals from developing context-dependent inflexibility when using a newly learned skill. Diller, Goodgold, and Kay[18] found that variable practice schedules were more effective than repetitive practice schedules in promoting retention of perceptual learning in

37 adults who had brain injuries with right hemispheric pathology.

Contextual Interference

Contextual interference refers to factors in the learning environment that increase the difficulty of initial learning. Limited KR feedback is one example of contextual interference that has already been discussed. As shown by studies of KR feedback, these factors tend to promote more effective retention and generalization. One explanation for this finding is that high contextual interference forces a person to "use multiple and variable processes to overcome the difficulty of practice."[29] In addition, people develop more elaborate memory representations of the underlying strategies that were used for task achievement during the acquisition phase of learning.

Blocked and random practice schedules are examples of low and high contextual interference respectively. During blocked practice, patients practice one task until they master it. This is followed by practice of a second task until it is also mastered. (Note that this differs somewhat from repetitive practice because task variety is ultimately introduced in treatment.) Random practice requires patients to attempt multiple tasks or variations of a task before they have mastered any one of the tasks. In addition, the various trials are performed in a random order.

Motor performance in an open-task context—a setting in which relevant objects in the environment are moving unpredictably—is another example of high contextual interference. Jarus[29] found that individuals who were trained to produce motor responses to an open-context computer task developed better performance flexibility and could better generalize their skills for use in carrying out a novel task as compared to subjects who were trained to respond to a closed, or self-paced, computer task.

Whole Versus Part Practice

Therapists may intuitively believe that it will be easier for a patient to learn small segments of a task than the task in its entirety. However, breaking a task into its component parts for teaching purposes is useful only if the task can be naturally divided into units that reflect the inherent goals of the task.[50,70] One reason for this is that continuous skills (or whole-task performance) are easier to remember than discrete responses.[51] For example, once people have learned to ride a bicycle or play tennis, they will retain these motor skills even without practicing them for many years. On the other hand, segmented, laboratory-type motor skills may be acquired easily but are less likely to be retained over time. Therefore therapists are advised to teach tasks in their entirety rather than in artificial segments. For example, for best retention and generalization, the task of putting on a shirt is best taught all at once rather than in different portions during consecutive therapy sessions. If it is difficult for a stroke survivor to master all the steps simultaneously, the therapist can cue the patient or provide manual guidance for selected aspects of the task. The patient will become accustomed to completing the task during each trial. The therapist's assistance can be gradually decreased as practice sessions continue.

Practice in Natural Settings

Transferring skills learned during training to real-life situations is significantly influenced by the degree of similarity between the practice environment and the actual environment.[50,70] Mathiowetz and Wade[34] studied the movement patterns of individuals with and without motor impairments as they performed selected tasks (eating applesauce, drinking from a glass, turning pages of a book) under three practice conditions. The impoverished condition was the least natural; subjects mimed the tasks with no access to the objects associated with task performance. The partial condition resembled partial simulations that are often used for practice during rehabilitation therapy. Subjects mimed the tasks with a limited array of the objects normally used. In the natural condition, subjects performed the actual tasks. Data collected through the use of a computerized motion analysis system revealed that each of the three practice conditions elicited unique kinematic profiles in both individuals with normal motor performance and individuals with movement impairments resulting from multiple sclerosis. This finding indicates that patients may be learning different motor skills when they practice contrived or partially simulated versions of tasks. There is no guarantee that a motor skill learned during artificial practice sessions will be generalized by the patient so it can be used for performing the actual task in its natural setting.

Skills that are learned to perform tasks such as dressing or bathing are best generalized when the skills have been acquired in a setting that resembles the environment in which the activity will ultimately be performed. Occupational therapy clinics with simulated home and community environments will promote better generalization of performance area skills than clinics in which practice of daily tasks is contrived. However, many stroke survivors can never generalize what they learn in simulated settings; in these cases, home-based occupational therapy is required.

Different Practice Conditions for Different Task Categories

Gentile[21,22] has postulated that motor activities can be classified into four general categories based on environmental pacing conditions and variability between successive trials. Practice conditions for learning will vary depending on the task category.

Closed tasks are activities in which the environment is stable and predictable and methods of performance are consistent over time. Brushing teeth or getting into and out of a bathtub are examples of closed tasks that may be goals for stroke survivors. The best strategy for developing skill in a specific closed task is to develop a narrow and consistent method of performance through repetitive practice of the task.

Variable motionless tasks also involve interacting with a stable and predictable environment, but specific features of the environment are likely to vary between performance trials. Drinking is an example of a variable motionless task because the type of mug, glass, or cup used, as well the amount the container is filled, will vary in different situations. Dressing is another example because people's wardrobes consist of clothing of varying fabrics, dimensions, and styles. To achieve independence in a variable motionless task a patient must learn more than one method of performance. The therapist must provide individuals with opportunities to solve the activity's motor problems in a wide variety of contexts.

In consistent motion tasks an individual must deal with environmental conditions that are in motion during activity performance; the motion is consistent and predictable between trials. Stepping onto or off of an escalator or moving through a revolving door are examples of consistent motion tasks. Patients need practice that will enable them to accurately match the timing of their actions to the predictable changes of the moving objects in the environment.

Open tasks require patients to make adaptive decisions about unpredictable events because objects within the environment are in random motion during task performance. These activities require appropriately timed movements as well as spatial anticipation of where the relevant objects will be moving. For example, a passenger who is sitting in a moving train must maintain balance when the supporting surface is moving unpredictably. When crossing a street, a person must anticipate the speed and rhythm of both pedestrians and oncoming traffic. When playing most ball games, people must predict the speed and direction of the ball to position themselves in the right place at the right time. Research has shown that the skills required for successful open-task performance cannot be learned through repetitive practice in a stationary environment.[26] Natural practice in an unpredictable environment seems to be the best strategy for developing skill in open-task performance.

ACTIVITY-BASED TREATMENT IN OCCUPATIONAL THERAPY

Activity-based intervention is a foundation of occupational therapy in stroke rehabilitation. During the evaluation process, an occupational therapist determines the following: (1) which activities are important to the stroke survivor as determined by the individual's roles, interests, and anticipated environment, (2) which activities the stroke survivor can or cannot perform, and (3) which performance component and performance context factors impede the survivor's ability to complete the identified activities.

During treatment, occupational therapists use activities in two major ways. Some activities may be designed to pro-

vide structured challenges to improve skills in specific areas of impairment. In the OT literature this is called *purposeful activity*[27] or *occupation-as-means*.[62] For example, an occupational therapist may engage a stroke survivor in a modified card game. Depending on the performance component goals for this individual, the occupational therapist may structure the activity so that it requires forward reach with a hemiparetic arm. Alternatively, the card game may require the person to place the cards along a wide horizontal surface while standing. This activity structure provides opportunities for learning balance strategies while shifting the center of gravity in a lateral direction.

Other activities are designed to provide practice in specific tasks or areas of disability. Examples include direct practice in performing a morning self-care routine or getting into and out of an automobile.

Effectiveness of Activities as Rehabilitation Interventions

Research literature provides strong support for the use of activity in occupational therapy treatment.[45,62] As discussed in the previous section, generalization of learning is facilitated when subjects practice in natural activities that provide opportunities to develop strategies for performance in a variety of contexts.

Nashner's[14,39,40] classic studies established that factors in the environmental context of task performance directly influence which motor strategies a person will use. Occupational therapists structure the environment during activity performance to elicit desired motor and cognitive strategies.

Mathiowetz and Wade[34] found that individuals use different movement patterns when actually performing an activity as compared to when they pretend to perform. This supports the use of activities rather than exercises or simulated movements when specific task performance is the treatment goal. In a similar study, Wu, Trombly, and Lin[73] also used computerized motion analysis to study movement patterns. They examined the kinematic strategies used by college-aged subjects without disabilities when they reach forward under three conditions. In the natural activity condition, subjects actually reached for a pencil in preparation for writing their names. In the imagery-based condition, subjects reached the same distance for an imagined pencil. In the exercise condition, they simply reached forward in a similar trajectory. Like Mathiowetz and Wade,[34] Wu, Trombly, and Lin[73] found that subjects used significantly different movement strategies in the three conditions. In addition, they found that the natural activity condition elicited significantly more efficient organization of movement as evidenced by reach patterns that were faster and straighter, used less force, and showed greater preplanning. These results indicate that activity performance facilitates motor control better than performance of contrived movements.

Van de Weel et al[66] had similar findings in their study of active forearm supination and pronation in children of average intelligence who exhibited right hemiparesis resulting from cerebral palsy. After the children had experienced full, passive ROM in pronation and supination, they were required to actively perform the movements under two conditions. In the first condition, they were instructed to use a drumstick to bang on drums that were positioned to require full forearm ROM. For the other condition, they were instructed to move the drumstick back and forth as far as they could in the frontal plane. Movement range was significantly greater when banging the drums than during the abstract exercise condition.

Sietsema et al[53] also had similar findings in their study of forward reach in adults with hemiparesis resulting from traumatic brain injury. Neurodevelopmental treatment strategies were used to prepare subjects for forward reach from the sitting position. In the exercise condition, subjects rotely reached out their hands as far as they could. In the activity condition, they reached forward to control "Simon," a popular computer-controlled game that challenges players to repeat its sequences of flashing lights and sounds by pressing colored panels. Data collected through computerized motion analysis revealed that subjects displayed significantly greater mobility when engaged in the activity as compared to when they attempted to reach forward in a purely exercise context.

Hsieh et al[28] found that adults with hemiplegia performed significantly more repetitions of an exercise to improve dynamic balance when the exercise was embedded in a bean-bag toss activity as compared to when the exercise was performed in isolation. Wu et al[72] found that an activity-based program effectively improved symmetrical posture in adults with hemiplegia. Data collected from The Balance Master system indicated that symmetric weight bearing and the midline position of center of gravity improved when an activity-based program consisting of structured wood sanding and bean-bag toss games was introduced and decreased when the activity-based program was withdrawn. Patients continued to receive physical therapy intervention during the baseline and withdrawal phases.

Other studies with a variety of populations have shown that subjects perform movement sequences for a longer duration or with greater numbers of repetitions when the movements are embedded in activities rather than composed of rote exercise routines.[4,37,43,56,74]

Activity Analysis

Occupational therapists are experts at analyzing activities and selecting and synthesizing activities that will serve as useful rehabilitation modalities. Activity analysis is the process of closely examining a selected task to determine its relevant performance components. In stroke rehabilitation, occupational therapists use activity analysis as a tool in three major ways:

1. In task analysis of performance areas
2. As an evaluation tool of performance components
3. As a treatment goal

Task Analysis of Performance Areas

An occupational therapist assesses tasks of daily living in the environmental context in which the individual plans to perform each task. The therapist determines which performance components are necessary for task performance and compares this analysis to the functional strengths and impairments exhibited by an individual stroke survivor. This task analysis enables the occupational therapist to plan an individualized treatment program that will improve relevant performance skills and enable the person to use compensatory strategies to overcome those performance components that show weak potential for significant improvement. When providing treatment to a stroke survivor, the occupational therapist is most concerned about performance components related to balance, motor control, and visual-spatial and cognitive skills.

Because the ability to preplan movements is often impaired after stroke, the occupational therapist determines the optimal "postural set" for performing a selected task. To perform the simple act of standing up, persons must posturally set themselves in several ways. Both feet must be positioned on the floor in an appropriate base of support. Perpendicular angles are established at the ankle and knee and hip joints, and the pelvis is tilted anteriorly to free the lumbar spine for forward movement.[11,15,16,19,47]

When standing, people automatically change the configuration of their bases of support in anticipation of the direction toward which they expect to shift their body weight. If they plan to shift forward, as is done when reaching ahead, they will establish an anterior-posterior base of support. If they plan to shift to the left or right, as is done when stepping laterally to position themselves in front of a bathtub, they will establish a medial-lateral base of support. Persons with hemiplegia often assume postural support bases that are inappropriate for the activity in which they are preparing to engage. The occupational therapist facilitates future task performance by determining and then instructing the individual in choosing appropriate postural sets for a performance area activity. For example, assuming the most efficient postural set for standing in front of a toilet can determine whether a man will be able to safely urinate independently.

Just as appropriate postural sets are important precursors to efficient motor performance, preplanning is also instrumental in determining the success of cognitively or visually challenging tasks. Activity analysis includes a determination of preliminary cognitive strategies that will facilitate task performance. For example, a person with right hemisphere dysfunction may experience difficulty in spatially orienting a blouse or slacks for independent dressing. The individual may be unaware that prior to the stroke a quick and automatic process was used to visualize and orient the garments in relation to the body segments. The occupational therapist's skill in activity analysis enables development of a workable strategy, such as lining up each garment before attempting to complete the additional steps of dressing.

The occupational therapist determines each task's requirements for shifting body weight in relation to center of gravity. Postural adjustments that normally serve as balance mechanisms during weight shift are often impaired after stroke.[9,15] Understanding a task's inherent balance challenges is critical for developing treatment goals and compensatory strategies. Success in shifting weight during activity performance can be facilitated greatly through the use of appropriate postural sets. The importance of this class of prerequisite skills is important when bathing. If patients will be using a tub bench, they will need to posturally set themselves for a posterior weight shift from stand to sit onto the bench. Once sitting, they will need to rotate their pelvis and bring both legs into the tub. The next step will be to shift their weight laterally, while sitting, to position themselves on the tub bench. A forward weight shift will often be required to adjust the water, and significant challenges to a lateral weight shift when sitting may be presented when patients must wash their genitals. If patients will be stepping into the bathtub and standing under a shower, they must posturally set themselves for a lateral weight shift for entrance and exit to and from the tub or shower. Reaching up and down from the standing position will be a critical performance component for safe, independent completion of this activity. These performance component skills may often be practiced in other contexts, such as in activities that require similar balance adjustments while sitting and standing. However, they must ultimately be practiced in the context in which the actual bathing activity will take place.

Difficulty with disassociation between body segments is a common secondary impairment associated with stroke.[6,16,19] The occupational therapist assesses the type and magnitude of such disassociations in each performance area task that is analyzed. For example, to put on shoes and socks, patients must be able to disassociate their pelvis from the lumbar spine to anteriorly and posteriorly tilt the pelvis to cross one leg over the other. They will also need to disassociate their lumbar from their thoracic spine to achieve the trunk rotation required to reach their left hand to their right foot. If they will be using their paretic arm to assist with the task, disassociation between the scapula and thorax will be required, as will disassociation between the humerus and scapula. Determination of these requirements through activity analysis guides treatment and helps the stroke survivor understand the therapist's rationale for choice of treatment methods.

Various tasks require different levels of motor planning and motor sequencing. For patients with impairments in these areas, the therapist will determine the nature of each of their challenges within specific performance area activities. Finally, when stroke survivors demonstrate impairments in visuospatial or cognitive skills, the occupational

therapist will carefully analyze each task's unique challenges and assist individuals in developing strategies to meet these specific performance component requirements.

Activity analysis also enables the occupational therapist to determine strategies for task performance that will promote efficient movement patterns and be least likely to contribute to the development of secondary impairments. Strategies for relaxing excessive skeletal muscle activity and preventing abnormal postures are described in Chapters 5, 6, and 19. The occupational therapist instructs the stroke survivor in the way to incorporate these strategies into the routine performance of daily activities. In addition, activity analysis assists the therapist in determining which compensatory strategies or adaptive equipment will be most effective for each individual stroke survivor. Figure 2-7 has a summary of the way occupational therapists apply their activity analyses of performance area tasks to the rehabilitation program for stroke survivors.

Activity Analysis as a Tool for Evaluating Performance Components

Skill in activity analysis enables occupational therapists to evaluate performance components through observation of patients as they participate in selected tasks. Arnadottir's A-One Evaluation[3] provides a systematic framework for assessing cognitive and perceptual function through structured observations of activities of daily living (ADL) performance. This tool is discussed further in Chapter 13.

Carr and Shepherd's Motor Relearning Program for Stroke[9-12] describes a therapeutic strategy for evaluating

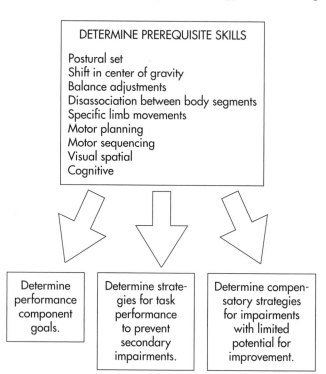

Figure 2-7 Activity analysis of performance area tasks.

motor skills in the context of task performance. The therapist analyzes a patient's performance of a specific task and compares it with the normal kinesiology associated with that task. As in the neurodevelopmental treatment approach,[6,16,23] a major focus of this analysis is to identify those factors that serve as obstacles (or blocks) to moving in efficient kinesiologic patterns. If patients with hemiparesis are trying to reach forward to grasp for a cup, they may tend to use the entire shoulder girdle as one tightly bound unit instead of disassociating the scapula from the thorax or the humerus from the scapula.

Intervention strategies are directly determined from task analysis. In the previous example the therapist would direct the patient's attention to the lack of mobility between structures at the shoulder girdle and seek to redevelop appropriate kinesiologic linkages for shoulder function. The patient will then practice reaching forward in a variety of contexts while the therapist provides manual guidance and KP feedback. Strong backgrounds in kinesiology and movement analysis are helpful to the therapist when implementing a motor relearning approach. In addition, Carr and Shepherd have provided descriptions of normal function for selected activities.[11,12] Occupational therapists may wish to compare their detailed observations of a patient's movement during task performance with these descriptions of normal functions for that activity.

Skill in Activity Analysis as a Treatment Goal

It was mentioned previously in this chapter that stroke survivors, as well as occupational therapists, benefit by developing skill in analyzing activities. An ultimate goal in stroke rehabilitation is for individuals to learn the strategy of analyzing activities in reference to their own functional strengths and impairments. During the occupational therapy process, the therapists share their strategies for activity analysis and challenge patients to develop their own skills in this area. Midway through the treatment process, therapists present new tasks and require the stroke survivors to analyze each task's inherent performance requirements. In addition, occupational therapists encourage individuals to develop their own alternative strategies for task performance. The therapist's major role at this stage is to provide feedback about the safety and efficacy of the person's ideas. Before treatment is terminated, stroke survivors should develop skill in activity analysis so that they have the confidence and capability to attempt an infinite variety of new tasks and roles.

Activity Selection and Synthesis

An occupational therapist determines the performance component goals for each stroke survivor based on the following: (1) activity analysis of performance areas that are important to the individual, and (2) the therapist's evaluation findings about the person's motor, cognitive, and perceptual functions. These goals are considered in addition to general background understanding of the individual's interests, roles, and remaining abilities in the selection and synthesis of purposeful activities that will be used as treatment modalities (Figure 2-8).

Activities as Treatment Modalities

The use of activities as treatment modalities to improve specific performance components is unique to the occupational therapy process. It differs from the use of activities by other professionals in the following ways:

1. *Each activity presents a set of two goals that are clear to the participant.* One goal is to satisfactorily complete a task, such as win a game or get desired items from the refrigerator. The activity will not be effective unless patients view the goal as being acceptable within the context of their age, environment, or interests. The second goal is the more critical goal when activities are used as modalities to improve performance components. This is the goal of developing skill in a specified aspect of motor, cognitive, or perceptual function. If this goal is clear and relevant to patients, they will often gladly participate in the activity, even if the activity itself is not one they would have chosen to engage in for other reasons. For example, a therapist may ask patients to play dominoes so that they can practice forward reach and lateral pinch movements. It is not essential that the patients were previously avid dominoes players. If they understand the therapist's rationale for choosing this activity and do not intensely dislike any particular element of the dominoes game, the activity can be synthesized into a highly effective therapeutic modality.

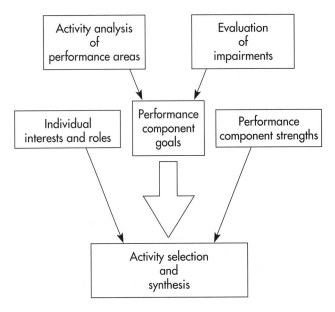

Figure 2-8 Factors influencing activity selection and synthesis.

2. *The therapist skillfully adapts selected aspects, or regulatory conditions, of the activity.* Regulatory conditions[21] are environmental features that directly influence a person's choice of motor or cognitive strategies. Nelson[41] has referred to these features as "occupational form." Occupational therapists adapt and grade the position of materials; the supporting surfaces and position of the individual; the size, shape, weight, or texture of materials; and rules and procedures that govern activity performance. In dominoes, an activity in which critical performance components are arm reach and grasp, the position of the patient in relation to the dominoes will be the most important regulatory condition. The height and distance of the table surface will be manipulated by the therapist to provide sufficient but not excessive challenges to shoulder control mechanisms. The dominoes themselves may purposely be on their sides, rather than flat, to encourage external rotation at the glenohumeral joint and supination at the forearm. The therapist will carefully consider the interaction between the person's balance adjustments and ability to control increasing numbers of degrees of freedom in movements of the hemiparetic arm. The choice of whether the person will perform the task while sitting or standing and the amount of shift in the individual's center of gravity that will be required will be determined on an individual basis and graded as the individual demonstrates improvements. In addition, inherent variations in reach patterns are incorporated into the activity so that the person has the opportunity to practice general motor strategies for reach and grasp rather than repetitions of a single movement.

3. *The therapist is used as a regulatory condition to activity performance.* Before initiating an activity, the therapist may facilitate enhanced performance by stretching shortened muscles or assisting the individual with aligning posture for more efficient movement. In addition, the occupational therapist provides vital cues to performance by manual, visual, and verbal guidance. These cues are gradually decreased over time until the stroke survivor can successfully perform the activity demands with no outside assistance. For example, manual guidance may begin proximally and proceed distally; the degree of "handling"[6,23] may decrease from significant support and guidance to mild cuing. Although the ultimate goal is for the stroke survivor to control and monitor personal actions, the therapist plays a crucial role in the early stages of learning and prevents the person from developing compensatory strategies that may lead to undesired secondary impairments.

4. *Activity synthesis is unique for each individual.* Although the occupational therapist applies carefully considered, general foundational concepts when planning treatment for stroke survivors and synthesizing activities, no textbook can provide specific activity formats that will be appropriate for large groups of individuals, even if they all have the same diagnosis. Each stroke survivor has an individual constellation of abilities, impairments, interests, roles, and personal goals. Occupational therapists synthesize activities by altering the regulatory conditions surrounding specific tasks in specific contexts so that environmental challenges to specific performance components can be presented. This requires flexibility, creativity, and sensitivity to individual needs.

REVIEW QUESTIONS

1. What are the similarities and differences between the major categories in AOTA uniform terminology and ICIDH terminology?
2. Why is it important to implement therapeutic procedures that will prevent abnormal muscle shortening after stroke?
3. In what way does metacognition affect a stroke survivor's ability to achieve rehabilitation goals?
4. From your knowledge of kinesiology, give specific examples of kinematic or kinetic linkages during normal movement.
5. Why is it useful for a stroke survivor to develop skill in task analysis?
6. Describe the factors that promote generalization of learning from the acquisition phase to the transfer phase.
7. How does an occupational therapist provide KP and KR feedback to stroke survivors during treatment?
8. State three examples of contextual interference that could occur during practice, and describe the research findings about the way these factors influence generalization of learning.
9. In what ways will practice conditions vary when stroke survivors are working to achieve skill in an open task as compared to when they are working to achieve skill in a closed task?
10. Describe the difference between "occupation as means" and "occupation as goal."
11. In what ways does the research literature support the use of activities as therapeutic modalities in stroke rehabilitation programs?
12. Which performance components are most important to consider when analyzing and synthesizing activities for stroke survivors?
13. What is unique about the way occupational therapists use activities for stroke rehabilitation as compared to the way they are used by other professionals?

■ COTA Considerations ■

- Treatment should focus on having the stroke survivor generalize new skills to activities beyond the context of the treatment session.
- Therapeutic practice of daily living tasks is most effective when performed in natural settings using variable and random practice schedules.
- When stroke survivors develop foundational strategies for performing functional tasks, they will be more likely to experience success with daily activities than if they are trained in specific techniques for task performance.

REFERENCES

1. Acquaviva J: *Occupational therapy practice guidelines for adults with stroke*, Bethesda, 1996, American Occupational Therapy Association.
2. Ada L, Westwood P: A kinematic analysis of recovery of the ability to stand up following stroke, *Aust Physiother* 38:135, 1992.
3. Árnadóttir G: *The brain and behavior: assessing cortical dysfunction through activities of daily living*, St Louis, 1990, Mosby.
4. Bakshi R, Bhambhani Y, Madill H: The effects of task preference on performance during purposeful and nonpurposeful activities, *Am J Occup Ther* 45:912, 1991.
5. Bernstein N: *The coordination and regulation of movements*, Elmsford, NY, 1967, Pergamon.
6. Bobath B: *Adult hemiplegia: evaluation and treatment*, ed 3, London, 1990, Heinemann.
7. Bobath B: *Adult hemiplegia: evaluation and treatment*, London, 1970, Heinemann.
8. Brunnstrom S: *Movement therapy in hemiplegia*, Philadelphia, 1970, Harper & Row.
9. Carr JH, Shepherd RB: A motor learning model for stroke rehabilitation, *Physiotherapy* 75:372, 1989.
10. Carr JH, Shepherd RB: A motor learning model for rehabilitation. In Carr JH et al, editors: *Movement science: foundations for physical therapy in rehabilitation*, Rockville, Md, 1987, Aspen.
11. Carr JH, Shepherd RB: *A motor relearning program for stroke*, ed 2, Rockville, Md, 1987, Aspen.
12. Carr JH, Shepherd RB: *Early care of the stroke patient: a positive approach*, London, 1983, Heinemann.
13. Catalano JF, Kleiner BM: Distant transfer and practice variability, *Percept Mot Skills* 58:851, 1984.
14. Cordo PJ, Nashner LM: Properties of postural adjustments associated with rapid arm movements, *J Neurophysiol* 47:287, 1982.
15. Davies PM: *Right in the middle: selective trunk activity in the treatment of adult hemiplegia*, New York, 1990, Springer-Verlag.
16. Davies PM: *Steps to follow—a guide to the treatment of adult hemiplegia*, New York, 1985, Springer-Verlag.
17. Dean C, Mackey F: Motor assessment scale scores as a measure of rehabilitation outcome following stroke, *Aust Physiother* 38:31, 1992.
18. Diller L, Goodgold J, Kay T: Project: R7 innovative intervention programs to rehabilitate perceptual, cognitive, and affective deficits of stroke patients (NIDRR Grant No G008300039), New York, 1988, New York University Medical Center, Institute of Rehabilitation Medicine.
19. Eggers O: *Occupational therapy in the treatment of adult hemiplegia*, London, 1984, Heinemann.
20. Fisher B: Effect of trunk control and alignment on limb function, *J Head Trauma Rehabil* 2:72, 1987.
21. Gentile AM: Skill acquisition: Action, movement, and neuromotor processes. In Carr JH, Shepherd RB, Gordon J, Gentile AM, Held, JN, editors: *Movement science: foundations for physical therapy in rehabilitation*, Rockville, Md, 1987, Aspen.
22. Gentile AM: A working model of skill acquisition with application to teaching, *Quest* 17:3.
23. Goodgold-Edwards S: Principles for guiding action during motor learning: a critical evaluation of neurodevelopmental treatment, *Phys Ther Practice* 2:30, 1993.
24. Gordon J: Assumptions underlying physical therapy intervention: theoretical and historical perspectives. In Carr JH et al, editors: *Movement science: foundations for physical therapy in rehabilitation*, Rockville, Md, 1987, Aspen.
25. Higgins S: Motor skill acquisition, *Phys Ther* 71:123, 1991.
26. Higgins JR, Spaeth RK: Relationship between consistency of movement and environmental condition, *Quest* 17:61, 1972.
27. Hinojosa J, Sabari J, Pedretti L: Position paper: purposeful activity, *Am J Occup Ther* 47:1081, 1993.
28. Hsieh CL et al: A comparison of performance in added-purpose occupations and rote exercise for dynamic standing balance in persons with hemiplegia, *Am J Occup Ther* 50:10, 1996.
29. Jarus T: Motor learning and occupational therapy: the organization of practice, *Am J Occup Ther* 48:810, 1994.
30. Jeannerod M: *The neural and behavior organization of goal-directed movements*, Oxford, 1990, Clarendon Press.
31. Lee TD, Swanson LR, Hall AL: What is repeated in a repetition? Effects of practice conditions on motor skill acquisition, *Phys Ther* 71:150, 1991.
32. Lindahl LG: Movement analysis as an industrial training method, *J Appl Psychol* 29:420, 1945.
33. Magill RA: *Motor learning: concepts and applications*, ed 4, Madison, 1993, Brown & Benchmark.
34. Mathiowetz V, Wade MG: Task constraints and functional motor performance of individuals with and without multiple sclerosis, *Ecol Psychol* 7:99, 1995.
35. Mathiowetz V, Bass Haugen J: Motor behavior research: implications for therapeutic approaches to central nervous system dysfunction, *Am J Occup Ther* 48:733, 1994.
36. McCoy AO, Van Sant AF: Movement patterns of adolescents rising from a bed, *Phys Ther* 73:182, 1993.
37. Morton GG, Barnett DW, Hale LS: A comparison of performance measures of an added-purpose task versus a single-purpose task for upper extremities, *Am J Occup Ther* 46:128, 1992.
38. Mulder T: A process-oriented model of human motor behavior: toward a theory-based rehabilitation approach, *Phys Ther* 71:157, 1991.
39. Nashner LM, McCollum G: The organization of human postural movements: a formal basis and experimental synthesis, *Behav Brain Sci* 8:135, 1985.
40. Nashner LM: Adaptation of human movement to altered environments, *Trends Neurosci* 5:358, 1982.
41. Nelson DL: Occupation: form and performance, *Am J Occup Ther* 42:633, 1988.
42. Norkin CC, Levangie PK: *Joint structure and function: a comprehensive analysis*, ed 2, Philadelphia, 1992, FA Davis.
43. Riccio CM, Nelson DL, Bush MA: Adding purpose to the repetitive exercise of elderly women through imagery, *Am J Occup Ther* 44:714, 1990.
44. Richter RR, Van Sant AF, Newton RA: Description of adult rolling movements and hypothesis of developmental sequences, *Phys Ther* 69:63, 1989.
45. Sabari JS: Motor learning concepts applied to activity-based intervention with adults with hemiplegia, *Am J Occup Ther* 45:523, 1991.
46. Salmani AW, Schmidt RA, Walter CB: Knowledge of results and motor learning: a review and critical reappraisal, *Psychol Bull* 95:355, 1984.
47. Schenkman MA et al: Whole-body movements during rising to standing from sitting, *Phys Ther* 70:638, 1990.

48. Schleenbaker RE, Mainous AG: Electromyographic biofeedback for neuromuscular reeducation in the hemiplegic stroke patient: a meta-analysis, *Arch Phys Med Rehabil* 74:1301, 1993.

49. Schmidt RA: *Motor performance and learning: principles for practitioners*, Champaign, Ill, 1992, Human Kinetics.

50. Schmidt RA: Motor learning principles for physical therapy. In Lister MJ, editor: *Contemporary management of motor control problems: proceedings of the II STEP conference*, Alexandria, Va, 1991, Foundation for Physical Therapy.

51. Schmidt RA: *Motor control and learning: a behavioral emphasis*, ed 2, Champaign, Ill, 1988, Human Kinetics.

52. Shumway-Cook A, Woollacott M: *Motor control: theory and practical applications*, Baltimore, 1995, Williams & Wilkins.

53. Sietsema JM et al: The use of a game to promote arm reach in persons with traumatic brain injury, *Am J Occup Ther* 47:19, 1993.

54. Singer RN, Cauraugh JHL: The generalizability effect of learning strategies for categories of psychomotor skills, *Quest* 37:103, 1985.

55. Summers JJ: Motor programs. In Holding D, editor: *Human skills*, New York, 1989, Wiley.

56. Thibodeaux CS, Ludwig FM: Intrinsic motivation in product oriented and non-product oriented activities, *Am J Occup Ther* 42:169, 1988.

57. Toglia JT: A dynamic interactional approach to cognitive rehabilitation. In Katz N: *Cognitive intervention: models for intervention in occupational therapy*, Stoneham, Mass, 1992, Butterworth-Heinemann.

58. Toglia JT: Generalization of treatment: a multicontext approach to cognitive perceptual impairment in adults with brain injury, *Am J Occup Ther* 45:505, 1991.

59. Toglia JP, Golisz K: *Cognitive rehabilitation: group games and activities*, Tucson, 1990, Therapy Skill Builders.

60. Toglia JT: Approaches to cognitive assessment of the brain-injured adult: traditional methods and dynamic investigation, *Occup Ther Practice* 1:36, 1989.

61. Toglia JP: Visual perception of objects: an approach to assessment and intervention, *Am J Occup Ther* 43:587, 1989.

62. Trombly CA: Occupation: purposefulness and meaningfulness as therapeutic mechanisms, *Am J Occup Ther* 49:960, 1995.

63. Trombly CA: Biofeedback. In Trombly CA, editor: *Occupational therapy for physical dysfunction*, ed 4, Baltimore, 1995, Williams & Wilkins.

64. Twitchell TE: The restoration of motor function following hemiplegia in man, *Brain* 74:443, 1951.

65. American Occupational Therapy Association: *Uniform terminology for occupational therapy*, ed 3, Rockville, Md, 1994, The Association.

66. van der Weel FR, van der Meer ALH, Lee DN: Effect of task on movement control in cerebral palsy: implications for assessment and therapy, *Dev Med Child Neurol* 33:419, 1991.

67. Van Sant AF: Rising from a supine position to erect stance: description of adult movement and a developmental hypothesis, *Phys Ther* 68:185, 1988.

68. Vereijken B et al: Freezing degrees of freedom in skill acquisition, *J Motor Beh* 24:133, 1992.

69. Winstein CJ: Knowledge of results and motor learning—implications for physical therapy, *Phys Ther* 71:140, 1991.

70. Winstein CJ: Designing practice for motor learning: clinical implications. In Lister MJ, editor: *Contemporary management of motor control problems: proceedings of the II STEP conference*, Alexandria, Va, 1991, Foundation for Physical Therapy.

71. World Health Organization: *International classification of impairment, disability, and handicap*, Geneva, 1980, The Organization.

72. Wu SH et al: Effects of a program on symmetrical posture in patients with hemiplegia: a single-subject design, *Am J Occup Ther* 50:17, 1996.

73. Wu CY, Trombly CA, Lin KC: The relationship between occupational form and occupational performance: a kinematic perspective, *Am J Occup Ther* 48:679, 1994.

74. Zimmerer-Branum S, Nelson DL: Occupationally embedded exercise versus rote exercise: a choice between occupational forms by elderly nursing home residents, *Am J Occup Ther* 49: 397, 1995.

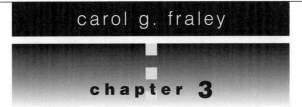

chapter 3

Psychosocial Aspects of Stroke Rehabilitation

key terms

quality of life
adaptation
coping
psychiatric conditions

depression
therapeutic relationship
empathy
caring

environment
context
therapeutic activities

chapter objectives

After completing this chapter, the reader will be able to accomplish the following:

1. Understand and appreciate the collective and personal experience of having a stroke and living with the consequences.
2. Recognize the importance of psychosocial factors in stroke recovery and function, including the following:
   Depression and other psychiatric diagnoses
   Social and psychological responses
   Quality of life
   Client-focused intervention
3. Identify theories and models of adaptation, coping, and adjustment with emphasis on the functional consequences.
4. Understand the development of a framework of practice skills based on the psychosocial core of occupational therapy, including the concepts of the following:
   Therapeutic relationship
   Empathy
   Caring
   Person-environment transaction
   Choice of therapeutic activities and approach
5. Understand potential models for practice (based on the psychosocial core) in the following treatment contexts: acute care, inpatient rehabilitation, subacute/nursing home, home care, outpatient, and community.

47

OVERVIEW OF COLLECTIVE ISSUES

Characteristics of the Population

Every year in the United States about 550,000 persons have an acute stroke. Men have at least 30% more strokes than women. Stroke rates are 50% higher in African-American men than white men and 130% higher in African-American women than white women.[42]

Persons who have had a stroke are at high risk of having another. Approximately 75% of strokes are first-time occurrences and 25% are recurrent.[88] Stroke is a leading cause of disability in older persons. The incidence of stroke doubles with every decade after 55 years of age.[42] Stroke is a major diagnostic group treated by occupational therapists practicing with adults who have physical disabilities.[8]

REALITY OF PROGNOSIS

Nearly 150,000 people per year in the United States die from strokes.[42] Although deaths from stroke have substantially decreased, the prevalence of stroke has increased. This means that there are more strokes and more stroke survivors.[16] About one half of people with first-time strokes live for 3 or more years, and more than one half of this group lives for 10 years. In 1991, there were approximately 3 million stroke survivors in the United States with varying degrees of impairment and disability.[42] For many of these survivors, their stroke marks a sudden and permanent change in who they are as defined by what they can and cannot do. Of the persons that survive stroke, it is estimated that 90% are left with some form of neurologic disability or deficit.[16] Most persons who survive a stroke experience a decrease in activity and decline in overall satisfaction with life.*

In the United States, 10% to 29% of stroke survivors are institutionalized after their stroke.[42] Women seem to be institutionalized more often than men,[41] and married men are less likely to be institutionalized than single men.[23]

The course of physical recovery after a stroke is most dramatic in the first 1 to 3 months, but it is not clear how long recovery continues. In the United States, data indicate that 75% of stroke survivors are able to walk after 6 months, but 24% to 53% are not independent in their activities of daily living (ADL) after 5 to 6 years.[42]

PSYCHOSOCIAL FACTORS IN STROKE RECOVERY AND FUNCTION

Factors influencing stroke recovery include type of stroke, severity of deficits, premorbid status, comorbidity, age, gender, living situation, and social support.† In the past 2 decades, there has been increased interest in the importance of psychologic and social factors in stroke recovery. Summaries of several studies follow:

- Published in 1979, The Framingham Study[41] provided an epidemiologic profile of 148 long-term survivors of stroke. Although much of the functional disability reported could be attributed to specific neurologic deficits, disability rates were highest for the disabilities in which psychosocial factors played a large role.
- In 1988, Evans et al[33] identified psychiatric comorbidity associated with increased hospital readmission rates for stroke patients. This was not the case for other medical conditions.
- In a study[89] published in 1989, multiple factors related to the adjustment of 40 stroke survivors were analyzed, and it was found that psychosocial factors predicted depression and motivation independent of the severity or site of the stroke.
- In 1992 a major prospective study in Sweden[12] addressed specific influences of different aspects of psychosocial function after stroke. Social network, functional ability, leisure-time activities, ill health, major depression, and life satisfaction were assessed over a 3-year period in a population of 50 long-term stroke survivors. The findings were that persons who had had a stroke had more psychiatric symptoms, lower functional ability, and reduced life satisfaction as compared with a general population of elderly.
- A 1993 study[21] of 87 stroke survivors in New Haven, Connecticut, found lower institutionalization rates in patients who had larger social networks and fewer limitations in physical function.
- Based on a 1994 qualitative study of a stroke survivor and her husband, Jongbloed[47] concluded that reactions to stroke are the result of physical, subjective, and environmental influences. Although the dominant occupational therapy professional view of stroke and its consequences emphasizes physical disability and ability, the physical and social consequences at home will influence adaptation in a more profound way than the ability or inability to perform specific tasks independently.[47]

PSYCHOSOCIAL ISSUES IN STROKE REHABILITATION

Occupational Therapy Concepts of Recovery and Function

The theoretical framework of occupational therapy is built on an acknowledgement that all people exist on multiple levels, including biologic, psychologic, sociocultural, and spiritual.[100] As defined by the American Occupational Therapy Association (AOTA),[5] occupational therapy is concerned with the function of people in their occupational roles. Occupational therapists use the word function interchangeably with performance (formerly occupational

---

*References 10, 12, 13, 16, 17, 21, 35, 41, 45, 48, 51, 53, 67, 76, 87, 89.
†References 10, 16, 23, 31, 41, 42, 48, 51, 87.

performance). "Occupational therapy practitioners help people address challenges or difficulties that threaten to impair their ability to perform activities and tasks that are basic to the fulfillment of their roles as worker, parent, spouse or partner, sibling, and friend to self or others."

Occupational Functioning

Trombly[92] proposes a model of occupational functioning as a framework for occupational therapy treatment of the whole person within the context of the physical disabilities setting. In Trombly's model the goal of occupational therapy is to develop a sense of competence and self-esteem. She feels that to engage satisfactorily in a life role, a person must be able to do the tasks that comprise that role. Tasks are performed within their natural context. Some are essential and some are not. Tasks are comprised of activities; to do a given activity a person must have abilities in the following areas:

- Sensorimotor
- Cognitive
- Perceptual
- Emotional
- Social

Trombly emphasizes that any and all human responses are complex and multifaceted and not responsive to separate treatment of the mind and body.

The model of human occupation (MOHO) expresses this complexity through a systems approach. The MOHO characterizes occupational function as a successful interaction between an individual and the environment, involving independent and hierarchical systems of volition, habituation, and performance.[49]

Psychosocial Variables for Occupational Therapists

Bonder[15] identifies psychosocial issues relevant to occupational therapy in a physical disabilities setting as those psychosocial variables that can help answer the following questions:

What do persons need and want to do?
What can they do and what can't they do?
What limits performance?

Bonder[15] divides psychosocial variables into psychologic and social variables. Psychological variables are internal, unobservable processes that provide the person's drive toward activity and those internal, unobservable processes that prevent activity. These psychologic variables include motivation, interest, and self-evaluation (self-concept and self-esteem) as well as depression, anxiety, and perceived stress. The occupational therapist's focus should be on those psychologic variables that are activity-related.

In Bonder's[15] model, social variables exist at two levels: (1) component skills (i.e., social skills), and (2) occupational performance (level in which social activities take place).

Social variables may be contrasted to psychologic variables, which are inferred from behavior or self-report.

Quality of Life

The editor of *Topics in Stroke Rehabilitation* (Kirschner[50]) in the issue on *Quality of Life in Stroke Recovery*, laments that ". . . our attempts to define, characterize, quantify, and understand quality of life have been extremely difficult and largely unsatisfactory." In the same issue, Tate et al[85] reflect that although physicians have defined health in terms of physical function, patients define it more broadly in terms of physical, social, emotional, and spiritual function.

Fidler[34] developed a lifestyle performance model based on her inherent belief that quality of life is the single most important theme in human performance. This model provides a framework for knowing and understanding a person's total activity repertoire within the context of the human world and the environment. Fidler hypothesizes that wellness and a sense of well-being are closely related to a state of being that is optimally satisfying to the self and significant others. The structure of the model contains four domains relevant to quality of life and occupational therapy:

1. Self-care and maintenance
2. Intrinsic gratification
3. Social contribution
4. Interpersonal relatedness

Cynkin and Robinson,[22] who developed an activity health perspective for occupational therapy assessment and intervention, share this view when they conclude that "The individual leads a most satisfying way of life if able to carry out the activities of everyday living in patterns and configurations that are acceptable to the group and also fulfill personal needs and wants."

In the *American Journal of Occupational Therapy, Special Issue on Stroke*, only one article addressed the psychosocial aspects of stroke. In this piece, Radomski[67] acknowledges that the occupational therapy profession has considered maintaining a good quality of life its goal from its beginnings. In spite of what professionals proclaim, stroke survivors, who are the most frequent recipients of occupational therapy services, generally appear to have a poor quality of life (as supported by studies outside of occupational therapy). Radomski suggests that occupational therapists make "erroneous assumptions about a causal relationship between a patients' physical recovery after a stroke and their quality of life."

Adjustment, Coping, and Adaptation

If ever achieved, adjustment to stroke is a long process; this was concluded by Holbrook[45] in a follow-up study of 180 patients from the unit at Frenchay Hospital in Bristol. "For a stroke patient, a successful rehabilitation is perceived as getting back to a formerly enjoyed way of life."

There are a number of theories about and trends in understanding psychologic adjustment to permanent physical disability. A review article by Shontz[82] reports that early assumptions about the source of a patient's psychologic distress revolved around the disability itself. Later psychoanalytic theory was used to explain psychologic reactions. Patients with physical disabilities were thought to utilize the same psychologic defenses as mentally ill patients. Reactions to illness and disability were described in terms of repression, projection, regression, displacement, reaction formation, and other familiar defense mechanisms.

Theories related to existentialism suggest that death is the ultimate disability and reactions to disability are less intense reactions to the prospect of dying. More sociologic models focus on the realistic problems—prejudice and public apathy toward disability—and suggest that the behavior of people with disabilities conform to social norms and expectations.

Wright[98] proposed that the behavioral reactions of people with disabilities were integrated responses to environmental pressures and internal mental processes. She did not consider the psychologic maladjustment of a person with a disability as a result of the disability itself but a result of the person's acceptance of society's devaluation of atypical people. A number of authors[14,94] have viewed the process of adaptating to traumatic disability as similar to the process of accepting death by a dying patient. The stages are summarized as follows:

1. *Denial:* The patient denies that the disability exists. This protects individuals from a reality that they are unprepared to accept.
2. *Mourning:* The patient mourns as a reaction to the reality of the disability. This stage often takes the form of hostility and anger or depression (which is internal anger).
3. *Adjustment:* The patient adjusts to the disability. At this stage the individual is self-accepting and capable of adjusting to the disability. The individual develops productive strategies for dealing with the potentially handicapping effects of disability.

Bishop and Pet[14] caution that disability is not death and adjustment is not just dealing with loss. They conclude that research studies have not supported the concept of progression through stages of mourning either when adjusting to the loss of a loved one or a disability. They see stroke and disability as different from death. Patients with disabilities are reminded of this each new day; every gain leads to a new challenge. Bishop and Pet think that rather than mourn, people who have survived a stroke need to address issues and adaptively compensate. "It is better to understand the individual stroke survivor's experience than to identify or anticipate preconceived, but unconfirmed, stages. Each person travels his or her own road at different speeds and with different detours and stopping points." In

their experience, adjustment problems can be most severe when a patient cannot use adaptive coping strategies that were used before the stroke. For example, one patient had used the hobby of building and repairing clocks to decrease stress in his life before his stroke. After the stroke, he could no longer use his right hand to engage in this significant and purposeful activity.[14]

The occupational therapist, Vargo,[94] writes that to truly adjust or learn to cope, a person with a physical disability must consciously and conscientiously combat society's devaluations. She recommends assisting patients with disability adjustment by the following:

- Admitting differences but distinguishing difference from inferiority
- Deemphasizing physique—emphasizing function and interpersonal skills
- Overcoming misconceptions associated with disability by persuading patients to pursue activities and be seen in public

Yerxa[100] provides a comprehensive discussion of the social and psychologic experiences of having a disability. She clarifies the differences between the medical model and traditional values supporting occupational therapy practice, including the importance of viewing the world from the patient's perspective.

Yerxa includes a number of personal accounts by persons with disabilities, including Vash,[95] who is a psychologist. Vash emphasizes that although society imposes certain stereotypes and preconceived notions of people with disabilities, there is a danger in identifying "the psychology of disability." She feels that people with disabilities are indeed people, and people have more similarities than differences. In Vash's opinion, responses to disability are as individual as people. Reactions to disability may be influenced by many factors including severity, visibility, stability, pain, gender, and affected activities. All reactions are affected by environmental influences and are highly dependent on the values, spiritual and philosophical beliefs of the person with the disability.

Kyllo,[52] who writes on spiritual topics related to stroke rehabilitation, clarifies that all people are spiritual (i.e., have values and life beliefs), although not all are religious. A stroke challenges the belief that life is fair, so anger in response to a disabling event is not uncommon. For religious persons, anger at God may seem appropriate because it is the only "safe anger" that has no ramifications. Some religious persons view increased or decreased faith as results of the stroke. As a religious counselor, Kyllo suggests that healing will not take place unless patients know that they have not been abandoned by God and they are not alone.

Gage[36] developed a coping appraisal model so that occupational therapists could explore the influence of coping on performance and maximize a patient's function through self-appraisal. *Coping* is defined as adaptation in a difficult situation. Gage's model is based on cognitive relational and social cognitive theories. She cautions that it is often incorrectly assumed that skill development alone will result in increased performance. Patients with the same skill levels may perform at entirely different levels, with one explanation being that different coping strategies produce variations in performance success.

Cognitive appraisal is the process during which people interpret what is happening in their environment (including stressful environments). The cognitive appraisal includes primary and secondary appraisals. During the primary appraisal, people determine their response to an occurrence by discerning whether it affects them. They determine this by asking themselves whether they have anything at stake. The quality and intensity of this emotional response is influenced by appraisals of the occurrence in terms of potential harm, threat, challenge, benefit, or importance. In the secondary appraisal the individuals evaluate their available resources to answer the question, "Can I handle this?" There is an appraisal of physical, psychologic, social, and material resources available to deal with the occurrence. Primary and secondary appraisals do not occur in any particular temporal order or sequence, and both are equally important. Factors that affect these appraisal processes include temporal issues, values and beliefs, physiologic arousal, age, social support, empowerment, efficacy, novelty, gender, mood, available information, and skills. A coping plan is developed as a result of the combination of the primary and secondary appraisals. Methods of coping can alter a response or change the situation. Coping interventions that alter an emotional reaction are considered emotion-focused coping interventions and include changes in the perception of a situation. Coping interventions that change the situation are problem-focused coping interventions. Utilizing a coping outcome appraisal process and performance feedback, primary and secondary appraisals can be influenced and adjusted. Coping interventions continue until the stressor or situation has been dealt with satisfactorily.[36]

Research on coping strategies used by people who had experienced traumatic life events, such as being in a severe accident, a victim of incest, or diagnosed with cancer, led to the development of cognitive adaptive theory. Taylor[86b] proposed a theory of adjustment based on work with women who had breast cancer. She argues that adjustment centers around three goals, and efforts to resolve these goals are highly dependent on the ability to form and maintain a set of illusions. These goals include the following:

1. A search for meaning
2. An attempt to regain mastery—over the event in particular and over life in general
3. An effort to restore self-esteem through self-embracing evaluations

Taylor[86b] suggests that the specific content of the cognitions that patients have about their situation matter less than the functions of these cognitions. When one response is blocked or found to be ineffectual, a patient may simply substitute another response with the same goal. For example, one patient felt she could avoid recurrences of her cancer by controlling her diet. When the cancer recurred, she was able to accept that her causal theory was wrong, and moved on to quitting her boring job and writing short stories. The goal of the behavior was control; in an attempt to control her life she moved from controlling her diet to her work life. She remained functional in spite of the reality that she could not control her cancer. Taylor concludes that rather than impeding adjustment, illusion may be helpful and even essential for adequate coping.

Another study centered around the cognitive adaptation perspective is a study on patient perceptions regarding postdischarge housing decisions after stroke rehabilitation. Despite functional limitations and rehabilitative team or family involvement, patients reported that they were primarily responsible for deciding where they would live after their stroke rehabilitation. The author[93] interpreted this exaggerated perception of control as an indication that patients who have had a stroke require additional assistance and interactive planning to determine the most appropriate housing. An alternative interpretation would be that the patients were adjusting to their disability by creating an illusion of mastery and control.

Psychiatrists Druss and Douglas[27] identified a cluster of adaptive traits that they decided was not accurately defined as "healthy" denial. Some patients who were well aware of their disability, illness, or impending death continued to emphasize the positive aspects of their situation and deliberately engaged in creative and productive activities.

Nancy Donaldson[26] incorporated many of these concepts when she told the story of adjusting to life after her 43-year-old husband had a stroke. Steve survived with a dense left hemiplegia and significant cognitive deficits. Donaldson thought their coping was greatly influenced by their capacity to assert power over a destiny that seemed out of control and be hopeful in spite of evidence that optimism might be inappropriate. She reflected that although they spent months grieving over what was lost, they learned to celebrate and cherish survival. They found new strength to live and adapt to their changed lives.

Depression

Incidence

Depression is the most commonly reported psychiatric condition after stroke. Depression is reported in 18% to 61% of patients after stroke. The highest level of reported incidence is from patient populations in acute and rehabilitation hospitals. The lowest levels are reported from community-based populations.[17] About half of patients diagnosed with depression suffer from major clinical depression and the other half have some other type of depressive disorder.[39] Some researchers consider depression following stroke a unique depressive syndrome (Post-Stroke Depression [PSD]), but others do not make this distinction. Several studies have found that at least 50% of PSD patients met the Diagnostic and Statistical Manual of Mental Disorders (DSM) criteria of major depression.[69,73]

Diagnoses: Signs and Symptoms

Signs of depression after a stroke may include erratic or abnormal performance or poor recovery, management difficulties, failure to participate fully in a rehabilitation program, or apparent worsening of neurologic deficits.[74] In some cases the only clue to a patient's depression are vegetative signs.[56] Although depression scales may be useful in screening patients for depression or as research tools, all definitive diagnoses of depression should be made by a mental health professional based on a complete clinical assessment.[42] Symptoms of major depression include the following[9]:

- Sadness—being in a depressed mood most of the day
- Markedly diminished interest or pleasure tension
- Fatigue or loss of energy
- Insomnia or hypersomnia
- Significant weight loss
- Psychomotor agitation or retardation
- Feelings of worthlessness or excessive or inappropriate guilt
- Diminished ability to think or concentrate or indecisiveness
- Recurrent thoughts of death

Etiology: Causes of Depression After Stroke

There is disagreement about whether depression after stroke is primarily reactive or organic in origin. The significance of lesion location and size has also not been resolved.[85a] Robinson and his colleagues have consistently found a higher incidence of depression after stroke in patients with left hemispheric lesions, particularly those that are more anterior in location.[69-71] Other researchers have not associated lesion location with incidence of depression after stroke.[30,35] Malec et al[57] found several problems with Robinson's research including the fact that most of his studies have been conducted on heterogeneous groups of stroke patients, some of whom had previous histories of psychiatric and substance abuse problems. Diagnoses of depression after stroke appears to be frequently complicated by previously existing conditions, additional brain pathology, marked language disturbances, additional severe illness, and/or social factors related to age. It is highly possible that depression after stroke includes both organic and reactive factors.[42,57,85a]

There is evidence that depression after stroke is related to other types of depression in the elderly. Sharpe et al[81] interviewed 60 stroke survivors at 3 and 5 years after stroke and concluded that depression in stroke survivors had the same associations as depression in an elderly population who had not had strokes. Depression was more likely in long-term stroke survivors who were old, lonely, functionally and cognitively impaired, and living in institutions. The strongest association found was between functional dependence and depression. The Perth community stroke study[17] found that a surprisingly high percentage of depression after stroke was correlated with existing depressive symptoms. House et al[46] compared 128 stroke patients at 12 months after stroke with a control group from the general population and concluded that undue emphasis has been placed on major depression following stroke.

Physical Impairments

There is evidence that there is not a direct correlation between physical disability and depression after stroke. A 2-year longitudinal follow-up study of stroke survivors in Maryland found no correlation between degree of upper or lower extremity weakness and depression.[87] Thompson et al[89] found that although stroke patients who were more impaired were more depressed, patients' interpretation of their situation was significantly correlated with the depression severity (with controls for the stroke type and severity).

Starkstein and Robinson[85a] concluded that the relationship between depression after stroke and physical impairment appears to be complex and interactive. Although depression after stroke does not cause physical impairment, once a patient is depressed, the depression may inhibit the patient's functional recovery and add to the physical impairment, which could lead to continued depression.

Social Withdrawal

There is a high correlation between depression after stroke and social withdrawal. Fiebel and Springer[35] found that the incidence of depression in 91 patients (26% at 6 months after their stroke) was significantly correlated with a failure to resume a premorbid level of social activities. Depressed patients lost a mean of 67% of their previous social activities, whereas patients who were not depressed lost a mean of 43%. In this study, depression was not positively correlated with age, sex, marital status, cognitive status, or the side of the brain lesion. Angeleri et al[10] found a close correlation between depression, social activity, and stress on family members when they compared 180 patients who had been hospitalized their first stroke with a control group of 167 age-matched subjects.

Patients with aphasia experience particularly marked social isolation.[76] Starkstein and Robinson[84] found that the frequency for depression after stroke was not higher in aphasic patients as compared to patients without aphasia. They did report that depression was more common in patients with nonfluent aphasias than patients with fluent or global aphasias attributing this to lesion location.

Treatment

Diller and Bishop[25] summarize current treatment approaches to depression. It is thought that supportive psychotherapy may be useful, especially for patients who hold distorted beliefs about themselves and their situations. No systematic studies of the efficacy of psychotherapy for depression after stroke have been conducted. The more cognitive impairment a patient has the more behavioral and less insight oriented an approach should be. Behavioral approaches may include environmental change and programs that activate a stroke survivor. Caregivers should also be sensitized to depression issues and be aware of helpful strategies to motivate the patient. Educational counseling, in groups and individually, to increase understanding of stroke and its consequences is also suggested. Patients may find encouragement in peer support groups (e.g., formal or informal stroke clubs or inpatient support groups). The use of antidepressants in treating major depression has been shown to be effective,[68] but caution must be exercised because of side effects, which can include delirium, sedation, and cardiovascular complications.[25,42,68] Andersen et al[11] found that second-generation antidepressants can be effective and well tolerated, especially in patients who become depressed 7 weeks or more after a stroke.

Prognosis

The course of depression is varied and specific to the individual. There is some evidence that dysthymia following stroke is more persistent than major depression. In a follow up of 37 patients at 1 year and 48 patients at 2 years, Robinson et al[72] found that by the end of 2 years, all patients with major depression improved whereas only 30% of the patients with dysthymic depression improved. More than one third of patients who were not depressed while in the hospital developed depression within 2 years after the stroke.[72] House et al[46] concluded that although symptoms of depression were more common in persons after stroke, it was not statistically significant. Many symptoms of depression disappear by 12 months after the stroke. Major depression persisted in only 3% of the 78 stroke patients studied. They found that although there was a high cumulative incidence of depression on a case-by-case basis, persistence of depression throughout the year was uncommon.

Mortality

There appears to be a significant association between depression after stroke and mortality after stroke. A follow-up study of 103 patients who had been identified as having major or minor depression 2 weeks after their stroke reported that depression and higher mortality rates were strongly associated.[60] Ten years after the initial stroke, information from 91 of the cases was available for

follow up. Of these 91 patients, 53% had died. Patients that were depressed were 3.4 times more likely to have died during this time than the stroke survivors who were not depressed. This finding was independent of other risk factors including age, sex, social class, type of stroke, lesion location, or level of social functioning. Although there were no suicides, depressed patients without social contact had an especially high mortality rate (90%).

Other Psychiatric Diagnoses

Although depression is the most frequently diagnosed psychiatric sequela of stroke, there are other psychiatric conditions that occur after stroke and potentially affect activity performance. Some of these fit DSM IV criteria,[14] and others are a clustering of symptoms more unique to stroke survivors. Diagnosis may be complicated by aphasia, perceptual deficits, or other neurologic symptoms. Although occupational therapists do not diagnose mental disorders, it is important to have an awareness of potential complications that can substantially interfere with function. Signs and symptoms of these conditions may be most apparent during activity performance.

Anxiety Syndromes: Agoraphobia

The Perth community stroke study[17] found that anxiety was significant in 26% of depressed men and 39% of women. Agoraphobia, or an abnormal fear of being in open or public places, was a particularly common associated anxiety disorder. House et al[46] reported that agoraphobia appeared to be a particularly persistent problem.

There is some debate as to whether depression with anxiety is a unique syndrome or a combination of the separate diagnoses of anxiety and depression. Patients who are both anxious and depressed have more chronic psychiatric problems and a poorer response to treatment than patients who have depression only. In a study of 24 patients in the first month after stroke, Starkstein et al[85b] found only a small number of patients with anxiety only. One half of the patients diagnosed with depression after stroke also met modified criteria for generalized anxiety disorder. They also found significance in the lesion location; anxious depressed patients had a significantly higher frequency of left cortical lesions, whereas the group of patients with major depression only showed a significantly higher frequency of subcortical lesions.

Symptoms of anxiety include the following[14]:

- A sense that something bad is going to occur
- A sense of tension, fear, or worry that is not proportional to the situation
- Racing thoughts
- Physiologic symptoms including a dry mouth, heart palpitations, cold hands and feet, "butterflies" in the stomach and if prolonged, diarrhea and urinary incontinence

Patients who have minor to moderate anxiety may respond to behavioral and cognitive approaches, whereas those with more severe anxiety disorders (moderate to severe) require medication. Relaxation training, such as deep breathing, creative visualization, and progressive muscle relaxation, is also potentially beneficial.[14]

Substance Abuse

Alcohol and cocaine abuse are significant premorbid risk factors for stroke. There is evidence that many persons who have had a stroke also have problems with substance abuse.[14,57] When relevant or suspected the complications of past abuse and the potential risks of future abuse should be addressed.

Sleep Disorders

Sleep disorders and disturbances are common after a stroke.[14,42] Problems contributing to sleep disturbances include drug reactions, problems with positioning and comfort, muscle spasms, depression and anxiety, urinary incontinence or frequency, and pain. If problems do not resolve, the person should have a complete assessment. Treatment may consist of reestablishing normal sleep patterns, eliminating causes of sleeplessness, or sleep medication. Sleep deprivation may cause slowed responses that mimic depression or lack of motivation in therapy.[42]

Secondary Mania

Secondary mania is less frequent than depression as a complication of stroke but does occur. Secondary mania refers to mania caused by toxic, metabolic, or neurologic conditions.[9] In a 1989 review article, Starkstein and Robinson,[85a] conclude that secondary mania is a rare psychiatric diagnosis that is made after stroke. They found secondary mania to be strongly associated with both a right hemispheric lesion in a limbic-connected area and a secondary predisposing factor, such as familial history of affective disorders, preexisting subcortical atrophy, or a seizure disorder.

Secondary mania following a stroke has the same symptoms and response to treatment as mania that develops without brain injury. The symptoms can include the following[14]:

Euphoria
Pressured speech
Flight of ideas
Grandiose thoughts and delusions
Insomnia
Hallucinations
Poor judgment
Paranoia
Hypersexuality

Mania can occur at any time after a stroke and can even occur more than 2 years after the stroke. Management of mania includes medications,[86a] and patients with mania are best treated in a low-stimulus environment with clear limits.[14]

Organic Mental Disorder

Persons who have had a stroke often have a premorbid history of dementia from multiple causes. There are also organically triggered behavioral responses to brain injury that may complicate a correct diagnosis of other psychiatric problems. For example, frontal lobe syndrome has symptoms of slowed mental processing and decreased arousal that may look like the symptoms of depression. Aprosody, or difficulty in expressing or recognizing emotions, is associated with nondominant parietal lobe lesions and can also be mistaken for signs of depression.[14,58]

Behavior Problems

Personality traits are magnified by the stress resulting from a stroke. In addition, patients may have cognitive deficits before and after their stroke that interfere with normal inhibition and modulation of behavior. The hospital or treatment environment can also contribute to problem behaviors. Problems reported by Bishop and Pet[14] include aggressiveness, sexual inappropriateness, verbal outbursts or yelling, avoidant/resistive behaviors, and dependent behaviors. The best interventions result from correctly assessing the etiology of the problem behavior. Interventions include medications, development of a consistent and structured routine and environment, symptom-focused behavioral modification, and a consistent team approach.[14]

Pathologic Laughing and Crying

When persons who have had a stroke have episodes of crying or laughing without feelings of sadness or happiness, the episodes are sequelae of brain damage. This syndrome has been recognized since the late nineteenth century and has been labeled by a variety of terms including *emotional lability, pseudobulbar affect, emotional incontinence*, and *pathologic laughing and crying*. The traditional explanation of this syndrome is that there is bilateral interruption of the upper motor neuron innervation of the bulbar motor nuclei that leads to the interruption of descending fibers to the brain stem.[73]

Some persons only experience isolated episodes of pathologic crying or laughing. The overlap between different types of emotional lability is great. Ross and Rush[74] suggested that pathologic laughing and crying may be a valuable marker for depression in patients who have a flat affect resulting from lesions in the right inferior frontal lobe; Robinson et al[73] concluded that depression and emotional lability are two distinct disorders that may coexist. Their study found that antidepressants were a useful treatment for pathologic laughing or crying regardless of whether the patient was depressed.

House et al[46] defined pathologic emotionalism by asking stroke survivors if they experienced the following conditions:

1. Increased numbers of crying episodes (or less often, laughing) since the stroke
2. Having little or no control over laughing or crying episodes
3. Having so little control over these emotional episodes that they occurred in front of others

All three of these conditions had to be present for the patient to meet the criteria for pathologic emotionalism. The syndrome appears to persist at least during the first year after a stroke. House et al found that 1 month after the stoke, 15% of 112 patients met this criteria, at 6 months 21% met the criteria, and at 12 months 12% met the criteria.

Stroke survivors and their significant others report that pathologic laughing and crying are particularly embarrassing in social situations. Bishop and Pet[14] emphasize that patients and their families need clear explanations of the nature and course of pathologic emotionalism. Families and others may view the symptoms as a sign of unhappiness, depression, or lack of cooperation (when the patient is laughing).

Personality Changes

Donaldson[26] wrote the following description of her husband's stroke recovery:

As we prepared to begin rehabilitation, given Steve's dense hemiplegia and significant cognitive effects, we were told the road back would be long—it is in fact endless. In critical care, I had been told I wouldn't "lose him," but of course I did. I lost my first Steve—my husband of 20 years as I had known him. Stroke is, after all, pervasive in its effects, wreaking havoc on motor, perceptual, cognitive, emotional, and sensory functions. Steve, the stroke survivor, is physically, intellectually, and emotionally changed.

House et al[46] reported that a common complaint of caregivers is that the stroke survivors are apathetic in comparison to their previous personality. This was reported in 11% of patients at 6 months and 3% at 12 months after stroke, indicating that this reaction is transient and usually resolves within the first year after the stroke. The most common psychologic symptoms after stroke House et al found were lack of energy and increased worrying characterized by tiredness, nervous tension, and delays in falling asleep. They also found a set of reactions that were not commonly reported or diagnosed because there was no satisfactory psychiatric nomenclature. This set of reactions consisted of anxiety, irritability, social withdrawal, and excessive concern about a range of mental (dementia) and physical symptoms. They felt that these reactions often made up the condition that was described by others as "personality changes," a term they considered unfortunate because the reactions are reversible. They are best described as an "adjustment reaction" rather than a personality change.

Miller[58] thinks that apraxias, agnosias, memory disorders, and cognitive deficits all affect personality. He explains that the generalized effects of brain damage include fatigue, decreased concentration, and impaired orientation. Left hemispheric brain damage tends to affect verbal, analytic, and mathematics abilities, whereas damage to the right hemisphere tends to impair visuospatial, musical, and some types of emotional functioning.

In a paper published in 1972, Gainotti[38] reported two types of emotional responses that correlated to the side of the brain lesion. He examined 160 patients, 80 with left-sided lesions and 80 with right-sided lesions. The subjects were given a battery of neuropsychologic tests to analyze their emotional reactions to failures. Patients with left-sided lesions had what Gainotti described as *catastrophic reactions*, and patients with right-sided lesions had what he labeled *emotional reactions*. Box 3-1 shows a summary of his findings.

Box 3-1

Characteristics of Catastrophic and Emotional Reactions

CATASTROPHIC REACTIONS	EMOTIONAL REACTIONS
Left brain damage	**Right brain damage**
Anxiety reactions	Indifference reactions
Bursts of tears	Tendencies to joke
Vocative utterances	Expressions of hate toward affected extremities
Depressed renouncements	Anosognosia
Sharp refusals to go on	Minimization
Found primarily in severely aphasic patients	

Data from Gainotti G: Emotional behavior and hemispheric side of the lesion, *Cortex* 8:41, 1972.

Gainotti[38] attributed these hemispheric differences to differences in the functional organization of sensory data in the two halves of the brain. "According to this view the left, verbal hemisphere should be considered as more important from the 'intellectual' point of view and the right, nonverbal hemisphere as more important from the 'emotional' point of view."

More recent research suggests that visual impairments may play an important role in what had previously been considered lateralized differences. In an article published in 1989, Egelko et al[31] reported a study of 58 cerebrovascular accident (CVA) patients from a rehabilitation unit. Subjects were tested on admission and 10 months after the stroke, and their scores were compared with scores of 22 age-matched control subjects. Performance was tested in the following domains: hemispatial neglect, reaction time, depression, affect, and comprehension. They found that when comparisons were made between right brain damaged and left brain damaged patient groups with normal visual fields, laterality differences were significantly reduced. Egelko et al caution against assessment bias based on assumptions of lateralized deficits. They also recommended increasing education of patients and family regarding the nature of residual deficits, expectations regarding resolution, and changed behavior after stroke.

Assumptions of rehabilitation potential should not be based on generalized theories of lesion location. Novack and associates[64] administered psychologic tests in an attempt to predict rehabilitation outcome of 134 stroke patients. Their findings, published in 1987, indicated that the best predictors of rehabilitation potential aside from admission status was the test of motor persistence and half-hour recall.

Teasell[87] concluded that although the location of the brain injury influences the psychologic reaction of the stroke survivor, no definitive evidence suggests that a specific lesion location is the sole factor in the determination of specific emotional reactions.

Social Consequences of Stroke

As discussed previously (see Depression) one of the most significant and long-lasting consequences of stroke is a decrease in social activities participation.[35,48] There is some question as to whether social isolation and severity of stroke residuals are related. No direct association seems to exist between social withdrawal and physical recovery. Labi and associates[53] found that a significant proportion of stroke survivors were socially disabled in spite of substantial physical restoration. This follow-up study was based on data from the 1972 to 1975 Framingham study group of 148 long-term survivors of stroke. In addition, 121 subjects who needed no more than minimal assistance in daily living activities and had satisfactory physical restoration were analyzed. Three parameters of social function were considered, including socialization in the home, socialization outside of

the home, and hobbies and interests. About one third of the survivors who had resumed most or all of their previous household responsibilities did not resume their previous social activities. Angeleri et al[10] reported in 1993 that even those patients who could walk and carry out ADL independently did not resume their social activities.

In a 1989 article, Atler and Cliner[13] found that although there was no relationship between the number of current residual deficits and self-care status, there was a significant relationship between current residual deficits and activity levels. They examined the relationship between family-based psychosocial variables and activity after stroke in 30 male stroke patients and their spouses. Patients reported an increase in the amount of time spent watching television, maintenance of socializing at home, and reading. Traveling and involvement in home maintenance were the two areas in which participation frequently discontinued. Participation in civic/collective and entertainment/social activities commonly declined. The area in stroke patients' lifestyles that changed the most was the hobbies and interests area. Atler and Cliner noted that a primary goal and focus of initial stroke rehabilitation is increasing independence in self-care; they questioned whether the relationship between the number of deficits and activity level would weaken if therapeutic intervention included more focus on work and leisure roles (see Chapter 23).

OCCUPATIONAL THERAPY INTERVENTION

Psychosocial Core of Occupational Therapy

Although most stroke rehabilitation occurs in what is by definition a physical disabilities setting, strokes frequently include psychiatric, psychologic, and social complications. Some of these complications are diagnosed as psychiatric conditions and others are considered reactive responses. If a psychiatric diagnosis becomes the primary diagnosis on which therapeutic intervention will be based, occupational therapy intervention by a mental health specialist may be indicated. A specialty of mental health practice includes specialized knowledge in the assessment and treatment of patients with a primary psychiatric diagnosis. Specialists have expertise in psychopathology and its impact on functional performance.[6]

A stroke is a traumatic event that may result in residual disability and can lead to a variety of responses both on the part of the stroke survivor and society. As Fidler writes in the *AOTA Position Paper on the Psychosocial Core of Occupational Therapy*,[6] psychosocial responses may be manifested as poor motivation; refusal to participate; and expressions of hopelessness, anger, or denial. Although these reactions may be secondary symptoms related to a primary diagnosis of stroke, they must be understood and addressed by occupational therapists to achieve treatment goals.

"Understanding the complex psychosocial dimensions of human performance, knowing which activities can best be expected to elicit the desired adaptive response, and the artful skill of enabling a trusting, reciprocal relationship are integral aspects of all occupational therapy practice."[6] These psychosocial foundations of occupational therapy are applicable to all practitioners.

The two major elements of any occupational therapy practice are (1) the psychosocial needs of the patient, and (2) the psychosocial competencies of the occupational therapist.[4]

The Relationship

Empathy and Caring

Peloquin[65,66] writes on the importance of occupational therapists having empathy. The medical model's emphasis on a rational "fixing mode" can be interpreted as a lack of caring by patients. Therapists may worry that empathy is not professional or is inappropriately intimate; from Peloquin's perspective, empathy forms connections in which helpers find similarities to their patients, and at the same time it also promotes a respect for differences. "Empathy does not exact a fusion but a connection. It implies an experience not only of the pain of another, but of the integrity and courage that dwell alongside the pain. In health care practice, empathy is the enactment of the conviction that empowered by someone's willingness to understand, the patient will gather the requisite measure of courage."[65]

Sachs and Labowitz[75] identified being caring as a central part of the occupational therapist's role. They write that caring is a complex concept including both labor (activity) and emotion (feeling) directed toward the preservation and growth of a person in need. As Peloquin[66] observes, patients argue that all helpers should care. "Helpers wrap themselves in their procedural authority, binding themselves so tightly in their concern for the right method, the latest technology, that it is no wonder that their actions seem constricted. Helpers can never be seen as personal if they offer knowledge and skills instead of themselves." Occupational therapists have to acknowledge that techniques and protocols can interfere with caring. Occupational therapists have traditionally endorsed a practice based on competence and caring. Both should be possible and ideally, compatible.

Defining the Purpose

Part of a practice built on competence and caring is an acknowledgement of collaboration in the therapeutic relationship. Occupational therapists have long valued a model of collaboration and active participation.[100,101] This process should start from the initiation of therapy. If the person who has had the stroke is able to understand the purpose of occupational therapy, they can also participate in establishing priorities for intervention. If the therapist focuses on component deficits in the absence of functional context, the patient may well assume that the goal of therapy is to restore lost abilities. Although this may be the appro-

priate goal in some areas, the reality may actually be that the patient will have to function in new ways because of permanent loss or impairment of component skills. One way to facilitate active participation and collaboration in the therapeutic process is to have the patient answer the question, "What do you need and want to do?" and "In what way can you accomplish this now that you have had a stroke?"

In 1993, Christiansen[18] wrote, "There is increasing agreement that occupational therapy's unique contribution to function is through emphasis on occupational performance. There is also recognition, although limited, that assessing function without regard to the patient's life tasks and roles has serious shortcomings."

In the same year, Trombly[91] acknowledged that occupational therapists frequently begin patient assessment by a bottom-up approach with an emphasis on component deficits before occupational performance. She thinks that although the therapist may make implicit assumptions about the connection between mastery of these components before performing an occupation or entire task, these connections are often not clarified for patients. Furthermore, the goals that the occupational therapist has in mind may or may not match or even be related to the patient's goals.

In contrast to the reductionistic bottom-up approach, a top-down assessment starts with an examination of role competency and meaning before assessment of functional components or disabilities. The occupational therapist focuses assessment on previous role performance as well as current and future roles. The patient may benefit from occupational therapy intervention if there is a discrepancy between past, present, and future role performance. This top-down approach makes treatment goals more apparent and relevant to the patient.[91]

Dunn[28] agrees that a contextual assessment approach is necessary to identify what a person seeking occupational therapy services needs and wants. Therapists should begin to apply the "so what" criteria to all evaluations and measurements: when considering a certain test, therapists should evaluate whether it is important to the person's life and function. If it is not, the therapist should use more relevant intervention.

Northen et al[63] studied 30 occupational therapists in an adult rehabilitation setting and determined that most therapists made some effort to involve patients and families in goal setting; however, most efforts were not the best they could be. Reasons that the therapists gave for less than optimal involvement of patients and families included time constraints and poor cognitive status. Evidence gathered by the researchers suggests these reasons may be based on false assumptions. They found that therapists who consistently involve patients and families at the maximum level took less (not more) time in the evaluation process. They also found that although patients' cognitive status may affect their ability to set realistic goals, it does not preclude involvement in the process of goal setting. Therapists with high scores used the following techniques to maximize involvement: probing for additional information about a patient's concerns and goals, giving situation-specific examples while explaining occupational therapy interventions, and telling the patient the way specific evaluative tests and measurements relate to potential treatment and outcomes.

Neistadt[62] surveyed 296 occupational therapy directors throughout the United States about whether occupational therapists were assessing patient priorities on admission and, if so, in what way. She found the majority were using interviews and that patient goals were vague and did not specify meaningful activities. She concluded that occupational therapists in the United States have not yet successfully translated core values, including the importance of patient-therapist collaboration, into formal procedures for practice in physical disabilities. Vague patient goals such as "I want to walk" or "I want to take care of myself" should not satisfy occupational therapists. The issue for occupational therapists is not whether patients want to walk but where they want to walk and what they want to do when they get there. Neistadt suggests that formal procedures do exist (specifically, the Canadian Occupational Performance Measure [COPM]).

The COPM is a patient-centered tool that is designed to help occupational therapists establish occupational performance goals based on patient perceptions of need. Roles and role expectations are considered within the context of the patient's own environment. It is also an outcome measurement tool that evaluates a patient's perception of change in defined problem areas. This approach helps the patient engage in the occupational therapy from the start of intervention and increases patient control of the therapeutic process[54] (see Chapters 15 and 27).

Choosing Therapeutic Activities: Meaning and Purpose

Clinical reasoning in occupational therapy includes both scientific as well as what has been called *narrative reasoning*.[77] As therapists put together the life stories of the patients they treat, a conditionally-reasoned new person emerges. This person may still have deficits but in spite of them functions at higher levels of autonomy and independence. Through engaging in therapeutic activities the patient and therapist test out the feasibility of this new person.

Schkade and Schultz[78] have proposed a therapeutic perspective of occupational adaptation in an effort to integrate the constructs of occupation and adaptation into a single interactive construct. In this construct, occupation is an interaction of the person and occupational environment. Occupational adaptation requires that the sensorimotor, cognitive, and psychosocial subsystems are involved in every occupational response.

At what point does a therapeutic activity address one functional component or life role as opposed to another? Like other occupational responses, therapeutic activities are simultaneously simple and complex. The choice of activities is crucial to the success of the therapeutic program and the satisfactory adaptation of the stroke patient. No prescriptive formulas of activities according to diagnoses or deficits exist. All activities include individual as well as sociocultural meanings.

Cynkin and Robinson[22] offer a systematic approach to assessing and improving a patient's state of activities health through the use of meaningful therapeutic activities. The activities health assessment consists of a series of activities schedules, information on the way patients perceive their lifestyles and functioning as revealed by the activities configuration, interview, and interpretation of findings. Based on this information the occupational therapist and the patient work together toward an agreed-on state of activities health.

Cynkin and Robinson[22] note that activities are chosen within the constraints of external and internal conditions. They must be appropriate, practical, versatile, and adaptive. Therapeutic activities, which are rehearsals for everyday living, can be real-life activities or simulated situations. The more closely they resemble the activities in the patient's real world the better. Although many basic self-care tasks and leisure activities may be closely approximated, most therapeutic activities are only simulations of situations encountered in the real world because of the great range of patient needs, the variations in individual and sociocultural activities configurations, and the constraints in many occupational therapy treatment settings. The use of simulated situations is justified by the assumption that learning can be transferred from one situation to another by generalization (see chapter 2). The more closely the simulations match the individual activities configuration of each patient, the more likely it is that generalization will occur. According to Cynkin and Robinson,[22] simulated activities will be effective only if they meet the following criteria:

1. They have meaning and relevance to the patient.
2. Their purpose is clear and acceptable to the patient.
3. There are enough elements of similarity between the simulated and actual situations to make transfer of learning likely.

Neistadt[61] addresses the issue of selecting therapeutic activities for persons with cognitive deficits. Her conclusion is that the decision about the amount of abstraction used in treatment approaches should be based on demonstrated learning capacities and not assumptions about brain damage.

Person-Environment Transaction

Law et al[55] propose a person-environment-occupation model of occupational performance that builds on concepts from the *Canadian Occupational Therapy Guidelines for Client Centered Practice* and environmental-behavioral theories. In the Canadian model the person is considered a combination of the mind, body, and spirit. The person has a set of performance components and life experiences, including self-concept, personality style, cultural background, and personal competencies, that influence occupational performance. Personal competencies include motor performance abilities, sensory capabilities, cognitive aptitude, and general health, as well as a set of learned and innate skills. The environment includes cultural, socioeconomic, institutional, physical, and social factors. In addition, the model considers the environment from the unique perspective of the person, household, neighborhood, or community. *Occupational performance* is defined as the outcome of the person, environment, and occupation. It is a dynamic experience in which a person is engaged in purposeful activities and tasks within a particular environment. The better the fit of the person, occupation, and environment the better the outcome.

Dunn et al[29] proposed a framework for considering the effect of context ("a lens from which persons view their world"[29]). Referred to as the *ecology of human performance*, the framework defines performance as both the process and result of the person interacting with context for the purpose of engaging in tasks. Therapeutic intervention is a collaboration between the person/family and the occupational therapist that is directed at meeting performance needs. Interventions are considered multifaceted and designed to accomplish any or all of the following:

1. Establish/restore a person's ability to perform in context
2. Alter the actual context in which people perform
3. Adapt contextual features and task demands so they support performance in context
4. Prevent the occurrence or evolution of performance errors in context
5. Create circumstances that promote more adaptive or complex performance in context.

Culture

In 1994, Mirkopoulos and Evert[59] wrote about the unmet challenge of addressing the importance of culture in occupational therapy practice. They concluded that in spite of numerous references to the importance of culture in our practice, there continue to be indications that occupational therapists as a group show a lack of sensitivity and awareness about cultural influences on human behavior and values including their own.

The first way to meet this challenge is on a case-by-case basis. A person who has a stroke should first be thought of as a person and not a stroke patient. In a patient-oriented practice the patient or family should be able to educate the therapist about cultural similarities and differences that are relevant to the person's needs and wants in regards to fulfilling culturally relevant occupational roles.

Mastery and Competence

For activities to be therapeutic, they must arouse and sustain what Bruner referred to as *the will to learn*. This will depends on a number of extrinsic and intrinsic motives. Intrinsic motives include curiosity, a desire for competency, aspiration to emulate a model, and a commitment to social membership and reciprocity.[22]

In an occupational adaptation perspective, Schkade and Schultz[78] assume that the human desire for mastery causes a person to adaptively respond to an occupational challenge. People commonly respond to challenges with already-existing modes of performance or behavior. This process occurs whether these existing modes are appropriate or functional. New or modified modes of performance develop only after existing modes fail or result in relative mastery. When people are confronted with occupational challenges that are beyond their current capabilities, they may engage in primitive behaviors. These behaviors can be normative, especially when they temporarily help restore balance. Relative mastery is defined as the extent to which the person experiences the occupational response as efficient, effective, and satisfying to self and society.

Gage and Polatajko[37] discuss the importance of perceived self-efficacy in determining a person's willingness to engage in activity. Perceived self-efficacy is a concept developed as part of social cognitive theory; it is individuals' beliefs in their ability to perform a specific activity. This self-assessment of efficacy helps determine which activities people will engage in and the amount of time they will attempt an activity in the face of previous failure. Discrepancies between perceived self-efficacy and skill competence may help explain discrepancies between attained skills and subsequent occupational performance. The concept of perceived self-efficacy supports the use of real-life contexts as much as possible in the choice of therapeutic activities. The closer patients' therapeutic performance relates to their own unique environments, the more likely they are to perceive themselves as able to perform that activity in their own life circumstances.

MODELS FOR INTERVENTION

Depressed, Medically Ill Patients

Watson[96] presents useful material on occupational therapy intervention for depressed, medically ill patients that is potentially applicable to depressed stroke survivors. The goals of therapeutic intervention include the following:

- Provide opportunities for mastery and control.
- Decrease emotional distress.
- Promote psychological competence.

• Help maintain and/or reestablish an active support network.

Watson writes that an important part of the assessment process is identification of previous methods of coping with stress. She states that the occupational therapist can provide support, and through establishment of therapeutic rapport, provide patients with an opportunity to redefine problems and identify positive aspects of their current situation so that solutions can be identified. To Watson, developing rapport means meeting patients at their own level. For a severely depressed patient this may initially mean limiting contacts to short, frequent interactions.

Watson believes that the therapist can provide patients with opportunities to express their perceptions of the stroke and its prognosis. Activities are selected to promote feelings of competence; treatment should initially focus on ability rather than disability. Activities that ensure success support feelings of mastery, control, and patient effectiveness.

Watson also suggests that depressed patients who may have difficulty feeling motivated to care for themselves may be asked to do things for others. Focusing on doing and giving may offer an opportunity to reengage in meaningful activities that contribute to nurturing significant relationships. Engaging in activity provides a structure for identifying strengths and gently challenging negative thoughts and self-perceptions.

Elderly, Mentally Ill Patients

Trace and Howell[90] describe the role of occupational therapy for elderly persons who have been diagnosed with a mental illness. They emphasize the importance of activity in reducing agitation and anxiety. They also report that engaging in activity can offer further opportunities for assessing the ways psychiatric symptoms interfere with function. Selecting activities for agitated patients requires consideration of the patient's motivation, cognitive abilities, and potential for risky, aggressive, or self-destructive behavior.

Trace and Howell state because withdrawal from a usual level of activity is often a major consequence of mental illness, patients may resist attempts to engage them in activity. Patients expect to fail; they then avoid activities and thus have a decreased performance ability. This cycle can be interrupted when the occupational therapist offers opportunities to succeed in part or all of an activity. The success contributes to an increased sense of competence, which then improves the chances of further participation.

Occupational therapists who work with depressed persons should be aware that anhedonia, or lack of pleasure in previously enjoyed activities, is a symptom of major depression. Persons with depression may have component skills to perform an activity but show little initial motivation or enjoyment of participation in activities. Occupational therapists should also monitor patients' functional progress when they are being treated with psychotropic drugs. Medication may improve performance or have adverse effects on mobility, attention, continence, communication, and cognition.[90]

According to Trace and Howell,[90] participation in therapy groups is an effective intervention, but psychiatric symptoms may require the skilled intervention of an occupational therapist to facilitate group participation. To intervene the therapist needs to understand the individual dynamics preventing full participation and support the patient in group participation. Patients with cognitive deficits may avoid tasks that expose deficits and make excuses rather than risk failure. Group activities offer a playful, safe arena in which to experience pleasure in interpersonal relationships, giving, and reciprocal interaction. Trace and Howell[90] conclude that psychosocial intervention is often not valued for its physical results. Although an additional 20° of shoulder motion may lead to independent dressing, improved self-concept and mood may motivate a patient to visit a senior center or prepare a meal.

DOCUMENTATION

The effects of psychosocial issues on occupational performance should be documented. Documentation should include the way in which symptoms, behaviors, abilities, and disabilities impact the patient's ability to perform. These performance components can be addressed through documentation in the form of treatment planning, intervention, progress reports, and discharge recommendations and summaries. The AOTA's *Uniform Terminology for Occupational Therapy—Third Edition*[3] includes a complete list of components and contexts that offer concrete guidelines for documentation (Box 3-2).

STAGES OF INTERVENTION AND ADAPTATION: CONTEXT OF TREATMENT

Although arguably regrettable[99] the majority of occupational therapy interventions occur during the more acute stages of stroke recovery. These interventions, which are largely reimbursed by Medicare, occur in acute care hospitals, subacute units, inpatient rehabilitation centers, nursing facilities, home care settings, offices, and outpatient departments.[8] Following is a summary of potential psychosocial issues presented within the context of existing treatment settings. These issues are by no means predictable, all inclusive, or mutually exclusive.

Acute Care

In an acute care setting, occupational therapists usually see a person almost immediately after a stroke. Some people are confused and have varying levels of consciousness and insight into their situation. A stroke is a potentially lethal event, so a reaction similar to that of a near-death experience is probable. Immediately after a stroke a major role

Box 3-2

Psychosocial Components: Domain of Practice

In addition to assessment and goal setting, occupational therapy intervention can address a number of psychosocial skills and psychologic components with attention to performance contexts. *AOTA Uniform Terminology for Occupational Therapy—Third Edition*[3] includes the following as performance components:

PSYCHOSOCIAL SKILLS AND PSYCHOLOGIC COMPONENTS

The ability to interact in society and process emotions

Psychologic

- Values: Identifying ideas or beliefs that are important to self and others
- Interests: Identifying mental or physical activities that create pleasure and maintain attention
- Self-concept: Developing the value of the physical, emotional, and sexual selves

Social

- Role performance: Identifying, maintaining, and balancing functions that are assumed or acquired in society (e.g., employee, student, parent, friend, religious participant)
- Social conduct: Interacting by using manners, personal space, eye contact, gestures, active listening, and self-expression appropriate to the environment
- Interpersonal skills: Using verbal and nonverbal communication to interact in a variety of settings
- Self-expression: Using a variety of styles and skills to express thoughts, feelings, and needs

Self-management

- Coping skills: Identifying and managing stress and related factors
- Time management: Planning and participating in a balance of self-care, work, leisure, and rest activities to promote satisfaction and health
- Self-control: Modifying behavior in response to environmental needs, demands, and constraints; personal aspirations; and feedback from others

PERFORMANCE CONTEXTS

Context in which activities are carried out—are equally as important as psychologic components

Temporal

- Chronologic: Age
- Developmental: Stage or phase of maturation
- Life cycle: Place in important life phases, such as career cycle, parenting cycle, or educational process
- Disability status: Place in continuum of disability, such as acuteness of injury, chronicity of disability, or terminal nature of illness

Environmental

- Physical
- Social: Availability and expectations of significant individuals, such as spouse, friends, and caregivers; in addition, larger social groups that are influential in establishing norms, role expectations, and social routines
- Cultural: Customs, beliefs, activity patterns, behavior standards, and expectations accepted by the society of which the individual is a member; includes politics, such as laws that affect access to resources and affirm personal rights, and opportunities for education, employment, and economic support

shift occurs—the person becomes a patient. The hospital culture has an entirely new set of conduct expectations built on dependence and compliance. Interpersonal and communication skills may not only be affected by brain damage but also by the hospital's lack of sensitivity to previously successful social behavior and conduct.

There are few opportunities for self-expression. Patients are rarely asked how they feel about their stroke, hemiplegia, or other related issues. A patient's ability to cope may depend on availability of past coping strategies and support networks. Time management becomes someone else's responsibility; there is little or no control over the daily schedule. Self-control may be impaired by sequelae of the stroke including emotional lability and/or major depression. Beliefs and values influence patients' ability to begin to cope with their situation. The patient may have a dramatic reaction to the sudden loss of function and physical integrity.

Early in the recovery process, patients may focus more on regaining lost physical function than accepting change and deficits.[44] Support may be best provided in the form of information and education. As occupational therapists work with patients, they may be confronted with questions regarding prognosis for recovery or what has happened. The anxiety and stress associated with an acute stroke often interfere with a patient's ability to comprehend what has occurred and the way to participate in rehabilitation. The goal of patient and family education should be to provide enough information to allow the patient and family to verbalize their understanding of the situation.

Patient accounts emphasize that the time after a stroke is one of confusion, passivity, and care by strangers.[66] At this point more than any other the patient's primary needs may be emotional support, empathy, and caring. The occupational therapist may be able to begin the process of helping the patient identify abilities, disabilities, and a changed situation. Questions about prognosis should be addressed with an appreciation of the potentially beneficial role of illusions in adjustment and adaptation. Therapists should determine whether the patient's beliefs are interfering with or facilitating functional performance. The smallest opportunities for control and mastery may make a significant difference in a patient's willingness to engage in therapy or self-care. Visitors and family members may also be struggling to understand the situation and the ways to engage and support the patient.

Depression is more common during the later rather than acute stage of treatment. Depression may be appear in the form of social withdrawal or expressions of hopelessness and self-hatred. If a patient is unable to participate in therapy because of depressive symptoms, the therapist should consult the physician or treatment team for a possible psychiatric referral. If a patient is put on antidepressant medication, the occupational therapist can help monitor the effect of the medication on occupational performance.

The occupational therapist can suggest environmental modifications to allow increased patient control and opportunities for social interaction. For example, the rooms of patients with severe neglect or visual impairment can be rearranged to allow them to attend to their door when visitors enter. Patients should be involved in their care as much as possible. A patient is often more reliable than rotating staff for following up a range of motion (ROM) program or instructions for use of a splint.

Therapeutic focus is a form of communication. If the occupational therapist only spends time working with an affected upper extremity, the patient may begin to equate therapeutic success solely with the performance of this extremity. All therapeutic activities should relate to real-life expectations of occupational performance. When simulations are used, the patient should understand, as much as possible, the purpose of the activity in relation to occupa-

tional performance and participation in previous occupational roles.

Inpatient Rehabilitation*

Penny remembered therapists as helpful and caring people. At that point, she believed that one day she would be "normal" again. She remembered being the center of attention but had little memory or appraisal of therapy as more than "little stuff."[19]

Patients treated in inpatient rehabilitation units have passed the most acute stage of stroke recovery and are spend their days participating in a rigorous training program. A patient's values and beliefs continue to influence attitudes toward recovery and treatment. Some patients may believe their illness and resultant disability are punishments for past behavior.

During inpatient rehabilitation the stroke survivor's self-concept is emerging. Patient's are asked to perform tasks and at times fail; failure is especially frustrating and embarrassing when it occurs in front of others. Patients can be traumatized by repeated reinforcement of their new limitations. Therapist intervention at this point is crucial to the patient's continuing motivation. Therapists who provide too much or not enough structure and support, push the patients too hard or too little, and discount or minimize the patient's feelings and emotional reactions can contribute to decreased patient motivation to accomplish the treatment team's goals.[44]

A patient's self-concept is shaped by stroke residuals as well as progress in therapy. Families and patients may think the progress is inadequate and more effort needs to be put forth, or they may fault the therapist or doctor. Both patients and significant others may require information and education about the uniqueness of individual strokes, deficits, and the complexity of recovery. Patients' feelings of failure can possibly contribute to depression, which decreases participation and further slows progress. This cycle of withdrawal further frustrates the patient, treatment team, and patient's significant others. Depression may be also be indicated during participation in activities by difficulty in initiation, a slow or anxious pace, and self-deprecating remarks.

Role shifts begin to be more relevant as plans are made for life after discharge from the hospital. The patient may ask, "Who am I now?" At this point the patient may appear to deny the presence of deficits or be unable to visu-

*The words of Penny Richardson, friend and colleague of Florence Clarke,[19] have been added to the recollections of other stroke survivors and their families. Penny Richardson was a professor and Chair of the Higher Education Department in the University of Southern California School of Education. In 1989 at 47 years of age, she suffered a stroke caused by a ruptured aneurysm. Penny died of a second brain hemorrhage in 1993, 5 weeks after Florence Clarke presented the Eleanor Clarke Slagle Lecture that was based on a narrative analysis of Penny's personal account.

alize the new self at home. Survivor accounts emphasize the importance of hope and encouragement at this stage.[19,26] Actual skills learned support the general concept that lost functions can be regained.

Social conduct in a rehabilitation unit is different than the patient has experienced in other settings and is often much more like school experiences than hospital or real life environments. Coping skills and adaptive strategies become more evident. Clarke et al[20] found that occupational therapists may not routinely address adaptive strategies that are successfully employed by much older Americans. These include maintaining spirituality, relationships with others, and support to continue community independence.

In addition to learning specific skills the patient is also developing a new identity—a person with a disability. An entirely new culture also exists that requires patients to adapt. They may feel threatened or reassured by membership in the disabled community. Patients who have more abilities than other patients have the opportunity to help them. Therapeutic groups can capitalize on the power of peer relationships and shared experience.

In an ethnographic study of a 30-year-old man with a spinal cord injury, researchers found that although the patient wanted help determining the way his future related to his past, therapists were more intent on teaching him new skills. They often discounted his past life experiences as having little significance and relation to his present and future.[83]

Subacute Facility or Nursing Home Care

Patients who do not meet the requirements for admission to an inpatient rehabilitation program and are not able to return home even after some rehabilitation may become residents of a subacute facility. This setting may be a temporary situation for patients who will eventually be able to return home or a permanent setting for those who do not have the ability or resources to return home. Rehabilitation services in this setting vary from substantial to sporadic.

The incidence of depression is known to be higher among the institutionalized elderly.[81] The facility itself can represent disability and abandonment to some patients. Residents must learn to adapt to an environment in which self-control and privacy almost always diminish. The social context is full of paid workers, disabled peers, and periodic visits from family and friends. Cultural values may influence the decision for placement as well as the individual's response to this environment.

The occupational therapist may be able to facilitate improvements in coping and adaptation by recognizing individual residents' interests and needs. A resident's self-concept may have been more positive in the past than it is in the present. Previously successful coping and adjustment strategies may offer the best indications of which strategies will be helpful in the future. Opportunities for self-

expression, creativity, and social interaction may promote development of increased self-esteem and efficacy.

Home Care

When stroke survivors return home, their interactions with the environment become crucial. The first few weeks after discharge from inpatient rehabilitation may be the most difficult for patients and those interacting with them.[42] The person's self-concept is affected even more by stroke residuals, which begin to play a part in everyday life. The stroke survivor may be embarrassed about being different or "less of a person." Society's reactions to stroke survivors will affect their self-concept. Drooling, incontinence, and flaccid or distorted extremities all signal to others that the person is not "normal." The American preoccupation with appearances may make this particularly difficult. Expectations of others may strongly influence role performance. Jongbloed[47] describes the way a stroke survivor's husband took over the kitchen duties and her struggle with him to resume cooking. The occupational therapist can help a patient identify possible roles according to abilities and deficits. Dickerson and Oakley[24] found participation in significantly fewer life roles among persons with physical or psychosocial disabilities than among adults without reported disabilities. Hallett et al[43] found that in an adult population of 28 persons who had experienced traumatic brain injuries (TBIs), there were significant decreases in the number of life roles assumed by each person. The most commonly lost roles included major organizing roles, such as employee, hobbyist, and friend. Although not as common, participation in additional roles such as home maintainer, family member, and religious participant were also documented.

Values can dictate a patient's ability to leave home or resume social participation. The occupational therapist can assist patients in the pursuit of social activities within their social context. Attempts to duplicate the hospital or rehabilitation environment may be counterproductive to reintegration. The therapist and patient can work together to set mutual goals that acknowledge deficits without removing hope of functional return.

Patients may be overwhelmed with their new sets of limitations and restrictions. Previously effective coping strategies may not work or may decrease adaptation. Returning to a schedule of activities that encompasses desired roles can maximize activity participation and function as well as help fight depression. The amount of support and structure required for successful performance is dependent on the complex interaction of the person, environment, and occupation.

Examples of therapeutic interventions that maximize this interaction include Schwartz's[80] work with brain-injured patients in the home setting. She describes home therapy with three patients who had significant cognitive deficits. Using models of psychosocial adaptation with decision-making and dynamic assessment, the occupational therapist was able to continuously review the patients' strengths and weaknesses as well as the psychosocial-environmental factors that affected treatment. Treatment intervention included saturation cuing with behavioral chaining and positive reinforcement, incorporation of the family or significant others as part of the treatment team, and environmental adaptions including tape-recorded messages and an appointment book of daily activities.

As time passes after the stroke, there is an increasing need to clarify goals of occupational therapy. A continued preoccupation with regaining lost abilities can leave patients feeling abandoned when therapy is discontinued. Therapists who are terminating therapy should be sensitive to the importance of patients' hopes and possible illusions about rehabilitation.

Donaldson[26] remembers when the following words from her husband made her realize the powerful role of hope in his day-to-day functioning: "I wake up every day and try to move my left arm, and every day when I can't, I'm disappointed—a little sad. And then I live that day and wake up again and try again. I hope that someday, somehow, I will be able to move my left arm. I expect you to join me in that hope." This hope for return of lost physical function helped Donaldson with assisting her husband to resume as many roles and activities as possible. He experienced failure, but this helped define the "new Steve" and his capabilities. Steve was not the same, but he and his wife managed to build a life together, although it was different than before the stroke. Donaldson particularly remembers how little support they received when attempting to return to previously enjoyed activities such as camping and traveling. Steve tried to return to work, but it prompted a complete neuropsychologic assessment. The results of this assessment were relevant to Steve and his wife because they indicated that he could not do everything he had done before. Learning—even if it is learning what you *can't* do so you can move on to what you *can* do—involves failure as well as success. When people fail at self-directed activities, they may be better able to tolerate this failure, as compared to failing at activities selected by someone else.

Outpatient Rehabilitation

Penny Richardson remembered outpatient therapy as seeming disconnected from her personal struggle to recover. When discharged, she explained: "I feel they abandoned me, and I feel that they did their thing. . . .but their thing was to do their things, not to help me do the things for myself. And so in a sense, they kept control of the situation. I was not empowered to do it on my own. They did it with me and in a sense, they flunked me."[19]

As patients become able to leave their homes (particularly Medicare patients), it is possible for therapy to continue for a limited duration in an outpatient setting. More than ever, goals should be developed according to the patient's role expectations. Psychosocial issues that should be addressed may include unrealistic expectations for the return of abilities that have been lost after the stroke. Although not absolute, most return of function occurs within 6 months after the stroke. The *Post-Stroke Rehabilitation, Clinical Practice Guideline*[42] suggests that continued rehabilitation should focus on areas of function and activities that are high priorities to the patient, including hobbies and recreational activities, social relationships, and family roles.[41] Use of the COPM can be helpful in identifying relevant areas of treatment.

Community Interventions

Occupational therapy's fullest promise may be delivered at the end of the spectrum of care when true adaptation and adjustment take place.[97] As health care becomes redefined and shifts from a model of treating sick people to a model of keeping people well, occupational therapists must find new opportunities for community intervention. Currently therapists may work with stroke survivors in established community programs such as senior centers, senior residences, and adult day health centers. Eilenberg[32] presents a model of a senior-center program to prevent depression in a high-risk senior population. The program was based on a sensory-integrative model that focused on the need for adequate, varied, and meaningful stimulation and social interactions. Eilenberg designed and implemented groups to help patients learn their own strengths, express their needs, and recognize their own roles in health maintenance. Groups of no more than 15 members attended an 8-week series of meetings. Each meeting included a 1-hour discussion on health-related topics and a half-hour session of movement activity, including posture, breathing, warmup activities, and dance. The members were enthusiastic about and supportive of the groups and appeared to receive at least some short-term benefits.

Another model of intervention, which is rarely used by occupational therapists under current reimbursement structures, is one that classifies someone other than the stroke survivor as "patient." The patient could be a spouse or an institution needing the intervention and expertise of an occupational therapist to help promote the stroke survivor's maximum occupational performance.

DISABILITY AND INCLUSION

In her 1994 Eleanor Clarke Slagle Lecture, Ann P. Grady[40] speaks about embracing the ideas of choice, relevance, and active participation in meaningful occupations to help build communities that include people with disabilities and allow them to live and function in the communities of their choice. "Occupational therapists have always recognized that disability was not an illness that could be cured by medicine. The challenge for us is to promote the *interactive model for practice* regardless of the venue of our practice. A concurrent challenge is to increase support for *more practice venues* in the community where engagement in *real occupation* takes place."

AOTA supports the Americans with Disabilities Act (ADA)[2] and "urges all occupational therapy practitioners to embrace opportunities to empower individuals with disabilities in the following five areas specified by the ADA: (1) employment, (2) public accommodation, (3) state and local government, (4) public transportation, and (5) telecommunications."

A final consideration involves the politics and economics of disability and rehabilitation. Disability rights activists have organized to redefine the meaning of disability for themselves and others. Schlaff[79] states that occupational therapists can actively contribute to this redefinition of disability through self-reflection and advocacy training. A civil rights movement advocating independent living promotes self-determination and a self-directed lifestyle. Individuals with disabilities who are independent are permitted to make their own decisions and choices and construct their own solutions to problems. Persons with disabilities, not the professionals helping them, are considered to be the best judges of their own interests and best qualified to organize and operate their programs.

In his book, *The Disability Business—Rehabilitation in America*, Gary Albrecht[1] examines the shift in the way rehabilitation services are viewed and delivered. In our society, rehabilitation has not been viewed as an indisputable right. Historically, services were provided through charitable organizations or government programs at no cost to the individual. The overall goal of rehabilitation was often to be capable of obtaining gainful employment. This goal negated those with less valued occupations and members of less valued segments of society. In contemporary society and today's health care environment, rehabilitation has shifted to being a service that is potentially beneficial to multiple individuals, even in the short term. Rehabilitation has become a business—a consumable commodity in demand by individuals with a variety of impairments. To Albrecht the critical questions are these: To whose benefit has this market been created, products developed, and profits made? Have political and economic issues taken precedence over the value of independence in society? Has the individual become lost in the business of rehabilitation? Persons with disabilities must be consulted if these questions are to be answered.

■

Case study*

The following vignette serves to stress how important it is to be attuned to the individual's activities background, not only in its outward trappings but in the nuances that give it significance. For graphic illustration, an extreme case of cultural variation has been chosen, although the sensitivity

*From Cynkin S, Robinson A: *Occupational therapy and activities health: toward health through activities,* Boston, 1990, Little, Brown.

and awareness required of the occupational therapist are not less even when the differences are not so obvious.

He is wheeled into the occupational therapy department, a thin small figure, slumped to one side, head lolling, a trickle of saliva at the corner of his drooping mouth, right arm hanging flaccidly. His eyes are dull, his furrowed skin ashy gray.

Newly recruited from his tribal home to work in the mines near the big city, he has awakened, after weeks of unconsciousness caused by a blow on the head, to a terrifyingly unfamiliar world. All attempts to communicate with him have failed. He seems to be quite unaware of the returning function in his right lower limb and trunk, so physical therapy has had to continue solely with its program of passive exercise. There is no objective way to determine whether he is aphasic or has deteriorated mentally, although he is regarded as a half-wit, probably bewitched, by his compatriots.

In the occupational therapy department his bewilderment is compounded by the strange apparatus and yet another white-coated "nurse" who gesticulates incomprehensibly and moves him as if he were a stuffed doll. The attendant with him, attempting to translate, shrugs his shoulders and rolls his eyes upward to indicate that the case is hopeless.

Outside on the lawn in the bright sunshine a group of other white-coated attendants on their lunch break and outpatients waiting their turn in the clinic are clustered around two players intent on outmaneuvering each other on a makeshift board (a discarded box lid) with "men" represented by soda bottle caps beaten flat. Loud chatter and frequent outbursts of laughter indicate that the bystanders are an essential element in this game of marabaraba, an African pastime so popular that it is played with improvised equipment in any available city spot during any break in the day's work.

One of the bystanders is an attendant, one foot encased in a walking cast, who is hopping about excitedly. The light dawns on the occupational therapist—a tribal game . . . a handicapped opponent . . . lower limb motion . . . adapted checkers . . . improvisation . . . an African way of life . . . time enough to enlist the ready-made crowd of spectators. Checkers adapted for lower limb exercises are available at the large general hospital across the road. A messenger, hastily dispatched, returns with 4-inch square wooden blocks, to which wire hoops are affixed for slipping over the ankle. A greatly enlarged board is marked out in chalk on the paved path outside the occupational therapy department. The patient is transferred from his clumsy wheelchair to an office chair with armrests and smoothly gliding castors. The puzzled attendant with the cast is coaxed into a similar chair. The opponents are wheeled into place, facing each other. Slowly the attendant slips the wire hoop, adjusted to accommodate to the size of the cast, over his foot. He flexes his hip, knee extended, lifting the block in the process; he pauses, surveys the board, extends his hip, and drops his "man" onto the appointed place. The bystanders, their curiosity aroused, crowd around, clicking tongues and shaking heads in pity and disbelief. Now it is the patient's turn. The block is slipped over his right ankle. With gentle pressure over the patient's hip joint the therapist draws the chair and extended leg back and forth alongside the board, then waits for a sign. The patient's eyes brighten, his head straightens, he focuses on the board, moves his hip independently, hovers over the board, frowns in concentration, and then, with visible effort, drops the block onto the exact spot he has selected. A roar of approval from the bystanders brings a crooked smile, a gleam in his eyes, a renewed frown of concentration, and the game is on . . .

■

CASE STUDY*

JJ, a 66-year-old widow with right hemiplegia, is working with a certified occupational therapy assistant (COTA)/registered occupational therapist (OTR) team in a community hospital's outpatient program. Sensorimotor function, as it relates to the performance of self-care and homemaking tasks, has been the primary focus of occupational therapy intervention. After a difficult treatment session where JJ became tearful and unwilling to engage in the activities, the COTA and the OTR consulted to do some joint problem solving. Both practitioners had worked with JJ over the course of her inpatient and rehabilitation programs. They discussed the need to talk with JJ about her feelings and listed possible contributing factors to JJ's tearfulness. Their list included:

- Depression and frustration with her lack of return to full upper-extremity function.
- Loss of valued roles, including homemaker, baker, and member of a recipe club.
- Quality of life issues due to above losses and lack of meaningful activities that she could do at home independently.
- Loss of confidence in her abilities and lack of recognition of her intact skills, with resultant lack of identity.

The COTA/OTR team discussed possible strategies to use when working with JJ at her next session, depending on her feelings and desires. These strategies incorporate the psychosocial skills of the occupational therapy practitioner:

- Reflecting JJ's feelings by saying, "It must be hard to contend with new limitations," and asking her for her view.
- Reviewing, with JJ, her past history relative to how she coped with difficult past situations.
- Collaborating with JJ to develop a clear plan for doing a meaningful activity that would be achievable and give her a positive sense of self.
- Helping JJ make a list of the skills she has, and working with her on developing a self-statement she would find affirming.
- Asking JJ if any family or friends could be more involved in her therapy, so that follow-up activities at home could include the type of joint activities that she enjoyed in the past.

*From American Occupational Therapy Association: Statement: Psychosocial concerns within occupational therapy practice, *Am J Occup Ther* 49:1011, 1995.

- Considering a psychiatric referral for possible clinical depression.
- Considering a referral to a community support group.
- Considering the need for assistive technology.

■

REVIEW QUESTIONS

1. Discuss examples of empirical evidence of the importance of psychosocial variables on functional stroke outcomes.
2. How significant is depression as a condition that occurs after stroke?
3. Which occupational therapy models of assessment are most relevant to a collaborative therapeutic relationship?
4. Describe several models of adjustment and coping that may be relevant to persons who have had a stroke.
5. In what ways might context influence an occupational therapist's choice of therapeutic activities?
6. What are some of the categories of adaptive strategies utilized by healthy elderly?

■ COTA Considerations ■

- Emotional reactions following stroke are common and may be directly related to physical or organic problems.
- If you notice a patient is depressed, notify the other team members. The person may require other additional psychologic intervention or drug therapy to effectively participate in a therapy program.
- Successful engagement in activities can assist in adjustment and adaptation to life after stroke.
- Functional activities should be chosen in collaboration with the patient so that the intervention has meaning to the patient.
- Most stroke survivors experience a decrease in activity involvement and life satisfaction.
- Therapeutic groups are effective in helping patients address psychosocial aspects of their stroke.

REFERENCES

1. Albrecht GL: The disability business—rehabilitation in America, Thousand Oaks, Calif, 1992, Sage Publications.
2. American Occupational Therapy Association: Position paper: Occupational therapy and the Americans with Disabilities Act (ADA), *Am J Occup Ther* 47:1083, 1993.
3. American Occupational Therapy Association: Uniform terminology for occupational therapy—third edition, *Am J Occup Ther* 48:1047, 1994.
4. American Occupational Therapy Association: Statement: Psychosocial concerns within occupational therapy practice, *Am J Occup Ther* 49:1011, 1995.
5. American Occupational Therapy Association: Position paper: Occupational performance: occupational therapy's definition of function, *Am J Occup Ther* 49:1019, 1995.

6. American Occupational Therapy Association: Position paper: The psychosocial core of occupational therapy, *Am J Occup Ther* 49:1021, 1995.

7. American Occupational Therapy Association: The philosophical base of occupational therapy, *Am J Occup Ther* 49:1026, 1995.

8. American Occupational Therapy Association: *Occupational therapy practice guidelines: stroke*, Bethesda, Md, 1996, The Association.

9. American Psychiatric Association: *Diagnostic and statistical manual of mental disorders*, ed 4, Washington, DC, 1994, The Association.

10. Angeleri F et al: The influence of depression, social activity, and family stress on functional outcome after stroke, *Stroke* 224:1478, 1993.

11. Andersen G, Vestgaard K, Lauritzen L: Effective treatment of post-stroke depression with selective serotonin reuptake inhibitor Citalopram, *Stroke* 25:1099, 1994.

12. Astrom M, Asplund K, Astrom T: Psychosocial function and life satisfaction after stroke, *Stroke* 23:527, 1992.

13. Atler K, Cliner J: Poststroke activity and psychosocial facts, *Phys Occup Ther Geriatr* 7:13, 1989.

14. Bishop DS, Pet R: Psychobehavioral problems other than depression in stroke, *Top Stroke Rehabil* 2:56, 1995.

15. Bonder B: Issues in assessment of psychosocial components of function, *Am J Occup Ther* 47:211, 1993.

16. Boynton De Sepulveda LI, Chang B: Effective coping with stroke disability in a community setting: the development of a causal model, *J Neurosci Nurs* 26:193, 1994.

17. Burvell PW et al: Prevalence of depression after stroke: the Perth community stroke study, *Br J Psychiatry* 166:320, 1995.

18. Christiansen C: The issue is—continuing challenges of functional assessment in rehabilitation: recommended changes, *Am J Occup Ther* 47:258, 1993.

19. Clarke F: Occupation embedded in a real life: interweaving occupational science and occupational therapy, 1993 Eleanor Clarke Slagle lecture, *Am J Occup Ther* 47:1067, 1993.

20. Clarke F et al: Life domains and adaptive strategies of a group of low-income, well older adults, *Am J Occup Ther* 50:99, 1996.

21. Colantonio A et al: Psychosocial predictors of stroke outcomes in an elderly population, *J Gerontol* 48(Suppl):261, 1993.

22. Cynkin S, Robinson A: *Occupational therapy and activities health: toward health through activities*, Boston, 1990, Little, Brown.

23. DeJong G, Branch LG: Predicting the stroke patient's ability to live independently, *Stroke* 13:648, 1982.

24. Dickerson A, Oakley F: Comparing the roles of community-living persons and patient populations, *Am J Occup Ther* 49:221, 1995.

25. Diller L, Bishop D: Depression and stroke, *Top Stroke Rehabil* 2:44, 1995.

26. Donaldson NE: Stroke outcomes: a consumer perspective, *Top Stroke Rehabil* 2:1, 1995.

27. Druss RG, Douglas CJ: Adaptive responses to illness and disability: Healthy denial, *Gen Hosp Psychiatry* 10:163, 1988.

28. Dunn W: The issue is—measurement of function: actions for the future, *Am J Occup Ther* 47:357, 1993.

29. Dunn W, Brown C, McGuigan A: The ecology of human performance: a framework for considering the effect of context: *Am J Occup Ther* 48:595, 1994.

30. Ebrahim S, Barer KD, Nouri F: Affective illness after stroke, *Br J Psychiatry* 154:195, 1989.

31. Egelko S et al: First year after stroke: tracking cognitive and affective deficits, *Arch Phys Med Rehabil* 70:297, 1989.

32. Eilenberg AO: An expanded community role for occupational therapy: preventing depression, *Phys Occup Ther Geriatr* 5:47, 1986.

33. Evans RL, Henricks RD, Lawrence KU: Effect of mental disorders on readmission for medical/surgical patients, *Psychol Rep* 62:519, 1988.

34. Fidler GS: Life-style performance: from profile to conceptual model, *Am J Occup Ther* 50:139, 1996.

35. Fiebel JH, Springer CJ: Depression and failure to resume social activities after stroke, *Arch Phys Med Rehabil* 63:276, 1982.

36. Gage M: The appraisal model of coping: an assessment and intervention model for occupational therapy, *Am J Occup Ther* 46:353, 1992.

37. Gage M, Polatajko H: Enhancing occupational performance through an understanding of perceived self-efficacy, *Am J Occup Ther* 48:452, 1994.

38. Gainotti G: Emotional behavior and hemispheric side of the lesion, *Cortex* 8:41, 1972.

39. Goldberg G, editor: Stroke rehabilitation, *Phys Med Rehabil Clin North Am* 2:547, 1991.

40. Grady AP: Building inclusive community: a challenge for occupational therapy, *Am J Occup Ther* 49:300, 1995.

41. Gresham GE et al: Epidemiologic profile of long-term stroke disability: the Framingham study, *Arch Phys Med Rehabil* 60:487, 1979.

42. Gresham GE et al: *Post-stroke rehabilitation*, Clinical practice guideline No 16, Agency for Health Care Policy and Research Pub No 95-0662 Rockville, Md, 1995, US Department of health and Human Services.

43. Hallett JD et al: Role change after traumatic brain injury in adults, *Am J Occup Ther* 48:241, 1994.

44. Harrell M, O'Hara CC: Meeting the emotional needs of brain injury survivors: an empowerment approach to psychotherapy, *Cognitive Rehabil* 9:12, 1991.

45. Holbrook SE: Stroke: social and emotional outcome, *J R Coll Physicians Lond* 16:100, 1982.

46. House A et al: Mood disorders in the year after stroke, *Br J Psychiatry* 158:83, 1991.

47. Jongbloed L: Adaptation to a stroke: the experience of one couple, *Am J Occup Ther* 48:1006, 1994.

48. Kettle M, Chamberlain AM: The stroke patient in an urban environment, *Clin Rehabil* 3:131, 1989.

49. Kielhofner G: A model of human occupation: theory and application, Baltimore, Md, 1985, Williams & Wilkins.

50. Kirschner K, editor: Ethics in practice—quality of life: is it in the eye of the beholder? *Top Stroke Rehabil* 2:58, 1996.

51. Kotila M et al: The profile of recovery from stroke and factors influencing outcome, *Stroke* 15:1039, 1984.

52. Kyllo DO: Spiritual topics in stroke rehabilitation, *Top Stroke Rehabil* 2:38, 1996.

53. Labi MLC, Phillips TF, Gresham GE: Psychosocial disability in physically restored long-term stroke survivors, *Arch Phys Med Rehabil* 61:561, 1980.

54. Law M, Baptiste J, Mills J: Client centered practice: what does it mean and does it make a difference? *Can J Occup Ther* 62:250, 1995.

55. Law M et al: The person-environmental occupational model: a transactive approach to occupational performance, *Can J Occup Ther* 63:9, 1996.

56. Lipsey JR et al: Phrenological comparison of post-stroke depression and functional depression, *Am J Psychiatry* 143:527, 1986.

57. Malec JF et al: Types of affective response to stroke, *Arch Phys Rehabil* 71:279, 1990.

58. Miller L: The "other" brain injuries: psychotherapeutic issues with stroke and brain tumor patients, *Cognitive Rehabil* 9:10, 1991.

59. Miropoulos C, Evert MM: Nationally speaking—cultural connections: a challenge unmet, *Am J Occup Ther* 48:583, 1994.

60. Morris PLP et al: Association of depression with 10-year poststroke mortality, *Am J Psychiatry* 150:124, 1993.

61. Neistadt ME: The neurobiology of learning: implications for treatment of adults with brain injury, *Am J Occup Ther* 48:421, 1994.

62. Neistadt ME: Methods of assessing clients' priorities: a survey of adult physical dysfunction settings assessment, *Am J Occup Ther* 49:428, 1995.

63. Northen JG et al: Involvement of adult rehabilitation patients in setting occupational therapy goals, *Am J Occup Ther* 49:214, 1995.

64. Novack T, Haban G, Satterfield W: Prediction of stroke rehabilitation outcome from psychological screening, *Arch Phys Med Rehabil* 68:729, 1987.

65. Peloquin S: The fullness of empathy: reflections and illusions, *Am J Occup Ther* 49:24, 1995.

66. Peloquin S: The patient-therapist relationship: beliefs that shape care, *Am J Occup Ther* 47:935, 1994.

67. Radomski MV: Nationally speaking—there is more to life than putting on your pants, *Am J Occup Ther* 49:487, 1995.

68. Redding MJ et al: Antidepressant therapy after stroke—A double-blind trial, *Arch Neurol* 43:763, 1986.

69. Robinson RG, Price TR: Post stroke depressive disorders: a follow up study of 103 outpatients, *Stroke* 13:635, 1982.

70. Robinson RG et al: A two year longitudinal study of post stroke mood disorders: findings during the initial evaluation, *Stroke* 14:736, 1983.

71. Robinson RG et al: A two-year longitudinal study of post-stroke mood disorders: dynamic changes in associated variables over the first six months of follow-up, *Stroke* 15:510, 1984.

72. Robinson RG, Boldue PL, Price TR: Two-year longitudinal study of poststroke mood disorders: Diagnoses and outcome at one and two years, *Stroke* 18:837, 1987.

73. Robinson RG et al: Pathological laughing and crying following stroke: validation of a measurement scale and a double-blind study, *Am J Psychiatry* 150:286, 1993.

74. Ross ED, Rush AJ: Diagnosis and neuroanatomical correlates of depression in brain-damaged patients—implications for a neurology of depression, *Arch Gen Psychiatry* 38:1344, 1981.

75. Sachs D, Labowitz DR: The caring occupational therapist: scope of professional roles and boundaries, *Am J Occup Ther* 48:997, 1994.

76. Sarno MT: Management of aphasia. In Bornstein RRA, Brown GG, editors: *Neurobehavioral aspects of cerebrovascular disease*, New York, 1991, Oxford University Press.

77. Schell BA, Cervero RM: clinical reasoning in occupational therapy: an integrative review, *Am J Occup Ther* 47:605, 1993.

78. Schkade JK, Schultz S: Occupational adaptation: toward a holistic approach for contemporary practice—Part I, *Am J Occup Ther* 46:829, 1992.

79. Schlaff C: Health policy from dependency to self-advocacy: redefining disability, *Am J Occup Ther* 47:943, 1993.

80. Schwartz SM: Adults with traumatic brain injury: three case studies of cognitive rehabilitation in the home setting, *Am J Occup Ther* 49:655, 1995.

81. Sharpe M et al: Depressive disorders in long-term survivors of stroke—associations with demographic and social factors, functional status, and brain lesion volume, *Br J Psychiatry* 164:380, 1994.

82. Shontz FC: Psychological adjustment to physical disability: trends in theories, *Arch Phys Med Rehabil* 59:251, 1978.

83. Spencer J et al: Socialization to the culture of a rehabilitation hospital: an ethnographic study, *Am J Occup Ther* 49:53, 1995.

84. Starkstein SE, Robinson RG: Aphasia and depression, *Aphasiology* 2:1, 1988.

85a. Starkstein SE, Robinson RG: Affective disorders and cerebral vascular disease, *Br J Psychiatry* 154:170, 1989.

85b. Starkstein SE et al: Relationship between anxiety disorders and depressive disorders in patients with cerebrovascular injury, *Arch Gen Psychiatry* 47:246, 1990.

86a. Tate DG, Dijkers M, Johnson-Green L: Outcome measures in quality of life, *Top Stroke Rehabil* 2:1, 1996.

86b. Taylor SE: Adjustment to threatening events—a theory of cognitive adaptation, *Am Psychol* 38:1161, 1983.

87. Teasell RW editor: Long-term consequences of stroke, *Phys Med Rehabil* 7:179, 1993.

88. Terent A: Stroke morbidity. In Whisnaant J, editor: *Stroke: populations, cohorts, and clinical trials*, Boston, 1993, Butterworth-Heinemann.

89. Thompson SC et al: Psychsocial adjustment following a stroke, *Soc Sci Med* 28:239, 1989.

90. Trace S, Howell T: Occupational therapy in geriatric mental health, *Am J Occup Ther* 45:833, 1991.

91. Trombly C: The issue is—Anticipating the future: assessment of occupational function, *Am J Occup Ther* 47:253, 1993.

92. Trombly C: Occupation: purposefulness and meaningfulness as therapeutic mechanisms—1995 Eleanor Clarke Slagle lecture, *Am J Occup Ther* 49:960, 1995.

93. Unsworth C: Clients' perceptions of discharge housing decisions after stroke rehabilitation, *Am J Occup Ther* 50:207, 1996.

94. Vargo W: Some psychological effects of physical disability, *Am J Occup Ther* 32:31, 1978.

95. Vash CL: *The psychology of disability*, New York, 1981, Springer Publishing.

96. Watson LJ: Psychiatric consultation—liaison in the acute physical disabilities setting, *Am J Occup Ther* 40:338, 1986.

97. Wood W: Delivering occupational therapy's fullest promise: clinical interpretation of "Life domains and adaptive strategies of a group of low-income, well older adults," *Am J Occup Ther* 50:109, 1996.

98. Wright BA: *Physical disability—psychological approach*, New York, 1960, Harper.

99. Yerxa EJ: Dreams, dilemmas, and decisions for occupational therapy practice in a new millennium: an American perspective, *Am J Occup Ther* 48:586, 1994.

100. Yerxa EJ: The social and psychological experience of having a disability: implications for occupational therapists. In Pedretti L, editor: *Occupational therapy skills for physical dysfunction*, ed 4, St Louis, 1994, Mosby.

101. Yerxa EJ: Nationally speaking—who is the keeper of occupational therapy practice and knowledge? *Am J Occup Ther* 49:295, 1995.

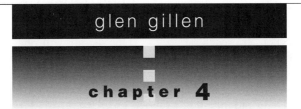

glen gillen

chapter 4

Trunk Control: A Prerequisite for Functional Independence

key terms

trunk   postural control   hemiplegia

activities of daily living

chapter objectives

After completing this chapter, the reader will be able to accomplish the following:

1. Understand the functional anatomy of the trunk.
2. Understand the control requirements for various movement patterns.
3. By activity analysis, understand key components of trunk control required for independence in various activities of daily living.
4. Understand treatment activities to improve and/or compensate for loss of trunk control.

Loss of trunk control is commonly observed in patients who have had a stroke. Impairment in trunk control may lead to the following:

- Dysfunction in upper and lower limb control
- Increased risk of falls
- Potential for spinal deformity and contracture
- Impaired ability to interact with the environment
- Visual dysfunction secondary to resultant head/neck malalignment
- Symptoms of dysphagia secondary to proximal malalignment
- Decreased independence in activities of daily living (ADL)

- Decreased sitting and standing tolerance, balance, and function

For a comprehensive review of this topic, see Chapter 2 for incorporating learning and environmental strategies into treatment plans focused on improving trunk control, Chapter 5 for a complete overview of the multiple variables that impact balance skills, Chapter 6 for a review on the interdependence of trunk control and upper extremity function, and Chapters 10 and 11 for an overview of mobility impairments.

Regaining trunk control has been a major focus of stroke rehabilitation for many years. The majority of the literature that focuses on trunk control/postural control is based on expert clinicians' observations of and treatment philosophies about trunk dysfunction after stroke. The neurodevelopmental treatment (NDT) approach[5,6,10,13,20] has traditionally emphasized improved trunk control as a key element of focus in the stroke population.

Well-controlled studies that specifically examine the impact of decreased trunk control on independence in ADL is lacking in the rehabilitation literature. Thus another goal of this chapter is that it will serve as an impetus for more studies that will ultimately enhance our ability to effectively treat the stroke population.

(See Chapter 6 for the available research related to trunk control during upper extremity tasks and Chapter 5 for research concerning trunk control and posture in relation to balance dysfunction.)

Bohannon and associates[9] have studied trunk muscle strength impairments after stroke (specifically forward and lateral trunk flexion strength). Their study included 20 patients with stroke and resultant hemiparesis and 20 control subjects. Trunk strength was measured with a hand-held dynamometer; subjects were seated upright during the study. Results indicated that trunk strength, whether lateral or forward, was significantly decreased in the patients relative to controls. The greatest difference in strength was in forward flexion strength. The patients demonstrated trunk weakness on the paretic side relative to the nonparetic side. The conclusion was that trunk muscle strength was impaired multidirectionally in the stroke population.

Bohannon[8] studied 11 stroke patients and evaluated (1) lateral trunk flexion strength and (2) the impact of trunk muscle strength on sitting balance and ambulation. His results indicated that the mean lateral flexion force on the paretic side was 32.1%, which was significantly less than the mean lateral flexion force on the nonparetic side. His study further demonstrated a statistically significant correlation between sitting balance and strength of the lateral trunk flexors.

Bohannon[7] also studied the recovery of trunk muscle strength after stroke in 28 subjects. Subjects' strength was tested in a variety of directions including forward flexion, movement toward the paretic side, and movement toward the nonparetic side. Statistical analysis demonstrated that trunk muscle strength increased significantly over time. The greatest recovery was in the direction of forward flexion. This study again verified a strong correlation between trunk muscle strength and sitting balance at both initial and final assessments.

In addition to the mentioned studies, several studies have been done that focused on documented electromyographic (EMG) activity in normal subjects during a variety of tasks including trunk displacements.* See Basmajian's and DeLuca's[4] text for a comprehensive review of EMG studies performed during functional tasks.

*References 1, 4, 12, 15, 26, 27.

FUNCTIONAL TRUNK ANATOMY

Skeletal System

This section will review the bony components of trunk anatomy including articulations and range of motion.

Vertebral Column

The vertebral column is made up of 26 vertebrae, which are classified as follows:

Cervical: 7
Thoracic: 12
Lumbar: 5
Sacral: 5 (fused into one bone—the sacrum)
Coccygeal: 4 (fused into one or two bones—the coccyx)

As a whole, the vertebral column from sacrum to skull is equivalent to a joint with three degrees of freedom[17] in the directions of (1) flexion and extension, (2) right and left lateral flexion, and (3) axial rotation. Kapandji[17] has documented the range of motion (ROM) throughout the vertebral column (Box 4-1).

An understanding of spinal alignment is necessary for effective evaluation and treatment planning. Normal alignment of the vertebral column implies that the appropriate spinal curvatures are present. In the sagittal plane the vertebral column shows four curvatures[17] (Box 4-2, Figure 4-1).

Pelvis

According to Kapandji,[17] "The bony pelvis constitutes the base of the trunk. It supports the abdomen and links the vertebral column to the lower limbs. It is a closed

---

Box 4-1

Range of Motion of the Vertebral Column

FLEXION	LATERAL FLEXION
Cervical: 40°	Cervical: 35° to 45°
Thoracolumbar: 105°	Thoracic: 20°
Total: 145°	Lumbar: 20°
	Total: 75° to 85°
EXTENSION	
Cervical: 75°	**ROTATION**
Thoracolumbar: 60°	Cervical: 45° to 50°
Total: 135°	Thoracic: 35°
	Lumbar: 5°
	Total: 90°

Box 4-2

Spinal Curvatures

Sacral curvature (fixed curvature): convex posteriorly
Lumbar curvature: concave posteriorly
Thoracic curvature: convex posteriorly
Cervical curvature: concave posteriorly

osteo-articular ring made up of three bony parts and three joints. . . ." The three bony parts include the two iliac bones and the sacrum. The three joints of the pelvis include two sacroiliac joints and the symphysis pubis.

It is critical to remember that because of the firmness of the sacroiliac and lumbosacral junctions, every pelvic movement is accompanied by a realignment of the spine predominantly in the lumbar region.[25]

Pelvic tilt can either occur anteriorly or posteriorly. In an anterior tilt the anterior superior iliac spines (ASIS) of the ilia migrate anteriorly to the foremost part of the symphysis pubis. This pelvic motion accentuates the lumbar curve and results in increased hip flexion. In contrast, posterior pelvic tilt results in a "flattening" of the lumbar curve as well as an increase in hip extension.

Lateral pelvis tilting results in a height discrepancy of the iliac crests and is accompanied by lateral spine flexion and a lateral ribcage displacement.

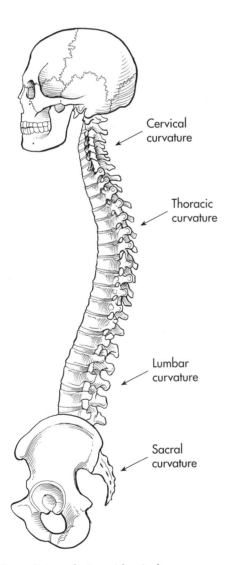

Figure 4-1 Lateral view of spine with spinal curvatures.

Ribcage

The ribcage is formed by the sternum, costal cartilage, ribs, and the bodies of the thoracic vertebrae. The ribcage protects the organs in the thoracic cavity, assists in respiration, and provides support for the upper extremities. During inspiration the ribs are elevated, and during expiration the ribs are depressed.

Although each rib has its own ROM (occurring primarily at the costovertebral joint), ribcage shifts occur with movement of the vertebral column. During column extension the ribcage migrates anteriorly and the ribs are elevated. During spinal flexion the ribcage moves posteriorly and the ribs depress. Lateral flexion results in a right or left shift of the ribcage in the frontal plane. Finally, rotation of the vertebral column results in one side of the ribcage moving posteriorly and movement of the opposite side anteriorly in the transverse plane.

Muscular System

Muscles of the Abdominal Wall

The general functions of the abdominal muscles are the following:

- Abdominal viscera support
- Respiration assistance
- Trunk control in the directions of flexion, lateral flexion, and rotation

Although these muscles are situated primarily on the anterior aspect of the trunk, they are also situated laterally and slightly posteriorly, forming a girdle around the abdomen. The abdominals consist of three groups of muscles; the rectus abdominus, the obliques (internal and external), and the transversus abdominus (Figure 4-2).

Rectus Abdominus

The rectus abdominus consists of right and left sides that are separated by a fibrous band called the *linea alba*, which runs from the xiphoid process to the pubis.

The proximal attachment is the xiphoid process of the sternum and adjacent costal cartilage, whereas the distal attachments are the pubic bones near the pubic symphysis.[25]

The muscle is easily palpated in the following two cases:

1. When the subject is supine and asked to lift the head and shoulders off the support surface in a straight plane ("sit-up")
2. During backward sway in sitting or standing position

When this muscle is activated and not opposed by the extensors, the pelvis and sternum are approximated, the pelvis is pulled into a posterior tilt, and the lumbar curves flatten. Because of its multisegmental arrangement, the rectus can contract in part or as a whole, making a variety of postures possible. De Troyer's[12] work demonstrated that ". . . abdominal muscle recruitment which naturally occurs

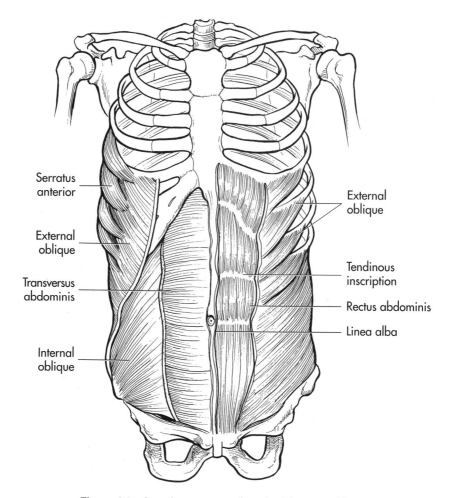

Figure 4-2 Anterior anatomy of trunk with resected layers.

in response to posture in most individuals does not uniformly involve the whole of the muscles. . . ."

The rectus abdominus (as well as the other muscles of the trunk) require a stable origin to function efficiently.[10] This stable origin can be the pelvis or thorax depending on the posture and which part of the trunk is moving. Davies[10] further explains, "The pelvis is stabilized in lying, sitting, and standing by the activity of the muscles around the hips, and in sitting and lying the stabilization is helped by the weight of the legs themselves. Stabilization of the thoracic origin for activities in which the abdominals contract to move or prevent movements of the pelvis requires selective extension of the thoracic spine." Davies further points out that the abdominals cannot function effectively when their origin and insertion are approximated (e.g., in patients with an exaggerated thoracic kyphosis).

The rectus abdominus can be self-palpated by assuming a recumbent posture in a chair (slumping in the chair) and then pulling up and forward to an aligned position. Notice that the burst of activity diminishes when leaning forward (shoulders move in front of hips).

Obliques

The obliques consist of three interwoven muscles: internal obliques, external obliques, and transversus abdominus.

The external oblique forms the superficial layer of the abdominal wall. Its fibers run an oblique course superoinferiorly and lateromedially.[17] The muscle is lateral to the rectus abdominus and covers the anterior and lateral regions of the abdomen. The attachments are as follows[25]:

Proximal attachment: Anterolateral portions of ribs where it interdigitates with serratus anterior and slips from latissimus dorsi
Distal attachment: Upper fibers—run down and forward and attach to an aponeurosis that connects them to the linea alba; lower fibers—attach to the crest of the ilium

If the external oblique contracts unilaterally, the trunk rotates to the opposite side. Therefore if you rotate to the left, the right external oblique is active and vice-versa. Bilateral contraction assists in trunk flexion and a resultant posterior pelvic tilt. This muscle is also active during straining and coughing.[25] The muscle is easily palpated while rotating the trunk to the opposite side.

The internal obliques are also located laterally and are covered by the external obliques. In essence the internal obliques constitute the second layer of muscles on the abdominal wall. This muscle basically covers the same area as the external oblique, but its fibers cross those of the external oblique. Attachments are as follows[25]:

Proximal attachment: Inguinal ligament, crest of ilium, and thoracolumbar fascia
Distal attachments: Pubic bone, an aponeurosis connecting to linea alba, and last three or four ribs

This muscle is again activated during trunk rotation, but contraction occurs toward the same side (i.e., rotation to the left occurs secondary to contraction of the left internal oblique). It becomes clear that the external and internal obliques are synergists in the action of trunk rotation. The right external and left internal oblique work together to rotate the trunk to the left and vice versa. "The efficient action of the muscles of one side of the abdominal wall is therefore very much dependent upon the fixation or anchorage provided by the activity of the muscles on the other side, particularly for activities involving rotation of the trunk."[10]

The internal obliques are difficult to palpate. However, tension may be felt under the fingertips when palpating the lateral abdominal wall on the side the trunk is rotating toward. This tension is due in part to activation of the internal obliques.

The transversus abdominus is the deepest layer of the abdominal wall. Its fibers run transversely, and it has been called the *corset muscle* because it encloses the abdominal cavity like a corset. Attachments are as follows[25]:

Proximal attachments: Lower ribs, thoracolumbar fascia, crest of the ilium, and inguinal ligament
Distal attachments: Via an aponeurosis fuses with other abdominal muscles into linea alba

This muscle's main action is forced compression; the muscle acts like a girdle to flatten the abdominal wall and compress the abdominal viscera. Weakness of this muscle permits bulging of the anterior abdominal wall thereby indirectly leading to an increase in lordosis.[18] This muscle may be palpated between the lower ribs and the crest of the ilium during forced expiration.

Posterior Trunk Muscles

This group of muscles includes quadratus lumborum, the erector spinae group, and latissimus dorsi (Figure 4-3). The actions of this group of muscles include trunk extension, lateral flexion, rotation of the trunk, and assistance with balancing the vertebral column.

Quadratus Lumborum

This muscle is lateral and posterior (i.e., on the posterior abdominal wall); it lies between the psoas major and the erector spinae group. The attachments are as follows[25]:

Proximal attachment: Crest of ilium
Distal attachments: Twelfth rib and transverse processes of L-1 to L-3

The main action of this muscle is to assist in "hiphiking." Therefore it is active during lateral trunk flexion. The easiest way to palpate this muscle is to have the subject prone; palpate superior and lateral to the iliac crest, and ask the subject to hike the hip.

Erector Spinae Group

This group of muscles is a large mass that fills the spaces between the transverse and spinous processes of the vertebrae and extends laterally covering a large portion of the posterior thorax. There are multiple muscles that make up this group, and they are named according to attachments, shape, and action. Muscles such as the transversospinalis, the interspinalis, the longissimus, and the iliocostalis are included in this group.

Collectively these muscles connect the back of the skull to the posterior iliac crest and sacrum. Unopposed contraction of the back extensors approximates the head and the sacrum. The pelvis is pulled into an anterior tilt (accentuating the lumbar curve), and the ribs are forced to flare. These muscles also contract during lateral flexion (to balance the abdominals), and they may assist in trunk rotation during unilateral contraction (e.g., assist the trunk with rotating to the ipsilateral side). This muscle group is easily palpated with patients in the prone position if the head and shoulders are lifted from the support surface[25]; it may also be palpated during forward sway in sitting or standing. The lower back extensors are easily palpated during low back extension (accentuating the lumbar curve) while the patient is sitting.

Latissimus Dorsi

This large muscle is superficial and covers the posterior/lateral trunk. Its attachments include the following[25]:

Proximal attachments: Spinous processes of T-6 down, dorsolumbar fascia, posterior crest of ilium, lower ribs, interdigitations with external oblique; fibers converge toward axilla, passing over inferior angle of scapula.
Distal attachment: tendon attaches to crest of lesser tubercle of humerus, proximal to teres major

Acting unilaterally, this muscle adducts, extends, and internally rotates the humerus as well as laterally flexes the trunk (approximates the shoulder and the pelvis). Bilateral contraction helps hyperextend the spine and anteriorly tilt the pelvis.

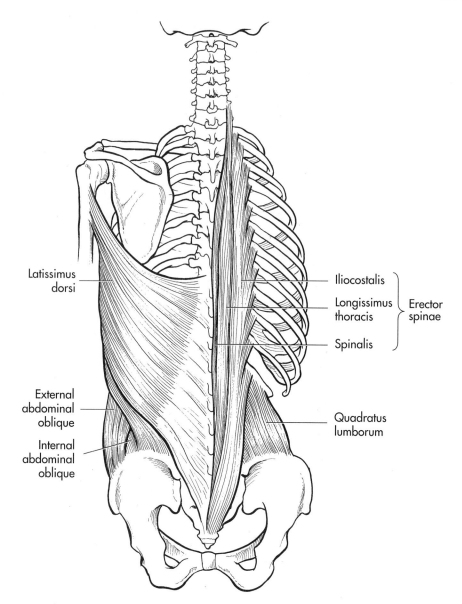

Figure 4-3   Posterior anatomy of trunk.

MOTOR CONTROL CONSIDERATIONS

Trunk Muscle Contractions

To achieve full trunk control and use this control during functional tasks, patients must regain the ability to contract their trunk muscles under three different circumstances outlined by Davies.[10] The task of lower extremity bathing from a seated position will be used to illustrate these points.

1. *Contracting to move opposite the pull of gravity:* When the trunk is moving in a direction that is opposite to gravitational pull, the muscles on the uppermost side of the trunk are contracting concentrically. For example, after washing feet, the trunk is straightened from a bent-over position by concentric contraction of the back extensors (the uppermost muscles). Therefore the muscles are actively shortening. The one exception to the rule that the uppermost muscles are active during this type of contraction is bridging. In this case, movement does occur in a direction opposite the pull of gravity (back and buttocks moving away from the support surface), but the underside muscles (the extensors) are contracting concentrically and are responsible for the success of this task.

Concentric contractions are used functionally to reposition the trunk during or after task completion.

2. *Preventing movement that would occur secondary to gravitational pull:* This type of muscle contraction (usually isometric) prevents falling toward the pull of gravity,

stabilizes the trunk for successful completion of tasks, and forms the basis of many balance reactions. During lower extremity washing, the back extensors will contract to stabilize (isometrically hold) the trunk as the lower leg is washed, allowing proximal stabilization for distal function. Note that when leaning all of the way forward (extreme flexion) the back extensors become inactive, and the vertebral ligaments become responsible for holding the trunk in this posture.[4]

3. *Controlling the speed of trunk movements in the direction of gravitational pull:* In this type of contraction the muscles are contracting eccentrically (in controlled and active elongation). The muscles responsible for this contraction are on the side of the trunk that is opposite the pull of gravity. When leaning forward to wash the feet during lower body washing, the back extensors contract eccentrically to control the speed and range of the forward trunk movement. This muscle contraction has a "braking effect" as the large mass of the trunk moves into the pull of gravity.

The previous examples show that functional independence requires control of all three trunk muscle contractions and combinations. Successful treatment plans must include activities that elicit a variety of trunk muscle contractions. Self-care training inherently challenges a variety of trunk postures and muscle contractions.

Musculoskeletal Components

Control of the trunk depends on several musculoskeletal variables including ROM, biomechanical alignment, strength, and muscle length. These variables are interdependent and can create a vicious circle in stroke patients.

Postural Malalignment

Stroke patients commonly assume postural malalignments that include the following:

Posterior pelvic tilt
Pelvic obliquity characterized by unequal weightbearing through the ischial tuberosities
Lumbar spine flexion (loss of the lumbar curve)
Increased kyphosis
Lateral spine flexion
Ribcage rotation (secondary to loss of abdominal control)
Head/neck malalignment (rotation away from and lateral flexion toward the involved side)

Prolonged postural malalignment results in muscle shortening on one side of the trunk and muscle overstretching on the opposite side. For example, a posterior pelvic tilt with lumbar flexion results in shortening of the anterior musculature and elongation (overstretching) of the posterior muscles. Lateral flexion on the right side results in muscle shortening on the right side and muscle elongation on the left side of the trunk.

Postural malalignment may be secondary to unilateral weakness (specifically around the pelvis), unbalanced skeletal muscle activity, perceptual dysfunction and an inability to perceive midline, and/or soft tissue shortening.

Prolonged postural malalignment can result in soft tissue shortening, loss of ROM, and an inability to generate enough force to contract the muscle group in question. The total force of muscle (active tension) is high at the muscle's rest length (i.e., when the trunk is properly aligned) and less when the muscle is tested at shorter lengths. Therefore the force-generating mechanism within the muscle works optimally at the muscle's rest length[19] (i.e., a symmetrical and aligned trunk).

Dissociation

Mohr[20] states, "Normal control in any body part demands the ability to dissociate (separate) different parts of the body." She gives the examples of dissociating the head from the body, one side of the body from the other, and the upper trunk from the lower trunk.

Examples of dissociation during functional tasks include upper trunk rotation with lower trunk stability while reaching for toilet paper, counter-rotation of the trunk during ambulatory activities, and upper trunk rotation with concurrent lower trunk lateral flexion to increase the range of reach beyond the arm span when reaching for a phone positioned on the left side of a desk with the right hand.

Difficulty with dissociation may be a result of soft tissue tightness, bony contracture, or efforts by the patient to decrease the degrees of freedom in the trunk[23] during functional activities (see Chapter 6).

Motor Adaptation

"Normal postural control requires the ability to adapt responses to changing tasks and environmental demands. This flexibility requires the availability of multiple movement strategies and the ability to select the appropriate strategy for the task and environment. The inability to adapt movements to changing task demands is a characteristic of many patients with neurological disorders. Patients become fixed in stereotypical patterns of movement, showing a loss of movement flexibility and adaptability."[24]

Motor adaptation can occur in response to an external perturbation or in anticipation of potentially destabilizing forces. Unexpected external perturbations include bumping into someone in a crowded lobby, being in a vehicle that unexpectedly turns or decelerates, and being on a moving platform, such as an escalator, that stops unexpectedly.

Activities that lead to trunk movements in anticipation of destabilizing forces include reaching for a heavy book off of a shelf, reaching beyond the arm span, and preparing to push or pull a chair into place. Shumway-Cook and Woollacott[24] point out that anticipatory postural control is heavily dependent on previous experience and learning.

Research focusing on anticipatory postural responses during reach activities will be presented in Chapter 6.

GENERAL CONSIDERATIONS WHEN EVALUATING AND TREATING THE TRUNK

1. Proper evaluation and treatment of the trunk result from use of keen observational skills. Patients should be undressed (shirtless or in sports bras or bathing-suit tops) so that movements are more easily observed during functional tasks. Clothing folds, wrinkles, and crooked seams can lead to incorrect observations.
2. The therapist must realize that the slightest change in posture can completely change trunk muscle activity and alignment.[10] For example, a subtle anterior shift of the shoulders will result in extensor activation, whereas a subtle posterior shift of the shoulders will result in trunk flexor activation.
3. The trunk should be evaluated in a variety of postures that coincide with ADL. Trunk adjustments are task specific, therefore a trunk evaluation of a patient who is supine should include activities such as rolling and bridging; evaluations of seated patients should include activities such as upper and lower extremity dressing and bathing; and evaluations of standing patients should include reaching for items in medicine cabinets, on bookshelves, and in kitchen cabinets.

EVALUATION PROCESS

Subjective Interview

Patients should be questioned about their perceived stability limits. Stability limits have been defined as the "boundaries of an area of space in which the body can maintain its position without changing the base of support."[24] Patients' perceived stability limits may or may not be consistent with their actual limits. If patients' perceived limits of stability are greater than their actual limits, they are at risk for falls. If their perceived limits of stability are less than their actual limits, they may be reluctant to attempt tasks with progressively greater demands on their postural system (e.g., lower extremity dressing without assistive devices, picking up objects from the floor without a reacher).

Perceived stability limits may have a direct correlation with observed neurobehavioral deficits. Body scheme disorders are commonly observed in the stroke population. These deficits include body neglect, somatoagnosia, and impaired right/left discrimination.[2] Ayres[3] has defined body scheme as a postural model on which movements are based. Knowledge of body parts and their relationships are necessary for deciding what and where to move and in what way to perform.[2] Spatial relations deficits including spatial neglect, depth perception, and spatial relations disorders may also have an impact on patients' perceived sta-

bility limits, (gaining and regaining midline orientation, position in space [see Chapter 13]).

Other components of the subjective interview include determining patients' insights into their trunk malalignments and their ability to perceive and assume midline positions. The therapist's goal in this interview is to gain insight into the patients' ability to make accurate observations about their postural dysfunction. This is difficult for many patients because trunk control does not occur at a conscious level in the majority of daily tasks.

Observations of Trunk Alignment/Malalignment

For the purposes of this chapter, observations will be reviewed in the seated posture.

The patient's trunk should be exposed as much as possible and the patient should be asked to, "Sit up nice and straight and gently rest your hands in your lap." (Table 4-1 outlines the ideal alignment of the trunk and extremities and common asymmetries observed after stroke during static sitting.)

Following the evaluation of postural malalignments during static sitting, the therapist should begin to hypothesize the cause of these malalignments. Causes may include increased skeletal muscle activity on one side of the trunk, inability to recruit muscle activity or weakness, soft tissue shortening, fixed deformity, body scheme disorder, and inability to perceive midline.

The therapist must remember that observed postures may be secondary to more than one impairment. For example, stroke patients tend to sit in a posterior pelvic tilt position with resultant hip extension and thoracic spine flexion. This posture may be a result of one of or a combination of the following:

1. Weakness or lack of activity in the trunk extensors, especially in the lower back
2. Fixed contracture of the hamstrings and/or thoracic spine
3. Abdominal weakness: The mentioned posture changes the center of gravity and decreases the potential to fall backwards. The abdominals are primarily responsible for preventing backward sway, therefore assuming a flexed posture reduces the chance of having to activate the abdominals to prevent falls.

Another example of a commonly observed malalignment is trunk shortening on the side affected by the stroke. This posture may be assumed for several reasons.

1. Inactive shoulder elevators on the side affected by the stroke that let the shoulder depress[10]
2. Increased muscle activity of the scapula depressors that pull the shoulder down on the affected side
3. Perceptual dysfunction resulting in an inability to find midline—bearing most weight on the stronger side resulting in a shortening of the affected side

Table 4-1

Normal Alignment and Common Malalignments After Stroke

NORMAL ALIGNMENT	COMMON MALALIGNMENT
Pelvis	
Equal weight bearing through both ischial tuberosities	Asymmetrical weight bearing
Neutral to slight anterior tilt	Posterior pelvic tilt
Neutral rotation	Unilateral retraction
Vertebral column	
Straight from posterior view	Scoliosis
Appropriate curves from lateral view	Loss of lumbar curve, increased thoracic kyphosis
	Shortening on one side, elongation on opposite side
Ribcage	
Neutral in terms of lateral tilt	Lateral tilt
Neutral rotation	Flaring on one side
Alignment over pelvis and under shoulders	Unilateral retraction
Shoulders	
Symmetrical height	Asymmetrical height
Alignment over pelvis	Unilateral retraction
Head/neck	
Neutral	Protraction
	Flexion to weak side
	Rotation away from weak side
Upper extremities	
Resting in lap; if weight bearing, effortless and symmetrical	Use of stronger extremity as postural support to maintain alignment
	Too little or too much activity in more involved extremity
Lower extremities	
Hips at 90°	Hips toward extension because of posterior pelvic tilt
Knee aligned with hips	Hip adduction resulting in knee contact
Feet in full contact with floor, accepting weight; feet under knees	"Windswept" hips
	Feet not equally bearing weight, or "pushing"; foot placed in front of knee

4. Increased muscle activity or shortening of the affected lateral flexors resulting in a shortening response
5. Fear of shifting weight to the affected side—majority of weight on stronger side resulting in shortening of the affected side

Following the observation of the patient in a static posture, the occupational therapist must observe trunk responses during functional activities. The two most effective methods of making these observations are observing patients during self-care and controlled reach pattern activities.

During functional reach patterns, trunk responses are required to (1) provide proximal stability for distal function, (2) enhance the ability to interact with the environ-ment by increasing reaching distance (i.e., extend the arm span with an appropriate trunk response), (3) and prevent falls.

An individual's reaching ability is limited by static trunk postures. As soon as an object is placed beyond arm length (e.g., on a floor, across a dining table, under a sink), a trunk response is required to successfully pick up the object.

In general, picking up an object from the floor or from in front of an individual requires an anterior trunk shift. Picking up objects placed beyond the arm span to the right or left of the individual requires a lateral weight shift from the trunk primarily onto one of the ischial tuberosities. Retrieving objects placed behind the trunk requires a posterior weight shift. Rotational trunk responses result from reaching across the midline or for objects posterior to the shoulders or hips. (For a more detailed review of weight shifting and trunk postures during reaching activities, see Table 6-1.)

The therapist's goals while observing the patient perform functional reach patterns are the following:

1. Ensure that trunk and upper extremity patterns are coordinated to result in successful task completion.
2. Note any fall potential.
3. Note asymmetries during reaching.
4. Objectively evaluate the perceived and actual stability limits of the patient.
5. Note in which directions the patient is or is not able to reach beyond the arm span.
6. Note factors such as trunk stiffness and decreased ROM.

Evaluating Specific Trunk Movement Patterns

In addition to performing each movement pattern, refer to the appropriate figures while reading this section. The following evaluation procedures are based on the work of Mohr,[20] Boehme,[6] Davies,[10] and Basmajian and DeLuca.[4]

Trunk Flexor Control

The trunk flexors are evaluated by the five different methods that follow:

1. Patients assume a seated, upright position. They are asked to move their shoulders behind their hips slowly and with control (Figure 4-4, *A*); this movement pattern occurs in the sagittal plane, is initiated from the upper trunk,[20] and elicits an eccentric contraction of the trunk flexors.[15,26] Holding the end range of this posture results in an isometric contraction of the trunk flexors. Observations should include resistance to movement, fall potential, and symmetry of the posterior weight shift. Unilateral weakness will cause the weak side to become posterior to the stronger side (i.e., will result in rotation of the trunk).
2. From the end position of the first movement pattern, patients are asked to move their shoulders forward so that they are sitting in proper alignment within the sagittal plane (Figure 4-4, *B*); this movement pattern is achieved by a concentric contraction of the trunk flexors.[15] Note symmetry during the movement pattern. Unilateral weakness will cause the stronger side to lead the pattern.
3. In an aligned, seated position, patients assume a controlled lumbar flexion posture (posterior tilt with flattening of the lumbar curve, spinal flexion) (Figure 4-4, *C*). Mohr[20] states that this movement pattern is initiated by the lower trunk and pelvis. If this pattern is performed actively, the final posture is assumed by concentric flexor contraction. This posture may also be achieved by a relaxation response of the low back

extensors, so the therapist should palpate the flexors to ensure the pattern is a result of active movement. At the end range of this pattern—posterior tilt and spinal flexion (a recumbent posture)—little to no muscle activity exists, and patients maintain this posture by support of their vertebral ligaments.[4]

4. Control of the trunk flexors should also be evaluated when the patient is supine (during rolling and bed mobility activities). While in a supine position the patient is asked to sit up in a straight plane. This movement pattern, which is primarily controlled by the rectus abdominus, allows the therapist to evaluate antigravity control of the trunk flexors.[18] The patient can also be asked to roll by lifting one shoulder up and across the trunk in a position of trunk flexion and rotation. This movement pattern also gives the therapist insight into the antigravity control of the flexors (primarily the obliques).[18]
5. Although the first four movement patterns to test flexor control were initiated by the patient, it is also

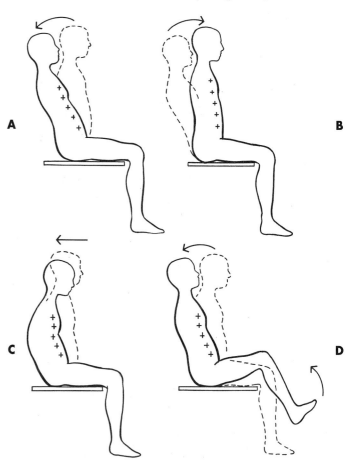

Figure 4-4 Trunk flexor control. Dotted lines indicate trunk starting position, solid lines indicate trunk final position, arrows indicate movement direction, and plus symbols indicate muscle groups primarily responsible for control of pattern. (Skeletal muscle activity occurs on both sides of the trunk [i.e., reciprocal innervation].)

useful to test the flexors' response to being moved by the therapist. The therapists lift the lower legs of the patient into a position of increased hip flexion. For the patient to refrain from falling backward, the trunk flexors must be activated isometrically (Figure 4-4, *D*).

As a rule of thumb, the trunk flexors are activated (1) in the seated position when the shoulders move posterior to the hips (backward sway), (2) when the trunk is moving away from the support surface (supine starting point), (3) and during rotational activities.

Trunk Extensor Control

The following four movement patterns are used to evaluate trunk extensor control during seated activities and bridging.

1. To start this movement pattern, the patient assumes a flexed spine posture with a posterior pelvis tilt (the resting posture for many stroke patients). The patient initiates the movement with the lower trunk and pelvis[20] and assumes an extended spine posture with a neutral to slight anterior tilt, which accentuates the lumbar curve (Figure 4-5, *A*). The movement pattern is completed by a concentric contraction of the trunk extensors which is the trunk pattern required for forward reach.
2. Patients assume an aligned, seated starting position and are asked to keep their spine straight as they lean forward, keeping the shoulders in front of the hips in the sagittal plane (Figure 4-5, *B*). This posture is assumed by an eccentric contraction of the trunk extensors,[4,15,26] and if the posture is held between the middle to end range the back extensors isometrically contract. The patient has unilateral weakness if the

trunk moves forward asymmetrically. Unilateral weakness causes the weaker side to lead the movement pattern (e.g., to fall into gravity). If the movement continues in a forward direction (e.g., patient reaches down to the floor), the back extensors become inactive at the end range and the position is maintained by the tension of the vertebral ligaments.[4]

3. While in the end posture of the second movement pattern, patients are asked to move their shoulders back to assume a seated, aligned position (Figure 4-5, *C*). To assume this posture the trunk extensors contract concentrically, although the hip extensors initiate the movement[4,26]; this movement occurs in the sagittal plane.
4. The back extensors should also be tested by observing the patient in a bridge posture. While in a supine position with the hips and knees flexed, the patient is asked to assume a bridge position, which is accomplished by a concentric contraction of the back and hip extensors[10] and maintained by an isometric contraction of the same muscles. The release of the posture is controlled by eccentric contraction of the back and hip extensors.

As a rule of thumb, in the seated posture the back extensors are active (1) during anterior weight shifts (in which the shoulders move in front of the hips), (2) when correcting posture to a position of alignment from an anterior weight shift, (3) during bridging activities.

Control of the Lateral Flexors

Lateral flexion occurs in the coronal plane, therefore a balance of control between the flexors and extensors is required to maintain movement. EMG studies have demonstrated that dorsal and ventral muscles coactivate during

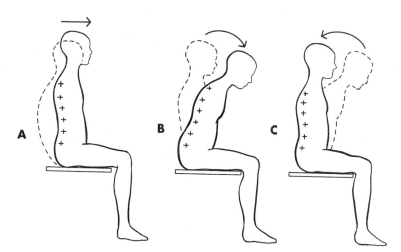

Figure 4-5 Trunk extensor control. Dotted lines indicate trunk starting position, solid lines indicate trunk final position, arrows indicate movement direction, and plus symbols indicate muscle groups primarily responsible for control of pattern. (Skeletal muscle activity occurs on both sides of the trunk [i.e., reciprocal innervation].)

lateral flexion.[26] EMG activity of the right and left erector spinae has been documented during lateral trunk flexion.[4,15]

Mohr[20] states, "Two different movement strategies occur when you reach down to the side: (1) the initiation may occur in the upper trunk and the ipsilateral spine shortens, or (2) the movement can be initiated with your lower trunk and pelvis, resulting in ipsilateral elongation." Three movement patterns are used to evaluate control of lateral trunk flexion.

1. The first movement pattern is initiated from an aligned, seated position. The pelvis remains stable, and the upper trunk initiates lateral flexion toward the floor with the shoulder approximating the hip (Figure 4-6, *A*). The end posture (one of ipsilateral trunk shortening) occurs by an eccentric contraction of the side of the trunk that is elongating.[20,26] In Figure 4-6, *A*, the right side of the trunk is shortening, but the predominant control is on the left side, which is elongating eccentrically. Holding this posture between the middle and end ranges allows evaluation of isometric lateral flexion control. Both sides of the trunk should be evaluated using this movement pattern.
2. While in the end position of the first movement pattern, patients are asked to realign themselves by sitting up straight (Figure 4-6, *B*). The trunk is realigned by a concentric contraction of the lateral flexors[26] (the left lateral flexors in Figure 4-6, *B*).
3. The last movement pattern is used to evaluate lateral flexion, which initiates the movement from the lower trunk and pelvis.[20] This movement pattern allows reach beyond the arm span in the frontal plane. During this movement the majority of weight is shifted to one ischial tuberosity; the shoulder and hip approximate in this pattern. In the resulting posture the trunk is elongated on the weight-bearing side and trunk shortening

on the non-weight-bearing side (Figure 4-6, *C*). The predominant control comes from concentric contraction of the lateral flexors on the shortening side. (Figure 4-6, *C* illustrates the contraction on the right side of the trunk.) Both sides of the trunk must be evaluated.

Rotation Control

"Rotation of the vertebral column is achieved by the paravertebral muscles and the lateral muscles of the abdomen. Unilateral contraction of the paravertebral muscles causes only weak rotation. . . . During rotation of the trunk, the main muscles involved are the oblique muscles. Their mechanical efficiency is enhanced by their spiral course around the waist and by their attachments to the thoracic cage away from the vertebral column, so that both the lumbar and lower thoracic vertebral columns are mobilised."[17] When rotating the trunk to the left, both the right external and left internal obliques are activated (Figure 4-7). The fibers of both of these muscles run in the same direction and are

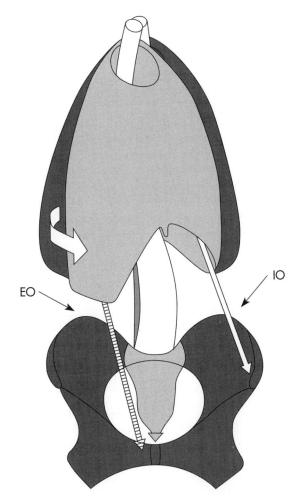

Figure 4-7 Rotation control. *IO*, Internal oblique; *EO*, external oblique. (From Kapandji IA: *The physiology of the joints: vol 3: the trunk and vertebral column*, New York, 1974, Churchill Livingstone.)

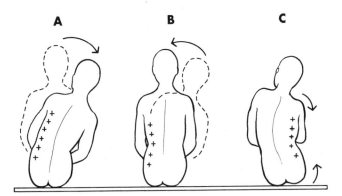

Figure 4-6 Lateral flexor control. Dotted lines indicate trunk starting position, solid lines indicate trunk final position, arrows indicate movement direction, and plus symbols indicate muscle groups primarily responsible for control of pattern. (Skeletal muscle activity occurs on both sides of the trunk [i.e., reciprocal innervation].)

synergistic. Basmajian's[4] review of the EMG literature demonstrates that bilateral activity in the extensors at the thoracic level is evident during rotation.

Mohr[20] states, "Stroke patients will very rarely rotate because normal rotation requires extensors and flexors to be active simultaneously on opposite sides of the trunk." Rotational trunk control depends on muscle fixation on one side of the trunk, resulting in efficient muscle action on the opposite side.[10]

Trunk rotation can occur in two positions: flexion with rotation and extension with rotation.[6] Mohr[20] points out that rotation can be initiated by the upper trunk or the lower trunk/pelvis. Rotation control is evaluated by five movement patterns.[6,20]

1. In the first movement pattern the patient sits upright, and the pelvis remains stable on the support surface. The patient reaches across midline so that the shoulder moves toward the opposite hip (e.g., reaching with the right arm across the body toward the floor). The result is a position of flexion and rotation. The primary control is by concentric contraction of the obliques as well as contraction of the back extensors (especially at the thoracic level). Both sides of the trunk must be evaluated.
2. In the second movement pattern the upper trunk remains stable, and the lower trunk and pelvis initiate a forward movement on one side (e.g., scooting forward). The result is a position of extension with rotation.
3. In the third movement pattern the patient reaches behind at the shoulder level (upper-trunk initiated), and the resulting posture is rotation and extension.
4. The fourth movement pattern involves initiating a backward shift with the lower trunk and pelvis (scooting backwards) while shifting to one side and rotating the opposite side posteriorly; this posture is flexion with rotation.
5. The final movement pattern is similar to a pattern reviewed in the section on trunk flexion control. The patient is supine and initiates a segmental roll by lifting the shoulders up from the support surface and toward the opposite side of the body. This pattern is controlled by a concentric contraction of the abdominals (the obliques).

Trunk Control During Basic Activities of Daily Living

The previous section focused on select movement patterns of the trunk. Evaluating the trunk in this manner is useful for identifying specific problem areas and focusing treatment plans. However, more relevant to all rehabilitation professionals is the impact that impaired trunk control has on functional tasks. Most if not all of the reviewed movement patterns (and combinations of them) are utilized dur-

ing ADL performance. Therefore the evaluation of trunk control can take place during skilled observations of ADL.

It must be clarified that there are an infinite number of variations in observed movement patterns during task performance. Therefore the focus of evaluation and treatment should be on observing, evaluating, and treating the patient in a variety of different environments and with tasks that include multiple variables. The situational context and task demands will determine which components of trunk control are necessary for successful task performance. Box 4-3 has an example of task variables that affect trunk control patterns.

The list of trunk control variations during ADL performance in the following section are not considered exhaustive but are guidelines for observating trunk patterns and inherent variations during various tasks. The reader should mimic performing each task to ensure understanding of the posture descriptions.

Upper Extremity Dressing
Pullover Shirt
- *Trunk flexion:* Required for the patient to manipulate the shirt in the lap and reach down toward the lap to insert an arm into the sleeve
- *Trunk extension:* Observed as the patient realigns the trunk, continues to pull up the sleeve, and inserts the head into the shirt
- *Trunk rotation with extension:* May be necessary for reaching posteriorly and adjusting the orientation of the shirt and/or tucking the shirt into the pants

Button-Down Shirt
- *Trunk flexion:* Used to orient the shirt correctly on the lap for preparation of donning and guide the arm into the sleeve when the trunk is inclined forward
- *Trunk extension:* Required to realign the trunk from the previous position
- *Trunk rotation with extension:* Used to reach with the more functional arm behind the head and to the opposite shoulder to grasp the collar of the shirt and pull it

Box 4-3

Variables While Eating That Affect Required Trunk Control Patterns

Size of table
Type of seating surface (presence of armrests or backrest, cushions, chair height, distance person is from table)
Placement of items such as condiments, utensils, and serving bowls (e.g., near or far, right or left)
Type of food (hot soup, cold fruit)
Solitary or group dining (may get assistance with passing needed items)
Errors (dropping fork, spilling beverage)

to the opposite side (Figure 4-8); also used to move the second arm through the sleeve and tuck the shirt into the pants

- *Trunk flexion:* used as the patient attempts to button the shirt; more often used as relaxation position (a slumped posture) rather than an active flexion pattern

Lower Extremity Dressing (Seated)
Pants, Underwear, Shoes, Socks

- *Trunk flexion:* Required to reach down toward the feet (Figure 4-9)
- *Trunk rotation with flexion:* Required to reach more functional arm toward the opposite foot
- *Trunk extension:* Required to realign the trunk from the previous positions
- *Lateral flexion:* Required when using a crossed-leg method to don/doff pants, underwear, or footwear; (The crossed-leg position shifts the patients' center of gravity posteriorly placing increased demand on the abdominals [i.e., controlling the trunk in flexion while preventing a posterior fall]; Figure 4-10.) Also required to successfully pull up or down the pants and underwear over the buttocks and hips

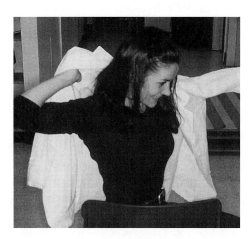

Figure 4-8   Trunk control during upper extremity dressing.

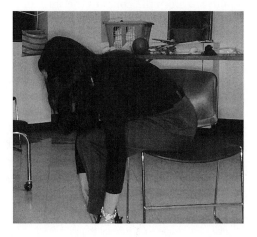

Figure 4-9   Trunk control during lower extremity dressing.

Grooming
Oral Care

- *Trunk flexion:* Isometric control commonly used to position the head over the sink to preventing spillage of paste and saliva onto clothing; increased trunk flexion for expectorating (paste, mouthwash) after completion of tooth brushing
- *Trunk extension:* Utilized to realign body from previous position; also utilized to reach for supplies in a medicine cabinet over a sink, as well as during gargling
- *Trunk rotation with flexion:* May be utilized to reach toward and adjust the faucet opposite the arm being used

Hair Care

- *Trunk flexion or extension:* May be utilized isometrically during hair washing; trunk flexion—utilized if patients prefer to lean forward and allow the lather to be rinsed off in front of them, trunk extension (and head/neck extension)—utilized if patients prefer to lean back and allow the lather to be rinsed off behind them; may both be utilized during hair combing to accentuate the position of the head and optimally position the brush or comb to make contact with the scalp
- *Lateral flexion:* May be utilized during hair washing or combing (initiated by upper trunk) as the head is tilted to the right or left side; may also be utilized for optimal head placement.

Eating

- *Trunk flexion and extension:* Utilized in varying degrees in conjunction with a hand-to-mouth pattern in which an anterior weight shift of the trunk toward the table occurs (Figure 4-11) to position the mouth over the plate as food enters; (The degree to which this weight shift occurs depends on the type of food being eaten. Food that is hot or liquid requires increased flexion toward the plate or bowl. The increased flexion reduces the distance the food must be transported thereby reducing spillage opportunities.)

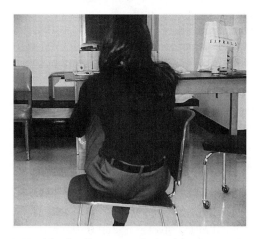

Figure 4-10   Trunk adjustments during lower extremity dressing.

- *Trunk rotation:* May be utilized in both flexion and extension to reach for condiments that are across the midline of the trunk
- *Lateral flexion:* Lower trunk initiated—may be utilized in reaching for condiments that are positioned to the side of the place setting and beyond arms length and may also be utilized in conjunction with trunk rotation postures (Figure 4-12); upper trunk initiated—may be utilized when reaching for an object that drops on the floor to the side of the patient

Bathing (Seated on a Tub Seat or Bench)
- *Trunk flexion and extension:* Required to reach toward the lower extremities and then realign
- *Trunk rotation:* Trunk rotation with flexion—utilized to reach down towards the opposite lower extremity for lower leg and foot washing; trunk rotation with extension—may be utilized when reaching posteriorly to wash back and neck; (In general, trunk rotation is utilized when reaching across the midline of the trunk. The amount of flexion and extension depends on the

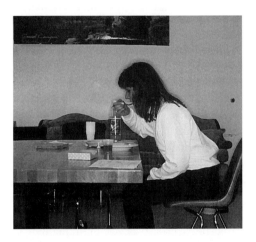

Figure 4-11 Trunk control while eating.

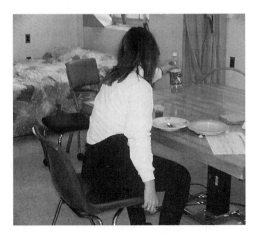

Figure 4-12 Trunk adjustments while reaching for utensils or condiments.

area of the body being washed [e.g., flexion for lower body washing, extension for upper body washing].)
- *Lateral flexion:* Lower trunk initiated—required to wash perineum and rectal areas; upper trunk initiated—may be utilized to wash the sides of the lower legs and/or to pick up a bar of soap from the bottom of the tub; (Bathing activities place extra demands on trunk control because of the slippery nature of the support surface.)

Toileting
- *Lateral flexion:* Lower trunk initiated—may be utilized depending on the sequence of clothing management for toileting and the type of transfer being utilized; (For example, if patients are performing a sit-pivot transfer, clothing is usually being managed from the seated position. Therefore lateral flexion is necessary so that pants and underwear can clear the hips/buttocks.) May also be utilized for wiping after toileting
- *Trunk rotation with extension:* Utilized to reach across the body for toilet paper
- *Trunk flexion:* May be used for self-catheterization, application of a condom-style catheter, management of feminine hygiene products, and wiping after toileting

Bridging
- *Trunk extension:* Necessary at trunk and hips to assume a functional bridge position; (The height of the bridge depends on the task. For example, bridging to utilize a bedpan requires more extension than bridging to don/doff pants.)

Scooting
- *Trunk flexion and extension:* Must be balanced for successful scooting; (The efficiency of the scooting pattern is compromised if the patient maintains a flexed trunk with a posterior pelvic tilt or a hyperextended trunk.)
- *Lateral flexion:* Lower trunk initiated—utilized to clear the buttocks from the support surface, which is required to advance the hip forward
- *Trunk rotation with extension:* Lower trunk initiated—allows the patient to achieve the goal of scooting forward

TREATMENT TECHNIQUES TO ENHANCE TRUNK CONTROL DURING TASK PERFORMANCE

Assuming an Appropriate Starting Posture

Before initiating tasks and retraining trunk control the trunk must be in a proper biomechanical alignment. The patient should be observed anteriorly, posteriorly, and laterally so that deviations from normal alignment can be detected (see Table 4-1).

Physically or verbally cuing patients to assume an appropriate starting posture should place them in a position of readiness for function optimal symmetry in the trunk that is usually in midline, depending on the task (Box 4-4).

This starting posture is similar to the position the trunk and lower extremities assume when a person begins a typing task.

An aligned and upright trunk posture has been shown to recruit muscle activity in the trunk. Floyd and Silver's[15] EMG studies demonstrated that a slumped position while sitting (simultaneous trunk flexion and extension of the hip joint) resulted in trunk extensor relaxation. In contrast, sitting upright in a chair without a backrest resulted in increased activity of the erector spinae muscle group. This muscle activity persisted as long as the trunk remained in extension despite adjustments of the head and shoulders. A slumped posture, which consists of trunk flexion, posterior pelvic tilt, and resulting hip extension, is commonly observed during evaluation of posture in the stroke population; it is a position of minimal skeletal muscle activity.

Andersson and Ortengren's[1] review of the literature demonstrated that the position of the feet had an impact on the myoelectric activity of the trunk extensors. Knee flexion (causing the feet to come toward the chair) increased muscle activity in the trunk, whereas knee extension resulted in a decrease in muscle activity. Stroke patients commonly assume a seated posture in which their feet (especially the more affected lower extremity) are positioned on the floor in front of their knees (e.g., in knee extension). The position of the feet tends to have an effect on pelvic tilt and resultant trunk postures. When the feet are positioned under the knees and toward the chair, an anterior pelvic tilt and trunk extension are enhanced. The opposite is also true: when the feet are positioned in front of the knees and the knees are extended, a posterior pelvic tilt and resulting trunk flexion are enhanced.

Patients should be encouraged to feel the difference between an aligned and a malaligned posture. The patient should be able to assume an appropriate posture automatically. It may be helpful to demonstrate the impact that a slumped posture has on reaching activities performed with the side less affected by the stroke. Patients may realize that the distance and quality of their reach is enhanced when they are sitting in a proper alignment.

Box 4-4

Seated Position of Readiness for Function

Pelvis is in neutral to anterior tilt
Equal weight bearing on both ischial tuberosities
Trunk erect and midline with appropriate spinal curves
Shoulders symmetrical and over the hips
Head/neck neutral
Hips slightly above the level of the knees
Knees in line with the hips
Feet equally weight bearing and underneath the knees

Although the use of mirrors for visual feedback may be appropriate for some patients, it should be used with caution in patients with neurobehavioral deficits. Another technique for assisting patients with gaining symmetry is to have the therapist positioned in front of the patient and assume the patient's postures to provide feedback for the patient. Therapists should slowly correct their posture, instructing the patient to mimic the movement. The therapist may state, "Keep your shoulders in line with mine" or "Keep your forehead at the same level as mine."

Mohr[20] emphasizes using activities that encourage rotation and lateral flexion to gain midline control: " . . . the active movements of the trunk into rotation and lateral flexion are caused by the same muscles that flex and extend the trunk. The different movements occur as a result of different interactions of these muscles with each other . . . . In order for patients to achieve midline postural control, the therapist must work with the patient in the higher levels of lateral and rotational planes of movement."

Maintaining or Increasing Trunk Range of Motion Through Mobilization and Movement

"If there is not full range in all trunk movements (flexion, extension, lateral flexion, and rotation), it will be more difficult to gain full control of the trunk. Any lack of range of motion in the trunk will lead to decreased function."[20]

Although limited ROM in the extremities is commonly evaluated and treated, the ROM in the spine is often overlooked. After acute strokes, patients lose the ability to shift their weight and make postural adjustments. Evaluating patients who have trunks that are completely influenced by gravity and demonstrate only static trunk postures is common. In these cases, prolonged immobilization of the trunk because of loss of control can result in loss of soft tissue elasticity, joint play, and ultimately function. These problems, compounded by inappropriate trunk positioning and support in upright postures, lead to a cycle of immobility, soft tissue changes, loss of range, and impaired functional abilities.

Specific trunk mobilization techniques are beyond the scope of this chapter but are discussed in the literature.[6,10,13,20] Just as we train patients to perform self-ROM activities for their extremities, we must promote patient awareness of trunk mobility and educate them about specific movement patterns that will maintain and/or increase their trunk ROM. Following are examples of movement patterns that patients can perform to meet this goal:

1. While supine, patients flex their hips and knees as if preparing to bridge. Patients are instructed to keep their shoulders flat on the bed and simultaneously allow their knees to fall slowly from one side and then the other. This movement pattern encourages dissociation from the upper and lower trunk (rotation).
2. While supine, patients keep their hips and knees straight while cradling their more affected upper ex-

tremity. The goal is to lift and rotate the upper trunk as if initiating a roll with the upper trunk *(rotation)*.

3. While sitting, patients cradle their more affected upper extremity against their chest. The therapist encourages patients to move the upper trunk in a twisting motion without letting the pelvis move *(rotation)*.

4. While sitting, patients practice moving from an upright posture to a posture of lateral flexion on one side so that they are weight bearing on their forearm to the side of their trunk. The pelvis should remain stable on the support surface for optimal stretch *(lateral flexion)*.

5. While sitting, patients hold their more affected wrist and reach to the floor between their feet. They are also encouraged to allow their head to drop and dangle *(flexion)*.

6. While supine, patients assume a bridge posture and hold the position as able *(extension)*.

7. While sitting, patients practice lifting their hip from the support surface. This movement can be enhanced by having the patient reach up and to the side with the opposite upper extremity. Reaching beyond the arm span in this posture requires lateral flexion for the reach pattern to be successful *(lateral flexion)*.

Utilizing Various Postures

The utilization of varying postures may be used as an adjunctive treatment during patients' performance of functional tasks. Postures should be selected based on specific patient needs. The chosen posture should accentuate and challenge the movement and control patterns that are interfering with independent performance of life activities. NOTE: If the patient is not engaging in a specific activity (self-care tasks, games, adapted sports), the utilization of these postures is not encouraged. Examples of varying postures include the following:

1. Seated with legs crossed: Use of this posture is appropriate for patients whose inability to control lateral flexion and flexion patterns and shift their weight is preventing functional independence. Working with patients in this posture encourages weight transference to one ischial tuberosity and has the added effect of challenging abdominal control. This occurs because the crossed leg is in a position of hip flexion. When the hips are flexed, the traction on the hamstrings tends to tilt the pelvis posteriorly,[17] resulting in a posterior shift in the center of gravity. Abdominal control is therefore required to prevent a posterior loss of balance.

   Participation in tasks such as lower extremity dressing, lower body washing, and/or activities such as modified volleyball will place extra demands on patients who are in this position.

2. Sitting in front of a table while bearing weight on both forearms: Ryerson and Levit[22] recommend this

posture during the acute stage of hemiplegia when little postural control is evident. In this posture patients use their upper extremities as a point of proximal stability. It should be stressed that the arm should be active, and the trunk should not be allowed to "hang" on an inactive arm.

   Patients are encouraged to practice anterior, posterior, and lateral shifting in this posture to reestablish postural control; coordinate trunk, scapula, and humerus patterns; and establish weight bearing of the upper extremities. Because both arms are engaged in a weight-bearing activity, it is difficult for the patients to participate in functional tasks. Immediately following utilization of this posture the therapist must engage the patient in a follow-up activity such as reaching to ensure the postures can be incorporated into daily living activities.

3. Prone on elbows: Although effective for gaining trunk extension, this position should be used with caution. It may compromise respiratory status, cause shoulder pain if upper extremity alignment is not considered, and be generally uncomfortable for older stroke patients. It may be effective for some patients and a required posture for some transitional movements such as floor-to-chair transfers.

4. Kneeling: This posture is appropriate for patients who are experiencing difficulty in gaining trunk/hip extension. Patients may also find this posture uncomfortable, but it may be necessary for transitional patterns.

5. Variations on the degree of hip flexion while seated: Changing the position of the lower extremities can challenge the performance of specific trunk patterns. Being in a position with the knees below the hips, such as sitting on a high stool, decreases the amount of hip flexion and has a tendency to place the trunk in increased extension.

   Conversely, positioning the patient with the knees above the hips (increasing the amount of hip flexion) results in a position of trunk flexion and a posterior weight shift, which places greater demands on the trunk flexors.

Treating the "Pusher Syndrome"

The "pusher syndrome" is a phrase coined by Davies.[11] Davies derived the name from what she felt was the most striking aspect of this syndrome—the patient pushes heavily toward the hemiplegic side in all positions and resists any attempt at passive correction (i.e., a correction that would bring the weight toward or over the midline of the body to the unaffected side).

Currently only one study[21] has focused on the rehabilitation of patients with the pusher syndrome. The study examined the syndrome's incidence, the relation of this syndrome to neurobehavioral deficits, and the impact of the syndrome on the rehabilitation process in 327 patients. The study revealed a 10% incidence. It also found no significant differences in hemineglect or anosognosia in patients with and without ipsilateral pushing. The study also found that patients who demonstrated ipsilateral pushing required 3.6 weeks longer to reach the same final outcome as patients who did not demonstrate ipsilateral pushing. Of note in this study are the Barthel Index scores at admission and discharge. On admission, patients who demonstrated ipsilateral pushing scored an average of 13.7 on the Barthel Index as compared to 46.8 for patients without evidence of pushing. On discharge the average score for pushers was 43.9 as compared to 66.8 for patients without pushing. In other words the discharge scores (in terms of ADL function) of the patients who were pushers were still below the admission scores for patients who did not push.

Davies[11] summarizes the typical signs of the pusher syndrome as the following:

- Head turned away from affected side and laterally flexed toward stronger side
- Decreased ability to perceive stimuli from affected side
- Lack of facial expression
- Poor breath control with monotone, hypophonic voice
- An elongated affected side
- Evidence of pushing with stronger leg while supine
- Holding onto side of bed or mat as if falling
- Shortening of stronger side of trunk with elongation of hemiplegic side while sitting
- Marked resistance to attempts to transfer weight to stronger side
- Pushing with stronger arm and leg to more affected side
- Difficulty transferring, especially to stronger side
- All weight shifted to affected side while standing; leaning against therapist's supporting arm or flexing forward at hips
- Hemiplegic leg adduction (scissors) when walking; difficulty taking a step with affected leg because of an inability to shift weight to stronger side

Davies[11] recommends the following specific treatments for the pusher syndrome:

- Restoring head movements: maintaining full passive range of motion (PROM), stretching, and encouraging active range of motion (AROM) by scanning activities
- Activating the side flexors (see activities described in previous sections)
- Using functional activities to regain midline while standing

A hands-on approach does not seem to be effective with patients who have the pusher syndrome; therapists' attempts to assist patients with gaining midline by handling is met by further patient resistance. Manipulating the environment and providing external cues (verbal) seem to be more effective. Examples include the following:

- Have patients reach with their stronger upper extremity for objects beyond their arm span to encourage a weight shift to the stronger side.
- Provide verbal cues to realign the trunk, such as, "Bring your head toward mine" and "Bring your left shoulder toward the wall."
- Provide a target toward which patients can move their trunk, and maintain the position as long as possible. For example, place a bolster on patients' stronger side, and cue them to lean against the bolster and hold the position (see Chapter 11).

Engaging in Reaching Tasks

Therapists can use placement of objects in reaching activities as a way to place a variety of demands on the trunk. The key to eliciting a trunk response is to place the object slightly beyond the arm's reach. Fisher[14] observes that when subjects without brain injuries reach, they anteriorly tilt the pelvis, slightly extend the upper back, and move the trunk in the direction of the arm. Patients with brain injuries do not incorporate trunk movements into arm movements and will reach only to arm's length as they maintain a slumped posture.

Therapists have the ability to control the desired response by the way they set up the activity. Setting up the activity includes placing items required during ADL in specific places, choosing the appropriate environment (e.g., kitchen with upper and lower shelves, bookcase, desk space, meal table), deciding how far beyond the arm span the activity should be placed, and deciding on the characteristics of the objects the patient is reaching for (number of objects, weight of the objects, whether objects require one or two hands). (See Table 6-1 for examples of activity placement and resulting trunk response.)

Using Moveable Surfaces

The use of moveable surfaces to challenge trunk control has been advocated by several authors.[6,10,16] Moveable surfaces utilized in treatment include items such as therapy balls, bolsters, and rocker boards. Moveable surfaces can be utilized in treatment in a variety of ways, including the following:

1. To grade the difficulty of the task
2. To challenge the patient to maintain control of the surface without outside assistance (challenge isometric patterns)
3. To allow the patient to respond to the therapist's perturbation of the moveable surface
4. To allow the patient to initiate moving the surface

5. To enhance stretching and mobilization of the trunk by using a particular surface such as a large ball
6. To add variety to treatment sessions
7. To focus on isolated trunk control

Although moveable surfaces are commonly utilized in the clinic, research concerning the effectiveness of this type of treatment compared to other types is lacking. It may be argued that when patients master trunk control on a moveable surface (a difficult situation), their control will improve on less demanding surfaces (surfaces that don't move). Unfortunately, this argument is not supported by current research that advocates task-specific training.

Use of moveable surfaces may be appropriate for patients who are experiencing difficulty controlling their trunk in environments with external perturbations (e.g., trains, automobiles, buses).

Adapting the Environment

Some patients may have very little improvement in trunk control. Environmental adaptations are necessary for these patients to enhance independent performance. Examples include the following:

1. Utilizing outside supports can help maintain trunk stability while the extremities are engaged in functional tasks. Supports such as lateral supports, anterior chest straps, arm chairs, utilizing pillows and cushions for propping, and lap trays are all examples of equipment used to compensate for compromised trunk control (see Chapter 19).
2. Rearranging the environment can decrease demands on the trunk. Placing required equipment within the patient's reach (arm reach) will not only increase independence but may prevent falls. Storing dishes on the counter instead of in a cabinet, placing utensils in front of the patient, and keeping grooming items on top of the sink instead of a medicine cabinet are examples of this strategy.
3. Providing adaptive equipment is a commonly used strategy to both increase independent performance and minimize safety risks. ADL equipment issued to compensate for poor trunk control may include the following:
     Long-handled shoe horns
     Elastic laces
     Adapted bath brushes
     "Soap on a rope"
     Reachers
     Tub seats
     Commodes
   (See Chapter 22 for more information on adaptive devices.)
4. Home modifications such as grab bars and bed rails

may also be indicated. (See Chapter 20 for a full review of home adaptations and equipment recommendations.)

Handling

Handling is a common technique utilized in the clinic. This intervention is commonly associated with the NDT approach. Handling may be utilized to allow the patient to feel the desired movement pattern, gain range, assist weak movement patterns, and provide external support to prevent falls. To be effective, the patient must be aware of the goal associated with handling, and the therapist should use handling within the context of a functional task. In addition, the handling from the therapist should be graded to allow the patient to perform as much of the movement pattern as possible. A variety of texts* are available that review specific techniques of handling. Although commonly used, this technique is not well supported by research.

Using Activities of Daily Living and Mobility Tasks

Clearly the most effective tools that occupational therapists can utilize to regain trunk control are self-care, instrumental ADL, and mobility tasks.

The therapist must first perform a thorough evaluation as described in previous sections. Following the evaluation, therapists and patients should identify the most problematic movement patterns that occur during the patients' daily activities. At this point, therapists utilize their activity analysis skills to choose appropriate tasks that incorporate the desired patterns and postures. For example, if the identified problematic patterns are lateral flexion and lateral weight shifts, therapists may choose the following activities for the patient to practice:

    Lower extremity dressing
    Weight shifting for pressure relief
    Scooting
    Assuming a sitting position from sidelying position
    Reaching for objects that are positioned above and to the side of the patient opposite the side where lateral flexion is desired
    Reaching for objects on the floor that are on the side of the patient

The majority of ADL and mobility tasks will encompass a variety of postures and movements. For the mentioned strategies to be effective, therapists should initially focus patients' attention on the desired components of trunk movements. As the patient progresses, the obvious goal is for the trunk responses to be relearned and become automatic.

*References 5, 6, 10, 11, 13, 16.

■
CASE STUDY

SG is a 64-year-old female who presented to the rehabilitation unit after a right middle cerebral artery CVA. The following data were collected from the initial evaluation (specific to the trunk):

- Sensation was intact.
- Static postural malalignments included posterior pelvic tilt, retracted left ribcage, increased weight bearing on left ischial tuberosity.
- Dynamic posture was difficult to assess because the patient was afraid to move. The patient could not reach beyond her arm span when reaching with her right arm. She had a tendency to fall backward and to the left during lower extremity dressing and when reaching for objects behind her.
- SG's personal occupational therapy goals were to (1) be able to independently don her shoes, (2) be able to reach for objects she had dropped without falling, and (3) decrease the amount of spillage that occurred during meals.

The initial treatment plan included adapting her wheelchair with lateral supports (which were removed when she was supervised by friends, family, and staff) and a lumbar roll to maintain optimal alignment while functioning in the wheelchair, trunk mobilizations (specifically in the directions of extension and lateral flexion to both sides), activities to recruit abdominal activity (rolling, games that encouraged trunk rotation, reaching for objects positioned overhead and behind her), and activities that presented unexpected challenges to her trunk control (e.g., balloon volleyball, catch). During the initial stages of treatment, the therapist sat behind SG in a straddle position, which increased feelings of security and allowed the therapist to provide outside assistance with difficult patterns as well as prevent falls. SG was observed while eating, and the therapist noted that she did not shift her weight anteriorly when bringing food to her mouth. Instead she kept her trunk supported against the back of the chair. Because of the increased distance the food had to travel to reach her mouth, their was marked spillage, especially of liquids on a spoon (e.g., soup, cereal milk). SG was trained to shift her weight forward as she brought food to her mouth. Although spillage still occurred, it happened less frequently, with the food falling to the plate or table and not in her lap.

As SG progressed the therapist was able to sit next to or in front of her during activities. She engaged in graded reaching activities in which the distance SG was required to reach was progressively increased. Activities included reaching to lower shelves in the refrigerator, reaching for objects positioned at specific levels (e.g., knee level, midshin level, floor level).

On discharge from inpatient rehabilitation, SG was able to (1) perform all basic ADL with distant supervision and without assistive devices, (2) reach to the floor when she propped her upper trunk with her more affected forearm against her knees, and (3) eat independently by using a rocker knife to cut her food, with spillage occurring only 10% of the time.

■

REVIEW QUESTIONS

1. What is considered an aligned posture in preparation for engagement in functional tasks? What are the common deviations from this posture after stroke?
2. Name three ADL tasks that require control in the rotation plane.
3. What are advantages and disadvantages of using moveable surfaces in trunk control treatment?
4. What are appropriate treatment activities for patients who lack trunk extensor control?
5. Explain the reason an appropriate starting alignment is considered a prerequisite for initiating functional activities.
6. Which trunk patterns are required for donning a button-down shirt?

■ ## COTA Considerations ■

- Trunk control impairments should be evaluated in the context of daily living skills to identify blocks to efficient and safe performance.
- Trunk range of motion must be evaluated and if necessary treated in the same way that ranges in the extremities would be evaluated.
- Utilize positioning devices to prevent postural malalignment when patients are not involved in activities.
- Vary task parameters to elicit a variety of trunk responses during functional tasks.

REFERENCES

1. Andersson BJG, Ortengren R: Myoelectric back activity during sitting, *Scand J Rehabil Med* 3:73, 1974.
2. Árnadóttir G: *The brain and behavior: assessing cortical dysfunction through activities of daily living*, St Louis, 1990, Mosby.
3. Ayres AJ: *Developmental dyspraxia and adult onset apraxia*. Torrance, CA: Sensory Integration International.
4. Basmajian JV, DeLuca CJ: *Muscles alive: their functions revealed by electromyography*, ed 5, Baltimore, 1985, Williams & Wilkins.
5. Bobath B: *Adult hemiplegia: evaluation and treatment*, ed 3, London, 1990, Butterworth Heinemann.
6. Boehme R: *Improving upper body control: an approach to the treatment of tonal dysfunction*, Tucson, 1988, Therapy Skill Builders.
7. Bohannon RW: Recovery and correlates of trunk muscle strength after stroke, *Int J Rehabil Res* 18:162, 1995.
8. Bohannon RW: Lateral trunk flexion strength: impairment, measurement reliability and implications following unilateral brain lesion, *Int J Rehabil Res* 15:249, 1992.
9. Bohannon RW, Cassidy D, Walsh S: Trunk muscle strength is impaired multidirectionally after stroke, *Clin Rehabil* 9:47, 1995.
10. Davies PM: *Right in the middle: selective trunk activity in the treatment of adult hemiplegia*, New York, 1990, Springer-Verlag.
11. Davies PM: *Steps to follow: a guide to the treatment of adult hemiplegia*, New York, 1985, Springer-Verlag.
12. De Troyer A: Mechanical role of the abdominal muscles in relation to posture, *Resir Physiol* 53:341, 1983.
13. Eggers O: *Occupational therapy in the treatment of adult hemiplegia*, New York, 1983, Springer-Verlag.

14. Fisher B: Effect of trunk control and alignment on limb function, *J Head Trauma Rehabil* 2:72, 1987.

15. Floyd WF, Silver PHS: The function of the erector spinae muscles in certain movements and postures in man, *J Physiol* 129:184, 1955.

16. Hypes B: *Facilitating development and sensorimotor function: treatment with the ball*, Hugo, Minn, 1991, PDP Press.

17. Kapandji IA: *The physiology of the joints: vol 3: the trunk and vertebral column*, New York, 1974, Churchill Livingstone.

18. Kendall FP et al: *Muscles testing and function*, ed 4, Baltimore, 1993, William & Wilkins.

19. Mitz AR, Winstein C: The motor system I: lower centers. In Cohen H, editor: *Neuroscience for rehabilitation*, Philadelphia, 1993, JB Lippincott.

20. Mohr JD: Management of the trunk in adult hemiplegia: the Bobath concept, *Top Neurol* 1990, APTA.

21. Pedersen PM et al: Ipsilateral pushing in stroke: incidence, relation to neuropsychological symptoms, and impact on rehabilitation. The Copenhagen stroke study, *Arch Phys Med Rehabil* 77:25, 1996.

22. Ryerson S, Levit K: The shoulder in hemiplegia. In Donatelli RA, editor: *Physical therapy of the shoulder*, ed 2, New York, 1991, Churchill Livingstone.

23. Sabari JS: Motor learning concepts applied to activity-based intervention with adults with hemiplegia, *Am J Occup Ther* 45:523, 1991.

24. Shumway-Cook A, Woollacott M: *Motor control: theory and practical applications*, Baltimore, 1995, Williams & Wilkins.

25. Smith LK, Weiss EL, Lehmkuhl, LD: *Brunnstrom's clinical kinesiology*, ed 5, Philadelphia, 1996, FA Davis.

26. Thorstensson A, Oddsson L, Carlson H: Motor control of voluntary trunk movements in standing, *Acta Physiol Scand* 125:309, 1985.

27. Woodhull-McNeal AP: Activity in torso muscles during relaxed standing, *Eur J Appl Physiol* 55:418, 1986.

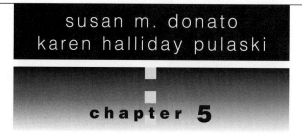

susan m. donato
karen halliday pulaski

chapter **5**

Overview of Balance Impairments: Functional Implications

key terms

balance	center of mass	base of support
posture	limits of stability	gaze stabilization

chapter objectives

After completing this chapter, the reader will be able to accomplish the following:

1. Identify the systems involved in balance as well as review the assessment and evaluation of component balance skills and balance during functional activity.
2. Provide examples of treatment plans and ideas based on specific balance dysfunctions to allow the therapist to implement focused intervention.
3. Participate in the development of goals and documentation systems with emphasis on the setting for service delivery and the impact of the current health care environment.

THEORY

Balance is the ability to control the center of mass over the base of support within the limits of stability; balance results in the maintenance of stability and equilibrium. A person's ability to maintain balance in any position depends on a complex integration of multiple systems. Many theories have been proposed to explain the ability to maintain balance. In the reflex or hierarchical model, balance is considered the interaction of reflexes and reactions, which are organized hierarchically, that result in the support of the body against gravity.[17,24] In this model, balance deficits are the result of eliminating higher central nervous system

control, resulting in the release of spinal and supraspinal reflexes. This model has declined in popularity in recent years because common opinion embraces the idea that the nervous system is more likely comprised of complex interactions of multiple systems rather than organized as a distinct hierarchy.

The systems or distributed control model introduced by Bernstein describes balance as a complex interaction of musculoskeletal and neural systems.[35] The ability to maintain balance is specific to and modified around the constraints of the environment and task. Within this system a disruption of balance (or instability) is the result of a malfunction in or disruption of any one or more of the elements of the postural control system. Likewise, balance is maintained through the interaction of sensory organization and postural control systems. The information is combined and integrated in the central nervous system.

SENSORY ORGANIZATION

According to the systems model, information from three sensory systems are utilized for maintaining balance. Information from the visual, vestibular, and somatosensory systems are of critical importance.

The visual system (see Chapter 12) provides information regarding vertical orientation and visual flow. Visual or optical flow information which describes movement of an image on the retina, is important input that aids in the detection of personal and environmental movement. Information provided by the visual system can be ambiguous and must be compared to other sensory information to determine accuracy. For example, a person sitting in a stationary car next to another stationary car at a red light may then receive optical flow information that indicates the other car is moving backward. This information alone is not adequate for determining which vehicle is moving; it only reveals that there is relative movement. The information must be compared to the other sensory information to determine which car has moved.

Somatosensory information is comprised of cutaneous and pressure receptors on the soles of the feet as well as muscle and joint receptors. It helps determine characteristics of and the relationship of the individual to the support surface. During most tasks, somatosensory information may be the most heavily relied-on input in the adult population. Like visual input, somatosensory input can be ambiguous. For example, dorsiflexion at the ankle indicates that the body is anteriorly displaced over the base of support. However, when standing on an incline, this ankle position may coincide with midline posture. The individual must take other senses into consideration to determine which position is accurate.

Information from the vestibular system helps determine head position and head motion in space relative to gravity. It generally plays a minor role in balance control, unless somatosensory and visual input are inaccurate or unavailable. It is the only sensory reference that is not ambiguous, because it depends on gravity, which is consistent in our environment.

The vestibular system is composed of the otolith and semicircular canals. The semicircular canals sense angular acceleration, which is a change in velocity along a curved path (e.g., shaking or nodding the head). The canals are capable of detecting movement in all planes because all three are oriented in different planes (Figure 5-1). Input from the semicircular canals is utilized to influence postural responses as well as drive compensatory eye movements.

The otolith is composed of the utricle and saccule. Together they are responsible for determining changes in head position in the linear plane, or translational movement of the head. Specifically, the utricle responds to head tilt and translations along the horizontal plane. In addition, it appears to play an important role in producing small, torsional eye movements, which keep the eyes level when the head is tilted laterally. This helps with maintaining postural control and vertical orientation in space. The saccule appears to be instrumental in detecting vertical translations of the head.

In addition to these three systems, individuals' internal representations or perceptions influence the interactions of information. Each individual possesses an internal perception related to the task, themselves, and the environment, which in turn influences sensory interactions and responses.

To appropriately utilize sensory information, each individual develops what is referred to as a *sensory strategy*. A

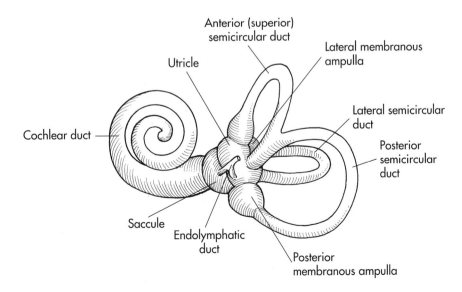

Anterior (superior) semicircular duct

Lateral membranous ampulla

Utricle

Lateral semicircular duct

Cochlear duct

Posterior semicircular duct

Figure 5-1 The semicircular canals.

Saccule

Endolymphatic duct

Posterior membranous ampulla

sensory strategy is formulated when the central nervous system integrates, evaluates, and selects information received from the visual, somatosensory, and vestibular systems. The information is evaluated according to internal and external constraints, including availability of sensory information and the accuracy of environmental information. Information evaluation may also depend on the movement strategy that is occurring. The development of a sensory strategy results in a sensory-motor interaction. The central nervous system determines the most efficient use of sensory input, which then allows for generation of appropriate motor output to complete the necessary task or reach a desired goal. This is an extremely rapid process that is not detectable when there are no deficits.

POSTURAL CONTROL

An individual's ability to maintain equilibrium depends not only on accurate evaluation and use of sensory information but also on the implementation of effective movement strategies. Movement strategies are stereotyped or synergistic patterns that are utilized to maintain the center of mass over the base of support. They are characterized as automatic, not reflexive or voluntary. They occur too quickly to be under voluntary control but are too slow to be considered reflexive.[34] Synergistic movement patterns are useful in that they reduce the degrees of freedom, thus decreasing the response time. Postural actions are reduced or absent when an individual utilizes an external support such as a cane or counter top to help maintain postural control. Automatic postural responses include ankle, hip, and stepping strategies.[34]

An ankle strategy is used to maintain the center of mass over the base of support when movement is centered around the ankles. Knee, hip, and trunk stability is necessary for this strategy to be effective. Ankle strategies are utilized to control small, slow swaying motions. They are effective when the surface area is firm and long in relation to foot length. Muscular activation while using the ankle strategy occurs in a distal to proximal sequence. Timing of muscular contractions is important to generate sufficient torque about the ankles and maintain adequate stability at the hips, knees, and trunk. Ankle strategies are frequently used during "quiet" standing. For example, this strategy is effective in controlling the small, slow swaying motions that occur when a person stands in line (e.g., at a bank or grocery store).

Hip movement that maintains or restores equilibrium is a hip strategy. This strategy is most effective in maintaining stability when the support surface is short in relation to foot length or is compliant. It is utilized to control large or rapid swaying motions or when an ankle strategy is ineffective (i.e., unable to occur rapidly enough or generate adequate torque). Muscle activation while using hip strategies occurs in a proximal to distal sequence. This strategy is used more frequently than ankle strategies when the center of mass approaches the outer limits of the base of support. It is more effective because of the ability to generate greater speed and range. An example of a situation in which people would use a hip strategy would be a circumstance that require them to stand on a narrow beam.

When ankle and hip strategies are or are perceived to be ineffective, the base of support is expanded in the direction of center of mass movement, resulting in the use of what is referred to as a *stepping strategy*. In this case a step is taken to widen the base of support. This is the strategy that is effectively utilized when taking each step while walking. Weight is shifted outside the existing base of support, and a step is taken to bring the base of support back under the center of mass.

Each of the preceding movement strategies are reactive responses to center of mass movement. Anticipatory control is postural muscular activity that precedes and decreases center of mass movement. Previous experience weighs heavily in the determination of the appropriate sequence and degree of muscle activity required to maintain stability when anticipating a perturbation. Because anticipatory activities precede destablization, misperceiving the needed amount of muscle activity may result in too much or too little correction. For example, when people pull a door open, they initiate a posterior weight shift to counteract the weight of the door. If the weight of the door is lighter than anticipated, too much correction might occur and may result in a posterior perturbation of balance.

CENTRAL NERVOUS SYSTEM STRUCTURES

Maintaining equilibrium involves the precise integration of sensory information as well as the generation of appropriate and effective motor responses. Specific central nervous system structures are responsible for performing these complex tasks.

The cerebellum is the primary integrating and modulating force in balance control. It receives information from structures such as the cortex, basal ganglia, spinocerebellar tract, vestibular nuclei, and vestibular pathways. Input is modulated, interpreted, and sent out to the cortex, basal ganglia, thalamus, fourth, fifth and sixth cranial nerves, vestibular nuclei and pathways, and indirectly to the spinal cord, providing the regulatory input needed to control movement. Damage to any one of these structures can result in difficulties with balance/postural control. Through this complex network of central nervous system interactions the cerebellum facilitates smooth coordination of movement. It influences the timing and synergy of muscle groups during synergistic movements as well as muscle tone, or stiffness. Symmetrical, appropriate, balanced skeletal muscle activity is necessary for maintaining postural alignment and is required for smooth, coordinated movements and stability. An example of a disorder involving the cerebellum is ataxia (poor coordination of agonist and antagonist muscles that results in jerky, poorly controlled movements). An individual with cerebellar dysfunction might have an unsteady gait or visual disturbances.

The basal ganglia are also involved in integrating information utilized for postural control. They are involved in a series of complex pathways—much of the exact nature of which is uncertain. The basal ganglia receive information from the cortex and cerebellum and then output information to the motor cortex via the thalamus. The basal ganglia work closely with the cerebellum and are believed to influence the sequencing of automatic postural reactions including the ankle, hip, and stepping strategies previously discussed. The continuous postural adjustments that play a role in smooth, coordinated movement are also controlled by the basal ganglia. Examples of disorders involving the basal ganglia include but are not limited to rigidity, bradykinesia (slowness of movement), akinesia, resting or intention tremors, chorea, and athetosis.

The brain stem is also involved in balance control because it houses the vestibular nuclei, which receive input from the cerebellum and the vestibular system. Information is output to the vestibulospinal tract, oculomotor complex, cerebellum, and parietal lobe. The brain stem is instrumental in the integration of the vestibular input and influences compensatory eye movements (Table 5-1).

COMPREHENSIVE EVALUATION

A comprehensive evaluation is crucial in helping the therapist understand specific balance problems patients may be experiencing. A comprehensive evaluation should always include a subjective client interview, an assessment of balance component skills, and an assessment of balance skills within the context of meaningful functional tasks. Evaluations may vary depending on the acuteness of the neurologic insult, severity of the cerebrovascular accident, and setting in which care is provided (e.g., in patient rehabilitation, outpatient rehabilitation, home health care).

Subjective Interview

It may not be possible for patients who have had an acute CVA to provide accurate information during the interview process. They may be able to provide more information later in treatment when they are outpatients or functioning in the home and community.

Subjective patient interviews allow patients to describe in their own words the way the CVA has affected their level of functioning. The interview should allow the therapist to obtain the following information about the patient:

1. *Premorbid health history*
   The patient's premorbid health history can have a significant impact on prognosis and thus appropriate goals. It is important for the therapist to have a thor-

Table 5-1

Central Nervous System Structures Involved in Balance Control

STRUCTURE	INPUT	OUTPUT	FUNCTION	INDICATION OF DYSFUNCTION
Cerebellum	Cortex Basal ganglia Spinocerebellar tract Vestibular nuclei Vestibular pathways	Cortex Basal ganglia Thalamus Cranial nerves—IV, V, VI Vestibular nuclei Vestibular pathways	Integrates and modulates information Regulates input to control movement Influences muscle tone/stiffness Inputs timing and synergy of muscle groups during synergistic movements	Ataxia Unsteady gait Visual disturbance
Basal ganglia	Cortex cerebellum	Motor cortex Thalamus	Sequences automatic postural reactions	Rigidity Bradykinesia Akinesia Tremors (resting/intention) Chorea Athetosis
Brain stem	Cerebellum Vestibular system	Vestibulospinal tract Oculomotor complex Cerebellum Parietal lobe	Integrates vestibular input Initiates compensatory eye movements	Dysfunctional compensatory eye movements Vestibular dysfunction

ough understanding of any premorbid conditions that could affect a patient's balance functioning. Examples include diabetic neuropathies, vision disturbances, vertigo, prior CVA or head injuries, prior lower extremity range of motion (ROM) or strength problems, or other orthopedic issues.

2. *Prior lifestyle*

As more details are added to this portion of the interview, the therapist will be better equipped to create an individualized treatment plan to meet the individual patient needs. The interview should include information such as the following:
- Waking time each morning
- Schedule of tasks used to prepare for the day
- Whether a bath, shower, or sponge bath is taken
- Bathing time
- Other household chores for which patient is responsible

It may be helpful (if the patient is able) to outline a schedule of a typical day at home. It is important for the therapist to attend the specifics of performing tasks as well as the order in which tasks occur.

3. *Prior functional status*

The therapist will need to have a thorough understanding of the patient's functional level prior to the CVA. This portion of the interview should include information such as the following:
- Whether the patient ambulated independently and what device if any was necessary for ambulation
- Whether the patient required any assistance with performing daily tasks
- Whether the patient was able to function independently in the community (including specifics about activities) and whether any change in activity was experienced in the past 6 months

4. *Patient's perspective of current functioning*

This area may be very difficult for patients who have just had a CVA, but it is important for the therapist to understand what patients consider as problems resulting from balance deficits. Early in the rehabilitation process, patients may cite self-care and mobility as problem areas. Later, when patients are receiving home health or outpatient services, they may no longer experience difficulty in these basic areas but may cite problems with household or community activities. This portion of the interview is important for determining patients' awareness level about the way their balance deficit limits their participation in normal activities as well as for determining appropriate and meaningful goals.

Component Assessment

When the subjective interview has been completed, objective data should be collected. It is important to evaluate the individual component parts of balance control before introducing more complex tasks. Thorough ROM testing of both active and passive ROM, particularly of the trunk and lower extremities, must be completed and will help determine whether a patient has any biomechanical constraints that might have an impact on postural control. Strength and appropriate patterns of skeletal muscle activity, particularly of the lower extremities and trunk, must be established to determine neuromotor influences on postural control. The sensory systems that play a role in maintaining equilibrium must also be examined. One such system is the visual system (see Chapter 12) and would include visual acuity and oculomotor function assessments. Oculomotor function is eye movements such as voluntary movements and gaze stabilization. Assessment of sensation is also critical and should include light touch, deep pressure, proprioception, and kinesthesia assessments. Sensation in the lower extremities is clearly one of the most critical factors affecting balance control. Vestibular system function is difficult to evaluate in isolation but will be discussed further in the context of sensory organization.

After evaluating balance components, more complex tasks that integrate the components must be examined. Patients' postural alignment should be evaluated while they are seated and standing. Observation skills are critical in performing these and subsequent assessments. Symmetrical alignment and appropriate positioning of body parts over the base of support are the goals. Any asymmetry in alignment or bias over the base of support should be noted. In general, the posture should be symmetrical—the head should be in midline, centered over the shoulders; the shoulders should be centered and aligned over the pelvis; under "normal" conditions the feet should be approximately hip distance apart; and the pelvis should be centered over the base of support created by the feet (Figures 5-2 and 5-3).

Each individual possesses an area about which the center of mass may be moved over any given base of support without disrupting equilibrium. This is referred to as the *limits of stability*. It is important to assess patients' ability to move within their limits of stability and note the symmetry and extent of those limits. Because of the biomechanical constraints of the foot and ankle the limits are greatest in the anterior/posterior direction and smaller in the lateral direction. The greatest degree of movement can occur anteriorly. The area created by the limits of stability is in the form of an ellipse (Figure 5-4). The limits of stability may be measured in a number of ways. An experienced evaluator with a strong understanding of typical limits of stability might ask patients to shift their weight as far as they can in all directions. The patients' ability to move over their base of support would be observed and noted. Patients may also be asked to perform a task that requires the center of mass to move over the base of support while the therapist observes their performance. Several computerized pressure plate systems on the market are able to com-

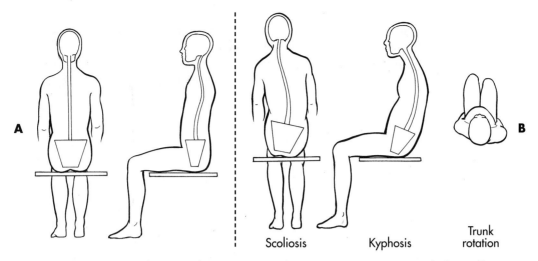

Figure 5-2 **A,** Correct alignment during sitting. **B,** Common asymmetries assumed after stroke.

Scoliosis   Kyphosis   Trunk rotation

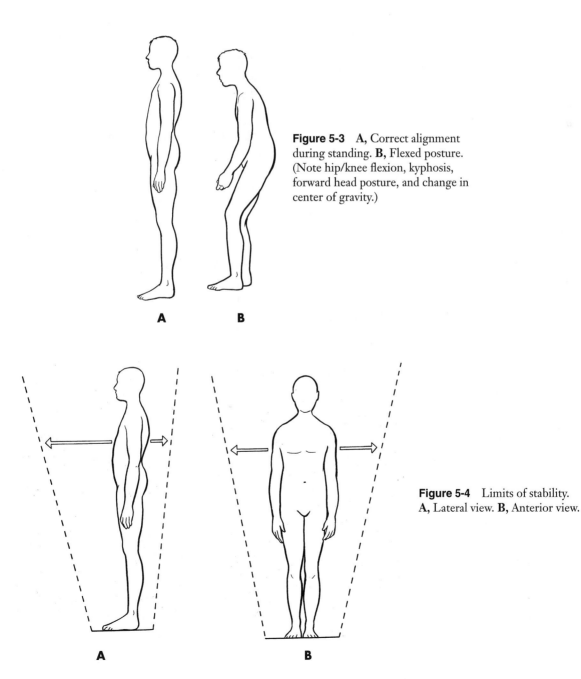

Figure 5-3 **A,** Correct alignment during standing. **B,** Flexed posture. (Note hip/knee flexion, kyphosis, forward head posture, and change in center of gravity.)

A   B

Figure 5-4 Limits of stability. **A,** Lateral view. **B,** Anterior view.

A   B

pute an individual's "normal" limits of stability based on height by force plate analysis. The normal and actual figures can then be compared. These pieces of equipment are quite costly and are not available in all clinics.

Postural Control System

Information regarding biomechanical and neuromuscular parameters available to the patient have been established through the comprehensive component evaluation. Integration and the effectiveness of these capabilities in the central nervous system are tested by assessing automatic postural responses; patients must be exposed to conditions that would normally elicit particular responses.

Ankle strategies[34] are most effective when used with a firm support surface that is long in relation to foot length. Ankle strategies are used to control small, slow swaying motions. For an initial assessment, the patient should be standing on a firm surface with the feet approximately hip distance apart. Oscillations about the ankles should be noted. If the patient is able to perform this task effectively, it may be necessary to increase the demands of the task by narrowing the base of support. Patients may be asked to place their feet together to decrease the size of the base of support, narrow the limits of stability, and increase the need to control center of mass oscillations. Increased use of ankle strategies should be noted. If swaying increases in speed or magnitude, a hip strategy[34] may be initiated. Individuals should be able to maintain their balance in this position with an ankle strategy and perhaps with minimal use of a hip strategy. Not using ankle strategies or using stepping strategies in this position indicates a disturbance in the ability to generate automatic postural responses.

Several methods exist for assessing hip strategies. Hip strategies are most effective when used with a support surface that is short in relation to foot length, the support surface is compliant, or ankle strategies are (or are perceived to be) ineffective. Simulating each of these conditions should result in the use of a hip strategy. The patient may be asked to stand on a 4-inch balance beam so that only the middle of the foot receives support. Ankle strategies are ineffective under these circumstances because adequate torque cannot be produced around the ankle when the support surface is this short. The use of primarily anterior/posterior hip strategies should be noted. Attempts to use ankle strategies only or any use of stepping strategies indicates a dysfunction in the ability to generate an appropriate hip strategy. Compliant support surfaces also result in use of hip strategies in "normal" subjects. This condition can be simulated by having the patient stand on a 4-inch thick piece of medium-density foam. Adequate torque around the ankles is not possible under this condition, and hip strategies are used in all planes/directions. As stated previously, excessive attempts to use ankle strategies or exclusive use of stepping strategies would indicate dysfunction.

Lateral hip strategies may be assessed by having the patient assume a tandem stance (a heel-toe position in which one foot is directly in front of the other). This position significantly narrows the lateral limits of the base of support; because ankle strategies have a limited lateral range of effectiveness, hip strategies are used. This position on a firm support surface would not be challenging enough to elicit hip strategy use in some patients. These patients could perform the same task on a 4-inch balance beam to further narrow the base of support.

When assessing use of hip strategies in any of these conditions, observation of strategy sequence is important. The effectiveness of the target strategy should also be noted. Use of ineffective strategies (i.e., loss of balance) indicates that a particular strategy has failed.

Use of the stepping strategy[34] may be elicited by further challenging the postural control system (e.g., by combining all of the previous test conditions). For example, patients may be asked to stand with feet together or in tandem on a compliant surface. A delay in or lack of a stepping strategy that results in a loss of balance indicates dysfunction.

Sensory Organization

In addition to automatic postural response assessments, assessments of sensory organizational abilities are also important. In other words, therapists must assess patients' abilities to organize and evaluate the orientationally correct sense used to generate appropriate responses. Six test conditions are considered acceptable for thoroughly assessing sensory organization.[32] Computerized tests of sensory organization are commercially available and are often combined with force plates that can measure motor responses to test conditions (to a degree). The sensory organization portion of the apparatus usually consists of a safety harness, moveable foot plate, and a moveable visual screen that surrounds the subject. Test conditions have also been simulated in the clinic by using 4-inch medium-density foam and a visual "dome" that encompasses the patient's visual field and is worn on the head.[32]

The first condition for testing sensory organization allows subjects to receive accurate input from all sensory systems. Patients stand on a firm support surface with their eyes open, and responses are recorded.

During the second condition, patients are asked to close their eyes, which deprives them of visual input. Therefore only somatosensory and vestibular input are available to help patients maintain equilibrium. Under this test condition, patients may have a postural response if conflicting information is received from the available sources, or the individual is accustomed to relying heavily on visual input.

In the third test condition, patients wear the visual screen or dome and thus receive conflicting visual information. The screen or dome is "sway referenced," which means that it moves along with the individual's naturally occurring sway and provides the visual system with the illusion that no sway is occurring—optical flow input indicates that the environment and the individual are stationary. In this test condition the support surface is firm and fixed, so somatosensory and vestibular information are accurate; although visual information is available it is inaccurate. The incoming sensory information must be checked and evaluated and only the accurate information utilized. Relying too heavily on visual input might result in increased sway caused by delayed identification of the need to adjust to spontaneous sway.

The fourth condition utilizes a sway-referenced support surface; the support surface is sway referenced to naturally occurring sway. The 4-inch foam may also be utilized to provide inaccurate somatosensory information. Under these circumstances, visual and vestibular information are accurate, and somatosensory information is available but inaccurate. Once again, an inappropriate postural response indicates an inability to utilize accurate information or identify and sensor inaccurate somatosensory information.

The fifth and sixth test conditions are the most complex and require patients to utilize vestibular information. During the fifth test condition, patients must close their eyes, which deprives patients of visual information. The support surface is sway referenced or foam is used, thus the only accurate information that helps maintain postural control is vestibular. Difficulty maintaining balance may result from a disturbance in the vestibular system or ability to integrate the information.

The sixth test condition utilizes sway-referenced visual and somatosensory information; vestibular information is the only accurate input. Disruption of the postural control may result because of the inability to evaluate the information (a more difficult process because two systems are providing inaccurate information) or a disruption of the central or peripheral vestibular system.[32]

This hierarchy of test conditions (Table 5-2) allows therapists to assess the central nervous system's ability to appropriately integrate information. It is also a method for determining whether a person is relying too heavily on a particular source of information. These tests can also pro-

vide preliminary information about vestibular system function and may indicate a need for further testing.

Assessment of Balance in Relation to Function

Occupational therapists should complete the initial assessment of function in relation to balance in the same way they assess all functional activities. A thorough understanding of normal movement and excellent observation skills are essential when assessing balance through functional activity. As with any skill therapists acquire, these abilities develop and improve as the therapists gain experience. Patients should attempt the activity, and therapists should determine (1) whether patients can do the task, (2) the quality of the performance, and (3) whether patients are unsuccessful and why. Therapists may not have determined the specific balance deficits yet, but they can look for a pattern of dysfunction. Observations during functional activities should focus on when patients lose and do not lose their balance. Therapists should determine what may be causing the loss of balance.

Specifically, therapists should observe what happens when patients have to move their center of mass over their base of support, move their head, stand on uneven surfaces, function in lower lighting, move from one type of surface to another, or function on a narrower base of support. Therapists should also observe patients' postural alignment, whether a bias in posture exists and in which direction that bias occurs, patients' limits of stability, the width between their feet during functional tasks, and what patients do after losing their balance (e.g., use ankle, hip, or step strategy or no strategy at all). The initial contact with patients engaged in functional tasks should only involve observations. Therapists must allow patients to "fail" in a safe way so that they can determine what patients will do during functional tasks.

The specific functional tasks that can be used during evaluation will depend on what the patient's goals are at the time of intervention. Acute and inpatient therapists usually focus on bathing and dressing; basic transfers including bed, toilet, and shower (if applicable); and basic home management tasks if indicated. Outpatient or home

Table 5-2

Test of Sensory Organization

TEST CONDITION	ACCURATE SENSORY INFORMATION	INACCURATE OR ABSENT SENSORY INFORMATION
1	Visual, vestibular, somatosensory	—
2	Somatosensory, vestibular	Absent vision
3	Somatosensory, vestibular	Inaccurate vision
4	Visual, vestibular	Inaccurate somatosensory
5	Vestibular	Absent vision, inaccurate somatosensory
6	Vestibular	Inaccurate vision, inaccurate somatosensory

health therapists usually focus on home management tasks such as meal preparation, cleaning, and doing laundry, as well as community tasks such as grocery shopping, banking, going to church, using public transportation, and participating in leisure activities.

After therapists have had an opportunity to observe patients during functional activities, they should begin to develop hypotheses about the reasons patients are losing their balance during various activities. The component evaluation as well as the diagnostic information can assist therapists determining whether their hypotheses are substantiated. For example, patients may lose their balance when attempting to put on their pants while standing. Therapists may hypothesize that the loss of balance is a result of a poor ability to shift weight accurately, poor postural alignment when attempting to shift weight, and a lack of lateral hip strategy use when standing on one leg. These hypotheses can be supported by testing patients' limits of stability, evaluating their postural alignment, and assessing whether they are using an available hip strategy. These steps allow therapists to develop individualized treatment plans and set realistic short-term and long-term goals for each patient.

It is important to remember that therapists do not treat balance deficits separately from other deficits a stroke survivor may have. The treatment of balance dysfunction is obviously affected by any existing cognitive or visual perceptual deficits such as memory deficits or left neglect. For example, patients with cognitive deficits will undoubtedly benefit more from a treatment program that incorporates familiar, repetitive functional tasks than an exercise program with activities that are meaningless to them. Therapists should incorporate multiple goals into each treatment session.

Because of current, ongoing changes in health care reimbursement, it is crucial for therapists to collaborate with patients on focusing treatment around goals for the home or at work. This approach allows patients to transition as quickly as possible to less restrictive environments. Failure to focus on goals may result in patients being discharged to more restrictive environments that allow less independent lifestyles (e.g., to a nursing home instead of home). Therapists should also focus on treating specific balance deficits to develop an individualized treatment plan that will assist patients with becoming independent as soon as possible.

ESTABLISHING GOALS AND TREATMENT PLANS

Setting goals for patients with balance disorders can be difficult. Therapists must have a thorough understanding of patients' specific CVA neuropathology. Although complete neuroanatomy review is beyond the scope of this chapter, appropriate resources are listed in the References. Several factors contribute to whether patients receive a positive or poor prognosis and may include size and location of the lesion and any secondary factors that have developed, such as extensions of the original CVA, brain edema, and anoxia. The previous medical history will also be important for determining eventual functional outcomes. Factors to consider include any prior CVAs, a history of alcohol use, any head trauma, diabetic neuropathies, age-related changes (such as the loss of inner ear hairs), and balance problems (such as vertigo). Prior problems may interfere with a patient's ability to compensate for the new neurologic insult.

Ideally a treatment team consists of an otolaryngologist (ENT) or neurologist, a physical therapist, an occupational therapist, the patient, and the patient's family (if applicable). It is not the responsibility of occupational therapists to prognosticate, but to set realistic goals and design an appropriate treatment plan they must have input from the otolaryngologist or neurologist concerning prognosis. If therapists are not fortunate enough to work directly with an otolaryngologist they should contact the neurologist treating the patient for the CVA. Occupational therapists must also work closely with physical therapists to ensure that the treatment plans of both disciplines support and reinforce one another rather than work against one another.

After receiving the prognosis, the therapist must decide whether to design a treatment plan that focuses on remediation, compensation, or both. This may be greatly affected by the setting in which the therapist provides treatment. If the prognosis indicates considerable improvement within 3 to 4 weeks, a therapist providing inpatient services may decide to emphasize remediation for the first few weeks and then compensation just before discharge to ensure that the patient is functional in basic tasks. A therapist providing outpatient treatment for the same patient may focus solely on remediation because the patient has already established a safe way to function in the environment and is now focusing on improving balance deficits. If a patient has a very poor prognosis for recovery of balance function, the therapist may emphasize compensation early in treatment to ensure success. A patient's cognitive status will also significantly affect when compensatory devices are introduced into treatment. A patient with memory loss requires more repetition and time to learn to use a walker while performing kitchen tasks than a patient with no memory loss. Introducing devices and training the patient in their use early in treatment is more likely to facilitate learning specific techniques.

Therapists need to understand the implications of prescribing use of compensatory devices for patients with balance deficits. When a walker or cane is introduced into treatment before a patient is even given a chance to function without it, the patient's ability to remediate the balance deficits cannot be accurately assessed. A walker or cane instantly increases the base of support and thus decreases the demand on the patient's balance system to improve. A walker or cane also greatly changes the way in which a patient moves during functional activities and alters normal movement. The patient no longer has to shift weight in a normal way. Instead, weight is shifted through the upper extremities during ambulation. Postural muscle activity has been shown to be altered even when light upper extremity support is used.

Therapists must make informed decisions about using equipment during treatment. All of the factors discussed previously must be taken into consideration when choosing a treatment plan. Tub seats and reachers may be appropriate for patients with orthopedic limitations or who have a poor prognosis for recovery of balance function; however, introducing too many devices too early in treatment may in fact hinder recovery of balance function. For example, if patients are given tub benches or shower seats before being given the opportunity to attempt to stand in the shower, they may not be able to reach their full level of independence. This is not to suggest that devices should not be considered or recommended—numerous patients are only able to function because of their adaptive equipment and devices—it is only to suggest that when planning treatment, therapists should be extremely aware of the implications of using each device. Therapists may consider allowing patients to use devices outside of therapy that provide greater independence but limit their use during actual therapy sessions. Patients can then maintain their independence while still working toward improving their balance. Therapists may be able to help patients function more safely and become more active, even if they are using a device.

Using functional activities and emphasizing functional outcomes have always been basic principles of occupational therapy, and they are now beginning to be embraced by many other disciplines. Hsieh et al[20] stated that using added-purpose occupation is motivating during performance. They add that numerous studies suggest using meaningful tasks in treatment improves both movement and performance.* Traditional treatment of balance disorders has been focused on exercise with the hope and assumption that patients would carry over what they learned in exercise into daily function. Although occupational therapists have always centered treatment around functional activities, during the past few decades therapists may have treated daily activities as secondary in their attempt to integrate older neurophysiologic treatment approaches. Currently available information supports the use of functional tasks as primary intervention tools (Boxes 5-1 and 5-2). The tasks should specifically address the balance component disturbances that have been identified during evaluation so that occupational therapists can provide treatment that is individualized and extremely functional.

*References 4, 19, 21, 22, 23, 27, 28, 29, 31, 36, 37, 42, 43.

Box 5-1

Sample Treatment Activities and Goals While in Standing Postures

Static standing (no engagement in activity) graded by timed tolerance for the posture
Static standing while holding a glass of water
Standing while fastening shirt closures
Retrieving an object (graded by size and weight of object) from a shelf at chest level
Retrieving an object from a shelf at knee level (graded by weight and size of object)
Pulling up pants from ankles while standing
Setting table, including covering table with table cloth
Opening refrigerator and retrieving object from top shelf
Opening refrigerator and retrieving object from bottom shelf
Removing shoes while standing
Donning pajama pants while standing
Picking up phone book from floor
Placing full pet food bowl on floor
Retrieving pot or pan from lower cabinet

The treatment activities above do not necessarily represent a progression of difficulty.

Box 5-2

Sample Treatment Activities and Goals for Ambulatory Patients

Carrying empty shopping bag 30 feet (graded by distance and surface)
Carrying bag of groceries 30 feet (graded by weight, distance, and surface)
Carrying a half-full glass of water 30 feet
Carrying a full glass of water 30 feet
Carrying a full cup on a saucer 30 feet
Walking upstairs without upper extremity support
Walking upstairs carrying laundry basket

The treatment activities above do not necessarily represent a progression of difficulty.

TREATING ASYMMETRIC WEIGHT DISTRIBUTION

Patients who have had a CVA often have an impaired ability to control their center of mass over their base of support.[41] These patients often assume an asymmetrical posture during activities that require both static and dynamic balance skills. Asymmetrical posture and poor upright stability have been correlated with an increased risk for falls.[41] In addition, an unstable upright posture has also been correlated with functional assessment on the Barthel index.[25] Wu et al[41] state the "one functional goal in rehabilitating persons with hemiplegia should be . . . to improve symmetrical characteristics of postural control." The most common form of treatment for asymmetrical weight bearing and poor postural control is using both passive and active weight shifting.[12] This treatment has traditionally been provided in the form of exercise or introduction of outside perturbations to encourage postural reactions. The underlying assumption is that practicing the repetition of postural adjustments will result in long-term improvements in balance during ambulation and functional activities.[12] Numerous authors have advocated the use of passive and active weight shifting as a viable treatment approach.[5,6,7,39] If patients are not able to actively shift their weight, they may initially need guidance from the therapist and assistance with moving in effective patterns. Patients must also be able to actively shift their weight. Active weight shifting requires postural adjustments that are intrinsic to the activity being performed.[12] Patients must be able to initiate and execute a skilled weight shift that is an appropriate response to the perturbation actually experienced to maintain balance. Patients who experience difficulty with perceiving weight shifts and limits of stability may overestimate or underestimate the amount of weight shift required to adjust to the perturbation. Other patients may know the needed weight shift but may not be able to execute the coordinated motor movements and timing to make it effective.

Treatment for patients should focus on value-added occupations specific to individual patients. Information gained during the patient interview can be used to determine in which performance areas a patient is experiencing balance deficits (e.g., donning pants while standing, reaching into a lower cabinet during meal preparation) as well as which activities are valued by the patient. Occupational therapists must perform task analyses to determine which weight shifts are required to complete the tasks patients want to perform. Information from the component evaluation (e.g., poor ability to shift center of mass laterally and anteriorly when reaching up to a high cabinet in the kitchen) should also be considered when making the treatment plan.

Incorporating active weight shifting into a specific activity allows patients to learn more normal postural responses to particular activities; therapists do not have to assume training has transferred from an exercise to an activity. Therapists can also be sure that the type of weight shifting they are asking patients to do are appropriate for particular tasks. Patients are then able to incorporate an anticipatory set based on the specific task, an important component of motor learning. Activities can be graded by the amount of weight shifting required, size of the base of support, and complexity of the task. Weight shifting can occur as a result of present anticipatory controls (e.g., shifting the center of gravity laterally to prepare to don pants while standing) or outside perturbations (e.g., getting on or off an escalator). Weight shifts can also occur in response to movement that is initiated by the upper extremities (e.g., putting a table cloth on a table). These activities can be made more difficult by gradually increasing the force required by the upper extremities to perform the task (e.g., picking up an empty suitcase and then a full suitcase). Activities can be broken down into a hierarchy of tasks ranging from simple to more complex. Tasks should be selected based on patients' abilities as well as their typical daily activities. For example, the task of making a bed requires numerous weight shifts but would not be an appropriate activity for a patient who did not make beds before the CVA.

Patients may be able to use a variety of feedback mechanisms to improve symmetrical postural alignment. They can be instructed to use somatosensory information about pressure they receive through their feet while weight shifting (if sensation is intact). If patients have a lateral bias, they may need to be cued by the therapist. For example, a therapist can cue a patient with an anterior or posterior bias to locate foot pressure in relation to the balls of the feet.

Patients may also be instructed to use visual information. Therapists may need to use a mirror for patients with a posterior bias so that the patients can see they are drifting away from the mirror. This method may be most appropriate when performing self-care tasks that normally involve the use of a mirror.

TREATMENT PLANNING

As stated previously, the central nervous system uses information from the visual, vestibular, and somatosensory systems to maintain balance. Shumway-Cook and Horak[32] state that the central nervous system uses this feedback to monitor the relationship between the position of the body in space and the forces acting on it. The therapist must incorporate information obtained from the component balance assessment (specifically, from the test of sensory organization) into the treatment planning process. The therapist will usually be able to establish a correlation between functional observations and assessments from the test for sensory organization. Therapists should be able to identify functional tasks that place patients at risk for loss of balance; these activities can become part of the treatment plan (Table 5-3). Patients who lose their balance while transitioning from linoleum to carpeting in their house usually perform poorly under testing conditions forcing patients to maintain balance on uneven surfaces. Likewise, patients who lose their balance while walking in a mall or busy area with a great deal of peripheral movement usually perform poorly under the testing conditions forcing patients to maintain their balance while receiving conflicting visual input. Therapists need to observe patients' performances during component testing as well as functional tasks. Therapists must also determine possible

Table 5-3

Correlation of Component Testing and Functional Activities

SENSORY INFORMATION	STRATEGIES	TASK
1. Difficulty with #4, 5, 6 (sway reference support)	Absent hip strategy	Standing on carpet while opening into lower drawer with flexed hips and knees, walking outside on grass or beach and picking up object off ground, getting on or off escalator or moving sidewalk
2. Difficulty with #2, 3, 5, 6 (visual conflict)	Excessive ankle/step strategies	Walking in mall, scanning items in kitchen cabinets, scanning items in grocery store, hanging clothes on line out of basket, rinsing shampoo out of hair while in shower with eyes closed and head tipped back
3. Difficulty with #5, 6 (must rely on vestibular input)	Delayed strategies	Getting up at night to go to bathroom (i.e., walking in low light down carpeted hallway and transitioning to linoleum in bathroom), walking in dark movie theater down incline while searching for seat
4. Difficulty with #4, 5, 6	None or delayed lateral hip strategies	Standing on one foot to don pants, standing in near tandem to reach up or down into cabinet, walking from one point to another, standing in near tandem to pick something up off of floor (e.g., cat's dish)

compensations or strategies patients may use when one or more systems are impaired. Patients with somatosensory dysfunctions usually become visually dependent whereas patients with visual disturbances usually become dependent on surfaces. Patients with vestibular dysfunctions may become either visually or surface dependent. These compensatory strategies can work for patients in isolated environments but will prevent true independence and result in a higher risk for falls for patients who are active in the home and/or community. Patients will often limit their participation in home activities or simply stop going out into the community as a way to compensate for balance deficits, resulting in social isolation or depression. This information can be obtained from the initial patient interview.

After determining which systems are impaired, therapists should identify activities that are important to the patient and involve those systems. Those impaired systems can be gradually challenged to relearn adaptation by controlling the conditions in which the activities are performed. Surface-dependent patients may be more likely to lose their balance when transitioning from one surface to another in the home (i.e., from the kitchen linoleum to the living room carpet). Carrying an object from the kitchen into the living room may be a functional task that places patients at risk for loss of balance. Therapists can develop a treatment plan that initially requires patients to practice holding an item while standing on an uneven surface. The next step would be to have patients reach for an item while standing on an uneven surface. Patients would then carry an item as they transitioned from an uneven surface to an even surface and vice versa. These particular patients would also be at risk for loss of balance during other func-

tional tasks that required community (beyond the household) ambulation. Curbs, sidewalks, gravel, grass, and sand are all uneven surfaces. The somatosensory information received from the feet of surface-dependent patients tells the central nervous system that the patients are falling. A balance reaction that is inappropriate to the task (e.g., walking on an uneven surface) but appropriate to the information the central nervous system receiving and processing may result. Therapists should first have patients practice simple functional tasks on uneven surfaces and then increase the challenge by asking them to engage in more complex tasks while transitioning to and from uneven and even surfaces. The tasks should be meaningful to patients and related to their lifestyles.

Visually dependent patients often are at risk for loss of balance when their vision is obscured for any reason (e.g., when they are in the dark or poorly-lit areas) or "false" visual information is received by the central nervous system (e.g., peripheral images of people walking past patients telling the central nervous system they are falling forward when they are not).

Patients may be at risk for losing their balance when getting up in the middle of the night to get a drink or go to the bathroom, walking in a movie theater, or taking a night-time stroll outside if they are too reliant on their vision. Treatment plans can be developed that require patients to perform various activities in low lighting or with obscured vision. Common examples of this include closing the eyes in the shower while rinsing out shampoo, stepping from a brightly lit environment into a darker environment, and carrying a glass of liquid while walking. (Patients must keep their eyes on the glass rather than on the floor and the environment to make sure they do not spill the contents). Even walking while engaged in conversation can be difficult for visually-dependent patients because people normally look at one another rather than the environment while talking.

Patients may also lose their balance during functional activities if they have difficulty with head-eye coordination and gaze stabilization. Activities such as walking in a busy mall, scanning the grocery store shelves for items, and placing groceries on various shelves can all cause loss of balance. The central nervous system is unable to override the false visual information that results from these tasks and thus the patients feel they are losing their balance. Patients then institute postural reactions that are incongruent with the actual events that are occurring. Treatment plans can be developed that challenge patients' ability to maintain gaze stability during functional activities requiring coordinated head-eye movements.

Patients with impaired vestibular function are generally visually and surface dependent, although they usually rely more heavily on one system. Patients with premorbid health issues may be more reliant on one system for a predetermined reason. For example, patients with diabetic neuropathies may be more visually dependent because they do not have access to somatosensory information through their lower extremities. Most traditional treatment approaches have relied on graded, repetitive head movements in the form of exercise to improve vestibular functions.[8,11] Cohen et al[10] outline a treatment approach that incorporates this basic premise into functional activity. They stress that treatment activities must include head movements and positions that elicit the vestibular dysfunction during assessment. They also stress that activities must be interesting to patients; their use may assist patients with relating to real-life experiences. Suggested activities include retrieving towels in a basket on the floor and hanging them on an overhead clothesline, ambulating in the hallways while scanning and describing objects placed at various heights,

playing badminton, and dribbling a basketball back and forth across the room. A thorough and accurate assessment of the specific impaired balance deficit is necessary to design the most efficacious treatment plan.

RETRAINING BALANCE STRATEGIES

As discussed previously, part of the balance assessment is assessing what patients do to regain their balance. Three strategies were outlined as normal balance strategies—ankle, hip, and step strategies. A component assessment allows therapists to determine whether a strategy is being used, the amount of delay in strategy use (and therefore its effectiveness), and whether the appropriate strategy is being used. Therapists must be able to complete skilled, accurate task analyses to determine which strategy should be employed in particular activities. Therapists should see a correlation between functional activity observations and the results of component testing. This information can be used to determine which functional activities may place patients at risk for loss of balance. The identified activities may then become part of the treatment plan (see Table 5-3).

Treatment plans can also be designed to elicit the use of appropriate balance strategies. Ankle strategies can be elicited by asking patients to engage in tasks requiring small weight shifts on solid support surfaces that are larger than their feet. For example, patients could reach up into a cabinet to put away groceries or put away laundry on a shelf in a closet. Hip strategies can be elicited by asking patients to engage in tasks requiring larger weight shifts on narrow bases of support. These tasks could include playing toss and catch on a balance beam. Hip strategies can also be elicited by asking patients to reach into drawers or cabinets without locking their knees in extension; hip flexion will be necessary to counteract the resulting anterior weight shift (Figure 5-5). Step strategies can be elicited by engaging patients in activities that require them

Figure 5-5 **A,** Knees are hyperextended and locked during functional activity, weight shifted forward onto the upper extremities. Upper extremities used as a base of support rather than for function. **B,** Hips and knees are flexed (as during hip strategy use) to allow center of mass to remain over lower extremity base of support. Upper extremities are free to be used for function.

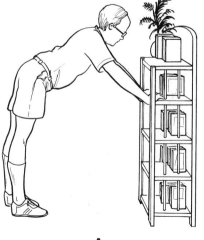

A

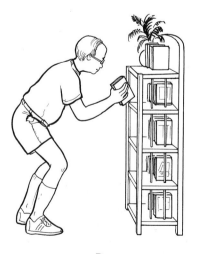

B

to make weight shifts outside of their base of support, such as hitting a tennis ball against a wall or reaching out of their base of support to pick up work boots off the floor.

OTHER FACTORS AFFECTING TREATMENT PLANNING

Therapists must consider other factors that may impair patients' balance while functioning. An extremely common factor that is often overlooked, especially in inpatient rehabilitation, is endurance. When patients are treated in an inpatient setting, they are often not asked to entirely complete tasks. For example, when bathing or dressing, the therapist may unintentionally "help" patients who are bathing or dressing by gathering their clothes or getting towels. Inpatients also often have large periods of time between therapy sessions when they are not engaged in activity. Therefore a rehabilitation day may have a great deal of therapy hours, but it does not accurately reflect patients' daily home life.

In the hospital, patients usually have breakfast brought to them and often eat it in bed. They may then have a break before occupational therapists arrive to address self-care tasks. Patients may then have another break before physical therapists arrive to address mobility activities. This type of schedule can result in an inaccurate picture of patients' independence and clearly does consider whether patients' endurance levels will affect their balance at home. Therapists need to devise a treatment plan that resembles the patients' typical day at home as closely as possible.

Other factors that can influence a patient's balance during functional activities are cognitive and visual perception impairments. Familiar, functionally based activities can help to reduce the effects of these impairments, but clearly occupational therapists must address these issues during treatment as well.

Medical factors such as infections, metabolic disturbances, and medications can also affect a patient's balance skills. Any significant changes observed by a therapist should be immediately reported to the physician.

■

CASE STUDY

MJ is 58-year-old female who was diagnosed with a right middle cerebral artery CVA. She was first assessed by an inpatient rehabilitation occupational therapist who determined that the patient had difficulty controlling her balance during bathing, grooming, and dressing. The patient stated that she wanted to independently perform all of these activities. The therapist noted that MJ had a postural bias to the right with both static and dynamic balance, used a very wide base of support during functional tasks, and was unable to control her center of gravity when shifting her leg to the left to complete a task. Component testing revealed left hemiplegia, but MJ was able to support weight on her left lower extremity. Sensation was impaired but not absent in her left lower extremity. MJ's per-

ceived limits of stability were not congruent with her actual limits of stability. She underestimated her ability to shift weight to the left and thus could not complete tasks that required her to shift weight to the left. When assisted with a left weight shift, MJ was not able to control the shift because of poor coordination and timing of muscle activation. Because she lost control whenever she shifted weight to the left, MJ compensated by maintaining an asymmetric postural alignment. When asked to actively shift her weight to the left, MJ altered her postural alignment by attempting to shift her shoulders rather than her center of mass.

Treatment initially centered on assisting MJ passively and then actively to achieve and maintain a symmetric postural alignment during static standing tasks. The therapist selected parts of self-care tasks that did not require large weight shifts (e.g., combing her hair, washing her face, selecting clothing from her closet) and focused on maintaining midline. The therapist helped MJ learn to use visual and somatosensory information when possible to provide information about her position in space.

As MJ improved her ability to achieve and maintain midline during additional static standing tasks, the therapist began to introduce tasks requiring a more significant weight shift from right to left (e.g., putting on her shirt while standing, reaching for objects on the sink, getting objects out of the closet that were placed to elicit a left weight shift). Emphasis was placed on assisting MJ with developing an awareness of her actual limits of stability. As MJ's control improved, the therapist also focused on narrowing her base of support to the more normal site dictated by particular activities. MJ improved to the point that she could maintain midline and actively shift weight laterally during self-care activities without assistance from the therapist.

■

DOCUMENTATION

Accurate documentation should include a full evaluation, description of the treatment plan, short- and long-term goals, and patient outcomes, which must be functional and measurable. Because of the current climate of managed health care, documentation should be as streamlined as possible and easily understood by any person who accesses the information, including other team members, case managers, third-party payors, and patients and family members. The documentation format should span the continuum of care and easily be adjusted to meet the patient's needs and for the setting in which intervention is being provided (e.g., inpatient rehabilitation, outpatient clinic).

Documentation can help structure thought processes as well as reinforce clinical reasoning skills in the areas of assessment, treatment planning, and establishment of goals. Documentation tools should be reliable, valid, sensitive, and specific and should reflect real-life situations. If possible, one multipurpose form should be used.

Specific balance component assessments can be accomplished by utilizing any of the assessments discussed previously, including sensory organization, balance strategy, and actual and perceived limits of stability testing. Documentation should also include an evaluation of physical status (e.g., ROM, strength).

One documentation tool is the functional independence day (FID) form.[14] Figure 5-6 is an example of a FID form that was used in an inpatient rehabilitation program. The FID form is used to generate a list of activities that can be adapted and individualized for patients based on one of their typical days. The example given in Figure 5-6 involves getting up in the morning, bathing, dressing, and carrying out simple homemaking tasks. The activity can be rated simply as pass or fail—that is, patients are either able to accomplish a task without losing their balance or are not. In this manner, the FID form could serve as the initial evaluation for function.

Assessments of function could be completed on a weekly, biweekly, or monthly basis, depending on the setting in which services are being provided. Four weeks of progress are included in Figure 5-6, so the FID information could also be the functional status portion of a weekly or monthly progress note. Progress could be further documented by distinguishing whether an activity was completed in a wheelchair or while ambulating level. A space for comments could be provided for observations, such as the number of times patients lose their balance, any devices used (such as a walker or tub bench), and cues provided during the task.

A FID form should be structured to measure the effect fatigue may have on patients' balance over a period of time. Therapists can adapt the FID form to reflect a "typical" day for an individual patient (this information should have been gained on the patient interview). The order in which activities occur should reflect the order in which they normally occur for patients. Activities can be added and deleted based on patients' daily activities. The FID format could be appropriate for inpatient, outpatient, home health and even extended care settings.

A FID form also allows therapists to quickly see which activities are difficult for the patient. Combined with the diagnosis, prognosis, and data from the evaluation, this information could assist the therapist in determining appropriate short- and long-term goals. The environment for therapy services will also have an influence on the choice of goals. Because of shorter lengths of stay, patients leaving inpatient settings may not even have independent goals for basic activities such as bathing and dressing if a family member is available to assist. Outpatient and home health therapists and clinicians providing treatment in subacute or extended care settings may be assisting the patient with basic activities as well as household management and community tasks. A FID form could readily assist the therapist with identifying specific problematic activities and allow the therapist can to directly address these activities without spending extensive time and effort reassessing the patient.

A FID form could also be used for patient and family education. The form is easy for patients and families to understand and clearly identifies activities the patient can complete independently or requires assistance with. The therapist could use the form during a hands-on demonstration of these tasks and show the family the way to assist the patient. Families and patients could be given a copy of this form so that they can see the progress that has been made as well as the type of assistance required.

A FID form could also be used for the discharge evaluation. It clearly tracks a patient's progress toward goals and status on discharge. The form could then be forwarded to the next care setting in the continuum and used as a source of information not only about initial evaluation and discharge status but also weekly or monthly progress. Specific skill component assessment information should also be forwarded.

One potential problem with using a FID format is the amount of time necessary to complete the assessment, especially if tasks are performed in the time frame described by the patient. One way to address the issue of time and ensure that all team members are working toward consistent, patient-centered goals is to share the responsibility of the evaluation among team members. This can be accomplished by arranging back-to-back therapy sessions (i.e., blocking off a large amount of time to assess one patient). Because task performance is rated on a pass/fail basis (and therefore the subjectivity involved when grading a test is not an issue), the assessment can be carried out by many team members. Once the assessment is complete, team members can collaborate to determine the treatment focus for the next week, set short- and long-term goals, and arrange discharge plans.

Another potential problem is that in some settings, such as subacute or extended care, performance of specific relevant tasks may be limited by space and/or equipment. Occupational therapists must improvise as much as possible to simulate a patient's typical day and work within the confines of the treatment setting.

The FID form is just one example of a documentation system that meets previously discussed criteria for documentation tools. Every setting is unique, so therapists should develop documentation formats that meet the needs of the patients served in each particular setting and must ensure documentation is focused on functional outcomes.

BALANCE ASSESSMENTS

In addition to those mentioned, numerous other functional balance assessments have been developed.[15,18,26,33] A brief overview of several of these assessments follows.

- The "get up and go" test requires the patient to stand up from a chair with armrests, walk a short distance,

Functional Independence Day

Patient name: _____

Diagnosis: _____

General comments (including general observations of balance, consistent direction of bias, reactions or loss of balance, cognitive/perceptual status, interfering factors): _____

_____

_____

_____

_____

Activity Evaluation date: Level: wheelchair (WC) or ambulatory (amb)				Comments (Note cues, assistive device, assistance, or # of loss of balance/posture)
Rolling				
Moving from supine to sitting				
Transferring out of bed				
Gathering necessary items for dressing				
Going to shower				
Undressing				
Transferring into shower				
Showering				
Transferring out of shower				
Drying off				
Dressing				
Going to room				
Putting away items				
Stripping bed				
Going to laundry				
Returning to room				
Making bed				
Gathering breakfast items				
Preparing meal				
Placing tablecloth				
Setting table				
Cleaning up (loading dishwasher)				
Vacuuming rug				
Going back to room				

Figure 5-6 Functional independence day. (Courtesy Susan Donato, Karen Pulaski, Diane MacKenzie, Karen McManus, Eileen Wusteny.)

turn around, return to the chair, and sit again.[26] Performance is rated on a somewhat nonspecific 5-point scale. This test is used with the older adult population and because of its vague rating criteria, the criteria should be established in a facility if used as an assessment tool.[30]

- The clinical test of of sensory organization and balance,[32] which was previously described, uses six test conditions to assess an individual's ability to access, utilize, and organize sensory information. Within this formalized procedure, tests are timed, the amount of sway is measured, and complete loss of balance falls are recorded. This test is also appropriate for use in children, patients with hemiplegia,[13] and patients with vestibular disorders.[9]

- The functional reach test[15] requires the patient to stand next to a wall with a yardstick placed parallel to the floor. The patient is asked to reach as far forward as possible, and the reach length is measured. This test is quick and easy to perform and does not require expensive equipment. Test/retest and interrator reliability are high.[15,40] It has been used with a variety of populations spanning children through the elderly.[15,16,40] The disadvantage of this exam is that it only measures one functional task and only assesses skills in the anterior direction.[30]

- The Tinetti test[38] assesses balance and gait. A specific scoring method is used and some education about the test is needed to administer it. For example, gait rating involves the observing of several aspects of gait, including step symmetry and step length. This test is also fairly quick and is easy to administer. It has been developed for and is used primarily with older adults.

- The Berg balance scale[2] test is more time consuming. A number of factors are examined, such as unsupported sitting and standing, transfers, reaching forward, picking objects up from the floor, turning 360°, and standing on one foot, and each is graded on a 5-point scale. The specific scoring criteria are outlined in the assessment. This test examines many aspects of balance and has been shown to have high interrelator reliability and validity in older adults.[1,2,3,30] This test has been primarily developed for and utilized with the older population and stroke patients.[2,3]

The assessment and treatment of balance disorders for recovering stroke patients are extremely complex. Therapists need to understand the balance system as well as have a comprehensive way to assess balance function and dysfunction. They then determine realistic short- and long-term goals that are appropriate for each patient based on diagnostic and evaluation information. A comprehensive treatment plan should be devised to improve specific balance deficits and ultimately assist the patient with transitioning to a more independent lifestyle.

REVIEW QUESTIONS

1. Name the three sensory systems involved in balance control and describe their roles.
2. What purpose do automatic postural responses serve in balance control?
3. What is the role of the cerebellum in balance control?
4. What comprises a component assessment of balance skills?
5. Describe three balance assessments.
6. Why should a therapist observe a patient during functional activity? What information should be gathered?
7. In what way does a therapist determine the focus of treatment (e.g., remediation or compensation)?
8. In what way does occupational therapy's treatment of balance deficits differ from traditional physical therapy treatment?
9. Describe the concept and benefits of using a FID flow sheet.

■ COTA Considerations ■

- Impairments of the visual, vestibular, or somatosensory systems may result in balance dysfunction.
- A subjective interview is critical for a stroke survivor with balance dysfunction. Questions should center on subjects such as premorbid health and function, lifestyle, and perceptions of past and current functioning.
- Balance evaluations should include both component evaluations and assessments of balance during functional tasks.
- A thorough evaluation and team approach must be utilized to determine whether a treatment plan should focus on compensation, remediation, or both.
- Graded functional activities that are meaningful to the patient and incorporate postural strategies and weight shifting are the treatments of choice for balance dysfunction.

REFERENCES

1. Berg K: Balance and its measure in the elderly: a review, *Physiother Can* 41:240, 1989.
2. Berg KD, Maki BE et al: Clinical and laboratory measures of postural balance in the elderly population, *Arch Phys Med Rehabil* 73:1073, 1992.
3. Berg K, Wook-Dauphinee S, Williams J: The balance scale: reliability assessment with elderly residents and patients with an acute stroke, *Scand J Rehabil Med* 27:27, 1995.
4. Block M, Smith D, Nelson D: Heart rate, activity, duration and affect in added-purpose versus single-purpose jumping activities, *Am J Occup Ther* 43:25, 1989.
5. Bobath B: *Adult hemiplegia: evaluation and treatment*, ed 2, London, 1978, William Heinemann.
6. Brunnstrom S: *Movement therapy in hemiplegia*, New York, 1970, Harper & Row.
7. Carr J, Shepherd R: *Physiotherapy in disorders of the brain*, Rockville, Md, 1980, Aspen.
8. Cawthorne T: The physiological basis for head exercises, *Charter Soc Physiother* 29:106, 1994.

9. Cohen H, Biathy CA, Gombash LL: A study of the clinical test of sensory interaction and balance, *Phys Ther* 73:346, 1993.

10. Cohen H et al: Vestibular rehabilitation with graded occupations, *Am J Occup Ther* 49:362, 1995.

11. Cooksey F: Physical medicine, *Practitioner* 155:300, 1945.

12. Daleiden S: Weight shifting as a treatment for balance deficits: a literature review, *Physiother Can* 42:81, 1990.

13. DiFabio RP, Badke MB: Extraneous eye movement associated with hemiplegic posture sway during dynamic goal-directed weight distribution, *Arch Phys Med Rehabil* 11:365, 1990.

14. Donato S et al: *Functional Independence Day.* Paper presented CanAm Occupational Therapy Association Annual Conference, Boston, 1994.

15. Duncan P et al: Functional reach: a new clinical measure of balance, *J Gerontol* 45:192, 1990.

16. Duncan PW et al: Functional reach: predictive validity in a sample of elderly male veterans, *J Gerontol* 473:93, 1992.

17. Easton T: On the normal use of reflexes, *Am Sci* 60:591, 1972.

18. Fregly A, Graybiel A: An ataxia battery not requiring rails, *Aerospace Med* 3:277, 1968.

19. Heck S: The effect of purposeful activity on pain tolerance, *Am J Occup Ther* 42:577, 1988.

20. Hsieh C et al: A comparison of performance in added-purpose occupations and rote exercise for dynamic standing balance in persons with hemiplegia, *Am J Occup Ther* 50:38, 1996.

21. Kircher M: Motivation as a factor of perceived exertion in purposeful versus nonpurposeful activity, *Am J Occup Ther* 38:165, 1984.

22. Lang E, Nelson D, Bush M: Comparison of performance in materials-based occupation, imagery-based occupation, and rote exercise in nursing home residents, *Am J Occup Ther* 46:607, 1992.

23. Licht B, Nelson D: Adding meaning to a design copy task through representational stimuli, *Am J Occup Ther* 44:408, 1990.

24. Magnus R: Some results of studies in the psychology of posture, *Lancet* 2:531, 1926.

25. Mahoney F, Barhel D: Functional evaluation: the Barthel index, *M Med J* 14:61, 1965.

26. Mathias S, Nayak USL, Isaacs B: Balance in the elderly patient: the "get up and go test," *Arch Phys Med Rehabil* 67:387, 1986.

27. Miller L, Nelson D: Dual-purpose activity vs. single-purpose activity in terms of duration on task, exertion level, and effect, *Occup Ther Ment Health* 7:55, 1987.

28. Morton G, Barnett D, Hale L: A comparison of performance measures of an added-purpose task versus a single-purpose task for upper extremities, *Am J Occup Ther* 46:128, 1992.

29. Mullins C, Nelson D, Smith D: Exercise through dual-purpose activity in the institutionalized elderly, *Phys Occup Ther Geriatr* 5:29, 1987.

30. Poole JL, Whitney SL: Can balance assessments predict falls in the elderly? 1995 American Occupational Therapy Association.

31. Riccia C, Nelson D, Bush M: Adding purpose to the repetitive exercise of elderly women through imagery, *Am J Occup Ther* 44:714, 1990.

32. Shumway-Cook A, Horak FB: Assessing the influence of sensory interaction on balance, *Phys Ther* 6610:1548, 1986.

33. Shumway-Cook A, Horak FB: Balance disorders assessment, *NERA*, 1992.

34. Shumway-Cook A, Horak FB: Balance rehabilitation in the neurological patient, *NERA*, 1992.

35. Shumway-Cook A, Olmscheld R: A systems analysis of postural dyscontrol in traumatically brain-injured patients, *J Head Trauma Rehabil* 5:51, 1990.

36. Steinbeck T: Purposeful activity and performance, *Am J Occup Ther* 40:529, 1986.

37. Thibodeaux C, Ludwig F: Intrinsic motivation in product-oriented and non–product-oriented activities, *Am J Occup Ther* 42:169, 1988.

38. Tinetti ME: Performance-oriented assessment of mobility problems in elderly patients, *J Am Geriatr Soc* 34:119, 1986.

39. Voss D: Proprioceptive neuromuscular facilitation, *Am J Phys Med* 46:838, 1985.

40. Weiner DK et al: Functional reach: a marker of physical frailty, *J Am Geriatr Soc* 40:203, 1992.

41. Wu S et al: Effects of a program on symmetrical posture in patients with hemiplegia: a single-subject design, *Am J Occup Ther* 50:17, 1996.

42. Yoder R, Nelson D, Smith D: Added-purpose versus rote exercise in female nursing home residents, *Am J Occup Ther* 43:581, 1989.

43. Yuen H: *The purposeful use of an object in the development of skill with a prosthesis*, master's thesis, Kalamazoo, 1988, Western Michigan University.

SUGGESTED READING

Badke MR, Duncan PW: Patterns of rapid motor responses during postural adjustments when standing in healthy subjects and hemiplegic patients, *Phys Ther* 63:13, 1983.

Black FO et al: Central vestibular disorders. In Bailey BJ, editor: *Head and neck surgery; otolaryngology*, Philadelphia, 1992, JB Lippincott.

Brook V: Motor control—how posture and movements are governed, *Phys Ther* 63:669, 1983.

Corab PJ, Nashner LM: Properties of postural adjustments associated with rapid arm movements, *J Neurophysiol* 47:287, 1982.

Crutchfield C, Shumway-Cook A, Horak FB: Balance and coordination. In Scully R, Barnes M, editors: *Physical therapy*, New York, 1988, JB Lippincott.

DiFabio R, Badke M: Relationship of sensory organization to balance function in patients with hemiplegia, *Phys Ther* 70:543, 1990.

Feldman AG, Levin MF: The origin and use of positional frames of reference in motor control, *Behav Brain Sci* 18:723, 1995.

Fergly A, Graybiel A, Smitty M: Walk on floor, eyes closed WFEC. A new addition to an alaxia test battery, *Aerospace Med* 43:395, 1972.

Forssberg H, Nashner LM: Otogenetic development of postural control in man: adaptation to altered support and visual conditions during stance, *J Neurosci* 2:545, 1982.

Gliner JA: Purposeful activity in motor learning theory: an event approach to motor skill acquisition. *Am J Occup Ther* 39:28, 1985.

Herdman S: Assessment and treatment of balance disorders in the vestibular-deficient patient, *Balance*, American Physical Therapy Association, 1994.

Horak FB: Clinical measurement of postural control in adults, *Phys Ther* 67:1881, 1987.

Horak F: Role of basal ganglia in posture and movement, *Neurology Newsletter*, 3:7, American Physical Therapy Association, 1979.

Horak FB: Set and gain control of posture in cerebellar and vestibular patients, *IEEE Trans Biomed Eng* 11:95, 1992.

Horak FB et al: The effects of movement velocity, mass displaced and task certainty on associated postural adjustments made by normal and hemiplegic individuals, *J Neurol Neurosurg Psychol* 47:1020, 1984.

Horak BF, Diener HC, Nashner LM: Influence of central set on human postural response, *J Neurophysiol* 62:841, 1989.

Horak GB, Nashner LM, Diener HC: Postural strategies associated with somatosensory and vestibular loss, *Exp Brain Res* 82:167, 1990.

Horak FB, Nashner LM, Nutt JG: Postural instability in Parkinson's disease: motor coordination and sensory organization, *Neurology Rep* 12:54, 1988.

Horak FB, Shupert C: Multitask tests of cerebellar operations, *Behav Brain Sci* 1992.

Horak FB, Shupert CL, Mirka A: Components of postural dyscontrol in the elderly, *Neurobiol Aging* 10:727, 1989.

Jeka J, Lackner JR: The role of haptic cues from rough and slippery surfaces in human postural control, *Exp Brain Res* 103:267, 1995.

Lee WA: A control system framework for understanding normal and abnormal posture, *Am J Occup Ther* 43:291, 1989.

Lee WA: Anticipatory control of postural and task muscles during rapid arm flexion, *J Motor Behav* 12:185, 1980.

Levine M, Lackner J: Some sensory and motor factors influencing the control and appreciation of eye and limb position, *Exp Brain Res* 36:275, 1979.

MacPherson JM, Horak FB, Dunbar DC: Stance dependence of automatic postural adjustments in humans, *Exp Brain Res* 118:557, 1989.

Martin JP: A short essay on posture and movement, *J Neurol Neurosurg Psychiatry* 40:25, 1977.

Nashner LM: Adaptation of human movement to altered environments, *Trends Neurosci* 5:358, 1982.

Nashner LM, Forssberg H: Phase-dependent organization of postural adjustments associated with arm movements while walking, *J Neurophysiol* 55:1382, 1986.

Nashner LM, Shupert C, Horak FB: Head-trunk movement coordination in the standing posture. In Pomperano O, Allum J, editors: *Prog Brain Res* 76:243, 1988.

Shumway-Cook A, Anson D, Haller S: Postural sway biofeedback: its affect of reestablishing stance stability in hemiplegic patients, *Arch Phys Med Rehabil* 69:395, 1988.

Shumway-Cook A, McCollum G: Assessment and treatment of balance disorders. In Montgomery T, Connolly B, editors: *Motor control for physical therapy*, 1991, Chattanooga Corporation.

Shumway-Cook A, Woollacott M: The growth of stability: postural control from a developmental perspective, *J Motor Behav* 1985.

Shupert CL et al: Automatic responses to head/neck pertorbations. In Brandt T et al, editors: *Disorders of posture and gait*, Stuttgart, 1990, Georgia Thieme Verlag.

Stein R: Peripheral control of movement, *Physiol Rev* 54:215, 1974.

Winstein CJ et al: Standing balance training: effect on balance and locomotion in hemiparetic adults, *Arch Phys Med Rehabil* 70:755, 1989.

Woollacott MH, Bonnet M, Yabe K: Preparatory process for anticipatory postural adjustments: modulation of leg muscle reflex pathways during preparation for arm movements in standing man, *Exp Brain Res* 55:263, 1984.

Woollacott M, Shumway-Cook A: Changes in posture control across the lifespan, *Movement Science*, American Physical Therapy Association, 1991.

Woollacott M, Shumway-Cook A, Nashner LM: Aging and posture control: changes in sensory organization and muscular coordination, *Int J Aging Hum Dev* 22:329, 1986.

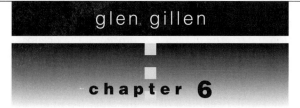

glen gillen

chapter **6**

Upper Extremity Function and Management

key terms

motor control	ADL/IADL	spasticity
subluxation	positioning	learned nonuse
pain	shoulder-hand syndrome	reaching
shoulder supports	activity analysis	manipulation
impingement	postural control	weight bearing
biomechanical alignment	contracture/deformity	orthopedic complications
function	weakness	

chapter objectives

After completing this chapter, the reader will be able to accomplish the following:

1. Identify the common biomechanical malalignments seen in the upper extremity and trunk after stroke, and recognize their impact on function.
2. Develop treatment plans to regain upper extremity function through the use of functional tasks.
3. Understand the application of adjunctive treatments for the upper extremity after stroke including treatments such as positioning, shoulder supports, biofeedback, and stretching programs.
4. Choose functional treatment activities appropriate to the level of available motor control.
5. Understand evaluation and treatment procedures for patients with symptoms of pain syndromes and implement pain prevention protocols into current treatment plans.

Impaired upper extremity function is one of the most common and challenging sequelae of a cerebrovascular accident (CVA). The most recent large-scale study to date, the Copenhagen stroke study, included 515 stroke patients, 71% of whom received occupational and physical therapy and 69% of whom had mild to severe upper extremity dysfunction on admission; all treatment plans included a focus on upper extremity function.[101] Obviously, numerous hours of therapy are spent on this area, as well as numerous dollars. This chapter highlights problems associated with upper extremity function after a CVA, research that has been published on upper extremity function/dysfunction after stroke, and suggested evaluation and treatment techniques that focus on acquiring functional use of the extremity and preventing pain syndromes and deformities. The problems that impede functional use of the upper extremity are complex, so a thorough understanding of Chapter 2 (Learning and Environmental Strategies) before reading this chapter is suggested. (See Chapters 12 and 13 for a discussion about the impact of vision and neurobehavioral deficits on upper limb function and Chapters 4 and 5 for a discussion about the impact of impaired balance and trunk control on upper extremity function.)

CONTROVERSIES SURROUNDING INTERVENTION

"I want to use my arm again"—a goal that occupational therapists hear from stroke survivors during almost every evaluation. For therapists to assist patients with meeting this goal, a thorough understanding of the various problems associated with upper extremity dysfunction after stroke is required. It is the therapist's responsibility to stay informed of (and contribute to) the new developments in and information about upper extremity function.

Since it began, the field of occupational therapy has been addressing human activity and performance and therefore motor control issues.[31] Therapists' interventions in the area of motor function have historically been and continue to be controversial. Instead of the traditional hierarchical/neurophysiologic models of motor function, current models encompass a variety of neuromotor, biomechanic, behavioral, cognitive, environmental, and learning processes. Mathiowetz and Bass Haugen[92] have compared and contrasted the various models of motor control therapy in the past and present. Although there are pros and cons associated with all of the approaches, research comparing the effectiveness of various approaches is lacking. However it is clear that current motor behavior research supports a treatment technique well known to occupational therapists—the use of function-based tasks.

The use of functional activities has formed the basis of occupational therapy since its inception.[95] However, the complex problems that interfere with upper extremity function may require an integrated treatment approach that uses functional tasks as the intervention foundation and hands-on approaches (e.g., handling, mobilization, soft-tissue elongation) as adjuncts to intervention. Examples of treatment techniques using current theories of motor behavior in therapy that is focused on improving performance of functional activities can be found in the literature.[50,61,114]

As the body of knowledge concerning motor behavior continues to grow, therapists must critically analyze research findings as well as their own clinical practices. Burgess[31] reminds us, "A danger in times of transition and rapid change is a distraction from basic principles. When faced with a choice between conventional and new approaches, the occupational therapist should consider the following questions: Is this treatment really effective? How does it work and on what principles is it based? Is it accomplishing what is needed for this patient? Are some of the older treatment methods more solidly based, more effective, or cheaper? Are there other better ways to meet this patient's needs?"

DEFINITIONS AND CLASSIFICATIONS

A review of the literature on upper extremity function reveals a consistent problem—the lack of a definition for the word *function*. This may be attributed to the fact that a variety of disciplines are contributing information. Improved upper extremity function has been defined in terms such as deviations from basic synergies, improved/sustained muscle contraction, and increased passive range of motion (PROM). The World Health Organization's (WHO's) International Classification of Impairments, Disabilities, and Handicaps (ICIDH)[135] (see Chapter 2) is a helpful classification system that includes the following categories:

1. *Disease:* underlying pathologic process (e.g., hemorrhage, emboli)
2. *Impairment:* dysfunction at the level of an organ or system (e.g., paresis, sensory loss, decreased postural control)
3. *Disability:* dysfunction in task performance (activities of daily living [ADL], instrumental ADL [IADL], reaching and manipulation during daily tasks)
4. *Handicap:* factor that limits or prevents fulfillment of a role (e.g., parent, worker)[4,110a,135]

Using this system of classification, occupational therapists' interventions should focus on improving upper extremity function by decreasing the levels of disability and handicap. Therefore a functional improvement is an improvement that enhances the occupational performance of patients and results in improvements in performance areas (ADL, IADL, work/productive activities, leisure activities) rather than performance components (ROM, strength, postural control). It is recognized that therapists must evaluate performance components and when needed intervene for improved performance.[5]

Patients should be engaged in a functional activity when evaluation and treatment take place, although the therapist and patient may be focusing on a particular performance component of the task (e.g., focusing on the postural adjustment that enables a patient to reach for a condiment on the opposite side of a lunch table during a meal).

Hughlings Jackson's classification of observed symptoms after a central nervous system lesion is another system that is helpful for evaluating and treating the upper extremity after stroke. Jackson, a nineteenth century neurologist, classified symptoms as either positive or negative.

Positive symptoms are spontaneous, exaggerated disturbances of normal function and react to specific external stimuli. They include symptoms such as spasticity, increased deep tendon reflexes, and hyperactive flexion reflexes.

In contrast the negative symptoms are deficits of normal behavior or performance. Negative symptoms include loss of dexterity, loss of strength, and restricted ability to move.[86,87]

In the past the major focus of therapeutic interventions was to decrease the positive symptoms associated with brain lesions. Therapists worked under the assumption that a cause and effect relationship existed between the two groups of symptoms. More recently, researchers have demonstrated that the alleviation of positive symptoms (e.g., spasticity) does not automatically result in an increased ability to move. Landau[86] states, ". . . there is no evidence that what I have inferred to be entirely negative symptoms can be helped directly by reflex suppression." Therapists must therefore take a broader view when identifying and treating upper extremity problems. Focusing on only the positive symptoms will not directly result in increased function.

ACTIVITY ANALYSIS OF SELECT UPPER EXTREMITY TASKS

The following examples illustrate the complexity of upper extremity function and should assist in the evaluation process.

Reaching Task

The reaching task described requires the patient to reach for a book on a shelf that is at forehead level. First and foremost, initiation of any movement pattern requires a motivational drive to perform; therefore the activity must have an inherent purpose. The motivation behind and purpose of this activity may be to further clinical knowledge, enhance leisure time, or pass a midterm. To successfully complete this activity the patient must appropriately process visual/perceptual information collected during the scanning process before initiating the reach pattern. Because the item is above eye level, neck extension with concurrent right and left lateral head and neck rotation as well as sufficient ocular ROM are required. A variety of visual information is collected during visual scanning, which help identify particular characteristics of the book (e.g., call number, title, color, size). This information is interpreted by several visual/perceptual processes (e.g., figure ground, color discrimination, depth perception).

Before the reach pattern is initiated, the lower extremities and trunk undergo several postural adjustments to provide stabilization. The antigravity shoulder muscles prepare to bring the arm to shelf level, and the hand is prepositioned and oriented to prepare for grasping. While the reach pattern is being performed, the scapula protracts and rotates upwardly by the combination actions of the serratus anterior and upper and lower trapezius muscles. The rotator cuff keeps the humerus in a position biased toward external rotation and seats the head of the humerus in the glenoid fossa. The lower extremities and trunk stay active and stable during the performance of the pattern and may assist with a weight shift toward the shelves depending on the body position.

When the hand makes contact with the book, it is molded to the book's spine and the pattern is reversed (eccentrically), which returns the book to the side of the body. After the book is removed from the shelf, the grasp and pattern of skeletal muscle recruitment may be adjusted depending on the weight of the book. Although this activity pattern is preplanned based on prior experience, the book may be lighter or heavier than anticipated, so adjustments must be made in response to the feedback. (For example, attempting to pick up a supposedly full suitcase that is actually empty results in an exaggerated lifting motion that may cause a loss of balance.) While the book is being returned to the side, a variety of adjustments may have to be made to allow the cover of the book or call number to be seen.

Weight-Bearing Task

The weight-bearing task described requires the patient to use one arm as a postural support (i.e., extended-arm weight bearing) on a kitchen table while the other arm and hand wipe the table. As mentioned previously motivation and purpose are required. The motivation may be hunger (so the table must be cleaned in preparation for a meal), extrinsic (e.g., visitors), or work related (e.g., table space needed to balance the check book or prepare a lecture). Because the weight-bearing arm is being used as a postural support, a variety of postural adjustments occur in the arm. The weight-bearing arm is active during the task—the active skeletal muscles include (but are not limited to) the scapula muscles biased towards protraction, the elbow extensors, and the trunk muscles. The amount of skeletal muscle activity in the arm may decrease because of fatigue, resulting in a "locked" elbow, an inactive scapula biased toward an elevated position and retraction, and the trunk inactive and "hanging" on the arm.

The arm that is wiping the table must stay active and endure the entire activity if the task is going to be successful. The shoulder complex of this arm glides the hand and sponge along the table surface, so it is technically weight-bearing and moving simultaneously. The amount of force and pressure exerted on the hand depends on the demands of the task (e.g., wiping crumbs, cleaning off dried syrup).

A variety of weight shifts occur during this activity, and they are affected by the size of the table and amount of pressure needed by the wiping hand to accomplish the task. The degree and variety of motor output is specific to the demands of the task.

As with all upper extremity tasks, multiple visual/perceptual processes are required for successful completion of this task. These processes are used to locate the crumbs on the table, clean both sides of the table, and determine when the task is complete (i.e., when the table is clean).

PROBLEM-ORIENTED APPROACH TO EVALUATION AND TREATMENT

Evaluation and treatment of the upper extremity are complex tasks that require an understanding of multiple systems. Because of its complex nature, upper extremity intervention does not lend itself well to using one particular treatment approach (e.g., neurodevelopmental treatment, proprioceptive neuromuscular facilitation, Margaret Rood's approach). Many therapists use an eclectic approach to intervention.[47] Regardless of their approach, therapists need to remain open minded about their interventions and consider the complexity of causes that interfere with upper extremity use (Figure 6-1). Many of the various problems associated with upper extremity function overlap and build on each other.

Impaired Postural Control

Improving proximal stability to enhance distal mobility has long been a tenet of occupational therapy interventions. Postural adjustments stabilize supporting body parts while other parts (i.e., the upper extremities) are being moved.[63] The following studies will describe the impact of postural adjustments on arm function.

In the classic study by Belenkii and associates,[12] unimpaired subjects who were evaluated while standing were asked to raise their arm to a horizontal position after they heard an external signal. Various electromyographic (EMG) studies were performed to trace the pattern of muscle activation. The results demonstrated that the pos-

tural muscle synergies of the trunk and lower extremities were activated *before* (by 90 ms) the anterior deltoid, the primary muscle used to perform this motion. The subjects were then evaluated in the supine position while performing the same task. No lower extremity activation was detected in this position (i.e., a different pattern of postural adjustments). The following conclusions can be inferred from this study:

1. Postural adjustments are task specific.
2. Training of the upper extremity in the supine position will not automatically carry over to activities performed while sitting or standing (if postural control is a limiting factor).
3. Having different disciplines treat one particular half of the body is detrimental to patients' progress because upper extremity function depends on postural support from the lower extremities and trunk.

Bouisset and Zattara[23] replicated the previous study and demonstrated that an upward and forward trunk movement resulting from spine and/or lower limb extension precedes upper limb movement. This movement pattern is a familiar one to therapists who cue their patients to focus on spinal extension and the associated anterior pelvic tilt while treating arm function.

Horak et al[72] compared postural adjustments of subjects with and without hemiplegia during a variety of tasks with different parameters. The hemiplegic subjects demonstrated the same sequence of muscle activation as the subjects without hemiplegia, although activity on the hemiparetic side was delayed. In addition, the hemiparetic individuals were not capable of making rapid movements with the unimpaired arm. This was hypothesized to be secondary to a delay in the anticipatory activity of the con-

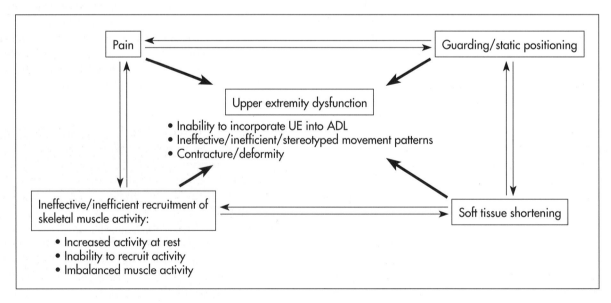

Figure 6-1 Complexity and interdependence of causes of upper extremity dysfunction.

tralateral hemiplegic muscles. This study dispels the myth that there are "good" and "bad" sides after a stroke, especially when postural control is compromised.

In their study of postural adjustments during arm movements, Cordo and Nashner[41] were able to demonstrate that when subjects' postural stability was increased (e.g., by outside shoulder support or placing a finger lightly on a support rail), postural activity was reduced and voluntary movement enhanced. This concept is crucial to understand when treating upper extremity dysfunction. As support is increased, the postural demands of the task are decreased and vice versa. The therapist can control the patient's level of postural stability by manipulating the following treatment environment factors:

- Positioning: supine to sitting to standing
- Type of support surface: stationary or unstable surfaces
- Positioning of objects used in activities: near or far

Cordo and Nashner also make a critical distinction between associated postural adjustments that *precede* voluntary movements (e.g., reaching) and automatic postural adjustments that *follow* external perturbations (e.g., standing on a bus that stops at a light, being moved by the therapist). Training in one type of adjustment cannot be assumed to carry over into other types of adjustments.

Woollacott and associates[134] demonstrated that their subjects' postural activity varied depending on the task being performed (pushing, pulling) and whether they received information in advance regarding the goal of the task.

Voluntary movements are "accompanied by postural adjustments which show three main characteristics: (1) they are 'anticipatory' with respect to movement and minimize the perturbations of posture and equilibrium due to the movement, (2) they are adaptable to the conditions in which the movement is executed, and (3) they are influenced by the instructions given to the subject concerning the task to be performed."[91]

Postural control disorders in CVA patients have been well documented.[1,13] Lee[88] emphasized the detrimental impact that postural dysfunction has on free arm movements and therefore activities of daily living (ADL). Although a variety of muscles can serve as postural stabilizers, postural control of the trunk is critical for upper extremity function[14] (see Chapter 4).

Trunk muscle strength correlates significantly with sitting balance, and extremity strength scores correlate with trunk control.[15] Trunk strength has been shown to be impaired in multiple directions including forward and lateral flexion.[17] Decreased trunk control forces patients to use their more functional upper extremity as a postural support during activities performed in the upright position, therefore making participation in functional activities more difficult or impossible.

Fisher[60] compared the postural adjustments of normal and brain-injured subjects made while reaching for objects. Normal subjects tilted the pelvis anteriorly, extended the upper trunk, and moved the trunk in the direction of the arm. In contrast, the brain-injured subjects did not incorporate trunk movements into arm movements; they only reached as far as arm length and maintained a slumped (flexed) posture.

Based on the previous information, trunk treatment cannot be separated from upper extremity treatment. Several authors have demonstrated that trunk control can be treated during reaching activities.[14,36,96] Therapists must remember that postural adjustments are context specific, so treatment plans must be developed accordingly. Occupational therapists must use their activity analysis skills to help patients develop the missing trunk control components. (See Table 6-1 for examples of the effects of object positioning on trunk control and weight shifting during reaching activities.) Functional mobility patterns requiring increased trunk control (e.g., scooting) should be incorporated into treatment plans for upper extremity function (see Chapter 10). Many authors[13,14,43,44,52] advocate the use of handling to elicit postural reactions. These techniques should only be used in conjunction with a functional task; the goal of improving occupational performance should not be considered secondary. Therapists must also realize that postural reactions elicited during handling are responses to movement (caused by the therapist's hands) and do not consider responses to anticipate movement (e.g., reaching during kitchen activities).

Postural control evaluations should be performed within the context of upper extremity tasks such as reaching or performing ADL and IADL. Evaluating postural control separately will not provide the therapist with sufficient information for intervention. To address this issue, Abreu[1] created the quadraphonic approach postural test (Figure 6-2). During this test, therapists observe body alignment and effect of self-initiated perturbations and external perturbations on movement. (See Chapters 4 and 5 for more information related to postural control.)

Spasticity

Spasticity, which is a positive symptom according to Jackson's classification system, has been a subject of debate by various authors. Patients with spasticity have been shown to spend 3 times longer in rehabilitation units than stroke patients without spasticity.[56] Although an abundance of research has been done on spasticity, disagreements still exist about its definition, physiologic basis, treatment, and evaluation.[56]

Duncan and Badke[50] point out that several different phenomena commonly observed in stroke rehabilitation including hyperactive stretch reflexes, increased resistance to passive movement, posturing of the extremities, excessive cocontraction, and stereotypical movement synergies

Table 6-1

Effects of Object Positioning on Trunk Movements and Weight Shifts During Reaching Activities*

POSITION OF OBJECT	TRUNK RESPONSE/ WEIGHT SHIFT
Straight ahead at forehead level, past arm's length	Trunk extension, anterior pelvic tilt Anterior weight shift
On floor between feet	Trunk flexion Anterior weight shift
To side at shoulder level, past arm's length	Left trunk shortening, right trunk elongation, left hip hiking Weight shift to right
On floor, below right hip	Right trunk shortening, left trunk elongation Weight shift to right
Behind right shoulder, at arm's length	Trunk extension and rotation (right side posteriorly) Weight shift to right
At shoulder level, to left of left shoulder	Trunk extension and rotation (left side posteriorly) Weight shift to left
On floor, to the left of left foot	Trunk flexion and rotation (left side posteriorly) Weight shift to left
Above head, directly behind	Trunk extension, shoulders movement to behind hips Posterior weight shift

*These examples are for a patient with left hemiplegia. The left column indicates where to position objects during a reaching task (using the right upper extremity). The column on the right indicates the resultant trunk position and weight shift.

are clumped together in the category of spasticity. Spasticity has become a catch-all term for a variety of problems. Rather than being a specific symptom, spasticity is related to a variety of neural and nonneural factors. Therefore spasticity cannot be treated uniformly by surgical, physical, or pharmacologic procedures.[48]

Spasticity has been defined as a type of hypertonus that increases with joint movement velocity (e.g., is velocity-dependent) and is attributed to hyperactive stretch reflexes mediated by muscle spindle stretch receptors.[32] In addition, a Babinski sign is characteristic, and hyperactive tonic neck or vestibular reflexes may be present.[89] "Spastic paresis" is a commonly used term that implies a cause and effect relationship (i.e., a cause and effect relationship between positive and negative symptoms). This belief has recently been challenged.

The Bobaths[13] stated that there is "An intimate relationship between spasticity and movement . . . spasticity must

be held responsible for much of the patient's motor deficit." Treatment techniques were based on "helping the patient gain control over the released patterns of spasticity by their inhibition." Patients were treated under the assumption that "Weakness of muscles may not be real, but relative to the opposition by spastic antagonists."[13] A variety of studies have been published that refute these assumptions.

Sahrmann and Norton[115] studied both normal subjects and subjects with upper motor neuron symptoms. The movement pattern studied was alternating flexion and extension of the elbow. The analysis of their EMG findings showed that the primary cause of impaired movement was not antagonist stretch reflexes but limited and prolonged agonist contraction recruitment and delayed cessation of agonist contractions after movement had stopped. Rather than focusing treatment on inhibiting spasticity, therapists should train patients to perform alternating movement patterns (e.g., hand-to-mouth patterns) efficiently.

Fellows and Thilmann[57] studied the importance of hyperreflexia and paresis on voluntary arm movements in normal subjects and subjects with spasticity resulting from a unilateral ischemic cerebral lesion. The subjects with spasticity showed a lower maximum movement velocity; the more marked the paresis, the greater the reduction in maximum velocity. No relationship was found between the degree of voluntary movement impairment and level of passive muscle hypertonia in the antagonist. The conclusion was that agonist muscle paresis, rather than antagonist muscle hypertonia, had the most significant effect on impaired voluntary movement.

In their study on overcoming limited elbow movement in the presence of antagonist hyperactivity, Wolf et al[132] concluded that functional elbow improvements could be made without first training the patient to specifically inhibit hyperactivity.

Landau[86] performed pharmacologic interventions that effectively abolished the hyperactive stretch reflexes in his patients. This intervention did not result in a corresponding improvement in motor behavior.

In the traditional evaluation of spasticity, the therapist moves the patient's limb. It is quickly moved in a direction opposite to the pull of the muscle group being tested, and the examiner feels for a resistance to the movement. The gold standard for rating resistance is the Ashworth scale,[9] which has a 5-point scale (Box 6-1).

It has been argued that a spastic muscle's response to stretch is not the same during passive and active movement. In addition, spasticity is a multidimensional problem that incorporates neural and nonneural components (e.g., altered soft tissue compliance). Therefore some authors[70] have questioned the usefulness of test measures such as the Ashworth scale and are investigating a more comprehensive evaluation of spasticity.

Although the research on spasticity does not support focusing treatment on suppressing stretch reflexes, it does

POSTURAL TEST AND SCORING SHEET

Occupational Therapy

Patient:	Handedness:
Date:	Lesion site:
Age:	Education:
Dx:	Native language:
Onset:	Therapist:

Period of observation:
From: AM/PM   To: AM/PM   Observation location:

Observe the dynamics of movement and the changes in body parts displacements, velocity, and joint angular movement. In addition, observe the apparent amount of forces and rotations that take place while engaging in the movement. Plot the circumference that describes the farthest point that a subject could lean without stepping, reaching for support, protection, or falling. Note the changes at the beginning of the movement, during the movement, and on completion of the movement.

Posture Observations: Limits of Postural Stability	Performance response				Instructions response	
	Anterior	Posterior	Right	Left	Cue used	Response to cue
A. Resting Posture						
1. Describe patient's resting posture sitting and standing.						
a. Head observation						
b. Upper trunk observation						
c. Lower trunk observation						
d. Upper extremity observation						
e. Lower extremity observation						
2. Describe patient's sitting and standing dependency on hand support.						
a. Postural support is hand(s) free						
At rest						
During function						
b. Postural support is hand(s) dependent						
At rest						
During function						
c. Postural support is non-functional						
At rest						
During function (needs external support)						

3. Pelvic tilt effect

Neutral pelvic tilt effect on hand reach

_____

_____

Anterior pelvic tilt effect on hand reach

_____

_____

Posterior pelvic tilt effect on hand reach

_____

_____

Figure 6-2   Abreu's quadraphonic approach postural test. (From Abreu B: The quadraphonic approach, *Occup Ther Pract* 3:4, 1992.)

Continued

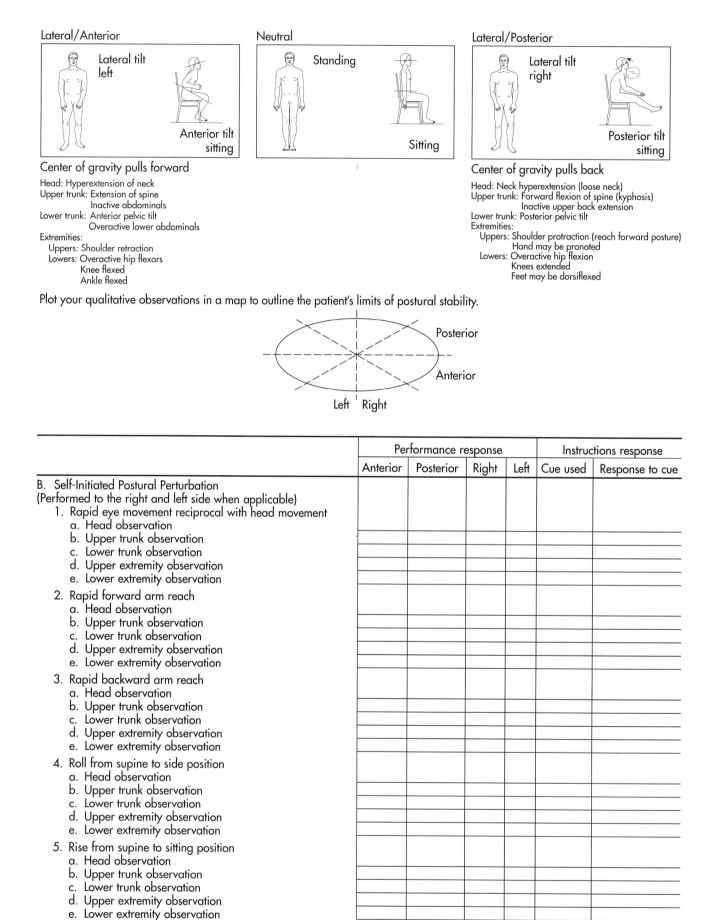

Lateral/Anterior

Lateral tilt left

Anterior tilt sitting

Center of gravity pulls forward

Head: Hyperextension of neck
Upper trunk: Extension of spine
　　　　　　Inactive abdominals
Lower trunk: Anterior pelvic tilt
　　　　　　Overactive lower abdominals
Extremities:
　Uppers: Shoulder retraction
　Lowers: Overactive hip flexors
　　　　　Knee flexed
　　　　　Ankle flexed

Neutral

Standing

Sitting

Lateral/Posterior

Lateral tilt right

Posterior tilt sitting

Center of gravity pulls back

Head: Neck hyperextension (loose neck)
Upper trunk: Forward flexion of spine (kyphosis)
　　　　　　Inactive upper back extension
Lower trunk: Posterior pelvic tilt
Extremities:
　Uppers: Shoulder protraction (reach forward posture)
　　　　　Hand may be pronated
　Lowers: Overactive hip flexion
　　　　　Knees extended
　　　　　Feet may be dorsiflexed

Plot your qualitative observations in a map to outline the patient's limits of postural stability.

Posterior

Anterior

Left　Right

	Performance response				Instructions response	
	Anterior	Posterior	Right	Left	Cue used	Response to cue
B. Self-Initiated Postural Perturbation (Performed to the right and left side when applicable)						
1. Rapid eye movement reciprocal with head movement						
a. Head observation						
b. Upper trunk observation						
c. Lower trunk observation						
d. Upper extremity observation						
e. Lower extremity observation						
2. Rapid forward arm reach						
a. Head observation						
b. Upper trunk observation						
c. Lower trunk observation						
d. Upper extremity observation						
e. Lower extremity observation						
3. Rapid backward arm reach						
a. Head observation						
b. Upper trunk observation						
c. Lower trunk observation						
d. Upper extremity observation						
e. Lower extremity observation						
4. Roll from supine to side position						
a. Head observation						
b. Upper trunk observation						
c. Lower trunk observation						
d. Upper extremity observation						
e. Lower extremity observation						
5. Rise from supine to sitting position						
a. Head observation						
b. Upper trunk observation						
c. Lower trunk observation						
d. Upper extremity observation						
e. Lower extremity observation						

Figure 6-2, cont'd　For legend see p. 115.

	Performance response				Instructions response	
	Anterior	Posterior	Right	Left	Cue used	Response to cue
6. Rise from prone to standing position						
a. Head observation						
b. Upper trunk observation						
c. Lower trunk observation						
d. Upper extremity observation						
e. Lower extremity observation						
7. Rise from sitting to standing position						
a. Head observation						
b. Upper trunk observation						
c. Lower trunk observation						
d. Upper extremity observation						
e. Lower extremity observation						
C. Externally Initiated Postural Perturbation						
1. Visual perturbation on stable support						
a. Head observation						
b. Upper trunk observation						
c. Lower trunk observation						
d. Upper extremity observation						
e. Lower extremity observation						
2. Visual perturbation on unstable support						
a. Head observation						
b. Upper trunk observation						
c. Lower trunk observation						
d. Upper extremity observation						
e. Lower extremity observation						
3. Visual occlusion on stable support						
a. Head observation						
b. Upper trunk observation						
c. Lower trunk observation						
d. Upper extremity observation						
e. Lower extremity observation						
4. Visual occlusion on unstable support						
a. Head observation						
b. Upper trunk observation						
c. Lower trunk observation						
d. Upper extremity observation						
e. Lower extremity observation						
5. Stepping reaction						
a. Head observation						
b. Upper trunk observation						
c. Lower trunk observation						
d. Upper extremity observation						
e. Lower extremity observation						
6. Equilibrium reaction—side to side						
a. Head observation						
b. Upper trunk observation						
c. Lower trunk observation						
d. Upper extremity observation						
e. Lower extremity observation						
7. Equilibrium reaction—back/forth (Remember to apply twice as great a force during the forward test.)						
a. Head observation						
b. Upper trunk observation						
c. Lower trunk observation						
d. Upper extremity observation						
e. Lower extremity observation						

Figure 6-2, cont'd For legend see p. 115.

Box 6-1

The Ashworth Scale

1—Normal tone
2—Slight hypertonus; noticeable catch when limb is moved
3—More marked hypertonus; but affected limb still moves easily
4—Moderate hypertonus; difficulty with passive movement
5—Severe hypertonus; rigid limb

Box 6-2

Treatment of Spasticity

- Prevent pain syndromes.
- Guide *appropriate* use of available motor control.
- Maintain soft-tissue length.
- Avoid using excessive effort during movement.
- Encourage slow and controlled movements.
- Teach specific functional synergies during tasks.
- Avoid use of repetitive compensatory movement patterns.

support treatment focusing on preventing secondary structural muscle changes in patients with spasticity.

Hufschmidt and Mauritz's study[74] suggests that spastic contracture is the result of degenerative changes (e.g., atrophy, fibrosis) as well as changes of the passive and contractile muscle properties.

In their study on spastic and rigid muscles, Dietz and associates[49] concluded that the actual muscle fibers undergo changes, which explains the increased muscle tone in spastic patients.

For treating patients with spasticity, Perry[106] emphasizes early mobilization and assistance with developing evolving motor control into effective function. These two interventions result in minimal contractures and prevent improper use of patients' available control mechanisms. Hummelsheim et al[74b] studied the results of sustained stretch in spastic patients. They found that sustained muscle stretch, according to Bobath principles, of approximately 10 minutes led to significant reduction in the spastic hypertonus in the elbow, hand, and finger flexors. They hypothesized that this benefit is a result of either stretch-receptor fatigue or adaptation to the new extended position.

Little and Massagli[89] also emphasize using a stretching program incorporating nocioception prevention and patient education focusing on the adverse effects of spasticity (contracture), use of slow movements, and importance of daily stretching.

In addition to the mentioned techniques, specific modalities and their physiologic bases have been described in the literature and include local cooling, vibration therapy, and electrical stimulation.[39]

Perry[106] summarizes the effective rehabilitation of a patient with spasticity by using five categories: contracture minimization, realistic planning, muscle strength preservation and restoration, enhancement of returning control, and substitution for permanent functional loss.

Carr and associates[35] summarized their treatment approach based on the assumption that clinical spasticity is a manifestation of both length-associated muscle changes and disordered motor control. "The development of spasticity will be less severe if soft tissue length can be maintained and if motor training emphasizes elimination of unnecessary muscle force and training muscle synergies as part of specific actions."

Again, it must be emphasized that many of the observed phenomena that occur during treatment should not automatically be attributed to spasticity and require more in-depth evaluations and treatment plans (Box 6-2, Table 6-2).

Loss of Soft Tissue Elasticity (Contractures and Deformities)

Contracture in CVA patients is the result of immobilization and may be attributed to spasticity, flaccidity, improper positioning, postural malalignment, a lack of variation in limb postures (e.g., prolonged sling use), or a combination of various factors. The formation of contractures indicates a poor prognosis for limb function.

Perry[106] discusses the vicious cycle of contracture and spasticity, "contractures stiffen tissues, immobility creates contractures. Spasticity preserves the contracture by excluding the intramuscular fibrous tissues from the stretching force."

Botte et al[22] have reviewed the literature correlating spasticity and contracture. As the CVA patient progresses to a state of spasticity, the increased activity of the spastic muscles may result in characteristic posturing of the limb, resulting in increased stiffness of the soft tissue surrounding the joint and the eventual formation of fixed contracture. Botte et al[22] further point out that contracture is associated with loss of elasticity and fixed shortening of involved tissues. Contracture may occur in a variety of soft tissues including the following:

Skin
Subcutaneous tissue
Muscle
Tendon
Ligament
Joint capsule
Vessels, nerves

Halar and Bell[68] categorize contracture as arthrogenic (resulting from cartilage damage, joint incongruency, capsular fibrosis), soft tissue related (skin, tendons, ligaments, subcutaneous tissue), and myogenic (shortening of the muscle by intrinsic or extrinsic factors). Ough et al[105] emphasize the importance of the difference between myogenic and joint contracture, especially if the muscle spans two or more

Table 6-2

Suggested Interventions for Problems Commonly Thought to be Caused by Spasticity*

OBSERVATIONS DURING TREATMENT	SUGGESTED INTERVENTIONS
Associated reactions or posturing upper extremity—usually consisting of retraction, posterior trunk rotation, internal rotation, elbow flexion, and wrist and digit flexion—during difficult tasks (e.g., gait, transfers, dressing)	Upper extremity posturing indicates that the task is difficult for the patient. Treatment should include increasing the efficiency of task performance by building in trunk and lower extremity control, incorporating the upper extremity into the task (e.g., by bilateral ironing or using arm as postural support), teaching patient to relax upper extremity after difficult tasks
Stereotypical flexor synergy patterns when attempting to move arm against gravity	Evaluate components of movement pattern and identify factors that limit efficient movement (e.g., weakness, postural dysfunction, malalignment, inappropriate task choice). Provide activities that elicit missing components of movement pattern.
Flexion posture when resting	Implement a contracture prevention program. Provide adequate positioning and teach safe, self-ROM exercises.
"Catch" felt during quick-stretch evaluation of upper extremity	Do not assume that this phenomenon is resulting in observed movement dysfunction. Instead, interpret it as a red flag warning that soft tissue shortening may be present or develop.

*This table represents a variety of functional limitations and problems traditionally considered to be the direct result of spasticity. Although sometimes interconnected, these problems stem from different sources and must be treated accordingly.

joints (e.g., the wrist and hand). The contractures can be differentiated by flexing the proximal joint and noting the resulting position of the distal joints. Joint contracture is not affected by changes in proximal joint position.

Booth[21] has reviewed the physiologic and biochemical effects of immobilization on muscle. His findings indicate that muscle strength rapidly declines during limb immobilization because of a decrease in muscle size; muscle fatigability increases rapidly after immobilization. His observations also indicate that muscle atrophy in immobilized limbs begins rapidly, and a decrease in muscle size is greatest in the early phases of immobilization.

Tabary et al[121] performed animal studies and studied structural changes of immobilized limbs. Muscles immobilized in their lengthened position showed no difference in their length/tension properties as compared to normal muscles. In contrast, muscles immobilized in the shortened position showed a considerable decrease in extensibility.

Passive Range of Motion

Soft tissue and joint mobilization are the treatments of choice for preventing contracture. The benefits of mobilization include maintenance of joint lubrication,[22] prevention of secondary orthopedic problems (impingements), maintenance of soft tissue length, and possible reduction of spasticity by acting on the nonneural components of spasticity.

Contracture is prevented by deliberate and frequent limb movement, with active movement being preferred over passive when possible. Perry[106] points out that it is essential to move the patient through complete ROMs and not just the middle ranges. Therapists must determine what is a full ROM for each individual patient, so age-related factors must be considered. Determining the full ROM on the less affected side may be helpful. A joint that goes through its full ROM once daily develops almost no deformities.[105] Although the ability to participate in all ranges of trunk and upper extremity activities should be maintained, particular attention should be paid to the following ranges:

- The mobility of the scapula on the thoracic wall with emphasis on protraction and upward rotation should be maintained because this range is critical in the prevention of soft tissue impingement in the subacromial space during overhead movements of the arm, as well as in preparation for forward reach patterns.[33,52] Overhead ranges should not be attempted unless the scapula is freely gliding in upward rotation.
- Maintaining external (lateral) rotation of the glenohumeral joint allows abduction of the arm as the humerus rotates laterally to permit the greater tuberosity of the humerus to clear the acromial process.[33] Bohannon et al[18] and Zorowitz et al[139] found that the range of external rotation was the factor most significantly correlated to shoulder pain.
- Elbow extension is important because the majority of stroke patients favor elbow flexion as a rest posture.
- Wrist extension with concurrent radial deviation should also be maintained. During wrist ROM exercises, therapists must realize that the range of wrist deviation is at a maximum when the wrist is slightly flexed and a minimum when the wrist is fully flexed.[80] Wrist extension is at a maximum during neutral deviation and a minimum during ulnar deviation.[80]
- Composite flexion of the digits leads to collateral ligament elongation.[33] This length must be maintained to prevent deformity and prepare the hand for return of motor function.

- Composite extension of the wrist and digits results in long flexor elongation.
- Digits ranged in both intrinsic plus (metacarpal phalangeal [MP] flexion and interphalangeal [IP] extension) and intrinsic minus (MP extension and IP flexion).

Halar and Bell[68] recommend active ROM (AROM) and PROM combined with a terminal stretch at least twice per day if contracture is beginning to develop. A sustained stretch lasting 20 to 30 minutes is effective for mild contracture. During the terminal stretch the proximal body part should be well stabilized. The therapist may slightly distract the joint during the stretch to prevent soft tissue impingement. The scapula position must be monitored during PROM activities. If necessary the therapist should support the scapula in a position of protraction and upward rotation. In addition, the therapist must support the humerus in an external rotation position. The elbow crease should be facing up (not medially toward the trunk) to ensure proper alignment (Figure 6-3).

Positioning

Positioning is another effective means of maintaining soft tissue length. Positioning needs of patients must be addressed while they are in bed or wheelchairs/armchairs (see Chapter 19) and anytime they are in a recumbent position. Effective positioning encourages proper joint alignment, variations in joint position, comfort, and the maintenance of stretch in areas at risk for contracture. Common areas of concern during patient positioning include head

and neck alignment, trunk alignment, glenohumeral joint alignment, scapula alignment, maintenance of abduction, external rotation, elbow extension, and maintenance of long flexor length.

A thorough literature review comparing authors' strategies on bed positioning has been published.[34] This review found no consensus on some issues and multiple discrepancies on strategies. Many of the positioning protocols are based on the principle of inhibiting primitive reflexes, a topic of considerable debate.

Patients are engaged in therapy only a portion of the day. Studies have shown that patients on rehabilitation units spend almost half of their days engaged in passive pursuits including sitting unoccupied and lying in bed. Therefore patients at risk for developing contracture secondary to limb immobilization are good candidates for participation in a positioning program in addition to therapy.

The positioning suggestions in Box 6-3 are based on Carr and Kenney's review[34] of the positioning literature and highlights the consensus of reviewed authors.

Although the positioning suggestions shown in Box 6-3 represent the consensus of many authors, major areas of intervention are missing, which result in the controversies surrounding this area of intervention. For example, glenohumeral joint support remains controversial. Although

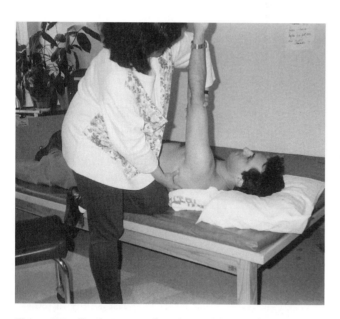

Figure 6-3 Passive range of motion activities with strict attention to the biomechanical alignment of the scapulothoracic and glenohumeral joints. Therapist's right hand assists with mobilization (upward rotation) of the scapula, while left arm keeps humerus externally rotated.

Box 6-3

Suggested Bed Positioning

POSITIONING OF PATIENTS ON UNAFFECTED SIDE

Head/neck: neutral and symmetrical
Affected upper limb: protracted and forward on pillow—wrist neutral, fingers extended, thumb abducted
Trunk: aligned
Affected lower limb: hip forward, flexed and supported; knee forward, flexed and supported

POSITIONING OF PATIENTS ON AFFECTED SIDE

Head/neck: neutral and symmetrical
Affected upper limb: protracted forward—elbow extended, hand supinated, wrist neutral, fingers extended, thumb abducted
Trunk: straight and aligned
Affected lower limb: knee flexed
Unaffected lower limb: knee flexed and supported by pillows

POSITIONING PATIENTS IN SUPINE

Head/neck: slight flexion
Affected upper limb: protracted and slightly abducted with external rotation—wrist neutral, fingers extended
Trunk: straight and aligned
Affected lower limb: hip forward on pillow, nothing against soles of the feet

most authors agree that the scapula should be protracted with a pillow, no consensus exists about support of the humerus. If only the scapula is protracted with a pillow, the humerus will take on a position of relative extension. Therefore support of both the scapula and humerus will achieve the original goal of proper joint alignment (Figure 6-4).

At this point, no definitive studies support one type of positioning more than another. Occupational therapists must decide what their intervention goals are and critically analyze their effectiveness. Therapists should not use general, generic strategies for bed positioning; instead,

each patient's positioning needs should be evaluated individually.

Patient Management of the Extremity

Strategies to teach patients safe ROM activities they can perform themselves need to be initiated as soon as patients are medically stable. Although the clasped hand position followed by overhead movements of both extremities have been advocated by some authors, this position may not be the most effective, especially for trauma prevention. This movement pattern does account for factors such as scapula-humeral rhythm (especially if weakness, malalign-

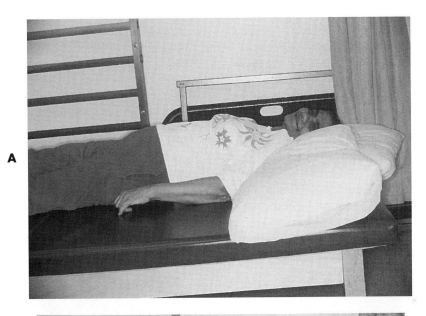

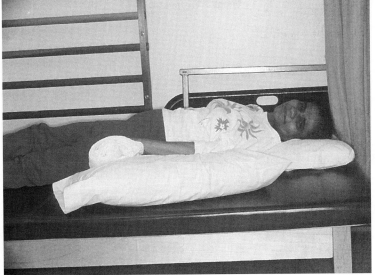

Figure 6-4 **A,** Bed positioning with only scapula supported. Note that humerus takes on a position of relative extension, with head of humerus migrating anteriorly. **B,** Proper support of scapula and humerus ensures proper biomechanical alignment of shoulder joint.

ment, or tightness around the scapula exists), overzealous patients who do not or cannot respect their pain, or critical shoulder biomechanics. Many patients observed performing this type of ROM activity have their trunk hyperextended, scapula retracted, and humerus internally rotated. This type of alignment does not correspond with ROM pattern that emphasizes forward flexion of the humerus; it promotes proximal patterns (e.g., retraction) that should be discouraged. Recommended techniques for patients performing ROM activities by themselves safely include the following:

1. The patient is seated at a table with both arms on top of a towel. The less affected arm guides the towel around the table, with the majority of movement occurring in the trunk and from hip flexion. The patient's goal is to "polish the table" while holding positions at the end of desired ROM. The further the patient's chair is positioned from the table, the greater the ROM. This technique not only enhances the range of the glenohumeral and elbow joint but encourages scapula protraction and weight shifting. Excessive effort is minimized because the towel assists the movement (Figure 6-5).

2. The patient's less affected arm cradles the more affected arm, lifts it to 90°, and places it into positions of horizontal abduction and adduction. Increased horizontal adduction on the more affected side encourages scapula protraction. This technique also encourages trunk rotation.

3. While seated or standing, the patient reaches down to the floor and allows both arms to dangle. This position encourages extension of the elbow, wrist, and digits and forward flexion of the humerus with scapula protraction. It is an especially useful technique for patients after they have performed an excessively difficult activity (e.g., gait, transfer, dressing) that results in stereotypical arm posturing (Figure 6-6).

4. While seated or standing, the patient places the more affected extremity onto a table or counter so that the forearm is bearing the weight. With the extremity in this position, the patient turns the trunk away from the supported extremity. As the trunk turns further away and is enhanced by the posterior reach of the less affected arm, the external rotation of the more affected shoulder increases (Figure 6-7).

5. Some authors[45] have advocated rolling over the protracted scapula (from supine to sidelying) several times to mobilize the scapula.

6. If the scapula of a patient is mobile and stays mobile, the range of abduction and external rotation may be increased by having the patient lie supine, placing the hands behind the head, and allowing the elbows to fall toward the bed (Figure 6-8). This is a common resting position for an individual who has unimpaired upper extremity function. This technique should be used judiciously and only for patients who move slowly, respect pain, and have a mobile scapula. The five techniques outlined previously may be used for almost all patients because they inherently follow biomechanical principles.

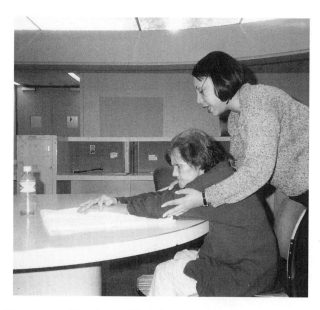

Figure 6-5 Towel-on-table. Therapist is training patient to perform safe self-range of motion. As patient pushes towel toward bottle, range of motion is gained in humeral flexion, scapular protraction, and elbow extension (which are ranges required for functional reach). Note that much of range is gained by hip and trunk flexion.

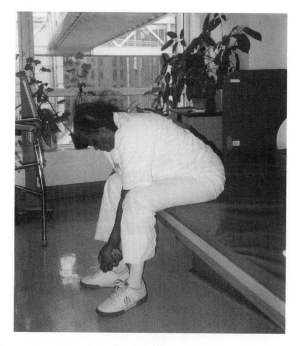

Figure 6-6 Patient performs self-range of motion activity by reaching to floor. This pattern is especially effective after a difficult task that results in stereotypical posturing.

The ultimate strategy used to decrease contracture and maintain ROM is encouraging functional use of the trunk and upper extremity. A person who has never had a stroke maintains ROM of an extremity by incorporating it into ADL. Eliminating maladaptive positions during activities, gaining balanced muscle activity on both sides of the joints, and focusing on activities that encourage ROMs that are commonly decreased in CVA patients (e.g., external rotation, forward flexion, abduction, protraction) should all be incorporated into a comprehensive upper extremity program. (See Chapters 8 and 9 for other adjunctive treatments to prevent or correct short tissue shortening.)

Shoulder-Hand Syndrome

Shoulder-hand syndrome (SHS) is classified as a reflex sympathetic dystrophy (RSD) disorder. The painful lesion that precipitates SHS is either a proximal trauma such as a shoulder, neck, or ribcage injury or a visceral source such as stroke.[85] The syndrome begins with severe pain and progresses to stiffness in the shoulder and pain throughout the extremity. Other symptoms include moderate to marked swelling of the wrist and hand, vasomotor changes, and atrophy.[85] If untreated, SHS may result in a frozen shoulder and permanent hand deformity.[27]

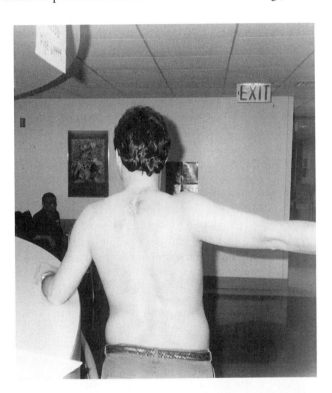

Figure 6-7 External rotation of left glenohumeral joint achieved by reaching to side and behind with opposite arm.

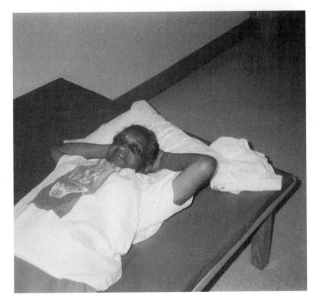

Figure 6-8 Bed positioning—to be used judiciously for patients who respect their own pain. This rest posture is effective at maintaining external rotation and abduction of the glenohumeral joint. If range is lacking, the humerus can be supported with a towel until patient gains increased external rotation and horizontal abduction.

Although the etiology of SHS remains obscure, most authors associate it with a change in the autonomic nervous system (primarily sympathetic).[40] A recent study by Braus and associates[27] suggests that the SHS in hemiplegic patients is initiated by a peripheral lesion (e.g., a tissue or nerve injury). The authors hypothesize that increased neural activity after a peripheral injury or inflammation leads to a central sensitization that is responsible for the severe pain associated with SHS. Autopsy data collected by the authors confirmed microbleeding in the area of the suprahumeral joint of the affected side. If the underlying cause is in fact peripheral in nature, then prevention programs would theoretically be effective.

The reported incidence of SHS ranges from 27%[27] to 25%[123] to 12.5%.[46] Males seem to be slightly more affected than females.[46,123] The majority of patients with SHS symptoms have partial motor loss, moderate or severe sensory loss, and varying degrees of spasticity.[46] Associated risk factors include subluxation, considerable weakness, moderate spasticity, deficits in confrontational field testing (secondary to hemianopsia or neglect), and altered shoulder biomechanics that may compromise the suprahumeral joint structures.[27]

Three stages of SHS have been described (Box 6-4).

Davis et al[46] outlined the major diagnostic criteria for SHS based on the following clinical symptoms:

- Shoulder: loss of ROM and pain during abduction, flexion, and external rotation movements
- Elbow: no signs or symptoms
- Wrist: intense pain during extension movements, dorsal edema, tenderness during deep palpation
- Hand: edema over metacarpals, no tenderness

Box 6-4

Stages of Shoulder-Hand Syndrome

STAGE 1

The patient complains of shoulder and hand pain, tenderness, and vasomotor changes (with symptoms of discoloration and temperature changes). Chances of reversal are high at this stage.

STAGE 2

The patient has early dystrophic limb changes, muscle and skin atrophy, vasospasm, hyperhidrosis (increased sweating), and radiographic signs of osteoporosis. At this stage, SHS becomes increasingly difficult to treat.

STAGE 3

Patients rarely have pain and vasomotor changes, but they do have soft tissue dystrophy, contracture (including a frozen shoulder and clawed hand), and severe osteoporosis. At this stage, SHS is irreversible.

- Digits: moderate fusiform edema, intense pain during flexion of the MCP and proximal interphalangeal (PIP) joints, loss of skin lines

The Tepperman et al[123] study concluded that MCP tenderness during compression was the most valuable clinical sign of RSD, with a predictive value of 100%. Vasomotor changes and IP tenderness had the next highest predictive value at 72.7%. Therapists must remember that many of the mentioned signs and symptoms can be found in stroke patients without SHS. If a patient has several characteristic signs and symptoms, a diagnosis can safely be made on clinical grounds alone.[40] Although the diagnosis for SHS is primarily clinical, the most effective way to confirm its presence is to use a differential neural blockade. A stellate ganglion block may be used to alleviate the symptoms. The block interrupts the abnormal sympathetic reflex; the diagnosis of SHS is confirmed if the symptoms are alleviated.

SHS should be prevented so that it will not have to be treated. Davis[45] has developed a prevention protocol that focuses on the following:

1. Therapists gaining full understanding of the anatomy and physiology of normal and hemiplegic shoulders
2. Proper handling of the upper extremity, including avoiding arm traction during mobility, ADL, and gait activities; supporting the arm as necessary, preventing prolonged arm dangling, and using the trunk and scapula rather than the arm as support during transitional movements
3. Staff education focusing on the mentioned handling techniques
4. Mobilizing the scapula to ensure gliding when raising or performing ROM activities with the arm
5. Family education focusing on proper extremity handling and transfer techniques; training families not to guard at the affected upper extremity during ambulation (because a balance loss would result in an automatic reflex—grabbing the patient's arm)
6. Edema control that begins as soon as signs of it are observed (see Chapter 7)
7. Training patients to take responsibility for protecting their affected arm.

Davis[45] hypothesizes that certain factors contributing to SHS can be controlled by therapists. One factor is the extravasation of intravenous fluids. Intravenous fluids should be infused into the less affected arm if possible; if not, they should be infused proximal to the wrist on the affected side. This strategy prevents infiltration around the needle and a possible edema syndrome. Another contributing factor is poor positioning. Patients should be positioned so that they cannot roll over onto the affected arm, pin it down, and compromise circulation. The other factor is immobilization of a painful shoulder by the patient. "In this sense, a painful shoulder (but not necessarily SHS) can evolve into SHS through immobility and consequent circulatory problems. Therefore, proper management of the hemiplegic patient in order to prevent trauma to the shoulder is critical."[45]

In a recent prospective two-part study performed by Braus and associates[27] a prevention protocol was implemented that focused on protecting the affected upper extremity from trauma. All patients, relatives, and members of the therapy and medical teams received detailed instructions when patients were initially hospitalized to avoid peripheral injuries to the affected limb. Wheelchair and bed positioning were modified to ensure no pain resulted from improper positioning. Passive movements of the upper extremity were not made unless the scapula was fully mobilized. Any activity or position that caused pain was immediately changed, and no infusions into the veins of the hemiplegic hands were performed. These strategies alone decreased the incidence of SHS from 27% to 8%.

If symptoms of SHS begin to develop, therapists should make an early diagnosis and begin aggressive treatment.[27,33,40,45,85] In the Braus[27] study, patients who already had definite SHS symptoms were placed either in an experimental group (that received a 14-day treatment with low doses of oral corticosteroids and "daily therapy based on the Bobath concept") or a placebo group (that received placebo medication and daily therapy). Of the 36 patients in the experimental group, 31 were free of symptoms after 10 days of treatment. The use of oral corticosteroids in conjunction with therapy has also been advocated by Chu[40] and Davis.[45]

Therapy intervention should be symptom specific. Edema must be alleviated immediately, and joint mobility must be maintained while preventing pain.[85,129] Davies[44] advocates using activities that result in increased upper extremity ROM but actually result from trunk and hip flexion (e.g., towel exercises, pushing away a therapy ball while seated, reaching to the floor). Mobilizing the scapula, which can be accomplished by the therapist or having the patient roll onto the protracted scapula from the supine to the sidelying position, have also been described.

Research is beginning to show that peripheral lesions are the cause of SHS in CVA patients, so interventions should incorporate this knowledge. Inappropriate ROM exercises (e.g., overhead ROM activities in patients without scapula mobility, overzealous exercise), mishandling during ADL (e.g., pulling on the affected arm during transfers, bathing, dressing, bedtime activities) are all factors to consider. In addition to evaluating and treating SHS, occupational therapists play a major role in staff education. All staff and family members who physically move patients need to be aware of appropriate techniques so that injuries can be prevented.

Andersen[6] suggests the following treatment strategies:

1. PROM, self ROM, and AROM activities several times per day with specific focus on movements that elevate the arm above the cardiac level (for edema control)
2. Bilateral activities during ADL if AROM is limited
3. Edema control
4. Prevention of prolonged static positioning

Weakness

The impact of weakness (a negative symptom) on CVA patients' functional status has long been ignored. The motor control deficits in patients were previously attributed exclusively to spasticity, which resulted in treatment focused on inhibiting the spasticity. Many therapists considered upper extremity muscle tests for strength difficult to interpret because of common "synergy patterns." Bourbonnais et al[24] demonstrated that the patterns of activity in the elbow flexor muscles were not consistent with established synergistic patterns. Weakness of the upper extremity musculature plays a major role in upper extremity dysfunction, probably more than the positive symptoms after stroke. Muscle weakness is reflected by the inability of patients to generate normal levels of muscle force.[25] Stroke survivors who have written about their experiences focus on the difficulty in force production. Brodal[28] reflected on his own stroke: "It was a striking and repeatedly made observation that the force needed to make a severely paretic muscle contract is considerable. . . . Subjectively this is experienced as a kind of mental force, a power of will. In the case of a muscle just capable of being actively moved the mental effort needed was very great."

Bourbonnais and Vanden Noven[25] reviewed the physiologic changes in the nervous system that contribute to muscle weakness in patients with hemiparesis. They summarized specific changes at the motor neuron and muscle levels that decrease a patient's ability to produce force. These changes are summarized in Box 6-5.

Bohannon et al[19] found that static strength deficits of the shoulder medial rotator and elbow flexor muscles did not correlate with antagonist muscle spasticity. They concluded that therapists may determine an agonist muscle's capacity for force production based on its own tone rather than that of its antagonist.

Box 6-5

Physiologic Changes Contributing to Weakness

Motor neuron changes: loss of agonist motor units, changes in recruitment order of motor units, changes in the firing rates of motor units
Nerve changes: changes in peripheral nerve conduction
Muscle changes: changes in the morphologic and contractile properties of motor units as well as in the mechanical properties of muscles

Gowland et al[65] studied agonist and antagonist activity during upper limb movements in stroke patients and concluded that treatment should be aimed at improving motor neuron recruitment rather than reducing antagonist activity. In their study, patients who could not perform select upper extremity tasks had EMG values that were significantly and consistently lower than those of patients who were successful at the task.

Bohannon and Smith[20] analyzed strength deficits in stroke patients and verified that muscle strength improves in stroke patients with hemiplegia who are undergoing rehabilitation. The most effective means of increasing muscle strength needs to be researched.

Flinn[61] presented a case study of a young female with left-sided hemiplegia. Her treatment program focused on participating in graded functional tasks that systematically increased the motor demands on the more affected upper extremity. Her task-oriented treatment program was augmented by resistive exercises using elastic tubing. Substantial results after 6 months of therapy included improved level of occupational performance in ADL and IADL, improved manual muscle test scores (which increased from 2/5 to the 4/5 and 5/5 ranges), improved hand function, and improved grip strength scores. Identifying the underlying problems (in this case, weakness and an inability to control excess degrees of freedom) is of utmost importance when planning treatment strategies.

There has been a long-standing debate about which type of muscle contraction (eccentric, concentric, or isometric) is the most effective in strengthening patients. Muscle groups need to contract in a variety of ways to successfully complete functional tasks. For example, when a person reaches for a can of soup on a high shelf, the shoulder musculature must contract (concentrically) to bring the hand to the level of the shelf, maintain the contraction (isometrically) to locate the correct item and control the weight of the arm and item in gravity (eccentrically) as the can is placed with control on the counter top.

Many patients are able to elicit an isometric contraction when placed in select positions; the Bobaths[13] called this the *placing reaction*. Muller[99] concluded that isometric contractions were most effective during strength training because they produced more tension than concentric contractions and were more efficient because they expended less energy.

In a study of dynamic muscle strength training in stroke patients, Engardt et al[53] found that eccentric contractions were more effective than concentric contractions. Twenty patients with hemiparesis resulting from CVAs participated in activities that elicited either concentric or eccentric contractions. After the treatment, significant improvements resulted in the relative strength of paretic muscles during eccentric and concentric actions in the group that was solely trained with eccentric contractions (i.e., eccentric training increased the strength of both types of

contractions); this was not true for the group that only received concentric-contraction training. Therefore eccentric-contraction training was determined to be more advantageous and efficient.

Another method for increasing skeletal muscle strength was proposed by Yue and Cole.[137] Healthy subjects were separated into three groups: those receiving imagining training (i.e., training in which the person imagines a muscle is contracting but is not activating the muscle), those receiving contraction training, and a control group. Training resulted in a maximum voluntary contraction force increase of 22% in the imagining group, 30% in the contraction group, and 3.7% in the control group. This study demonstrated that strength increases can be achieved without muscle activation. Early strength increases appear to be the result of practice efforts on central motor programming. This study adds to the increasing evidence that the neural origin of strength increases before muscle hypertrophy.

Superimposed Orthopedic Injuries

Orthopedic problems associated with stroke have been well documented. These complications have a negative impact on functional outcomes, prolong rehabilitation, and are one of the main causes of upper extremity pain syndromes after stroke.

Rotator Cuff and Biceps Tendon Lesions

The rotator cuff guides and leads the movements of the shoulder joint. The cuff supplies the strength needed to complete the ROM in the shoulder joint[78] and seats the head of the humerus into the glenoid fossa.

Najenson and associates[100] studied 32 hemiplegic patients with severe upper limb paralysis; 18 patients served as controls by having their less affected side evaluated. Forty percent of the patients (13 out of 32) had a rotator cuff tear on the affected side. None of the patients had complaints about the affected shoulder before the stroke. Only 16% of the patients in the control group (3 out of 18) had ruptured rotator cuffs on the less involved side; all three seemed to be long-standing tears.

Najenson and colleagues also discussed the pathophysiology of a rotator cuff tear in hemiplegic patients. Many older patients are predisposed to rotator cuff ruptures because of degenerative changes associated with aging. Cuff tears commonly result from impingement of the cuff between the greater tuberosity and acromial arch (Figure 6-9), which occurs when the humerus is forced into abduction without external rotation (e.g., during inappropriate PROM activities or activities that are not sensitive to shoulder biomechanics [e.g., reciprocal pulleys]). Impingement can be prevented by therapists who have a thorough understanding of joint alignment during treatment.

Nepomuceno and Miller[103] found seven rotator cuff tears and one a transverse bicipital tendon tear in 24 sub-

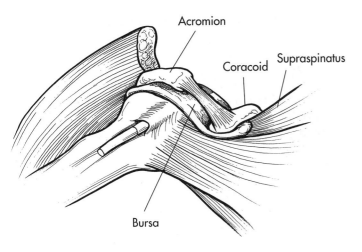

Figure 6-9 Impingement of soft tissues located in subacromial space. Impingement occurs between the head of humerus and acromion/coracoid. Impingement occurs during forced humeral flexion/abduction without concurrent upward rotation of scapula and/or external rotation of humerus.

jects with painful hemiplegic shoulders. None of the patients had premorbid shoulder pathology. With one exception, all patients with soft tissue lesions had left-sided hemiplegia. (This study did not evaluate the presence of visual field loss or neglect.)

Therapists should note that a relationship between rotator cuff age and wear has been documented. After age 50 the percentage of lesions significantly increases, reaching 60% after 60 years of age.[104]

Adhesive Changes

Adhesive changes in the hemiplegic shoulder are considered to be results of immobilization, synovitis, or metabolic changes in joint tissue. Hakuno[67] studied adhesive changes in hemiplegic shoulders and found that hemiplegia had a significant influence on the prevalence of adhesive changes in the shoulder. Adhesive changes were found in 30% of patients' affected glenohumeral joints as opposed to 2.7% on the less involved side.

Rizk et al[109] examined 30 hemiplegic patients with shoulder arthrography and found that 23 patients had capsular constriction typical of frozen shoulder (adhesive capsulitis). Therefore early passive shoulder ROM was advocated.

Roy and associates[111] use the following clinical criteria for adhesive capsulitis: shoulder pain, external rotation of less than 20°, and abduction of less than 60°.

Brachial Plexus Injury

Brachial plexus injury was identified in five of twelve patients in the study by Kaplan et al.[81] All five had EMG evidence indicating neuropathy of the upper trunk of the brachial plexus on the side affected by the stroke. The deltoid, biceps, and infraspinatus muscles were all involved. Moskowitz and Porter[98] also summarized the findings in five CVA patients with "traction neuropathies" of the upper trunk of the brachial plexus.

Merideth and associates[94] reviewed the diagnostic and treatment procedures for CVA patients presenting with brachial plexus injuries. Physical examination findings included flaccidity and atrophy of the supraspinatus, infraspinatus, deltoid, and biceps muscles in the affected upper extremity with increased muscle tone or distal movement (an atypical pattern of recovery). EMG criteria for diagnosing brachial plexus injuries include the finding of fibrillation potentials in the muscles that are innervated by the upper trunk of the brachial plexus.

Treatment of these patients included positioning and passive and active ROM activities. During AROM activities, effects of gravity were monitored to prevent further traction. Using a positioning pillow, the affected upper extremity was positioned as follows: externally rotated 45°, 90° of elbow flexion, and forearm neutral. Patients used slings while ambulating and were educated not to sleep on their affected side, which could result in compression and traction injuries to the upper trunk. (Many authors encourage sleeping on the affected side if this pathology is not present.) A major component of the treatment program was the education of the patient, staff, and families regarding proper care and positioning of the upper extremity.

Pain Syndromes

Although pain syndromes have previously been discussed in the context of orthopedic injuries and SHS, their impact on functional recovery is significant, so this section will specifically review the literature on hemiplegic shoulder pain.

The incidence of shoulder pain in hemiplegic patients has been reported to be as high as 72%.[18,111,127] Roy and associates[111] identified strong associations between hemiplegic shoulder pain and prolonged hospital stays, arm weakness, poor recovery of arm function, ADL, and lower rates of discharge to the home. It is the onus of those responsible for stroke patients to be aware of hemiplegic shoulder pain and to diagnose, relieve, and prevent this syndrome. Although shoulder pain is obviously not the only variable leading to prolonged hospital stays, it is a potentially preventable variable over which occupational therapists have some control.

Andersen[6] reminds therapists that a "painful shoulder can limit the patient's general mobility, because when a patient protects his or her arm, this restricts both active and passive movements. This limits the patient's activities such as rolling in bed, transferring, putting on a shirt or blouse, and bending to reach his or her feet to put on shoes and socks." The occurrence of shoulder pain has also been linked to depression.[116]

The literature concerning hemiplegic shoulder pain is confusing at times and often contradictory. The following review was obtained from a selection of articles from a variety of disciplines. The focus of the review is clinical correlations associated with hemiplegic shoulder pain.

In their study of 55 patients, Roy and associates[111] found positive correlations between hemiplegic shoulder pain and "glenohumeral malalignment without descent of the humeral head" as well as between hemiplegic shoulder pain and RSD (SHS). The study did not confirm a strong association between spasticity (measured by the Ashworth scale) and hemiplegic shoulder pain.

Joynt[79] found significant correlations between loss of motion and shoulder pain and questioned the relationship between neglect/perceptual dysfunction and pain. His left-sided hemiplegic subjects had a higher incidence of shoulder pain, which led him to question whether there was increased incidence of trauma. He found no correlation between shoulder pain and subluxation, spasticity, strength, or sensation.

Joynt identified the subacromial area as a pain-producing location in a significant number of cases. Of 28 patients who received a subacromial injection of 1% lidocaine, over half obtained moderate or marked pain relief and improved ROM. The author suggested that physical agent modalities, steroid injections, and careful ROM activities focusing on impingement prevention were significant in reducing pain.

The subacromial area is prone to trauma during therapy and patient handling. The subacromial space includes the supraspinatus tendon, long head of the biceps, and subacromial bursa[33] (Figure 6-10). All of these structures are prone to impingement and inflammation. Andersen[6] suggests that structure impingement can easily develop in hemiplegic patients during ROM activities because the normal scapulohumeral rhythm becomes impaired. If the scapula is not rotated upward (either by therapist's manipulation or active control), the humerus becomes blocked by the acromion and causes impingement, inflammation, and pain (see Figure 6-9). Combined motions of scapula retraction with forward flexion should be avoided to prevent impingement. Instead, the scapula should glide freely and be protracted and upwardly rotated during upper extremity activities. Objects for reaching activities should be placed in front or below waist level of the patient to encourage humeral forward flexion with scapular protraction.

Some patients may develop inflammation around the biceps tendon and supraspinatus insertion because of impingements. Palpation skills are important for determining which structures are involved (Figure 6-11). To palpate the biceps tendon, palpate the acromion and drop one finger to the anterior shoulder; the biceps tendon lies in the groove between the greater and lesser tuberosities of the humerus. If pain is felt when pressure is applied, the biceps tendon has probably been affected. (Passively rotating the humerus while palpating will assist the therapist with locating the tuberosities.)

To palpate the supraspinatus tendon, palpate the acromion, but this time drop one finger to the lateral shoulder right below the center of the acromion. If pain is

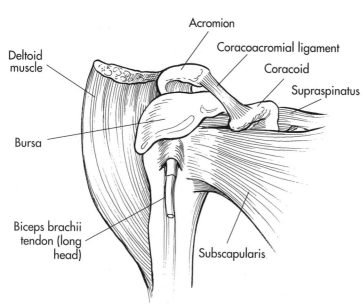

Figure 6-10   Subacromial space.

elicited by pressure or slight friction, the supraspinatus has most likely been affected.

Bohannon et al[18] studied the relationship of five variables (age, time since onset of hemiplegia, range of external rotation of the hemiplegic shoulder, spasticity, and weakness) to shoulder pain. In their study of 50 patients, 36 had shoulder pain. Range of shoulder external rotation was considered the factor related most significantly to shoulder pain. They hypothesized that hemiplegic shoulder pain was in part a manifestation of adhesive capsulitis. In this study only patients with full external rotation were free of pain. The suggested treatment was elimination of inflammation and maintenance of ROM.

Hecht[71] treated 13 patients with limited ROM and shoulder pain with percutaneous phenol blocks to the nerves of the subscapularis (a major shoulder internal rotator). Immediate and significant improvements were observed in the flexion, abduction, and external rotation ROMs; pain relief was also noted. This study indicates that the subscapularis is a key muscle and should be addressed during treatment focusing on maintaining soft tissue length. The subscapularis muscle may tighten in patients with the previously mentioned pain syndrome. If the humerus resists external rotation with the arm at the side during evaluation, the subscapularis can be presumed to be a factor contributing to the deformity.[105] This study adds

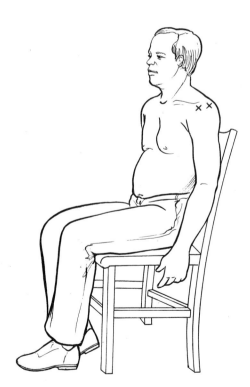

Figure 6-11 Palpation point. The *x* on left (more anterior) is palpation point for long head of biceps. The *x* on right (more lateral) is palpation point for supraspinatus tendon.

more support to the concept of focusing on maintaining the range of humeral external rotation to prevent resulting complications.

Bohannon and Andrews[16] studied 24 patients in an effort to establish a relationship between subluxation and pain. Despite the emphasis placed on reduction of subluxation, the relationship between shoulder pain and subluxation has not been established. Their study did not find an association between shoulder pain and subluxation (which was defined in this study as the separation between the acromion and the humeral head). A study by Arsenault et al[8] also found no significant relationship between subluxation and shoulder pain.

A more recent study by Zorowitz et al[139] also focused on the correlation between subluxation and pain. Results showed that shoulder pain did not correlate with age, vertical or horizontal subluxation, shoulder flexion, abduction, or Fugl-Meyer scores, but it did correlate with the degree of shoulder external rotation.

Kumar et al[84] demonstrated a positive correlation between shoulder pain and therapy programs that did not consider biomechanical shoulder alignment during treatment. Patients were assigned to one of three exercise groups: ROM initiated by the therapist, skateboard treatment, and overhead pulley treatment. Of the patients who developed pain during the treatment programs, 8% were in the ROM group, 12% in the skateboard group, and 62% in the overhead pulley group. The probable cause of this discrepancy was soft tissue damage resulting from forced abduction without external rotation. This study showed that poorly prescribed activities by the therapist can be the cause of pain syndromes. This study found no significant relationship between subluxation and pain.

In a 3-year study of 219 hemiplegic patients, Van Ouwenaller and associates[127] found that 85% of the patients who developed pain had spasticity (an increased myotatic reflex) as compared to 18% of flaccid patients. They also found that 50% of the patients who developed pain had anteroinferior subluxations (which were not defined). The authors advocated use of muscle relaxation techniques for the shoulder girdle as outlined by Bobath. These techniques resulted in "clear cut reductions of pain when applied judiciously and for long durations."

Jensen[78] attributes shoulder pain to traumatic tendonitis resulting from unskilled and strenuous joint treatment during ADL (e.g., bathing, dressing, bed mobility) and bilateral ROM activities of more than 90° resulting in "jamming [of] soft tissue against the acromion resulting in lesions." Jensen suggests the following precautions: educating all staff members, placing signs over patients' beds to warn staff of the shoulder instability, supporting the arm during the acute stage, avoiding treatment that may cause soft tissue impingement, having a thorough understanding of shoulder anatomy, and dissuading use of pulley exercises and self-ROM activities.

Loss of Biomechanical Alignment

Immediately after a stroke, patients lose their ability to maintain upright control and become malaligned because of the effects of gravity, weakness, and muscle imbalance.

Occupational therapists must be able to identify malalignments to effectively treat upper extremity dysfunction. Following are common trunk and upper extremity alignment problems and a review of activities to counteract the adverse effects of malalignment.

Loss of Pelvic/Trunk Alignment

After a stroke, patients commonly lose their ability to perform postural adjustments and maintain postural alignment because of weakness, a loss of equilibrium, and righting reactions; the trunk assumes an asymmetrical posture.[13,14,43,52]

The first area to observe is the patient's pelvis and its effect on spinal alignment. Patients typically bear weight asymmetrically through their pelvis (by one ischial tuberosity accepting more weight than the other), which results in lateral spine flexion.[52] This lateral flexion causes the trunk musculature to become shortened on the non–weight-bearing side and lengthened on the weight-bearing side[43] (Figure 6-12). At the same time, patients tend to assume a posterior pelvic tilt, which results in spinal flexion. Again the result is a muscle imbalance, with the anterior musculature (abdominals) becoming shortened and the posterior muscles (extensors) becoming elongated. Davies[43] hypothesizes that patients sit with posterior pelvic tilt to compensate for weak abdominals. Patients assume this "safe" posture to prevent themselves from falling backward. The spinal flexion that results from the posterior tilt leads to loss of natural lumbar spine lordosis and accentuated thoracic spine kyphosis.

Abdominal weakness (especially the obliques) results in a destabilization of the ribcage. A lack of balance between the obliques results in trunk and ribcage rotation[80] (see Chapter 4).

Loss of Scapula Alignment

Upper extremity malalignment is commonly a result of pelvic and trunk malalignments. When in a resting position the scapula is flush on the ribcage (the scapulothoracic joint) and upwardly rotated.[80] When the scapula is palpated, the distance between the inferior angle and the vertebral column should be greater than the distance between the medial border of the scapular spine and the vertebral column[80] (Figure 6-13). In the resting position the glenoid fossa of the scapula faces upward, forward, and outward.[33] Therefore the trunk and ribcage must be stable to properly support the scapula. In hemiplegic patients, the scapula loses its orientation on the thoracic wall and assumes a position of relative downward rotation.[33,44,52]

Cailliet[33] describes several events that result in a downwardly rotated scapula (Figure 6-14), such as lateral flexion toward the hemiparetic side. The lateral flexion may be a result of trunk weakness, perceptual dysfunction that results in an inability to perceive midline, or excess activity in unilateral trunk flexors (i.e., latissimus dorsi). Downward rotation can also be caused by unopposed muscle activity that depresses and downwardly rotates the scapula (i.e., rhomboids, levator scapula, latissimus dorsi) or by generalized weakness in the muscles that orient the scapula in a position of upward rotation (i.e., serratus anterior, upper and lower trapezius).

Loss of Glenohumeral Joint Alignment

Thus far the loss of pelvic/trunk, ribcage, and scapula control have been reviewed. All of the aforementioned alignment changes have an impact on the stability and alignment of the glenohumeral joint. The mechanisms of glenohumeral joint subluxation as reviewed by Cailliet[33] and Basmajian[11] will be used as working models to describe this problem.

The following factors assist in maintaining glenohumeral joint stability: the angle of the glenoid fossa when facing forward, upward, and outward; the support of the

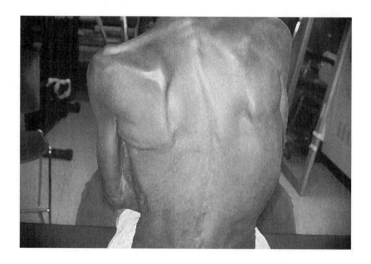

Figure 6-12 Asymmetrical trunk posture in patient with left hemiplegia. Note the left trunk shortening, right trunk elongation/overstretching, ribcage shift, loss of scapula stability on ribcage, relative downward rotation of scapula, increased weight bearing on right ischial tuberosity, and shoulder asymmetry (left hemiplegia).

scapula on the ribcage; the seating of the humeral head in the fossa by the supraspinatus; possible support from the superior capsule; and contraction of the deltoid and cuff muscles when passive support is eliminated by slight abduction of the humerus.[33] Cailliet states that any change in these factors may play a role in causing subluxation (Figure 6-15).

Basmajian's EMG studies[11] confirm that downward migration of the humeral head is prevented by the supraspinatus when a downward load is applied to the upper extremity (e.g., when a person holds a briefcase). Authors previously believed that the deltoid performed this function, but the deltoid actually shows no activity during this function. Basmajian points out that the supraspinatus is a horizontally positioned muscle that runs through the supraspinous fossa and can only be effective if the scapula is correctly oriented on the thorax.

The upward orientation of the glenoid fossa creates a "cradle" for the humeral head. As the humerus is pulled downward, it is forced to move laterally by the slope of the fossa.[11] The supraspinatus (and superior portion of the capsule) prevent this lateral movement and therefore downward migration. Basmajian also points out that this mechanism is not effective if the humerus is abducted. This position predisposes patients to subluxation by eliminating the described mechanism. Many patients are positioned so that their humerus is slightly abducted because of the lateral trunk flexion toward the more affected side or as a result of passive positioning.

Chaco and Wolf[38] confirmed that the supraspinatus did not respond to loading in the hemiplegic patients they studied. Although not immediate, subluxation did develop later in the study in the patients who remained flaccid. It was inferred that the joint capsule holds the head of the humerus in relation to the glenoid fossa but unless the supraspinatus starts responding, it cannot prevent subluxation indefinitely.

Ryerson and Levit[112,113] have described three patterns of subluxation in the glenohumeral joint. They emphasize that the therapist must assess trunk posture, determine the scapula's position on the trunk, evaluate scapula mobility and rhythm, and examine the alignment and mobility of the glenohumeral joint, before setting treatment goals for the shoulder. (Table 6-3 reviews Ryerson and Levit's subluxation classifications, including inferior, anterior, and superior subluxations.)

Hall and associates[69] assessed the validity of three clinical measures (palpation, arm length discrepancy, and thermoplastic jig measurement) for evaluating shoulder subluxation in adults with hemiplegia resulting from a stroke. These measures were combined with anterior/posterior X-rays of the hemiplegic shoulder; results indicated that palpation had the highest correlation with successful subluxation evaluation. In their technique for palpating subluxation, the patient is seated with the upper extremity un-

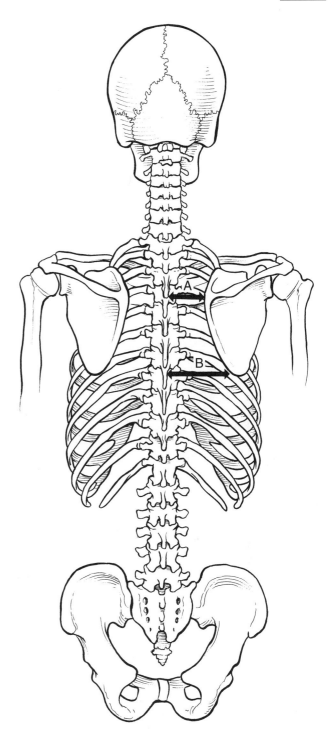

Figure 6-13 Normal resting posture of scapula in upward rotation. *A,* distance (in finger breadths or centimeters) from medial border of the spine of the scapula to the vertebral column; *B,* distance from the inferior angle of scapula to vertebral column. Distance *B* should be greater than distance *A* if the scapula is appropriately aligned. If *A* equals *B* or *A* is greater than *B,* scapula has assumed a position of relative downward rotation.

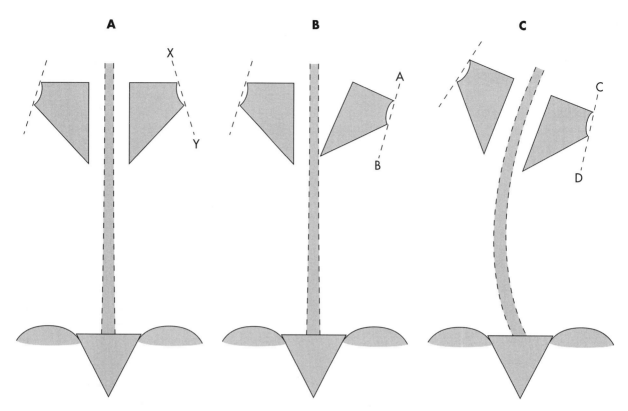

Figure 6-14 **A,** Scapular alignment with a straight spine (x-y glenoid angle). **B,** Paresis with downward rotation of scapula (A-B glenoid angle). **C,** Relative downward rotation of scapula with functional scoliosis (C-D glenoid angle). (From Cailliet R: *The shoulder in hemiplegia*, Philadelphia, 1980, FA Davis.)

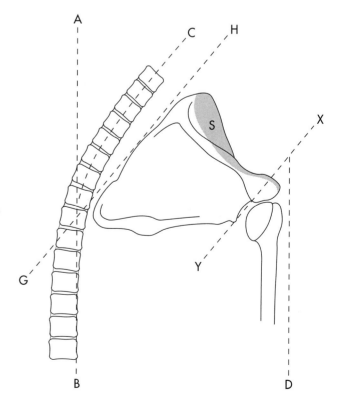

Figure 6-15 Biomechanics of subluxation secondary to malalignment. *AB* indicates an aligned spine (the goal of treatment). Instead the spine assumes a position of lateral flexion (*CB*). The scapula downwardly rotates (*GH*), resulting in a downward angulation of the glenoid fossa (*XY*). Because of the scapula position, the supraspinatus (*S*) loses its mechanical line of pull, making it ineffective and prone to overstretching. The final result is a subluxation of the glenohumeral joint. (Modified from Cailliet R: *Shoulder pain*, Philadelphia, 1990, FA Davis.)

Table 6-3

Subluxation/Malalignment Patterns in the Upper Extremity After Stroke

	TRUNK ALIGNMENT	SCAPULA ALIGNMENT	HUMERAL ALIGNMENT	DISTAL EXTREMITY ALIGNMENT	MOVEMENT AVAILABLE
Inferior subluxation	Lateral flexion to weak side	Downwardly rotated	Relative abduction and internal rotation, humeral head below inferior lip of fossa	Elbow extension and pronation	Scapula elevation and internal rotation
Anterior subluxation	Increased extension, lateral flaring or rotation of ribcage	Downwardly rotated and elevated, winging	Hyperextension and internal rotation, humeral head inferior and forward relative to fossa	Elbow flexion and pronation or supination	Shoulder elevation, humeral internal rotation and hyperextension, elbow flexion
Superior subluxation	Elements of flexion and extension, ribcage flaring	Elevated and abducted	Internal rotation and abduction, humeral head lodged under coracoid	Supination and wrist flexion	Shoulder elevation, abduction, and internal rotation; elbow/wrist flexion

Data from Ryerson S, Levit K: Glenohumeral joint subluxations in CNS dysfunction, *NDTA Newsletter* November, 1988; Ryerson S, Levit K: The shoulder in hemiplegia. In Donatelli RA, editor: *Physical therapy of the shoulder,* ed 2, New York, 1991, Churchill Livingstone.

supported at the side in neutral rotation; trunk stability was maintained during the evaluation. During palpation, subluxation was measured by palpating the subacromial space (the distance between the acromion and the superior aspect of the humeral head) with the index and middle fingers of the therapist. The authors concluded that their findings provided cautious optimism in terms of measuring and identifying subluxation. Prevost et al[107] also validated that palpation is a reliable measurement tool, in the evaluation of subluxation. It should be noted that the evaluator should palpate both shoulders for comparison.

Hall and associates[69] used a 0 (no subluxation) to 5 (2½ finger-widths subluxation) scale during their study. Bohannon and Andrews[16] used a 3-point scale to demonstrate interrater reliability for measuring subluxation: none = 0, minimal = 1, and substantial = 2.

Loss of Distal Alignment

Shoulder alignment problems directly impact the alignment and control of the distal extremity. Boehme[14] states that rotational movements of the forearm "occur at the proximal end with the radius rotating on a vertical axis . . . the ulnar head is displaced, . . . the mechanics are made possible by concurrent external rotation of the humerus." The typical alignment of the humerus after stroke is one of internal rotation, which blocks forearm rotation.

Kapandji[80] states that when the elbow is flexed (a typical posture), pronation is reduced to 45°. Boehme[14] points out that when the wrist is bound by flexion and ulnar devia-

tion (the typical posture of the CVA patient), control of forearm rotation is also blocked.

Wrist motion can become limited by virtue of its own alignment. The range of deviation is at its minimum when the wrist is in flexion and at its maximum when the wrist is in a neutral position or slight flexion.[80] Flexion and extension ranges of the wrist are at a minimum when the hand has an ulnar deviation, and at a maximum when the hand has a neutral deviation.[80]

A loss of palmar arches in the hand results in an inferior movement of the metacarpals followed by a distal hyperextension of the MCPs and flexion of the PIPs and distal interphalangeals (DIPs), the typical claw-hand posture (see Chapter 8).

Interdependence of Trunk and Limb Alignment

Anatomically, therapists must remember that only one bony attachment connects the entire limb to the axial skeleton—the sternoclavicular joint.[82] (The scapulothoracic joint is not a true joint; the scapula rides on the thoracic cage and is maintained by muscular attachments only.[82]) Therefore the clavicle serves as an anatomic link between the shoulder complex and trunk. This point should solidify the interdependence between the trunk and upper extremity. Any malalignments in the proximal segments will have deleterious effects on the upper extremity (Figure 6-16).

The musculature acting on the shoulder has proximal points of attachment. A group of upper extremity muscles

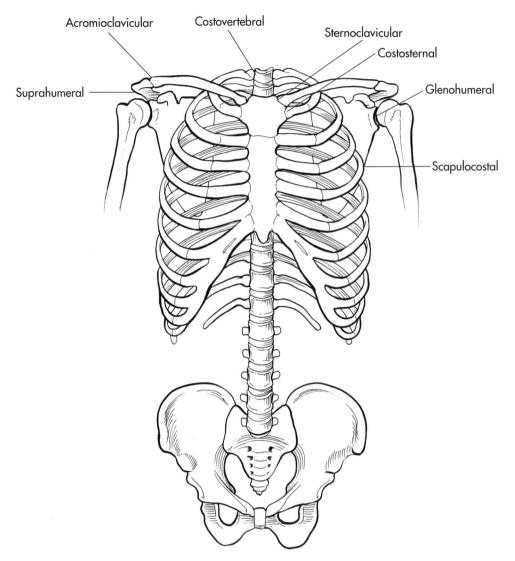

Acromioclavicular   Costovertebral
                                                    Sternoclavicular
                                                         Costosternal
Suprahumeral   Glenohumeral

                                                              Scapulocostal

Figure 6-16 Shoulder anatomy. Note seven joints that make up shoulder complex. The
sternoclavicular joint is the only bony attachment of shoulder to trunk, with the clavicle serving as
bridge between trunk and shoulder. Skeletal alignment of shoulder joint depends on trunk alignment
and stability. For example, if the pelvis becomes malaligned (pelvic obliquity), the vertebral column,
the ribcage, and other components lose their alignment (see Figure 6-12).

(the trapezius, rhomboids, serratus anterior, and levator scapula) runs between the trunk and scapula and another (the pectoralis and latissimus dorsi) runs between the trunk and humerus. Another group of muscles (the deltoid, rotator cuff, and coracobrachialis) attaches from the humerus to the scapula.[82] These attachments emphasize the interdependence of trunk alignment and extremity control.

Mohr[96] points out that biomechanical malalignment produces a pattern of movement that looks like stereotypical patterns used by patients with spasticity. For example, patients who gain early control of scapula elevation and humeral abduction continue to use this pattern and also flex the trunk, resulting in more elevation and abduction. As the scapula tips forward, it predisposes the humerus to internal rotation and extension because of its position in the fossa.[96] The distal arm follows into elbow flexion, pronation, and wrist and digit flexion. Mohr points out that if a normal individual only activates the scapula elevators with humeral abductors, the resulting pattern looks very similar to the patterns used by CVA patients.

These alignment problems need to be addressed before and throughout the treatment session. They should be corrected by mobilization techniques, positioning, and appropriate activity choices. The therapist needs to ensure alignment during ROM activities and maintain appropriate alignment during functional activities. For example, the alignment of the trunk and pelvis of patients who are trying to feed themselves will have a direct impact on the quality of the extremity movement pattern. Even in persons without known neuropathology, the quality of the eating activity is clearly compromised if they assume a forward flexed and laterally flexed static posture rather than an aligned and active trunk posture.

Ryerson and Levit[113] suggest patients perform activities that maintain enhanced trunk alignment and simultaneously coordinate movements of the scapula, trunk, and humerus.

Learned Nonuse

The term *learned nonuse* was coined by Taub.[122] The learned nonuse phenomenon was originally found in primate studies and later applied to chronic stroke patients. When a single forelimb of a monkey was deafferented, the animal would not use that limb in an unrestricted (free) environment. The monkeys' initial attempts to use the limb resulted in failures (e.g., dropping food, losing balance, falling). The monkeys in this study soon found that they could function in their environment with three limbs instead of four. Continued attempts to use the affected limb led to repeated failures at attempted tasks; the effect was suppression of any desire to use that limb. The monkeys *learned* not to use the limb to avoid failure, which masked any future recovery of limb function. Taub et al pointed out that in a free situation, the monkeys did not learn that they could regain use of the forelimb as they recovered function. When the intact forelimb was restrained, the monkeys were forced to use the affected side. This technique converted a useless limb into one capable of extensive movement.

Taub hypothesized that the nonuse or limited use of an affected upper extremity in humans after stroke could in some cases be a result of a similar phenomenon of learned suppression.

To test this hypothesis, Taub studied nine patients with chronic (i.e., greater than 1 year after stroke) hemiplegia. To be included in this study, patients had to demonstrate the ability to extend the MCPs and IPs at least 10°, extend the wrist 20°, and walk without an assistive device. They had to have grossly intact cognitive function, no excess spasticity, be right-arm dominant, and be less than 75 years old.

Patients were assigned to a control or an experimental group. The experimental group underwent forced-use treatment in which the intact limb was placed in a sling and resting-hand splint. The restraint was worn at all times during waking hours except when toileting, when napping, and at times when balance might be compromised. The restraint was worn for 14 days. Each weekday, patients received therapy and were given a variety of tasks, such as eating with utensils, playing ball, playing Chinese checkers and dominoes, writing, and sweeping, to perform with the paretic limb for 6 hours throughout the day.

The control group's treatment focused on increasing attention to the paretic limb. This group was verbally told that they had more potential in their extremities than they were using. Therapists performed PROM activities, and self-ROM activities were performed daily for 15 minutes. The affected limb was not given any training for active movement.

Each group was evaluated before and after intervention with a variety of arm function evaluations and a self-reported motor activity log. The restraint group had significantly faster mean performance speeds from the evaluations, increased quality of movement, and an increased ability to use the extremity in ADL. These improvements were reevaluated 2 years later; they were at least maintained if not increased. Although the comparison group made subtle gains after intervention, the gains were not retained for the follow-up evaluation. Taub et al[122] concluded that the motor ability of stroke patients who met their inclusion criteria could be significantly increased by the interventions effective for overcoming learned nonuse.

Wolf et al[133] researched forced-use treatment in 25 chronic hemiplegic and stroke patients with minimal to moderate extensor muscle function. The forced-use program lasted for 2 weeks, with the intact limb being restrained during waking hours. Significant changes were noted in performance of 19 of the 21 tasks that were evaluated, with most changes persisting for 1 year after the study. The authors concluded that learned nonuse does occur in select neurologic patients and that this behavior can be reversed through application of a forced-use paradigm.

Taub et al[122] summarize by stating that if the "neural substrate for a movement is destroyed by CNS injury, no amount of intervention designed to overcome learned nonuse can be successful in helping recover lost function. However, many stroke patients . . . have considerably more motor ability available than they utilize. The suppression of this additional motor capacity is set up by unsuccessful attempts at movement in the acute poststroke phase . . . increased motor activity should then become increasingly possible, but the suppression of movement remains unabated and inhibits use of the limb. However, if individuals are correctly motivated to use this unexpressed ability, they will be able to do so."

When attempting to incorporate a forced-use method into a treatment program for their own patients, therapists should note that to date this technique has not been used with patients who have had acute strokes. Therapists should refer to Taub's inclusion criteria for treatment. If this technique is to be used, the patients' level of motor function (both gait and upper extremity) should be relatively high, and both studies indicate that distal extensor control is needed for this treatment to be successful.

Inefficient and Ineffective Movement Patterns

Being unable to move effectively and therefore unable to interact with the environment is one of the most devastating sequelae of stroke. The loss of the ability to move effectively is a negative stroke symptom.

The movement patterns of CVA patients have long been discussed in the literature. There continues to be controversy over the nature of these patterns. These movement patterns have been described as reflex based, a release of abnormal synergies, the result of reversed inhibition or the release of lower patterns of activity from higher inhibitory control, and as learned patterns of movement. Mathiowetz[92] points out that more contemporary models of motor control describe patterns developing after central nervous system damage as results of attempts to use remaining resources to achieve occupational performance. He gives the example of a typical flexor pattern in the upper extremity; the pattern can stem from factors other than spasticity, such as the inability to recruit appropriate muscles, weakness, soft tissue tightness, and perceptual deficits.

Carr and Shepherd[36] state that "muscles that are held persistently in a shortened position not only develop contracture but also appear 'easier' for the patients to activate. . . . In the stroke patient such activity appears to become habitual, certain muscle groups, apparently those whose mechanical advantages are greatest (because of their shortened length), contracting persistently to the disadvantage of others." This phenomenon can easily be observed if a patient is observed reaching out to a target. Many patients have difficulty with the protraction, elbow extension, and wrist and digit extension patterns of this task. If the therapist observes the patients who have been in a resting posture (e.g., seated in a wheelchair) for a prolonged time period, the shortened muscles will include the retractors, elbow flexors, and wrist and digit flexors.

Ada et al[3] hypothesize that muscle weakness or paralysis effectively immobilize the upper limb, which results in soft tissue contracture. The immobility causes length-associated changes in muscles, and persistent positioning results in contracture. These changes in the upper limb result in compensatory movements that generate strong neural connections after frequent repetition, ensuring that the compensatory or adaptive movement patterns become learned rather than more effective and efficient.

A Russian neurologist, Nicoli Bernstein, emphasized a task-oriented view of motor performance and introduced the concept that purposeful movement is organized to solve motor problems.[114] Bernstein introduced the concept of degrees of freedom. He hypothesized that the principal problem faced by the central nervous system was the large number of joints and muscles in the human body and the infinite combinations of muscle action.[64] For example, in the upper extremity there are multiple degrees of freedom if the number of planes through which each joint moves are combined. When contemplating the combinations of degrees of freedom in the trunk, scapula, and shoulder to the hand, it becomes evident that task of controlling them is phenomenal. Bernstein states that "The coordination of a movement is the process of mastering redundant degrees

of freedom of the moving organ, that is, its conversion to a controllable system." Bernstein views motor control as a person's ability to coordinate kinematic linkages that limit degrees of freedom (see Chapter 2).

Flinn[61] uses the example of gymnasts learning a new maneuver to apply the concept of degrees of freedom to a task. Gymnasts limit the degrees of freedom in the task by holding some joints rigid while focusing on one specific body part (e.g., foot placement). Although the gymnasts may initially appear stiff, as they become able to control more degrees of freedom, the stiffness disappears and movement relaxes. This example can be applied to learning how to rollerblade, ice skate, or perform a new swimming stroke. Sabari[114] discusses a patient with hemiplegia who does not dissociate the pelvis from the lumbar spine or scapula from the thorax, which may be an effort to decrease the degrees of freedom.

With this concept in mind, many of the ineffective movement patterns we see in our patients can be attributed to attempts to control the degrees of freedom. This needs to be considered during treatment planning when choosing activities. The degrees of freedom must be carefully controlled by stabilizing or eliminating use of some of the joints and therefore decreasing the number of joints involved (e.g., supporting the distal extremity on a table, substituting flat-hand stabilization for a hand grasp).[61]

Many of the inefficient movement patterns we see in CVA patients may be a result of attempting tasks beyond their level of motor control (Figure 6-17). Many therapists have watched patients with newly developed motor control proudly show how they can "lift their arm." Of course, the resulting movement is a stereotypical pattern used by CVA patients. Mathiowetz and Bass Haugen[92] suggest that the use of these movement patterns is evidence of attempts to use remaining systems to complete tasks. They give the example of a patient with weak shoulder flexors trying to lift an arm. The patient flexes the elbow when trying to raise the arm because this movement strategy shortens the lever arm and makes shoulder flexion easier.

Based on these concepts the roles of the occupational therapist in treating inefficient and ineffective upper extremity patterns are the following:

1. To use skills of activity analysis to guide patients' participation in functional upper extremity tasks that correspond to their level of motor control
2. Through this process, to enable our patients to interact with the environment using their more affected upper extremity
3. To use evaluation skills to narrow down which performance components (e.g., postural control, weakness, pain, a combination of components) related to upper extremity function are blocking improvements in occupational performance (e.g., ADL, IADL, work, leisure)

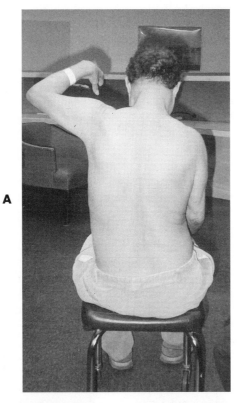

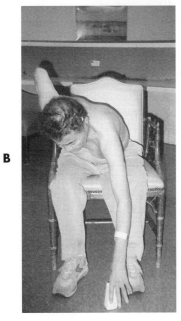

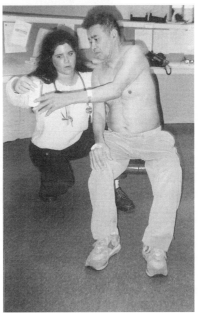

Figure 6-17 **A,** When asked to reach, this patient utilizes a stereotypical flexor pattern. Note trunk lateral flexion, scapula adduction, humeral abduction, and distal flexion. **B,** When position of activity is changed to correspond with available motor control and patient is given a goal (e.g., "Pick up the bottle"), movement pattern is more effective and efficient. **C,** Another position change of same activity results in forward reach with less impact of compensations seen in **A.** Note that patient reaches with wrist extension and his hand is prepositioned for successful task completion. Purpose of activity drives motor output.

4. To provide function-based activities that focus on improving the identified problem area in an effort to improve task performance

Mathiowetz and Bass Haugen[92] suggest using an intervention system that the therapist can employ when using a task-oriented approach. Evaluation must focus on occupational and role performance. The therapist should collaborate with patients to decide which tasks are presenting problems and should be evaluated (e.g., using the Canadian Occupational Performance Measure [COPM]) in relation to the patients' roles. Next, the therapist should observe the patient performing the selected tasks in varied contexts. This observation would give the therapist information regarding the way the environment impacts task performance as well as which components are contributing to the observed functional deficit. With this information the therapist could evaluate the specific components that are interfering with task performance.

In terms of treatment, Mathiowetz and Bass Haugen suggest that therapists help the patients "find the optimal strategy for achieving functional goals." Goals can be achieved by altering the task requirements, altering the environmental context, and by guiding remediation of the component deficits that interfere with functional performance. The most powerful tools occupational therapists have for intervention are functional activities. Although functional activities have formed the basis of treatment since the profession was developed, only recently has the true impact of functional tasks been evaluated in this area of intervention.

USE OF FUNCTIONAL TASKS TO MAXIMIZE UPPER EXTREMITY FUNCTION

The foundation of occupational therapy is built on patients taking an active role in their own recovery by participating in functional activities. In the recent past, many therapists, while attempting to apply neurophysiologic principles to treatment, have limited their use of this modality in favor of more passive techniques that are applied to the patient (e.g., brushing, icing, neurodevelopmental treatment-based handling techniques performed separately from functional tasks). We have now come full circle, with the most current research on motor control supporting the use of tasks performed in context-specific situations. This is not to say that treatments based on the older neurophysiologic theories are not useful, even if their theoretical bases are outdated. Many of the more traditional treatment techniques (e.g., the neurodevelopmental treatment [NDT] approach) are focused on more current problems such as alignment, length-associated changes, and postural control. Some authors are combining the more traditional approaches developed in the 1950s with techniques based on current research.[114] Carr and Shepherd's motor relearning

program for stroke[36] is based on basic principles of activity analysis and the use of tasks combined with current motor learning research. Many of the techniques seem similar to the Bobath[13] concept (i.e., bearing weight on the affected side, teaching movement with patients in upright postures, eliminating unwanted muscle activity, and weight shifting) but are based on current research studies and a modern understanding of the nervous system.

There is a trend in the literature to avoid basing stroke interventions on one person's major contribution to the field of neurologic rehabilitation (e.g., Bobath, Rood, Brunnstrom); instead, interventions should be based on current science without losing sight of basic occupational therapy principles. Use of a comprehensive and holistic approach to the evaluation and treatment of CVA patients would therefore be encouraged.

Functional tasks in therapy include tasks that incorporate weight bearing for postural support, reaching, carrying, lifting, grasping, and manipulating of common objects. These types of activities clearly carry over into daily life tasks and are comprehensive enough to treat a variety of problem areas.

Reaching and Manipulation

The events leading up to a simple voluntary movement such as reaching for a glass of water involve multiple complex processes. Ghez[62] classifies these processes as follows.

First, the glass needs to be identified and its position located in space. This first step encompasses a variety of visual and perceptual processes. Second, a plan of action needs to be selected to bring the glass to the mouth. Ghez points out that this step involves specifying which body parts are needed and in which direction they should move. To do this, the location of the glass must be evaluated in relation to the position of the hand and body. The information collected allows the motor system to determine the appropriate trajectory of the hand. The last step is the execution of the response. Multiple commands are sent to the motor neurons specifying the temporal sequence of muscle activation, the forces to be developed, the changes in joint angles, the orientation of the hand to fit the glass, and the coordination of the shoulder with the distal arm to ensure that the glass will be grasped on contact and without delay. Multiple problems can interfere with these three steps including the issues discussed in the previous section, visual dysfunction, and praxis deficits.

Two components of upper extremity function have been described by Jeannerod.[75,76] The transportation component, which includes the trajectory of the arm between the starting position and the object, and the manipulation component, which is the formation of grip by combined movements of the thumb and the index finger during arm movement.

In her study of reaching deficits in subjects with left hemiparesis, Trombly[126a] used kinematic analysis and

EMG to document impairments in voluntary arm movements. Her analysis demonstrated that the ability to reach smoothly and with coordination was significantly less in the impaired arms than in the unimpaired arms. The continuous movement strategy used during reaching activities was lost, movement time was longer, peak velocity occurred earlier, and indications of weakness were present.

In a follow-up study, Trombly[125] documented the observed improvements in her subjects' reaching abilities. Her findings indicated that the amplitude of peak velocity improved over time. The level of muscular activity did not improve, but the discontinuity of movements decreased. From her findings, Trombly hypothesized that therapy allowing relearning of sensorimotor relationships is warranted for some patients. She stated that the "level and pattern of muscle activity of these subjects depended on the biomechanical demands of the task rather than any stereotypical neurological linkages between muscles."

Van Vliet et al[128] studied subjects in the early months after a stroke. The subjects were able to improve their reaching kinematics during a 3- to 4-week period; they progressed toward normal performance. Providing the subjects with a meaningful task (e.g., drinking from a cup) helped them perform the reach-to-grasp movement considerably.

Jeannerod[76] states that "Formation of the finger grip during the action of grasping a visual object involves two main functional requirements, the fulfillment of which will determine the quality of the grasp. First, the grip must be adapted to the size, shape, and use of the object to be grasped. Second, the relative timing of the finger movements must be coordinated with that of the other component of prehension by which the hand is transported to the spatial location of the object." Jeannerod observes that finger posturing anticipates the real grasp and occurs during transportation of the hand. This shaping of the hand is a mechanism that is independent of the manipulation itself. If treatment programs focused on improved function of the upper extremity are to be designed, then they must include a variety of common objects with different shapes, sizes, and textures to affect this reaching component.

Exner,[54] who defines in-hand manipulation as the process of adjusting objects being grasped in the hand, has developed a classification system that can be used to assist the therapist in activity choice. (Exner's classification system is outlined in Box 6-6.)

Wu and associates[136] demonstrated that using material-based occupation (e.g., picking up a pen and preparing to write your name) enhanced quality of movement performance more than imagery-based occupation (e.g., pretending to pick up a pen and preparing to sign your name) and exercise (e.g., moving your arm forward). Their data suggest that material-based occupation resulted in decreased reaction time, movement time, and movement units. Although this study was performed on normal sub-

Box 6-6

Exner's Classification of Manipulation Tasks

TRANSLATION

The object in the hand moves from the finger surface to the palm or vice versa.

SHIFT

Movement occurs at the finger and thumb pads by alternating thumb and radial finger movements (e.g., moving a coin near the DIP joints further out to the pads of the fingers).

SIMPLE ROTATION

The object is turned or rolled between the finger pads and thumb pad by alternating thumb and finger movements (e.g., unscrewing a jar lid).

COMPLEX ROTATION

The object is rotated, which requires isolated, independent movements of the finger or thumb. The object is turned between 180° and 360° (e.g., turning a paper clip so that correct end can be placed on a piece of paper).

jects, they inferred that material-based occupation may be used to elicit efficient and economical preprogrammed movement for performing tasks.

In a study of fine motor coordination training, Neistadt[102] examined the effects of constructing puzzles and performing kitchen activities on fine motor coordination in a group of brain-injured men. Her results demonstrated that the subjects in the functional meal preparation group showed significantly greater improvements in dominant hand dexterity, which is used for picking up small objects than the subjects in the tabletop puzzle activity group. Her findings suggest that functional activities are more effective (not to mention more meaningful) than tabletop activities for fine motor coordination training in the brain-injured population.

Sietsema et al[118] studied brain-injured patients engaged in rote exercise tasks and occupationally embedded tasks (e.g., reaching out to control a computer game). Their subjects presented with "mild to moderate spasticity" on evaluation. Their results indicated that the game elicited significantly more ROM during the reach pattern performance than the rote exercise. Their study supports the hypothesis that occupationally embedded interventions promote increased performance. The authors hypothesized that the the game provided motivating feedback that enhanced performance.

At this point, research has confirmed that the demands and goals of the task influence motor output. For example, the characteristics of an item being carried across a kitchen will influence factors such as how fast a person will move, whether one or two hands will be used to grip the object, how close to the body the items will be carried, and how stable the arms will be held. In daily life there are many examples of the ways in which movement in daily activities is influenced by the environment (e.g., carrying empty ice trays or full trays, a half-glass of wine or a full cup of coffee, one paper plate or a stack of china plate).

Rosenbaum et al[110b] have demonstrated that the goal of the task influences motor output. His subjects were asked to reach for a cylinder and stand it on one end or the other. Depending on the goal of the task (i.e., which side they were to stand the cylinder on), his subjects reached with either a pronated or supinated grasp pattern. (Sample activities used to retrain reach patterns are provided in Box 6-7.)

Weight Bearing

The use of weight-bearing tasks has long been advocated in patients after CVA. Upper extremity weight bearing has been suggested for achieving a variety of therapeutic goals, including inhibiting hypertonus by moving the body proximally against the distal upper extremity[44] and stimulating upper extremity extension during protective responses.[14] Brouwer and Ambury[30] concluded that upper extremity weight bearing normalizes corticospinal facilitation of motor units in stroke patients. They hypothesized that the mechanism responsible for their results was a sustained increase in motor cortical excitability through augmented afferent input.

McIllroy and Maki[93] Marsden and associates[90] documented that if the upper extremity is used as a postural support (e.g., during weight bearing), postural responses to the opposite arm's movements occur throughout the weight-bearing upper extremity as well as to other perturbations of posture. Their paper also demonstrated that postural responses from the triceps only occurred when the hand was in contact with a firm object.

Although from a neurophysiologic perspective the effect of weight bearing on upper extremity control (i.e., the "normalization of tone" and "inhibition of spasticity") remains controversial, the use of weight-bearing patterns is still necessary for treating the upper extremity after a stroke if the goal of treatment is to improve functional performance. Examples include using the more affected upper extremity in a weight-bearing pattern and as a postural support while manipulating clothing during toileting activities or to enhance participation in IADL (e.g., using the more affected extremity as a postural support during activities requiring standing such as doing the laundry or preparing a meal).

Weight-bearing activities can also be used to address performance components that interfere with function. The problem of soft tissue shortening in the long flexors can be prevented or reversed by bearing weight on extended wrists with extended digits to maintain or increase tissue length. If evaluation reveals that weakness in the extremity is having a limiting effect on function, extended-arm

Box 6-7

Activities to Retrain Reach Patterns

- The patient is positioned in a supine posture while the therapist supports the weight of the distal extremity with a "hand-hold" position. The patient attempts to hold various positions and/or follow the movements of the therapist's hand (guiding). This activity is appropriate for the early motor recovery stage. The degrees of freedom are minimized (with trunk and scapula being supported by the supine posture), and the therapist eliminates the weight of the patient's extremity, maximizing the potential for skeletal muscle recruitment. This activity is easily taught to family members.

- The patient stands or sits in front of a table with a hand resting on a dust cloth that is on top of the table. The patient focuses on gliding the hand across the table. The critical pattern consists of humeral flexion, scapula protraction, and elbow extension. The cloth reduces friction, and the weight of the arm is supported on the table (e.g., weight bearing with superimposed motion).

- The patient is seated, and objects are positioned on the floor in front of patient. The patient reaches for objects on the floor. This downward reach pattern enhances scapula protraction, humeral flexion, and elbow extension by nature of the position of the objects. As the patient gains more control, the objects are raised up to the midshank level, then the knee level, and then the waist level, systematically increasing the motor demands of the task.

- The patient is engaged in the above reach patterns while therapist provides resistance to the functional pattern by tying an elastic band around the palm. The therapist is behind the patient holding the opposite end of the band and is able to grade the level of resistance.

- During the reach activities the demands of the distal components of movement are systematically increased (e.g., increasing manipulation requirements) (Figure 6-18).

weight bearing activities can be used to strengthen the triceps and scapula musculature (i.e., the protractors) if the weight-bearing activities are performed in appropriate alignment and the weight-bearing pattern remains active during the activity.

To ensure appropriate alignment, severe internal rotation, forced elbow extension, and an inactive trunk should be avoided.[113] During weight-bearing activities, maintenance of palmar hand arches is important for maintaining biomechanical alignment and enhancing active patterns. The points of contact between the weight-bearing surface and the hand include the thenar eminence, hypothenar eminence, metacarpal heads, and palmar surfaces of the phalanges.[80] The arch should be maintained so that therapists can insert a finger between the web space and the first

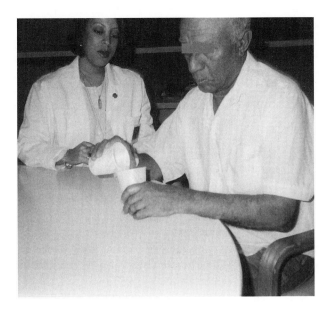

Figure 6-18 Increasing distal demands of task.

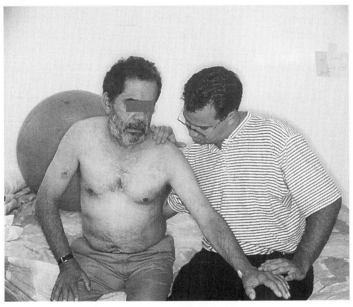

Figure 6-19 Aligning extremity and trunk in preparation for weight-bearing activities. Weight bearing into the therapist's leg allows therapist to detect muscle activity, grade the weight bearing, maintain palmar arch, and maintain alignment.

metacarpal head and slide it under the hand until they make contact with the hypothenar eminence.

Although the more affected arm is in a weight-bearing position, the less involved extremity should be engaged in activities that promote weight shifting in all directions (Figure 6-19). Weight-bearing activities can be performed by the forearm or an extended arm, depending on the demands of the task and the level of available motor control.

SELECTED ADJUNCTIVE INTERVENTIONS AND TREATMENTS

Shoulder Supports

Shoulder supports include any devices used to align, protect, or support an affected proximal limb. Shoulder supports include bed-positioning devices, adaptations to seating systems,

and slings. The use of shoulder supports, especially slings, has been debated in the literature for at least 30 years.

Much of the debate is fueled by the variety of available slings, the controversy over their effectiveness, when and how they should be used, and whether they add to the already numerous complications resulting from an extremity affected by stroke.

Boyd and Gaylard[26] published the results of their survey of Canadian occupational therapists who prescribe slings. The respondents most frequently indicated that the goals of using a sling were to decrease and prevent subluxation and pain. The respondents frequently measured the effectiveness of their interventions by the level of resulting pain relief, subluxation assessments, and the amount of hand swelling. Less frequent measures of effectiveness included ROM, spasticity, and body awareness.

Considering the previously proposed cause of subluxation (see Biomechanical Alignment section), Cailliet[33] suggests that if the goal of treatment is to provide glenohumeral joint stability, then the device must support the scapula on the ribcage with the glenoid fossa facing upward, forward, and outward and must compensate for a lack of support by the rotator cuff and possibly the superior capsule. At this point, no slings are available on the market that assist in realigning the scapula on the ribcage. Therefore slings cannot be prescribed to "reduce a subluxation." They may lift the head of the humerus to the level of the glenoid fossa, but the scapular and trunk alignments (the key to correcting shoulder malalignment) remain impaired. This "reduction" may be seen as treating a symptom of a larger problem. It must be realized that there may be cases in which treating this symptom is appropriate. Analysis is critical for determining which goals certain interventions are achieving. Palpating the subluxation before and after the sling is donned is not sufficient. The effect (if any) of the sling on the more proximal segments needs to be evaluated.

In their review of the literature, Smith and Okamoto[119] identified desirable and undesirable features of slings. Proper positioning of the humeral head in addition to humeral abduction, external rotation, and elbow extension are cited as desirable positions as opposed to humeral adduction, internal rotation, and elbow flexion. The latter positions typically cause problems in the maintenance of tissue length in the stroke population. The sling should also permit the impaired extremity to provide postural support when the patient is seated and should allow self-ROM. In terms of positioning, the sling should provide neutral wrist support, unobstructed hand function, finger abduction, and scapula protraction and elevation.

Smith and Okamoto emphasize that if a therapist expects compliance with sling use, comfort, cosmetic appeal, and easy donning and doffing are crucial. The authors published a checklist to assist therapists in analyzing the slings they provide.

The percentage of therapists using slings has been reported to be as high as 94%,[26] despite the fact no definitive studies support or reject the use of slings.

Several studies have compared and contrasted the effectiveness of various supports. Zorowitz et al[138] compared the following four supports:

1. *The single strap hemisling:* The strap has two cuffs that support the elbow and wrist. The arm is held in a position of adduction, internal rotation, and elbow flexion.
2. *The Bobath roll:* This strap includes a foam roll that is placed in the affected axilla beneath the proximal humerus. The shoulder is maintained in a position of abduction and external rotation with elbow extension.
3. *The Rolyan humeral cuff sling:* This figure-eight strap system has an arm cuff that is sized to fit distally on the humerus of the affected arm. The shoulder is positioned in slight external rotation.
4. *The Cavalier shoulder support:* This type of support provides bilateral axillary support and consists of bilateral straps that are positioned along the humeral head and integrated posteriorly into a brace that rests between the scapula.

In this study, 20 patients were evaluated in the listed supports with anteroposterior shoulder radiography. The authors evaluated the vertical, horizontal, and total asymmetries of glenohumeral joint subluxation compared to the opposite shoulder. In terms of vertical asymmetry, the single strap hemisling corrected the vertical displacement, the Cavalier support did not alter vertical displacement, and the remaining supports significantly reduced but did not correct vertical displacement.

Although as a group, the subjects had no significant horizontal asymmetry when no supports were used, the Bobath roll and the Cavalier support produced a significant lateral displacement of the more affected shoulder's humeral head. This fact is of interest because one proposed goal of a sling is to decrease or prevent subluxation; this study demonstrated that equipment that is not well researched may actually cause shoulder asymmetry in patients who previously had none.

In terms of total asymmetry, the Rolyan humeral cuff sling was the only support that significantly decreased (although it did not eliminate) total subluxation asymmetry.

Moodie and associates[97] evaluated the effectiveness of five shoulder supports: the Bobath roll, a plexiglass lap tray on a wheelchair, a wheelchair-mounted arm trough, a conventional triangular sling (which is much like an arm cast support), and the Hook Hemi Harness (which has two adjustable shoulder cuffs with a suspension strap that are tightened while the affected arm is lifted, resulting in shoulders of equal height). Anteroposterior radiographs of 10 subjects demonstrated that the conventional sling, lap tray, and arm trough were effective in decreasing the width of the glenohumeral space to normal. The Bobath roll and the Hook Hemi Harness were not effective in reducing the subluxation. The authors pointed out that although the conventional sling decreased the subluxation, it reinforced the flexor pattern found in the upper extremity.

Brook et al[29] compared the effects of three supports: the Bobath sling, an arm trough/lap board, and the Harris hemisling (which has two straps and cuffs that cradle the elbow and wrist, holding the arm in a position of adduction, internal rotation, and elbow flexion). The Harris hemisling resulted in good verical correction; in comparison, the Bobath sling did not correct the subluxation as well, the arm trough/lap board was less effective and tended to overcorrect, and the Bobath sling tended to distract the joint horizontally.

It is important to note that none of the mentioned studies discussed scapula or trunk alignment; they only addressed the glenohumeral joint.

Hurd and associates[73] alternately placed 14 patients into a control group (which used no sling) or treatment group (which used a sling). These patients were treated identically in all other respects. The patients were initially evaluated and then evaluated again 2 to 3 weeks later and 3 to 7 months later. No appreciable difference in shoulder ROM, shoulder pain, or subluxation was found between the treated or control groups. No evidence of increased incidence of peripheral nerve or plexus injury was noted in the control group. The authors concluded that the hemisling does not need to be uniformly used by all patients with a flaccid limb after a CVA. They suggested that a sling may be useful when used with discrimination but did not elaborate on this point.

Several authors have published designs for other supports including a "splint jacket"[51] to decrease shoulder pain, the Varney Brace (which was originally designed for acromioclavicular separations) to put downward pressure on the shoulder and upward pressure on the elbow,[83] a modified Bobath sling that provides distal support,[120] and a shoulder-forearm custom support.[108]

Some authors have suggested that slings be prescribed to prevent overstretching soft tissue. Chaco and Wolf[38] suggested that permanent subluxation of the glenohumeral joint could be prevented by avoiding loading on the joint when the limb is flaccid. They concluded that the joint capsule holds the head of the humerus in relation to the fossa when the supraspinatus is not responding but cannot prevent subluxation for an unlimited time unless the cuff responds.

Other authors[6,10] also suggest that if the joint capsule is prevented from stretching during the stage in which the limb is flaccid, patients would have a better opportunity to develop adequate muscle function to maintain joint alignment. Kaplan et al[81] suggest using a sling during the flaccid stage to prevent distraction of the joint resulting in a possible brachial plexus injury.

Some therapists have suggested that sling use may increase body neglect and interfere with body image, although this hypothesis has not been researched. Although they have not been specifically related to sling use, Taub's learned nonuse studies[122] may influence therapists' decisions about whether to prescribe a sling, especially for a patient in the acute phase.

Zorowitz states that "although supports are commonly used during the rehabilitation of stroke survivors, there is no absolute evidence that supports prevent or reduce long-term shoulder subluxation when spontaneous recovery of motor function occurs, or that a support will prevent supposed complications of shoulder subluxation. Without proper training in the use of a support, stroke survivors may face potential complications such as pain and contracture."[138] Although the literature does not give definitive answers about when or whether to use slings, the following guidelines can be inferred:

- Sling use should be minimized during the rehabilitation process.
- Slings may be useful for supporting the more affected extremity during initial transfer and gait training.
- Slings that position the extremity in a flexor pattern should never be worn unless the patient is in an upright posture; in these cases, they should only be worn for select activities (initial mobility training) and short time frames. This type of sling should never be worn by patients in recumbent postures.
- Therapists should continue to investigate the use of alternative means to support the more affected extremity during activities performed in the upright position, such as putting the hand in a pocket, receiving support from an over-the-shoulder bag, adding scapula taping protocols to present treatment plans,[7] or using functional electrical stimulation.[55]
- Each patient's clinical picture must be evaluated on an individual basis. The pros and cons of slings need to weighed, and the goal of sling use needs to be clarified (Box 6-8). Following prescription of the sling, the therapist must reevaluate the effectiveness of the sling (i.e., determine whether the sling is truly meeting the predetermined goal).
- Therapists must become familiar with a variety of slings. One particular sling will not meet the needs of every patient (Figure 6-20).

It may be inferred from the literature that the most effective way to reduce the level of subluxation is to provide the patient with activities that enhance trunk and scapula alignment, activate the rotator cuff, and enhance functional use of the extremity during weight-bearing and reach patterns.

Biofeedback

EMG biofeedback is increasingly being studied for its potential use in the treatment of upper extremity dysfunction after stroke. Biofeedback is provided by electronic instruments that measure and give information about neuromuscular or autonomic activity in the form of auditory or visual feedback signals.

Tries' review[124] of the literature includes a variety of rationales for integrating EMG biofeedback, including training voluntary inhibition of spastic muscles and restoring muscle balance, into an upper extremity program. Tries outlines specific techniques for scapula mobility and stability; humeral rotation; integrating scapular and humeral rotation with a forward reach pattern; and reinforcing functional patterns in the elbow, forearm, and hand.

Tries presents a case study outlining the applications of biofeedback for a left-sided hemiplegic patient. Her case

Box 6-8

Considerations When Prescribing a Sling

PROS

- Protects patient from injury during transfers
- Allows therapist freedom to control trunk and lower extremities during initial gait, transfer, and upright function training
- May prevent soft tissue stretching (e.g., capsular stretching)
- Prevents prolonged dangling of extremity
- May relieve pressure on neurovascular bundle (brachial plexus/brachial artery)
- Supports weight of arm

CONS

- May contribute to neglect or body scheme disorders
- May contribute to learned nonuse
- May hold upper extremity in a shortened position (e.g., internal rotators, adductors, elbow flexors)
- Fosters dependence on passive positioning
- May initiate shoulder-hand syndrome development (i.e., immobility leading to swelling, shortening, pain)
- May predispose patient to shoulder pain from short-ened internal rotators
- Does not reduce the amount of subluxation because the alignment of the scapula and trunk are not affected
- Approximates head of humerus to malaligned scapula
- Prevents reciprocal arm swing while walking
- Prevents arm function (e.g., postural support, carrying) in upright postures
- Blocks sensory input
- Prevents balance reactions of the upper extremity
- May block spontaneous use of the upper extremity
- Places no motor demands on the upper extremity

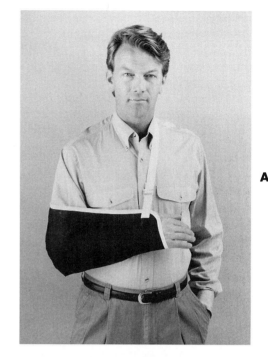

A

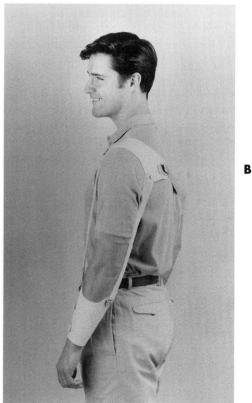

B

study illustrated that despite sensory, cognitive, and per-ceptual impairments, this patient had significant, clinical upper limb functional improvements when combining EMG biofeedback and traditional occupational therapy.

Greenberg and Fowler[66] compared kinesthetic biofeed-back (feedback information pertaining to actual movement of a body part rather than the activity of muscle fibers) to conventional occupational therapy. Their results indicated that kinesthetic biofeedback was equally as therapeutic as but no more effective than conventional occupational ther-apy for increasing elbow extension in hemiplegic subjects.

Crow et al[42] studied two groups (a group receiving biofeedback and a control group) of 20 patients. The pa-tients were studied before and after 6 weeks of treatment and during a follow-up visit 6 weeks later. Although the groups did not significantly differ before treatment, the biofeedback group improved significantly on arm-function evaluations. At the 6-week follow up, it was discovered that the beneficial effects did not persist in the experimental group.

Figure 6-20 **A,** Pouch sling. Sling is only to be used with patients in upright postures and frees therapist's hands to control trunk and lower extremities. This sling may be appropriate for initial phases of walking, transfer, and upright function training. (Courtesy of Sammons, Inc., Bolingbrook, Ill.) **B,** Shoulder saddle sling. Sling supports distal weight of extremity and can be worn under clothing. This style of sling can be worn all day because it does not block distal function or hold extremity in a flexor pattern. (Courtesy of Sammons, Inc., Bolingbrook, Ill.)

Schleenbaker and Mainous[117] concluded from their meta-analysis that biofeedback is an effective tool in neuromuscular reeducation for executing ADL. The use of EMG biofeedback warrants further investigation into its use as an adjunctive tool to enhance upper extremity function in select patients with hemiparesis.

SAMPLE GOALS AND ACTIVITY CHOICES

The following goals are examples of treatment activities for different levels and combinations of functional recovery. Using goals and treatments interchangeably ensures a task-specific approach to intervention. These examples should not be interpreted as progression in recovery. Although previous assumptions were that proximal recovery of abilities precede distal recovery of abilities, this is not always the case. The activities below are graded by increasing the degrees of freedom (e.g., increasing the number of planes of movement that are controlled, integrating hand use), the level of antigravity control, and the objects used in the task. It is important to note that the cognitive demands of the task will have a substantial impact on the level of upper extremity function.

Focusing attention on the more affected upper extremity (no active movement)
- Patient washes upper extremity during upper body bathing activities
- Patient attends to upper extremity while rolling by passively guiding upper extremity across trunk when preparing to roll
- Patient prevents arm from dangling while seated in chair
- Patient positions upper extremity on table during mealtime

Prevention goals
- Patient stretches arm correctly by reaching to floor and maintaining this position after difficult tasks result in arm posturing
- Patient's family demonstrates proper guarding techniques for a mobile patient
- Patient's caretaker demonstrates proper positioning of patient in bed

Forearm weight bearing as a stabilizer
- Patient stabilizes check book with upper extremity while writing checks
- Patient stabilizes cutting board with upper extremity during meal preparation
- Patient holds magazine open with upper extremity while doing crossword puzzle

Using upper extremity for assistance during transitions
- Patient utilizes upper extremity for assistance with assuming sitting position from sidelying position

- Patient uses upper extremity to push up into standing position
- Patient uses upper extremity to reach back before sitting
- Patient uses upper extremity to lower trunk to mat when assuming supine posture from sitting posture

Incorporating upper extremity as a postural support when sitting and standing (extended arm weight bearing with stablized hand on support surface)
- Patient uses upper extremity to assist with lateral shifting while relieving pressure
- Patient stabilizes upper body with affected upper extremity while wiping and dusting table or ironing with less affected upper extremity
- Patient uses more affected upper extremity as a stabilizer on a grab bar while manipulating clothing with less affected upper extremity during toileting
- Patient stabilizes upper body with upper extremity while grooming at sink

Weight bearing with superimposed motion (i.e., hand does not leave support surface but slides and pulls objects)
- Patient irons and dusts with more affected upper extremity while stabilizing upper body with less affected upper extremity
- Patient uses affected upper extremity to lock wheelchair brakes with brake extensions
- Patient uses more affected upper extremity to smooth out laundry
- Patient uses more affected upper extremity to wax and buff car
- Patient uses more affected upper extremity to push shopping cart or rolling walker

Antigravity shoulder movements without hand function
- Patient initiates roll with more affected upper extremity
- Patient lifts more affected upper extremity into shirt sleeve
- Patient lifts more affected upper extremity to counter top
- Patient pushes drawer closed with back of more affected hand
- Patient turns off light switch with side of more affected hand

Initial hand movement (static grasp) with limited shoulder movement (in lap or on work-surface activities)
- Patient adjusts shirt cuff with more affected upper extremity
- Patient holds book in lap with both hands while reading
- Patient stabilizes fruits or vegetables with affected hand while cutting with less affected hand
- Patient holds shopping bag with more affected upper extremity during ambulation
- Patient holds washcloth with more affected upper extremity and washes mid to lower body

Reach patterns with hand activity
- Patient picks up sock from floor with more affected upper extremity
- Patient retrieves item from under sink cabinet with more affected upper extremity
- Patient opens medicine cabinet with more affected upper extremity
- Patient retrieves item from top shelf of medicine cabinet with more affected upper extremity
- Patient drinks out of a cup with more affected upper extremity

Advanced hand
- Patient holds coins in affected palm and slides them to finger tips
- Patient types 15 words per minute with both upper extremities
- Patient signs check with more affected upper extremity
- Patient picks up and reorients paperclip with affected upper extremity.

SELECTED EVALUATION TOOLS

Evaluation tools that are standardized, reliable, and valid can no longer be overlooked. Many therapists continue to use piecemeal evaluations that do not incorporate the use of functional tasks and rely too heavily on evaluating performance components. Trombly[126b] states that ". . . occupational therapists need to develop standardized instruments that relate motor function to occupational performance . . . and to demonstrate the validity and reliability of the instruments to document improved functioning after occupational therapy by patients who have had a stroke."

The Fugl-Meyer Test (Upper Extremity Motor Function)

Becoming familiar with this test is helpful because it is used in many research papers to document improvement in function. It is based on the motor recovery model developed by Twitchell and on Brunnstrom's idea that motor recovery occurs in a specific sequence of steps. Improved motor function is considered a deviation from stereotypical synergies defined by Brunnstrom in this test. It does not involve the use of functional tasks and is not a useful tool for use by occupational therapists to document improved arm function.

Assessment of Motor and Process Skills

Motor and process skills[58,59] are evaluated within the context of IADL. This evaluation allows the occupational therapist to assess a variety of motor (and process) skills within the context of occupational performance—specifically, during observation of IADL. Evaluated motor skills include posture, mobility, coordination, strength, reach,

manipulation, grip, lifting, effort, and energy expenditure. This is a model occupational therapy evaluation (see Chapter 15).

Jebsen Test of Hand Function

This evaluation[77] includes the performance of seven test activities including writing a short sentence, turning over index cards, picking up small objects and placing them in a container, stacking checkers, simulating eating, moving empty large cans, and moving weighted large cans during timed trials. The original paper is based on data collected from 360 normal subjects and patients, including patients with hemiparesis resulting from a CVA. The mean times and standard deviations for normal subjects (with their dominant and nondominant hand) are published in the paper. The test is standardized, reliable, and does not have a practice effect. Therapists must be aware that some of the tasks are simulated activities, and some tasks cannot be considered ADL tasks.

Motor Assessment Scale

Developed by Carr and Shepherd,[37] this test has been found to be highly reliable, with an average interrater correlation of .95 and a .98 average test/retest correlation. This evaluation includes sections on upper arm function, hand movements, and advanced hand activities. The upper arm function section includes movement patterns without tasks; the hand sections incorporate the use of objects.

The Functional Test for the Hemiplegic/Paretic Upper Extremity

Although this evaluation[131] is based on Brunnstrom's view that motor recovery takes place in a specific sequence, it does involve the use of functional tasks that are associated with daily living. This test has been found to be highly correlated with scores on the Fugl-Meyer Test. The test requires approximately 30 minutes to administer. Examples of tasks evaluated include folding a sheet, stabilizing a jar, hooking and zipping a zipper, screwing in a light bulb, and placing a box on a shelf.

GENERAL TREATMENT PRINCIPLES

- Maintain a patient-centered approach to the treatment of upper extremity dysfunction.
- Evaluate and plan treatments that focus on improving occupational performance.
- Focus treatment on task-specific training.
- Maintain mobility (upward rotation and protraction) of the scapula and humeral external rotation to prevent pain syndromes and prepare for return of function.
- Maintain soft tissue length and joint mobility in the trunk, head and neck, and more affected upper extremity.

- Provide appropriate positioning strategies for times when patients are not involved in activities and are in recumbent postures.
- Train all caregivers (staff and family) in the appropriate handling of the more affected upper extremity during ADL and mobility.
- Evaluate and treat any pain syndrome immediately and consistently until symptoms are alleviated.
- Guide appropriate usage of available motor control by providing functional activities that correspond to the patient's level of recovery. Discourage participation in activities that require extra effort.
- Grade activities systematically and with control to increase level of control and functional use.
- Prevent learned nonuse by incorporating the upper extremity into daily life immediately after the CVA.
- Encourage patients to take responsibility for the protection, maintenance, and improvement of their more affected upper extremity.
- Incorporate principles of learning and environmental strategies into the upper extremity treatment plan (see Chapter 2).

■

CASE STUDY

JC is a 60-year-old male who suffered a right middle cerebral artery CVA 1 week before referral. JC was in his usual state of good health until he experienced a sudden onset of left-sided weakness. Before this incident, JC had just sold his antique store to enjoy retirement. JC lives alone, and his interests include reading, gardening, watching movies, wine tasting, and restoring furniture. JC's evaluation and occupational therapy treatment plan (focusing on improved upper extremity function for this study) were as follows.

Initial evaluation

JC was alert and oriented, followed complex commands, had no evidence of cognitive-perceptual deficits with the exception of questionable difficulty with activities incorporating spatial relations components, and had intact sensation. His resting sitting posture consisted of a posteriorly tilted pelvis with minimal functional kyphosis, increased weight bearing on the left ischial tuberosity, right trunk shortening, and a posteriorly rotated left ribcage. JC required minimal assistance with postural adjustments while performing reaching tasks with the right upper extremity. At rest, his left scapula was downwardly rotated and had minimal winging. There was an anterior-inferior subluxation of the left glenohumeral joint.

When asked to demonstrate any arm function, JC attempted to lift his arm against gravity with a resulting pattern of active lateral trunk flexion to the right, active scapula retraction and elevation, and active humeral abduction; during this attempted movement, the distal extremity fell passively into gravity with a resulting pattern of humeral internal rotation, pronation, and wrist flexion.

PROM was within normal limits after the scapula was mobilized and gliding with the exception of lacking 20° of external rotation. There was no evidence of spasticity upon quick stretch. JC's muscle grades were grossly 2−/5: scapula and humerus (except external rotation 0/5), elbow: 3−/5, forearm: 2−/5, wrist: 1/5, finger flexion: 3+/5, finger extension: 2−/5, and finger abduction/adduction: 1/5. JC did not have selective control of his extremity; instead he moved in gross patterns. He was not able to incorporate his left upper extremity into his ADL on initial evaluation. Limitations to JC's ability to use his upper extremity were identified as inefficient movement patterns ("stereotypical") as a result of loss of postural control, weakness, and trunk and upper extremity malalignments.

Week one goals and treatments

1. Roll independently while protecting left upper extremity.
2. Stretch independently (using the towel-on-table program).
3. Independently position the left upper extremity on a table while eating and performing leisure activities.
4. Independently relieve pressure by lateral weight shifting in the wheelchair. (JC was instructed to perform this in front of dining table with both forearms supported on table.)

At this stage, JC was also provided with a half swing-away lap tray and bed positioning items including a pillow for under his left scapula and left elbow.

Treatment focused on left upper extremity protection during transitional movements as well as reaching activities using the right upper extremity in all directions, with a focus on trunk responses and inclusion of rotational activities to recruit abdominal muscle activity. Activities such as repotting plants were used because they required a variety of reach patterns and were previously enjoyed by JC. At this point the left upper extremity was used to stabilize objects (e.g., the bag of soil).

JC was given a styrofoam cup and asked to support his forearm on his lap tray, place the cup upside down into his left hand, and practice releasing it. As the task became easier, he turned the cup right side up to increase the difficulty level. During therapy, treatment focused on controlling the distal arm from the mouth to the table (eccentrically) with his elbow supported on the table and the therapist supporting the humerus with JC's hand empty.

Weeks two and three goals and treatments

1. Independently hold toothpaste tube in left hand while unscrewing the cap with the right hand.
2. Lift arm from lap to the lap tray without right upper extremity assisting.
3. Independently stretch left wrist and digits into extension.

At this stage, JC progressed to assuming standing postures in front of a work surface. Activities included buffing tables and sliding papers across the table past arm's length with the left upper extremity to encourage scapula protraction. Wiping the table (hand-over-hand) and focusing on patterns to the far left were used to maintain soft tissue length and encourage external rotation. As the task became easier, JC held the towel in his left hand and wiped the table using only his left upper extremity.

Weeks three, four, and five goals and treatments

1. Locking wheelchair brakes independently with left upper extremity.
2. Use both upper extremities to pull pants up from midthigh to waist while standing with close supervision.
3. Independently support left upper extremity in pants pocket while walking.

Week five (the final week of inpatient treatment) goals and treatment activities included the following:

1. Independently opening kitchen drawer with left upper extremity while standing
2. Holding an over-the-shoulder bag with left upper extremity while walking
3. Using both hands to don a sock
4. Turning sink faucets on and off with left upper extremity while standing

Note that the goals and treatment activities were not considered different entities. Treatment was task and goal specific.

When discharged from inpatient rehabilitation, JC was able to use his left upper extremity as a postural support during forearm and extended arm weight-bearing activities, integrate use of his left upper extremity during self-care activities (but limited to movement patterns below chest level [e.g., in lap activities, reaching below hips]), integrate use of his left hand into fine motor activities, and carry items in his left hand while walking. Movement patterns that required further antigravity shoulder patterns, increased hand control, and strengthening with resistance were the focus of outpatient occupational therapy.

■

REVIEW QUESTIONS

1. Which factors contribute to glenohumeral joint subluxation?
2. Why are handling techniques only considered adjuncts to function-based therapy?
3. Which factors contribute to a painful shoulder condition after a stroke?
4. In what way does biomechanical malalignment of the trunk and upper extremity contribute to ineffective and inefficient movement patterns?
5. Describe the learned nonuse phenomenon and treatments aimed at its prevention or reversal.
6. Why are weight-bearing activities considered critical treatments for patients after a stroke?
7. Which factors contribute to a malaligned scapula?
8. Describe a treatment progression aimed at increasing manipulation patterns.
9. According to the World Health Organization classification system, what is considered effective occupational therapy intervention in terms of improved upper extremity function?

■ COTA Considerations ■

- Prevent soft tissue shortening by appropriate ROM, positioning, activity placement, and educating the patient about limb management.
- Notify team members immediately if symptoms of a pain syndrome develop.
- Incorporate weight-bearing, reach, and manipulation activities into upper extremity treatment plans.
- Prevent learned nonuse by immediately incorporating the more affected extremity into ADL.
- Appropriately position patients (specifically, their shoulders) immediately and as needed.

REFERENCES

1. Abreu B: The quadraphonic approach: management of cognitive-perceptual and postural control dysfunction, *Occup Ther Pract* 3:12, 1992.
2. Abreu B: Perceptual motor skills: assessment and intervention strategies, *Cognitive Rehabilitation: Self-Study Series*, 1994, American Occupational Therapy Association.
3. Ada L et al: Task-specific training of reaching and manipulation. In Bennett KMB, Castiello U, editors: *Insights into the reach to grasp movements*, 1994, Elsevier Science.
4. Agency for Health Care Policy and Research: *Post-stroke rehabilitation clinical practice guideline*, Washington DC, 1994, The Agency.
5. American Occupational Therapy Association: Uniform terminology for occupational therapy-third edition, *Am J Occup Ther* 48:1047, 1994.
6. Anderson LT: Shoulder pain in hemiplegia, *Am J Occup Ther* 39:11, 1985.
7. Andeway K: Scapular malalignment in upper quadrant dysfunction, *Phys Ther Mag* pp. 60-65, 1994.
8. Arsenault AB et al: Clinical significance of the V-shaped space in the subluxed shoulder of hemiplegics, *Stroke* 22:867, 1991.
9. Ashworth B: Carisoprodol in multiple sclerosis, *Practitioner* 192:540, 1964.
10. Baker LL, Parker K: Neuromuscular electrical stimulation of the muscles surrounding the shoulder, *Phy Ther* 66:1930, 1986.
11. Basmajian JV: The surgical anatomy and function of the arm-trunk mechanism, *Surg Clin North Am* 43:1471, 1963.
12. Belenkii VY, Gurfinkle VS, Paltsev YI: Elements of control of voluntary movements, *Biophysics* 12:135, 1967.
13. Bobath B: Adult hemiplegia: evaluation and treatment, ed 3, Oxford, 1990, Butterworth-Heinemann.
14. Boehme R: *Improving upper body control: an approach to assessment and treatment of tonal dysfunction*, Tucson, 1988, Therapy Skill Builders.
15. Bohannon RW: Recovery and correlates of trunk muscle strength after stroke, *Int J Rehabil Res* 8:162, 1995.
16. Bohannon RW, Andrews AW: Shoulder subluxation and pain in stroke patients, *Am J Occup Ther* 44:507, 1990.
17. Bohannon RW, Cassidy D, Walsh S: Trunk muscle strength is impaired multidirectionally after stroke, *Clin Rehabil* 9:47, 1995.
18. Bohannon RW et al: Shoulder pain in hemiplegia: a statistical relationship with five variables, *Arch Phys Med Rehabil* 67:514, 1986.
19. Bohannon RW et al: Relationship between static muscle strength deficits and spasticity in stroke patients with hemiparesis, *Phys Ther* 67:1068, 1987.
20. Bohannon RW, Smith MB: Assessment of strength deficits in eight paretic upper extremity muscle groups of stroke patients with hemiplegia, *Phys Ther* 67:552, 1987.
21. Booth FW: Physiologic and biochemical effects of immobilization on muscle, *Clin Orthopaed Related Res* 219:15, 1987.

22. Botte MJ et al: Spasticity and contracture: physiologic aspects of formation, *Clinical Orthopaed Related Res* 233:7, 1988.

23. Bouisset S, Zattara M: A sequence of postural movements precedes voluntary movement, *Neurosci Lett* 22:263, 1981.

24. Bourbonnais D et al: Abnormal spatial patterns of elbow muscle activation in hemiparetic human subjects, *Brain* 112:85, 1989.

25. Bourbonnais D, Vanden Noven S: Weakness in patients with hemiparesis, *Am J Occup Ther* 43:313, 1989.

26. Boyd E, Gaylard A: Shoulder supports with stroke patients: a Canadian survey, *Can J Occup Ther* 53:61, 1986.

27. Braus DF, Krauss JK, Strobel JS: The shoulder-hand syndrome after stroke: a prospective clinical trial, *Ann Neurol* 36:728, 1994.

28. Brodal A: Self observations and neuro-anatomical considerations after a stroke, *Brain* 96:675, 1973.

29. Brooke MM et al: Shoulder subluxation in hemiplegia: effects of three different supports, *Arch Phys Med Rehabil* 72:582, 1991.

30. Brouwer BJ, Ambury P: Upper extremity weightbearing effect on corticospinal excitability following stroke, *Arch Phys Med Rehabil* 75:861, 1994.

31. Burgess MK: Motor control and the role of occupational therapy: past, present, and the future, *Am J Occup Ther* 43:345, 1989.

32. Burke D: Spasticity as an adaptation to pyramidal tract injury, *Adv Neurol* 47:401, 1988.

33. Cailliet R: *The shoulder in hemiplegia*, Philadelphia, 1980, FA Davis.

34. Carr EK, Kenney FD: Positioning of the stroke patients: a review of the literature, *Int J Nurs Studies* 29:355, 1992.

35. Carr JH, Shepherd RB, Ada L: Spasticity: research findings and implications for intervention, *Physiotherapy* 81:421, 1995.

36. Carr JH, Shepherd RB: *A motor relearning programme for stroke*, ed 2, Rockville, Md, 1982, Aspen Publishers.

37. Carr JH et al: Investigation of a new motor assessment scale for stroke patients, *Phys Ther* 65:175, 1985.

38. Chaco J, Wolf E: Subluxation of the glenohumeral joint in hemiplegia, *Am J Phys Med* 50:139, 1971.

39. Chan WY: Some techniques for the relief of spasticity and their physiological basis, *Physiother Can* 38:85, 1986.

40. Chu DS et al: Shoulder-hand syndrome: importance of early diagnosis and treatment, *J Am Geriatr Soc* 29:58, 1981.

41. Cordo PJ, Nashner LM: Properties of postural adjustments associated with rapid arm movements, *J Neurophysiol* 47:287, 1982.

42. Crow L et al: The effectiveness of EMG biofeedback in the treatment of arm function after stroke, *Int Disabil Studies* 4:155, 1989.

43. Davies PM: *Right in the middle: selective trunk activity in the treatment of adult hemiplegia*, New York, 1990, Springer-Verlag.

44. Davies PM: *Steps to follow: a guide to the treatment of adult hemiplegia*, New York, 1985, Springer-Verlag.

45. Davis J: The role of the occupational therapist in the treatment of shoulder-hand syndrome, *Occup Ther Practice* 1:30, 1990.

46. Davis SW et al: Shoulder-hand syndrome in a hemiplegic population: a five year retrospective study, *Arch Phys Med Rehabil* 58:353, 1977.

47. DeGangi GA, Royeen CB: Current practice among neurodevelopmental treatment association members, *Am J Occup Ther* 48:803, 1994.

48. Denny-Brown D: Preface: historical aspects of the relation of spasticity to movement. In Feldman RG, Young RR, Koella WP, editors: *Spasticity: disordered motor control*, Chicago, 1980, Year Book.

49. Dietz V, Quintern J, Berger W: Electrophysiological studies of gait in spasticity and rigidity, *Brain* 104:431, 1981.

50. Duncan PW, Badke MB, editors: *Stroke rehabilitation: the recovery of motor control*, Chicago, 1987, Year Book.

51. Egan JM: An aid for the management of shoulder pain in hemiplegia, *Br J Occup Ther* 53:362, 1990.

52. Eggers O: *Occupational therapy in the treatment of adult hemiplegia*, Oxford, 1983, Butterworth-Heinemann.

53. Engardt M et al: Dynamic muscle strength training in stroke patients: effects on knee extension torque, electromyographic activity, and motor function, *Arch Phys Med Rehabil* 76:419, 1995.

54. Exner CE: In-hand manipulation skills. In Case-Smith J, Pehoski C, editors: *Development of hand skills in the child*, Rockville, Md, 1992, American Occupational Therapy Association.

55. Faghri PD et al: The effects of functional electrical stimulation on shoulder subluxation, arm function recovery, and shoulder pain in hemiplegic stroke patients, *Arch Phys Med Rehabil* 75:73, 1994.

56. Feldman RD, Young RR, Koella WP, editors: *Spasticity: disordered motor control*, Chicago, 1980, Year Book.

57. Fellows SJ, Thilmann AF: Voluntary movement at the elbow in spastic hemiparesis, *Ann Neurol* 36:397, 1994.

58. Fisher AG: The assessment of IADL motor skills: an application of many-faceted rasch analysis, *Am J Occup Ther* 47:319, 1993.

59. Fisher AG: *Assessment of motor and process skills*, Colorado, 1995, Three Star Press.

60. Fisher B: Effect of trunk control and alignment on limb function, *J Head Trauma Rehabil* 2:72, 1987.

61. Flinn N: A task oriented approach to the treatment of a client with hemiplegia, *Am J Occup Ther* 49:560, 1995.

62. Ghez C: Voluntary movements. In Kandel ER, Schwartz JH, Jessell TM, editors: *Principles of neural science*, ed 3, New York, 1991, Elsevier.

63. Ghez C: Posture. In Kandel ER, Schwartz JH, Jessell TM, editors: *Principles of neural science*, ed 3, New York, 1991, Elsevier.

64. Gordon J: Assumptions underlying physical therapy intervention: theoretical and historical perspectives. In Carr JH, Shepherd RB, editors: *Movement science: foundations for physical therapy in rehabilitation*, Gaithersburg, Md, 1987, Aspen Publishers.

65. Gowland C et al: Agonist and antagonist activity during voluntary upper-limb movement in patients with stroke, *Phys Ther* 72:624, 1992.

66. Greenberg S, Fowler RS: Kinesthetic biofeedback: a treatment modality for elbow range of motion in hemiplegia, *Am J Occup Ther* 34:738, 1980.

67. Hakuno A et al: Arthrographic findings in hemiplegic shoulders, *Arch Phys Med Rehabil* 65:706, 1984.

68. Halar EM, Bell KR: Contracture and other deleterious effects of immobility. In DeLisa JB, editor: *Rehabilitation Medicine: Principles and Practice*, Philadelphia, 1993, JB Lippincott.

69. Hall J, Dudgeon B, Guthrie M: Validity of clinical measures of shoulder subluxation in adults with poststroke hemiplegia, *Am J Occup Ther* 49:526, 1995.

70. Harburn KL et al: Spasticity measure in stroke: a pilot study, *Can J Public Health* (suppl)83:41, 1992.

71. Hecht JS: Subscapular nerve block in the painful hemiplegic shoulder, *Arch Phys Med Rehabil* 73:1036, 1992.

72. Horak FB et al: The effects of movement velocity, mass displaced, and task certainty on associated postural adjustments made by normal and hemiplegic individuals, *J Neurol Neurosurg Psychiatry* 47:1020, 1984.

73. Hurd MM, Farrell KH, Waylonis GW: Shoulder sling for hemiplegia: friend or foe? *Arch Phys Med Rehabil* 55:519, 1974.

74a. Hufschmidt A, Mauritz KH: Chronic transformation of muscle in spasticity: a peripheral contribution to increased tone, *J Neurol Neurosurg Psychiatry* 48:676, 1985.

74b. Hummelsheim H et al: Influence of sustained stretch on late muscular responses to magnetic brain stimulation in patients with upper motor neuron lesions, *Scand J Rehabil Med* 26:3, 1994.

75. Jeannerod M: The formation of finger grip during prehension. A cortically mediated visuomotor pattern, *Behav Brain Res* 19:99, 1986.

76. Jeannerod M: The timing of natural prehension movments, *J Motor Behav* 16:235, 1984.

77. Jebsen RH et al: An objective and standardized test of hand function, *Arch Phys Med Rehabil* 50:311, 1969.

78. Jensen EM: The hemiplegic shoulder, *Scand J Rehabil Med* (suppl)7:113, 1980.

79. Joynt RL: The source of shoulder pain in hemiplegia, *Arch Phys Med Rehabil* 73:409, 1992.

80. Kapandji IA: *The physiology of the joints, vol 1, the upper limb*, New York, 1982, Churchill Livingstone.

81. Kaplan PE et al: Stroke and brachial plexus injury: a difficult problem, *Arch Phys Med Rehabil* 58:415, 1977.

82. Kent BE: Functional anatomy of the shoulder complex, *Phys Ther* 51:867, 1971.

83. Krempen JF et al: The use of the Varney brace for subluxating shoulders in stroke and upper motor neuron injuries, *Clin Orthopaed Related Res* 122:204, 1977.

84. Kumar R et al: Shoulder pain in hemiplegia: the role of exercise, *Am J Phys Med Rehabil* 69:205, 1990.

85. Lankford LL: Reflex sympathetic dystrophy. In Hunter JM et al, editors: *Rehabilitation of the hand: surgery and therapy*, ed 3, St Louis, 1990, Mosby.

86. Landau WM: Spasticity: the fable of a neurological demon and the emperor's new therapy, *Arch Neurol* 31:217, 1974.

87. Landau WM: Spasticity: what is it? What is it not? In Feldman RG, Young RR, Koella WP, editors: *Spasticity: disordered motor control*, Chicago, 1980, Year Book.

88. Lee WA: A control systems framework for understanding normal and abnormal posture, *Am J Occup Ther* 43:291, 1989.

89. Little JW, Massagli TL: Spasticity and associated abnormalities of muscle tone. In DeLisa JA, editor: *Rehabilitation medicine: principles and practice*, ed 2, Philadelphia, 1993, JB Lippincott.

90. Marsden CD, Merton PA, Morton HB: Human postural responses, *Brain* 104:513, 1981.

91. Massion J: Postural changes accompanying voluntary movements. Normal and pathological aspects, *Hum Neurobiol* 2:261, 1984.

92. Mathiowetz V, Bass Haugen J: Motor behavior research: implications for therapeutic approaches to central nervous system dysfunction, *Am J Occup Ther* 48:733, 1994.

93. McIllroy WE, Maki BE: Early activation of arm muscles follows external perturbation of upright stance, *Neurosci Letters* 148:177, 1995.

94. Merideth J, Taft G, Kaplan P: Diagnosis and treatment of the hemiplegic patient with brachial plexus injury, *Am J Occup Ther* 35:656, 1981.

95. Meyer AZ: The philosophy of occupational therapy, *Am J Occup Ther* 31:639, 1977.

96. Mohr JD: Management of the trunk in adult hemiplegia: the Bobath concept, *Topics in Neurology*, 1990, American Physical Therapy Association.

97. Moodie NB, Brisbin J, Grace Morgan AM: Subluxation of the glenohumeral joint in hemiplegia: evaluation of supportive devices, *Physiotherapy Can* 38:151, 1986.

98. Moskowitz E, Porter JI: Peripheral nerve lesions in the upper extremity in the hemiplegic patient, *New Engl J Med* 269:776, 1963.

99. Muller EA: Influence of training and of inactivity on muscle strength, *Arch Phys Med Rehabil* 449, 1970.

100. Najenson T, Yacubovic E, Pikielni SS: Rotator cuff injury in shoulder joints of hemiplegic patients, *Scand J Rehabil Med* 3:131, 1971.

101. Nakayama H et al: Recovery of upper extremity function in stroke patients: the Copenhagen stroke study, *Arch Phys Med Rehabil* 75:394, 1994.

102. Neistadt ME: The effect of different treatment activities on functional fine motor coordination in adults with brain injury, *Am J Occup Ther* 48:877, 1994.

103. Nepomuceno CS, Miller JM: Shoulder arthrography in hemiplegic patients, *Arch Phys Med Rehabil* 55:49, 1974.

104. Olsson O: Degenerative changes of shoulder joint and their connection with shoulder pain: morphological and clinical investigation with special attention to cuff and biceps tendon, *Acta Chir Scand* 181(suppl):1, 1953.

105. Ough JL et al: Treatment of spastic joint contractures in mentally disabled adults, *Orthoped Clin North Am* 12:143, 1981.

106. Perry J: Rehabilitation of spasticity. In Feldman RG, Young RR, Koella WP, editors: *Spasticity: disordered motor control*, Chicago, 1980, Year Book.

107. Prevost R et al: Shoulder subluxation in hemiplegia: a radiologic correlational study, *Arch Phys Med Rehabil* 68:782, 1987.

108. Rajaram V, Holtz M: Shoulder forearm support for the subluxed shoulder, *Arch Phys Med Rehabil* 66:191, 1985.

109. Rizk TE et al: Arthrographic studies in painful hemiplegic shoulders, *Arch Phys Med Rehabil* 65:254, 1984.

110a. Rogers JC, Holm MB: Accepting the challenge of outcome research: examining the effectiveness of occupational therapy practice, *Am J Occup Ther* 48:871, 1994.

110b. Rosenbaum DR, Jorgensen MJ: Planning macroscopic aspects of manual control, *Hum Movement Sci* 11:61, 1992.

111. Roy CW, Sands MR, Hill LD: Shoulder pain in acutely admitted hemiplegics, *Clin Rehabil* 8:334, 1994.

112. Ryerson S, Levit K: Glenohumeral joint subluxations in CNS dysfunction, *NDTA Newsletter* November, 1988.

113. Ryerson S, Levit K: The shoulder in hemiplegia. In Donatelli RA, editor: *Physical therapy of the shoulder*, ed 2, New York, 1991, Churchill Livingstone.

114. Sabari JS: Motor learning concepts applied to activity-based intervention with adults with hemiplegia, *Am J Occup Ther* 45:523, 1991.

115. Sahrmann SA, Norton BJ: The relationship of voluntary movement to spasticity in the upper motor neuron syndrome, *Ann Neurol* 2:460, 1977.

116. Savage R, Robertson L: Shoulder pain in hemiplegia: a literature review, *Clin Rehabil* 2:35, 1988.

117. Schleenbaker RE, Mainous AG: Electromyographic biofeedback for neuromuscular reeducation in the hemiplegic stroke patient: a meta-analysis, *Arch Phys Med Rehabil* 74:1301, 1993.

118. Sietsema JM et al: The use of a game to promote arm reach in persons with traumatic brain injury, *Am J Occup Ther* 47:19, 1993.

119. Smith RO, Okamoto G: Checklist for the prescription of slings for the hemiplegic patient, *Am J Occup Ther* 35:91, 1981.

120. Sullivan BE, Rogers SL: Modified Bobath sling with distal support, *Am J Occup Ther* 43:47, 1989.

121. Tabary JC et al: Physiological and structural changes in the cat's soleus muscle due to immobilization at different lengths by plaster casts, *J Physiol* 224:231, 1972.

122. Taub E et al: Technique to improve chronic motor deficit after stroke, *Arch Phys Med Rehabil* 74:347, 1993.

123. Tepperman PS et al: Reflex sympathetic dystrophy in hemiplegia, *Arch Phys Med Rehabil* 65:442, 1984.

124. Tries J: EMG feedback for the treatment of upper extremity dysfunction: can it be effective? *Biofeedback Self-Regulation* 14:21, 1989.

125. Trombly CA: Observations of improvements of reaching in five subjects with left hemiparesis, *J Neurol Neurosurg Psychiatry* 56:40, 1993.

126a. Trombly CA: Deficits of reaching in subjects with left hemiparesis: a pilot study, *Am J Occup Ther* 46:887, 1992.

126b. Trombly CA: Clinical practice guidelines for post-stroke rehabilitation and occupational therapy practice, *Am J Occup Ther* 49:711, 1995.

127. Van Ouwenaller C, Laplace PM, Chantraine A: Painful shoulder in hemiplegia, *Arch Phys Med Rehabil* 67:23, 1986.

128. Van Vliet P et al: The influence of functional goals on the kinematics of reaching following stroke, *Neurol Report* 19:11, 1995.

129. Waylett-Rendall J: Therapist's management of reflex sympathetic dystrophy. In Hunter JM et al, editors: *Rehabilitation of the hand: surgery and therapy*, ed 3, St Louis, 1990, Mosby.

130. Williams R, Taffs L, Minuk T: Evaluation of two support methods for the subluxated shoulder of hemiplegic patients, *Phys Ther* 68:1209, 1988.

131. Wilson DJ, Baker LL, Craddock JA: Functional test for the hemiparetic upper extremity, *Am J Occup Ther* 38:159, 1984.

132. Wolf SL et al: Overcoming limitations in elbow movement in the presence of antagonist hyperactivity, *Phys Ther* 74:826, 1994.

133. Wolf SL et al: Forced use of hemiplegic upper extremities to reverse the effect of learned nonuse among chronic stroke and head-injured patients, *Exp Neurol* 104:125, 1989.

134. Woollacott MH, Bonnet M, Yabe K: Preparatory process for anticipatory postural adjustments: modulation of leg muscles reflex pathways during preparation for arm movements in standing man, *Exp Brain Res* 55:263, 1984.

135. World Health Organization: *International classification of impairments, disabilities, and handicaps*, Geneva, 1980, The Organization.

136. Wu C-Y, Trombly CA, Lin K-C: The relationship between occupational form and occupational performance: a kinematic perspective, *Am J Occup Ther* 48:679, 1994.

137. Yue G, Cole KJ: Strength increases from the motor program: comparison of training with maximal voluntary and imagined muscle contractions, *J Neurophysiol* 67:1114, 1992.

138. Zorowitz RD et al: Shoulder subluxation after stroke: a comparison of four supports, *Arch Phys Med Rehabil* 76:763, 1995.

139. Zorowitz RD et al: Shoulder pain and subluxation after stroke: correlation or coincidence? *Am J Occup Ther* 50:194, 1996.

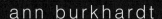

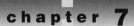

ann burkhardt

chapter **7**

Edema Control

key terms

edema	massage	pain syndromes
entrapment	congestive heart failure	compression therapy
vascular	renal failure	deep venous thrombosis
lymphatic		

chapter objectives

After completing this chapter, the reader will be able to accomplish the following:

1. Describe causes and underlying medical conditions that result in clinical symptoms of edema.
2. Provide clinical reasoning for edema treatment.
3. Describe types of evaluations used to detect edema and the success of edema treatment.
4. Describe types of treatments for edema, and provide specific information concerning possible indications and contraindications for the use of specific treatments.

Edema is a condition that results in an enlargement of a body part such as a limb or one of the various compartments of the body. Edema that develops after a stroke may be related to sequelae of the stroke underlying organ dysfunction. It is therefore important for therapists to use their clinical reasoning skills to determine (1) which factors may be causing the edema, (2) whether the underlying cause of the edema is related to failure or decreased functioning of an organ or system of the body (such as the heart, lungs, circulatory system, or kidneys), (3) whether contributing factors are present (such as a blood clot) that could worsen the patient's condition if treated in certain

ways, and (4) whether the edema treatment will increase the patient's function and quality of life.

PATHOPHYSIOLOGY AND MEDICAL MANAGEMENT

Upper extremity edema first seen unilaterally in a limb may be the result of (1) an entrapment from a postural change that causes impingement, (2) decreased activity of the vascular muscle pump, which is normally active during movement and functional use, (3) development of an abnormal sympathetic nerve response (e.g., reflex sympa-

152

thetic dystrophy), or (4) a blood clot in the involved limb. Although rare, if the patient has another malignant condition, such as cancer, that obstructs the lymphatic vessels, the unilateral upper extremity condition may be a result of tumor involvement.

Several entrapment syndromes can result in upper extremity edema, including (1) scalenus anticus syndrome, (2) first rib syndrome (costoclavicular syndrome), (3) thoracic outlet syndrome, and (4) reflex sympathetic dystrophy. These syndromes may develop with postural changes after stroke. The alleviation of some of these disorders through treatment may focus on changing seating behaviors through positioning, exercise, and modifications of the way activities are done.

Scalenus anticus syndrome[10] is characterized by neck and shoulder discomfort and a tingling sensation in the hand and fingers. The pain is vague and achy, and although the person may occasionally complain of shooting pain, it is not the prominent complaint associated with this condition. The scalenus anticus muscle is a strap muscle of the neck that originates on the cervical vertebrae (3 through 6) and inserts on the scalenus tubercle of the first rib. The subclavian artery and brachial plexus are normally behind the muscle. The scalenus anticus is often used for minor postural adjustments of the head such as nodding during a conversation. It assists with suspending the head over the trunk and is also an accessory muscle used during breathing, but its dysfunction is never life threatening from a respiratory perspective. The most significant clinical test for scalenus anticus syndrome is one which tests the patient's response to manual pressure on the muscle while the patient's head is rotated, laterally flexed, and posteriorly tilted to the opposite side. The area is tender to palpation.[7] The person may feel warmth or an exacerbation of the tingling as the muscle is stretched (during palpation). These symptoms are vascular in origin and related to neurovascular bundle impingement. The scalenus anticus syndrome evolves because the person assumes a position in which the shoulders are internally rotated (commonly referred to as *round shouldered*), head is flexed forward, and cervical spine is hyperextended. Although the scalenus anticus muscle attaches to the first rib, this condition is different than first rib syndrome because it does not result in rotation of the first rib.

The first rib syndrome is characterized by shoulder pain radiating proximally to distally. It may impinge the neurovascular bundle as well, but it is less likely to occur than it is with scalenus anticus syndrome. The first rib is normally tilted down and forward. If the person develops an abnormal posture of the cervical spine, the soft tissues accommodate over time, causing the anterior end of the rib to migrate into a position of upward rotation,[7] which impinges on the thoracic inlet of the neurovascular bundle. The symptoms usually arise later in the course of the disease because the body tends to adapt initially when the soft tissues are pliable and may be stretched. Over time, as contracture of the soft tissues occurs, the condition worsens.

Thoracic outlet syndrome (TOS) after a stroke may result from a narrowing of the space through which the neurovascular structures leave the chest cavity (the thorax) and descend to the peripheral structures in the arms. TOS may be associated with trauma or repeated trauma of the thoracic outlet at the shoulder. After repeated transient compressions, the brachial plexus may become scarred (i.e., develop neurofibrosis).[1] TOS is a compression syndrome and may result when a person with a hemiparetic upper extremity and decreased proprioceptive and kinesthetic sensation bears weight on the extended limb while the shoulder girdle is unsupported. It could also be exacerbated by bilateral overhead lifting (which often occurs when a person with hemiparesis is advised to passively assist the arm affected by the stroke with the other arm, especially when the affected arm has no protective position sense. That is, there is a lack of normal arm suspension as the head of the humerus glides down into overhead flexion and abduction with external rotation. The humeral head slides down so far that the normal counterbalance provided by the shoulder depressors is disturbed, resulting in impingement on the thoracic outlet). Repeated banging of the humeral head against the clavicle could narrow the thoracic outlet and irritate and inflame the brachial plexus.[1] Over time and with repeated trauma the acute inflammatory response, the cytokine reaction (which at the cellular level results in abnormal collagen formation and a loss of elastin in soft tissue) evolves into a chronic condition with permanent hypertrophic scarring of the nerves and permanent narrowing of the thoracic outlet.[1,8] The usual clinical complaints associated with TOS are pain, paresthesia, and arm weakness that worsens with activities requiring overhead reaching (overhead activities). This complaint is also usually associated with persons who had a history of being sedentary and then suddenly or abruptly increased their overhead activities. The usual pain distribution is tingling and numbness in the ulnarly innervated hand digits (the ulnar border of the middle, and ring, and little fingers). The underlying cause for this clinical symptom is the direct trauma to the medial cord of the inferior trunk of the brachial plexus.

Reflex sympathetic dystrophy (RSD) is a pain disorder that results from an injury but clinically appears to be out of proportion to the extent of the injury. It usually results from trauma, fractures, crush injuries, and sprains but also has been known to develop after a myocardial infarction; after a stroke; in patients with cervical disk disease, phlebitis, tuberculosis infection, or cancer; and after animal bites or frostbite.[9] It has also been observed in a patient who received an intramuscular influenza vaccine in a hemiparetic extremity and in another patient who had a repetitive strain injury after overusing an upper extremity bilateral exerciser (UBE). Typically, the patient is first seen with recalcitrant pain that worsens when the limb is touched or moved. Although a number of studies have attempted to link laboratory findings with the presence of RSD, the only laboratory anomaly that appears to be consistent is an elevated erythrocyte sedimentation rate in 70% of patients in one group.[9] The results of one animal study suggested that this anomaly may be linked to an increased number of Langerhans' cells in the skin, resulting in altered capillary innervation and eventual degeneration of motor end plates.[9] This has not yet been demonstrated in humans. RSD is a complex disorder and is probably formed by intricate neurophysiologic pathways that form an organic basis for the disorder. A preexisting psychologic condition was once thought to cause or predispose a person to RSD. Current thought is that chronic pain and debilitating body changes probably cause psychologic responses.

RSD is a systemic disease that usually begins in an affected extremity (e.g., an extremity affected by a stroke). There are three stages of RSD. Stage I is characterized by burning pain that worsens in severity and paresthesia resulting from light touch. Pitting edema of the dorsum of the hand is also common.[5] Digital and wrist motions progressively decrease, in part as a result of the edema, which acts as an internal splint and prevents full active motion, possibly resulting in overstretching the extensor muscles of the hand and a loss of extrinsic muscle-generated power (tenodesis). Motion is also diminished when the patient avoids using the limb because of anticipated pain exacerbation. The hand color is initially pale to bluish (cyanotic), but erythema of the metacarpal phalange joints eventually develops at the conclusion of stage I. The typical trophic changes of the skin are increased sweating and coolness. Vasospasm and peripheral vasoconstriction are common in this stage. Osteoporotic changes may be detected after 3 weeks and are characterized by the bone's moth-eaten appearance on X rays. This stage usually lasts approximately 3 months[5] (Figure 7-1).

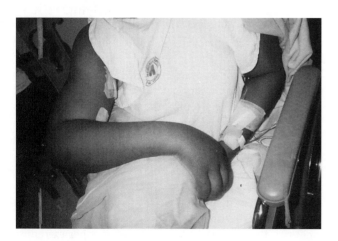

Figure 7-1 RSD edema.

Stage II may last for 9 months. It is characterized by worsening pain, decreases in the sweating response, shiny skin, erythema, and increased localized heat—in the portion of the limb where the pain is most intense. Progressively worsening stiffness is a prominent feature. Osteoporotic changes may affect the long bones of the arm. Edema persists, but rather than being fluid and causing pitting, it changes and causes the limb to become firm and brawny.[5]

Stage III, sometimes referred to as the *atrophic stage*, may last more than 2 years. The edema progresses from brawniness to periarticular thickening of the joint lining. For example, the digital ligaments and joint capsules may become thick and scarred as the soft tissues lose elastin after a cytokine response to a chronic inflammation. The fingertips take on a typical pencil-point appearance as the subcutaneous tissue and muscles atrophy. Osteoporosis is profound at this stage[5] (see Chapter 6).

In contrast to the entrapment syndromes, a stroke survivor may also develop peripheral edema associated with deep venous thrombosis (DVT) or phlebitis.[6] These conditions usually develop in individuals who have clots or vascular disorders and often have embolic stroke syndromes. Blood clots form when there is an increase in the number of platelets (blood cells that assist with blood clotting). A thrombus often forms in a blood vessel region that has had vessel-wall trauma. Areas with more plaque are prone to developing clots (e.g., carotid arteries). However, limbs are also very prone to clot formation when trauma to their vascular structures is related to prolonged vessel compression (e.g., resulting from bed rest, being unconscious, or being immobile during surgery. The intraoperative use of pneumatic pumps is a method used to prevent the development of DVT during or after surgery. Thromboembolic disease stockings (TEDS) also help prevent clots from developing in sedentary persons. Persons with hemiparesis of an upper extremity may also develop DVT in the arm.

DVT in any limb may result in edema. The most common clinical sign of DVT in the lower extremity is calf tenderness, and in any extremity is tenderness when a muscle compartment is lightly squeezed.[6] Initially the edema accompanying DVT is compartmentalized. If undetected for a day or two, the edema will progress distally to the clot. The person may experience distal vasomotor changes because the vascular flow is diminished mechanically by the loss of intravessel space caused by obstruction by the clot. The goal in the overall management of a blood clot is to dissolve and not cause movement of the clot, because the clot may travel to life-sustaining body organs and result in a secondary complication. For example, if a clot migrates to the heart, it may result in a heart attack. If the clot migrates to the lungs, it may result in a pulmonary embolus and perhaps respiratory distress. If the clot migrates to the brain, it may result in repeated cerebrovascular accidents (CVAs). If the clot remains in the limb but continues to increase in size, it could potentially cause a compartment syndrome (i.e., the circulation may be fully obstructed to the peripheral portion of the limb). The distal limb loses oxygen, and the tissue begins to necrose, or die. In this situation, it may be necessary to surgically extract the clot and decompress the intramuscular limb compartment, or the patient could lose the limb or die. The most frequent clinical sign of a compartment syndrome is acute loss of motor function followed by vascular signs such as cyanosis. Additional weakness in a person with preexisting hemiparesis could be difficult to detect, yet the therapist is often the first team member to detect the change in functional status.

Generalized edema that involves the trunk of the body or edema that involves bilateral limbs of the body may be a result of major organ dysfunction rather than the aforementioned impingement syndromes. Most commonly, patients with generalized edema are first seen with bilateral pedal edema involving both feet. In a patient with no history of stroke, pedal edema may develop for a number of reasons that are completely unrelated to stroke risk. For the purposes of this chapter, the edema discussion will be limited to edema in stroke survivors.

Bilateral pedal edema (Figure 7-2)—swelling of the feet and ankles—may be a sign of preexisting peripheral vascular disease (PVD), congestive heart failure (CHF), chronic renal failure (CRF), diabetic-related small vessel disease, inactivity resulting in understimulation of the internal large muscle pumps, or lymphedema tarda (an edema to which people are genetically predisposed that develops in adulthood). PVD may involve either (or both) the vein or artery systems of the limbs.[6] When a person is sitting with the legs in a dependent position, such as when the person is sitting on a bed with the feet resting on the floor, gravity encourages interstitial fluid to circulate toward the feet. If vascular disease is present, the vessels are either narrowed by plaque (e.g., from hypercholesterolemia), dam-

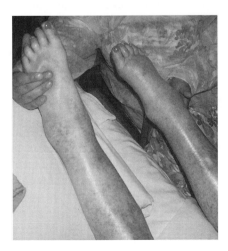

Figure 7-2   Bilateral pedal edema.

aged by tar and nicotine (e.g., from cigarette smoking), or atrophied because of hyperglycemic circulation (e.g., from diabetes). Whether the dysfunction is a result of vascular valve dysfunction, atrophy of vessel musculature atrophy, or internal vessel flow resistance (from a number of factors that result in vessel constriction), the edema results from impaired hemodynamics. One concern is the lack of assisting muscle pumping. A simple increase in active muscle contraction of the legs is sometimes sufficient to decrease pedal edema. Regardless of whether activity level has increased, if edema persists, further evaluation and treatment may be indicated. When patients have heart and lung or kidney dysfunction, medications may allow them to be able to use activity to resolve the edema. For example, diuretic medications may improve kidney function and mobilize the fluids abnormally retained by the body.[2]

If major organ system dysfunction persists or septicemia develops (a widespread infection in the blood stream), the edema may develop in the trunk (*ascites*) or throughout the entire body (*anasarca*). Treatment for ascites usually includes medications to enhance organ function and mobilize the fluids.[2] A patient with ascites or anasarca may have to stay in bed because the body may need all its energy for central hemodynamic and homeostatic processes rather than for the peripheral mechanical hemodynamic function potential that may be gained through gross mobilization and stimulation of cardiopulmonary function. When septicemia is the main cause of anasarca or ascites,[2,6] an antibiotic may be the most important treatment of the underlying cause of the edema. In this situation, the edema is caused by a lymphatic response to the potentially unbeatable antigen (bacteria, fungus or virus) resulting in a white blood cell-, protein-rich edema rather than a fluid-like blood plasma. In today's hospital environment, decades of fighting infections with broad-spectrum antibiotic agents has resulted in increasing numbers of resistant infections that will be tougher to control until another drug or method is devised.

In addition to diuretics, other drugs that enhance function of specific organs may be used to mobilize fluid as well. For example, patients with CHF may be receiving a diuretic (e.g., Lasix) while they are also receiving a drug to stabilize blood pressure (e.g., a β-blocker) and possibly even a drug to stabilize their arrhythmia (e.g., digoxin). Therefore internal medicine physicians often attempt to achieve homeostasis in an individual who has major organ failure by many methods. Rehabilitation may only be a small part of the initial treatment picture for these individuals.

EVALUATION METHODS

The most commonly used method to measure edema is taking circumferential measurements. The method for taking circumferential measurements is often not standardized from clinic to clinic, possibly resulting in haphazard approaches to measuring edema and its response to treatment. Therapists who work in settings in which edema is consistently measured or treated usually choose one of two methods of measurement: (1) measuring the limb consistently a certain distance (in centimeters) above and below an anatomic landmark (e.g., an upper extremity such as the elbow), (2) measuring the limb at certain anatomic landmarks (e.g., the insertion of the triceps or the midbelly of the biceps), the distance of which will vary according to the anatomic distribution in the individual. As with goniometry and manual muscle testing, the outcomes of these measurements will probably be most consistent when the same therapist measures and remeasures the person each time (i.e., relies on intrarater versus interrater reliability). A specific type of tape measure may also be appropriate to control the degree of pull against the tape (e.g., a measurement made with a weighted pull).

Another method used to measure the girth of a limb is volumetrically displacing water by submersing the limb in water that is contained in an enclosed space. The container has a spill-off valve from which the displaced water is collected and measured. Commercial volumeters may be purchased for the clinical setting. If volumetric measurements are used, consistent positioning must be used each time, and the limb must always be submerged to the same point; otherwise the measurement will be skewed.

Computer-generated measurements have also been developed but are currently too expensive for most clinics to own. These are probably the most reliable forms of volumetric measurement, but they presently are not consistently applicable.

Tonometry is another method used to detect or measure edema in a limb. The difficulty with using tonometry is that it does not accommodate for quality differences in edema. For example, a brawny limb may have measurements that are similar to a normal limb because the tone of the soft tissue is firmer, like toned muscle. In contrast, fluid and pitting edemas would result in greater girth.

Clinical observations are also used in the evaluation of edema. Examples of observations include the following:

1. Skin temperature
2. Skin moisture: moist or dry
3. Skin color: red (erythema), pale, cyanotic (bluish tint)
4. Firmness on palpation (soft, fluid-like, pitting, brawny, firm and woody)
5. Presence, quality and distribution of pain (tingling, numbness, coolness, heaviness, cramping, electrical or shocking)
6. Weeping of the edema through the skin
7. Loss of mobility or motion by increased girth versus motor weakness

8. Blood pressure (although care should be taken to avoid inflating a blood pressure cuff on a limb suspected of having DVT or phlebitis or that has had a lymphatic impairment)

Monitoring blood tests may also be helpful in the overall management of the edema. Erythrocyte sedimentation rate (ESR),[9] platelet level, white blood cell count (WBC), prothrombin time,[6] blood glucose levels, and creatinine and bilirubin counts may be helpful to follow, depending on the underlying medical conditions. Platelet levels and prothrombin time indicate the possible presence of or response to treatment of clotting disorders. WBC indicates the possible presence of an infection by stimulation of an immune response. Blood glucose levels in a diabetic patient will be extremely elevated if WBC is elevated. Creatinine and bilirubin counts are indicators of renal function.

Sensory assessment is a key component in the determination of the level of the entrapment[7] (i.e., the nerve root—following the distribution of the dermatome, the plexus—following the sensory loss of the pattern of the plexus trunk, or the peripheral nerve). In addition, diabetic patients may have entrapment neuropathies of rapidly adapting nerve fibers (A fibers—moving two point and vibratory sense) superimposed on a limb that has a diabetic large fiber (C fiber—pain and temperature sense) neuropathy. If patients have a lesion affecting the cerebellum, their position sense may also be impaired. If sensation is impaired, patients may tend to avoid or underuse the involved limb. The inactivity can generate edema through understimulation of the internal muscle pumps in the limb.[2] In addition, trauma caused by imperception of pain in the involved limb could result in posttraumatic edema. Documentation of type, distribution, and quality of pain perceived in the limb may provide clues to potential pain syndrome evolution (e.g., RSD). Cramping muscle pain is common at the proximal attachment of the extremity of the limb, as well as intracompartmentally in the extremity, especially in the forearm and lower leg when edema is present.

Active range of motion assessment is also important because distention of a limb area may decrease the available range of motion through overstretching one group of muscles (e.g., the extensors of the hand and wrist in a person with an edematous hand). Increased girth of a limb will also limit full active movement of the limb into flexion (e.g., the elbow in an arm or the knee in a leg). Passive range of motion activities should not be aimed at forcing an edematous compartment through full range of motion because it could result in additional chronic deformity. For example, overstretching the extensor digiti minimi can result in ulnar slippage and displacement of the tendon over time.

TREATMENT METHODS

Edema associated with entrapment syndromes—scalenus anticus syndrome, first rib syndrome, and TOS—may be relieved by treating the posture, positioning, and habits that have contributed to the development of these conditions. Strengthening weak muscles may also assist in correcting imbalances, which result in assuming positions of comfort that may contribute to decreased function by limiting ability to participate in activities. For example, a person with hemiparesis who sits in a posterior tilt may have flattening of their lumbar and thoracic curves and abducted scapulae, internally rotated and adducted humeri, and a hyperextended cervical spine. As a result of this posture, the soft tissues (e.g., muscles, tendons, nerves, ligaments, blood and lymphatic vessels, fascia and skin) have assumed a shortened position. Prolonging this position results in reflex muscle spasms to accommodate overstretching or shortening. As the muscles contract, the fascia tightens and the skin shortens, all entrapping the nerves and vascular structures and causing sensory changes and edema.

If the person weight shifts into a neutral pelvic tilt, the spinal curves are often restored, the head is suspended up over the spine, the scapulae adduct, and the humeri abduct and externally rotate.[3] Once repositioned, the individual can inhale more deeply, possibly enough to rotate the rib into a normal position. Teaching the person to self-cue and adjust the posture using techniques such as the Alexander technique may also improve postural habits.

With release of the soft tissues, hemodynamic flow improves because other structures, such as overstretched, reflex-spasming, posturally compromised muscles, were impinging the vessel flow. Impingement on vascular structures results in restriction of hemodynamic flow. Impaired vascular return results in local backflow, venous and lymphatic stasis, and edema. Myofascial release is a manual technique that is often helpful for stretching out and elongating (restoring normal length to) the soft tissue structures.

Positional elevation, compression and gentle massage techniques, pneumatic compression, and compression bandaging and gradient compression garments may be indicated for edemas resulting from impingement syndromes and major organ dysfunction. There are indications for and contraindications to the use of some of these techniques that do influence clinical reasoning and treatment modality choice. Awareness of the way the treatment causes change may provide the necessary underpinnings of the clinical reasoning process.

Positional elevation uses gravity to assist the hemodynamic flow in the limb backward and down toward the heart. The right side of the heart propels deoxygenated blood from the peripheral vascular system into the left side of the heart, where it becomes reoxygenated. Therefore if the stroke survivor has any right-sided heart failure, this technique would not be advisable. Encouraging backflow may overstress the heart and contribute to a life-threatening event. A person who has DVT would also not be encouraged to elevate the limb. Elevation could transport the clot toward the central organs—the heart, lungs, and brain in particular. A person with arterial dysfunction cannot tolerate positional elevation because it will produce Raynaud's phenomenon and can decrease viability of the distal ends of the limb (the fingers or toes); the person will develop dysesthesia within a short time.

When used, elevation only needs to suspend the distal portion of an extended limb 9 cm above the right side of the heart.[2] The person's extremity will need to remain elevated for 45 minutes to an hour at a time. Active movement is encouraged to prevent limb stiffness and stimulate the muscle pump to return the excess fluid to central circulation. Elevating the limb too much can contribute to traction or compression of the brachial plexus if the limb is improperly positioned. This could result in a change in the sensory and motor status of the limb and prolong the rehabilitative period. Elevation can help to mobilize fluid, but the edema returns when the limb returns to a dependent position.

Compression garments or wraps must be used to prevent backflow and limb refilling. Temporary compression garments, such as tubular support bandages, Isotoner gloves, self-adherent (e.g., Coban) wraps and compression wrapping bandages (e.g., Ace bandage, Comprilan) can be used. Stroke survivors are more prone to cyanotic changes when using compression wrapping. Changes in capillary refill and subtle somatic complaints of tingling and numbness may necessitate removal of the support. When compression wraps are tolerated, they assist in stimulating the internal muscle pump while the person is actively using the limb. They also provide neutral warmth, which can help relax the skeletal muscle response.

External supports such as air splints (which are static) and pneumatic massage pumps (which are dynamic: sequential or gradient sequential) can also be used to create a pressure gradient in the limb. These devices utilize air-filled sleeves to provide the pressure gradient. The air splint is inflated by mouth or a pump while the limb is in the sleeve; a valve is closed and the pressure remains in the device. Pneumatic pumps rely on a continuous airflow system generated by a motor (an air compressor), which inflates the pneumatic sleeve. Some pumps have one chamber or cell that inflates and then deflates around the limb; other pumps have multiple cells per sleeve. The distal cell fills first, and the remaining cells continue to fill distally to proximally, creating a "milking" motion that dynamically decongests the edematous limb. Pneumatic massage and air splints should not be used by stroke survivors who have DVT or active phlebitis, are receiving anticoagulant medications that drop their platelet levels below 120,000 mm³, have active, untreated, moderate to severe CHF or CRF.

Manual massage may also help decrease limb edema. The most popular massage technique in current use is manual lymphatic massage. The superficial lymphatics in the trunk and uninvolved extremity are stimulated first. The involved extremity is then massaged lightly using a combination of scooping, vibratory, and wedging strokes. The proximal extremity is massaged first, the middle portion second, and the distal portion last. Other popular techniques that may also be helpful are retrograde massage and accupressure massage (Figure 7-3).

The treatment of RSD is more complex because edema stemming from RSD may stimulate the pain response and increase the intensity of, while decreasing the tolerance for, the recalcitrant pain. Techniques that may be useful in treating RSD include (1) stressloading an activity, (2) combining rehabilitative treatment with nerve blocks (saline, Baer, lidocaine and/or marcaine ganglion blocks) and pharmacologic treatment (e.g., Amytriptilline, Nortryptilline, Tegretol, Dilantin). Electrical ganglion blocks, such as high-volt galvanic stimulation (HVGS) or transcutaneous nerve stimulation (TENS), may also be helpful as long as the affected limb is not ipsilateral to the region of a pacemaker or the individual does not have active, suboptimally controlled arrhythmia. Acupuncture may also be helpful in treating RSD pain. In stage II or stage III RSD, heavy sedation may be indicated to begin treatment depending on the patient's pain and psychologic response.[4]

RSD may also be treated with ice baths and contrast baths. One technique is to plunge the limb with RSD into an ice-slush bath for 3 to 5 seconds and repeat 2 to 3 times (Figure 7-4), causing quick vasomotor restriction. This should be followed by active or active assistive overhead motion (with respect for the patient's pain). The activities should be graded over time and progressed to include

stressloading activities within the context of ADL. No single technique will work for every person with RSD. Knowledge of and training in the aforementioned techniques may provide more options for the therapist and the patient with edema and pain to try until the correct combination of techniques or modality is determined. Creativity, ingenuity, and compassion are all important for effectively treating persons with pain syndromes.

■

CASE STUDY

VL is a 52-year-old woman who developed edema and worsening pain during a rehabilitation unit stay after a stroke that caused residual right hemiparesis. A "go-getter," VL performed five times the number of repetitions of all exercises and activities prescribed by her therapist. She says she assumed that "doing more and more would make her better sooner."

VL (who was right-hand dominant) complained of pain in her right shoulder that increased in intensity whenever she used the UBE machine. She was instructed to use the machine 3 times per day. In hopes of speeding up her recovery, she had been doing her repetitions 6 times per day.

VL is married and has a young child, and before her stroke, she worked full-time as a manager. Her avocational activities were skiing, ice skating, and walking. She enjoyed going to the theater, visiting museums, and trying new restaurants.

On evaluation, VL complained of middeltoid and clavicular pain. After obtaining a brief history, it was revealed that she had neck and shoulder discomfort for more than a decade before to her stroke. Her arm was moderately edematous, dusky in color, and cool in the distal portion. During active, overhead range of motion activities, she experienced a stabbing feeling that progressed to burning pain in the middeltoid. She also complained of reflex muscle spasm in her neck and shoulder

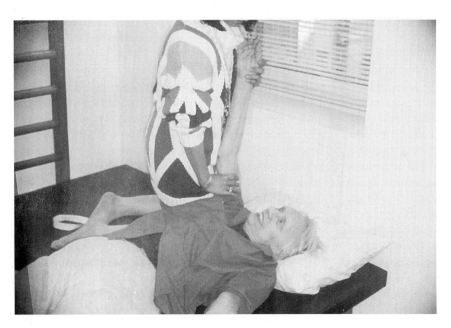

Figure 7-3 Manual massage techniques may assist with decreasing edema in a limb.

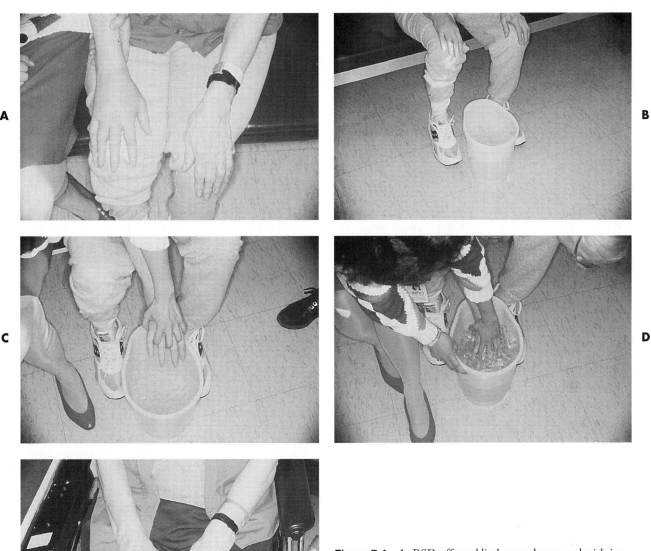

Figure 7-4 A, RSD-affected limbs may be treated with ice baths **(B, C, D)** for a noticeable decrease in edema **(E).**

girdle. Her active range of motion of her elbow was within functional limits, but she had an incomplete grasp/release and nonfunctional fine motor skills; for example, she could not hold money, a pen, or a piece of paper. If she tried to continue to move, she felt a cramping sensation. She was unable to use her arm for any self-care activities, such as washing or brushing her hair, toileting, fastening her brassiere, writing, holding utensils and cups, and handling her child.

Her evaluation included measurement of her active range of motion, documentation of the circumferential measurements of both upper extremities, observations of the trophic changes in her skin and her right arm circulatory status, and documentation of functional strength and skill level.

Treatment included active assistive range of motion activities for the neck and entire right arm; lymphatic massage; compression bandaging; elevation and distal muscle pumping; stressloading activities (e.g., using her arm as a support, cleaning the table with her affected arm); massage of and myofascial release techniques for the neck, trunk, and right upper extremity; guided imagery to decrease her anxiety about treatment possibly exacerbating her pain, and activities of daily living (both basic and instrumental).

Within a month, VL could use both arms to embrace her child when she sat on VL's lap. She could also prepare a cup of tea and carry a plate from the kitchen to the dining room table and could brush the right side of her hair with her arm supported on a table. Her edema decreased significantly with a combination of elevation, massage, and improved vascular return resulting from functional use of the arm. The relaxation response evoked by the guided imagery helped to decrease her concern about potential pain. Her therapy, combined with acupuncture treatment and HVGS on acupuncture meridians on days when she did not receive acupuncture treatment, all contributed to a positive outcome for this patient with RSD.

■

SUMMARY

Edema after a stroke may be caused by a number of underlying pathologic conditions, poor posture or positioning, or trauma to a limb that is weak or has diminished sensation or may accompany major organ failure. Knowledge of the underlying conditions and the side effects of their treatment helps the therapist make an informed recommendation for and implement a treatment plan.

Edema treatment is closely tied to the medical model. Rehabilitative strategies contribute to the resolution of the condition but not without the medical and other complementary techniques that may assist recovery. Patience, creative problem-solving, and perseverance are characteristics that commonly contribute to successful treatment of this population. More research, qualitative and quantitative, is needed to document successful functional outcomes in the management of edema and pain in the stroke population. RSD is an expensive and disabling condition when not treated early and when treatment choices are not grounded in procedural clinical reasoning.

REVIEW QUESTIONS

1. Explain the differences among scalenus anticus syndrome, first rib syndrome, and TOS. Discuss sensory findings and patterns of weakness including the contribution of poor posture to the development of these syndromes and the edema that results.
2. If a stroke survivor has symptoms of bilateral pedal edema, how would you choose the rehabilitation treatment?
3. Which drugs are used to treat neuropathic pain?
4. Describe the stages of RSD.
5. How would you treat hand edema in a person who has DVT in their hemiparetic upper extremity? Which precautions would you take?

■ COTA Considerations ■

- Edema can be caused by a variety of factors. The cause and type of edema will influence the rehabilitation treatment.
- Edema in a single limb may be caused by impingement on the vascular structures (blood vessels), which, after stroke, may occur from poor posturing or positioning after stroke.
- Edema in both legs, the trunk, or the entire body is usually associated with organ failure. Care must be taken not to overload the heart, lungs, or kidneys by mobilizing the fluid toward the failing organ.
- Edema can be treated by positional elevation, gradient compression bandages or garments, and pneumatic or manual massage.
- A review of the indications and contraindications for rehabilitation treatment measures is important for ensuring that the patient receives the appropriate treatment, which depends on multiple medical factors.
- Reducing edema can prevent pain, increase ease of gross mobility, and support participation in activities of daily living.

REFERENCES

1. Barbis J: Therapist's management of thoracic outlet syndrome. In Hunter JM et al, editors: *Rehabilitation of the hand: surgery and therapy*, ed 3, St. Louis, 1990, Mosby.
2. Brunwald E: Edema. In Wilson JD et al, editors: *Harrison's principles of internal medicine*, ed 12, New York, 1991, McGraw-Hill.
3. Davis PM: *Steps to follow: a guide to the treatment of hemiplegia*, Heidelberg, Germany, 1985, Springer-Verlag.
4. Davis Jan: The role of the occupational therapist in the treatment of shoulder hand syndrome, *Occup Ther Practice* 1:30, 1990.
5. Lankford LL: Reflex sympathetic dystrophy. In Hunter JM et al, editors: *Rehabilitation of the hand: surgery and therapy*, ed 3, St Louis, 1990, Mosby.
6. Moser KM: Pulmonary embolism. In Wilson JD et al, editors: *Harrison's principles of internal medicine*, ed 12, New York, 1991, McGraw-Hill.
7. Post M: *The shoulder: surgical and non-surgical management*, Philadelphia, 1988, Lea & Febiger.
8. Rote NS: Inflammation. In McCance KL, Heuther SE, editors: *Pathophysiology: the biological basis for disease in adults and children*, ed 2, St Louis, 1994, Mosby.
9. Shelton RM, Lewis CW: Reflex sympathetic dystrophy: a review, *J Am Acad Dermatol* 22:234, 1990.
10. Wilgis EF: *Vascular injuries and diseases of the upper limb*, Boston, 1983, Little, Brown.

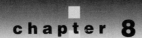

stephanie milazzo
glen gillen

chapter 8

Splinting Applications

chapter objectives

After completing this chapter, the reader will be able to accomplish the following:

1. Identify a variety of splinting options
2. Review positive and negative aspects of commonly used splints
3. Summarize the research that has been published on splinting and people who have had strokes
4. Present rationales for splinting that consider current concepts of motor control, including biomechanical principles
5. Critically analyze and reconsider the present approach to splinting, evaluating each extremity individually

Any discussion of splinting of the upper extremity after stroke produces debate among occupational therapists. The use of splints after stroke can be traced as far back as 1911.[32] Since then the debate about whether to splint and about the rationales for splinting has continued.

The following principles guide splinting decisions for patients after stroke:

• Splints are used to either maintain or increase the length of soft tissues (e.g., muscles, tendons, and liga-

ments) by preventing or correcting shortening of tissues and preventing overstretching of soft tissue.

• Splints are used to correct biomechanical malalignment, restoring muscles to normal resting length and protecting joint integrity. This biomechanical correction may result in a decrease in excessive skeletal muscle activity.

• Splints are used to position the hand to assist in functional activities.

- Splints compensate for weakness by providing external support, blocking the pull of muscle groups that have lost a balanced agonist-antagonist relationship, and altering the resting alignment of the joints to enhance functional postures.

The use of one rationale (i.e., never splinting, always splinting, only using resting splints) for splinting patients after stroke cannot be effective because of the variety of problems that occur after stroke. The sequelae of stroke are multilayered, encompassing a variety of symptoms and problem areas. The complexity of these problems has served as fuel for the splinting debate and the controversies surrounding splinting.

HISTORICAL PERSPECTIVE

Neuhaus et al[32] have published a review of the splinting literature over a 100-year period. Their review has documented two different approaches to splinting: the biomechanical approach and the neurophysiologic approach.

The biomechanical perspective considers issues such as soft tissue lengthening, prevention of contracture and deformity, maintenance of biomechanical alignment, and effects on the non-neural components of spasticity. In contrast the neurophysiologic perspective considers reflex inhibition, effects on the neural basis of spasticity, facilitation through sensory input, and inhibition through positioning and sensory input.

Earlier publications (from the early 1900s to the 1950s) emplasized a biomechanical approach, whereas literature after World War II emphasized a shift toward the neurophysiologic frame of reference. During this time, therapists (Rood, Bobath, Knott, Voss) developed theories based on neurophysiologic principles. Many of the neurophysiologic theorists were clearly opposed to splinting; others did not mention splinting at all as part of their treatment regimens. Rood (as cited by Stockmeyer[40]) stated that spasticity may be increased "by activating sensory stimuli of touch, pressure, and stretch, which result in undesirable contraction of muscle."

The neurophysiologic perspective currently is being questioned, and a shift is occurring toward a more comprehensive and current understanding of motor behavior. Nevertheless, many styles of splints and rationales are based on neurophysiologic principles.

To date, research does not support one treatment approach or style of splint as superior to another. Many of the statements and principles documented by the originators of the neurophysiologic theories have been accepted as fact. In light of current understanding of motor control, these statements need to be critically analyzed and researched before further splinting interventions are based on these concepts. See chapter 6 for a comprehensive review of these issues.

DORSAL VERSUS VOLAR SPLINTING

Splint fabrication and points of contact are areas of continuing debate. The following studies have investigated this controversy.

Zislis[46] compared the effects of two different wrist-hand splints on a patient with spastic hemiplegia. The author used simultaneous electromyographic (EMG) recordings of the flexors and extensors in the forearm to provide an objective measure of muscle activity. EMG readings were taken with no splint, with a dorsal-based splint (which kept the wrist neutral, fingers adducted and extended, and thumb free) used in hopes of facilitating the extensors, and with a volar-based splint (which kept the wrist neutral, fingers extended and abducted, and thumb free).

Zislis' results indicated that extensor muscle activity was not altered in any of the three situations, although flexor activity was varied. With no splint, flexor activity was exaggerated compared with extensor activity. The dorsal splint greatly increased the flexor activity, even more so than when no splint was worn. Finally, the volar-based splint diminished flexor activity and achived a state of "balanced physiologic activity between flexor and extensor muscle groups."

Zislis drew the following conclusions from the patient he studied:

1. Dorsal facilitation of the extensor was not evident, although dorsal facilitation of the flexors did occur.
2. Flexor inhibition from volar cutaneous receptors may occur.
3. Abduction and extension of the fingers may produce flexor inhibition.

Therefore Zislis recommended the use of volar-based splints with extension and abduction of the fingers.

Charait[7] observed 20 patients in her study of dorsal versus volar "functional position splints." In the splinted position the wrist varied from less than neutral to 30°, the thumb was abducted and opposed, and the fingers were positioned at 45° of finger flexion at the metacarpophalangeal (MP) and proximal interphalangeal (PIP) joints.

Charait observed the amount of spasticity and voluntary movement in both groups. In the group wearing volar splints, four patients showed no change in spasticity or voluntary motion and six experienced increased spasticity. In the group wearing dorsal splints, one patient showed no change, one experienced a considerable increase in spasticity, and eight had decreased spasticity (four of these also exhibited increased active finger and wrist extension). The author drew the following conclusions from her observations:

1. Volar pressure facilitates flexor muscles.
2. Dorsal pressure with decreased volar contact facilitates the extensors.
3. Prolonged stretch enhances inhibition.

Charait recommended splinting using dorsal-based appliances.

McPherson et al[26] compared dorsal and volar resting splints for the reduction of hypertonus. They assigned 10 subjects with hypertonic wrist flexors to the dorsal or volar group. For the purposes of the study, McPherson et al defined *hypertonus* as "the plastic, viscous, and elastic properties of the muscle resistant to stretch and with a tendency to return a limb to a particular abnormal resting posture." A spring-weighted scale was used to take measurements to assess the effectiveness of the splints in reducing hypertonicity. The results indicated no significant difference between the volar and dorsal splints in the reduction of hypertonus. As an aside, the authors found a correlation between age and reduction in hypertonus. The older subjects in the study demonstrated gradual but not statistically significant decline in hypertonus, whereas the younger adults demonstrated significant decline in hypertonus over 6 weeks.

Other studies have not specifically compared dorsal versus volar splinting but have instead evaluated the effects of one or the other. Kaplan[20] evaluated 10 patients who wore dorsal wrist splints. His study set out to "determine whether prolonged therapy with a dorsal splint will inhibit or diminish hyperreflexia or stretch reflex and at the same time increase muscular power by sensorimotor stimulation." The splint used in this study positioned the wrist and fingers in extension and supported the thumb in abduction. Most of the subjects wore the splints at least 8 hours per day, and Kaplan notes that many patients required several serial splints to gradually increase the stretch on the flexors. Patients were evaluated with EMG, strength testing, and hand function evaluation before and after splint application. The subjects in this study demonstrated "improvement in strength and function of muscle, with a decrease in the stretch reflex and spasticity . . . when a dorsal splint was properly applied in treatment of hemiplegia involving an upper extremity."

Brennan (as cited by Mathiowetz et al[25]) studied the effects of volar-based splints on his subjects. At the end of his study the patients who wore the volar-based wrist and hand splints demonstrated increased range of passive movement in which no resistance to stretch could be felt.

In their study of positioning devices on normal and spastic hands, Mathiowetz, Bolding, and Trombly[25] demonstrated that a volar-based resting splint increased EMG activity as the subjects performed a grasping activity on the contralateral side. They noted that the volar splint "is the least desirable positioning device while the hemiplegic subject is doing any activity that requires a comparable effort to squeezing 50% maximal voluntary contraction of grip."

The variability in the above studies makes decisions regarding dorsal versus volar-based treatment difficult to reach based on available research. Therapists must still evaluate individually the effect of variables on splinting outcomes. Moreover, the studies discussed in this chapter used a variety of outcome measures, varied in their methodologies, and implemented variable definitions and styles of splints.

REVIEW OF SPLINTS COMMONLY USED FOR PATIENTS AFTER STROKE

This section reviews positive and negative aspects of splints frequently used by occupational therapists; available research is discussed. Several of the following splints were developed based on the understanding of motor function gained after World War II, and some may still be useful and effective, although they may no longer be based on the original proposal of the splint.

Bobath Finger Spreader (Finger Abduction Splint)

The Bobath finger spreader (finger abduction splint) is fabricated of foam rubber and positions the fingers and thumb in abduction. A sturdier version of this splint (fabricated of low-temperature plastic) was proposed by Doubilet and Polkow.[9] According to Bobath the purpose of the splint is to "obtain extension of wrist and fingers. . . . Abduction not only facilitates extension of the fingers, but also reduces flexor spasticity throughout the whole arm. . . . It has a better and more dynamic effect than the use of a (standard) splint and reduces the possibility of edema."[3]

Doubilet and Polkow[9] recommended wearing the splint only during the day. Their paper includes anecdotal evidence of the splint's effectiveness:

The finger abduction splint is presently being worn by fifteen patients who are two to six months post CVA, these patients exhibited moderate to severe spasticity of the fingers and wrist, decreased range of motion, and edema in the wrist and hand. After one week of using the splint plus standard treatment in the therapy sessions a moderate reduction of spasticity was seen in these patients.

Doubilet and Polkow concluded that the splint results are promising and warrant continued trial and experimentation.

The finger abduction splint was objectively evaluated by Mathiowetz, Bolding, and Trombly[25] in a study investigating the effects of a variety of splints on the distal muscle activity of normal and hemiplegic subjects. Subjects wore the splints while performing resistive activities with the opposite hand. The results indicated "significantly *greater* EMG activity for the finger spreader compared to no device in the flexor carpi radialis of normal subjects during grasping" with the contralateral hand. In hemiplegic subjects the finger spreader did not evoke less EMG activity than no device. According to the authors the belief that this splint decreases spasticity shortly after application needs to be seriously questioned.

The finger spreader may be useful in maintaining the length of the flexors; however, wrist position is not considered with this splint, and the therapist must be aware of the wrist position. Because it is relatively subtle in terms of corrective forces, this splint may be indicated for patients with low tolerance for other, more cumbersome devices, and for patients with low pain thresholds. Donning and doffing procedures are straightforward for the confused patient (Figure 8-1).

Firm Cone

The firm cone can be fabricated of low-temperature plastic or purchased commercially; it is based on the theories of Rood. Rood's theory (as interpreted by Stockmeyer[40]) states that firm and prolonged pressure over the flexor surface of the palm and fingers results in an inhibition of the long flexors. The cone is positioned with the narrow end of the cone toward the radial side of the hand in the web space. It is positioned in this manner especially if the hand is tight. As the hand begins to relax, the ideal *biomechanical* position is for the cone to be positioned opposite to the initial position, that is, the wide end of the cone is placed in the radial side of the hand in the web space and the narrow end is placed in the ulnar side of the hand. Strapping material can be used to hold the cone in place. This device was included in the Mathiowetz, Bolding, and Trombly[25] study; the researchers found that the cone did not not evoke significantly less EMG activity during contralateral resisted function.

Neurophysiologic principles aside, the cone may be an effective positioning device for patients who have developed contracture in the long flexors. Combined applications of the cone with a standard wrist-extension splint, controlling the stretch on the wrist and digit flexors separately, are feasible. The size of the cone and the angle of wrist extension can be graded as the patient's status improves.

Another practical use of the cone is in the prevention of maceration of tissue in patients with moderate to severe flexion of the digits. The maintenance of flexor length is required for hygiene and cosmesis. Similarly to the use of the finger abduction splint, the use of the cone in isolation does not provide wrist support, thus predisposing the wrist to a flexed posture. Donning and doffing procedures are straightforward (Figure 8-2). First position the cone with the small end in the hand's web space. As the hand begins to relax, the wide end of the cone is placed in the web space and the narrow end is placed in the ulnar side, enhancing the natural biomechanical position.

Orthokinetic Orthotics

According to Neeman and Neeman,[28] the term *orthokinetic orthosis* "describes a cuff-shaped dynamic orthopaedic appliance which does not include rigid polymer or metal components. It does not apply any extraneous modulating force or constraint, in contrast to the typical splint. . . ." The orthokinetic cuffs designed by Blashy and Fuchs-Neeman[1] have been used for almost 40 years for patients with muscle weakness, muscle paresis, and resulting agonist-antagonist imbalance. The action of these orthoses is "exerted through internal restoration of neuromuscular balance between agonist and antagonist musculatures, by input of mild neural stimuli to mechanoreceptors in specifically targeted skin areas."[1] The designers state that the neurophysiologic mechanism involves activation of paretic agonist muscles and reciprocal inhibition of antagonist musculature.

The orthokinetic cuffs are fabricated of ribbed elastic bandage material applied circumferentially around various aspects of the patient's upper extremity. The cuffs are held on the arm by fasteners. Half of the cuff is designed to be elastic (the active field), and the other half of the cuff is sewn to reduce the stretch (the inactive field). The active field is worn over the muscle belly to be activated, and the inactive field is placed over the antagonist.

Neeman and Neeman have published several studies[28-31] on the effectiveness of these cuffs in the rehabilitation of the upper extremity after stroke. It was concluded that use of the cuffs results in pronounced restoration of agonist-antagonist muscle balance, increased active range of mo-

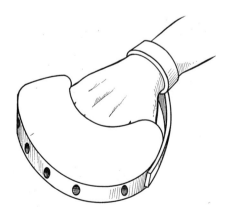

Figure 8-1   Bobath finger spreader (finger abduction splint).

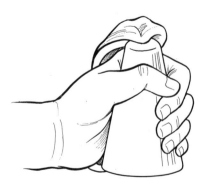

Figure 8-2   Firm cone.

tion throughout the extremity, and increased ability to participate in functional tasks.

The orthokinetic cuffs have been subjected to the greatest number of efficacy studies, all showing positive results. Fabrication guidelines are clearly stated in the cited studies and the cuffs are easily applied and comfortable.

The neurophysiologic rationale for the orthokinetic cuff has not been fully established. The active field may produce cutaneous stimulation and activate the exteroceptors of the skin and Ia afferent neurons of the muscle spindle. The inactive field seems to provide sustained deep pressure, which may produce an inhibitory response (Figure 8-3).

Orthokinetic Wrist Splint

The dynamic splint design of the orthokinetic wrist splint is based on the concepts of Rood.[40] Components of the splint include a firm cone in the palm of the hand, a volar-based forearm support, elastic straps to secure the forearm support by acting as orthokinetic cuffs, and a wrist hinge.[21] This splint has been recommended for patients with flexor hypertonicity who have at least minimal voluntary extensor activity. However, no data support the effectiveness of this splint (Figure 8-4).

Spasticity Reduction Splint

The spasticity reduction splint was developed by Snook[38] and is based on the Bobath[3] principle of reflex-inhibiting patterns. The splint is fabricated of low-temperature plastic. The forearm support is dorsal based and continues into a volar-based finger support. The wrist is positioned in 30° of wrist extension; the MPs are at 45° of flexion. The interphalangeal (IP) joints are fully extended, the fingers are abducted with separators, and the thumb is positioned in abduction and extension. Snook notes that if a flexion contracture is present, the wrist may be positioned at neutral or slightly less than neutral without producing a significant impact on the effectiveness of the splint.

Snook recommends an intermittent wearing schedule, observing that "a decrease in tone is usually seen almost immediately upon splint application; however, after an extended period of wearing time, tone tends to gradually increase."

Snook's original article describes fabrication and provides clinical observations and case studies. Research was not included in this article. Snook concluded that based on preliminary findings, the spasticity reduction splint has an impact "on the reduction and normalization of tone" and should be considered as a therapeutic tool when the therapist is dealing with a spastic hand.

McPherson[27] evaluated the effect of this splint on five severely and profoundly handicapped subjects (no patients who had strokes were included in this study). His results demonstrated a significant reduction in hypertonicity after 4 weeks of splint use. He further stated that the effects of the splint were not permanent; after the splints were removed, hypertonicity increased. The author measured "the force of spastic wrist flexors in pounds of pull on a spring weighted scale."

The fabrication guidelines for this splint are clearly outlined in Snook's[38] article. Compliance in wearing schedules may be problematic because the splint is bulky and the wrist and hand are held in an extreme range. Many patients require assistance donning the splint, depending on the level of flexion posturing in their hands.

Although this splint is based on Bobath's principles of positioning for reflex inhibition, the third edition of Bobath's text[3] states "We have discarded all static ways of treatment like 'reflex inhibiting postures' but have introduced a strong emphasis on movement and on functional activity." However, because this splint maintains a stretch to the musculature that traditionally becomes shortened in patients after stroke, it may be useful as an adjunct to treatment focusing on the maintenance of soft tissue length. Further research is required on patients after cerebrovascular accident to document this splint's effectiveness (Figure 8-5).

Inflatable Pressure Splints (Air Splints)

The use of inflatable pressure splints as adjuncts to therapy was first advocated by Johnstone[18]. These splints are commercially available and exert continuous or intermittent

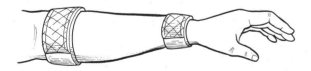

Figure 8-3   Orthokinetic orthotics.

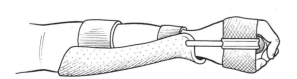

Figure 8-4   Orthokinetic wrist splint.

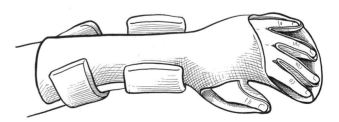

Figure 8-5   Spasticity reduction splint.

pressure to the area to which they are applied. The pressure of the splints should not exceed 40 mm Hg.[36] According to Poole,[36] "inflatable splints have been used with patients who have had a stroke to reduce tone, facilitate muscle activity around a joint, facilitate sensory input, control edema, and reduce pain." Poole's article includes a review of the neurophysiologic rationales for the use of inflatable splints.

Three studies have been published of investigations of the effectiveness of inflatable splints on patients who have had strokes. The earliest was a case study by Bloch and Evans[2]; its results indicated a reduction in spasticity and an increase in hand range of motion.

Nicholson (as cited by Poole and Whitney[37]) treated patients for 1 week with inflatable splints in conjunction with weight-bearing patterns. At the end of the treatment protocol, no improvements had occurred in sensation, strength, and range of motion.

Likewise, Poole et al[36] treated 18 people and assigned them to splint or no splint treatment protocols. The splinted group wore the splint for 30 minutes 5 days a week for 3 weeks. The splinted patients did not perform activities with the splinted extremity. Poole's results indicated no statistically significant differences in mean change in upper extremity sensation, pain, and motor function between the splinted and nonsplinted groups.

Although inflatable pressure splints do not seem to elicit the effects originally proposed, some therapists may consider using this style of splint to enhance functional performance during weight-bearing activities (Figure 8-6).

Resting Pan Splints

The resting pan splint can be dorsal or volar based. The suggested position is 20° to 30° of wrist extension, MP joints at 40° to 45° of flexion, IP joints in 10° to 20° of flexion, and thumb in opposition to the index finger.[24]

The resting pan splint is commonly used in clinics. Although it may be effective in the long term for patients after CVA, therapists must analyze critically the effects of this splint on the patient with acute and subacute impairments. This splint blocks any automatic and voluntary attempts at movement, completely covers the surface of the hand (thus preventing sensory input), and gives full passive support to the wrist and digits, which may be contrary to treatment programs attempting to train patients to be responsible for the positioning and ranging of their hands. Alternatives to this splint need to be considered.

Mathiowetz, Bolding, and Trombly[25] demonstrated that the use of a volar-based resting splint increased EMG activity in hemiplegic subjects who were performing grasping tasks with the opposite extremity. They concluded that this type of volar splint "is the least desirable positioning device while the hemiplegic subject is doing any activity that requires a comparable effort to squeezing fifty percent maximal voluntary contraction of grip."

Resting pan splints can be custom fabricated; they also are available commercially. Nighttime use of the resting splint may be considered for prevention of soft tissue contracture, but this style of splint should not be worn during daytime because it completely blocks spontaneous function, sensory input, and self-management of the hand (Figure 8-7).

Tone and Positioning (TAP) Splint

The tone and positioning (TAP) splint is semidynamic in nature; it is commercially available from Smith and Nephew Rolyan. It supports the thumb in abduction and extension with a neoprene glove. The TAP splint includes an elastic strap that is spirally wrapped up the forearm, providing a dynamic assist into pronation and supination. Data supporting the effectiveness of this splint are not available.

Casey and Kratz[6] have published a paper on the thumb abduction supinator splint (TASS). This splint is similar in design to the commercially available TAP splint. Their paper includes fabrication guidelines and recommends a wearing schedule of 3 to 4 hours on then 30 minutes to 1 hour off to allow the skin to be exposed to the air. They recommend using the splints on patients with mild to moderate spasticity without severe contractures—those

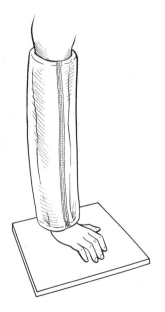

Figure 8-6   Inflatable pressure splints.

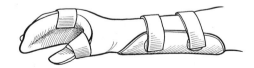

Figure 8-7   Resting pan splint and submaximal range splint.

who posture in a pattern of forearm pronation, with a fisted hand, and with the thumb in the palm.

Both the TAP and TASS splints may present difficulties to patients learning to donn and doff splints independently. These splints are designed to be used to enhance positioning and worn during functional activities. They may be particularly effective if worn during activities that result in stereotypical posturing of the limb (e.g., gait, transfers). They also may be effective during upper extremity activities because the digits are free to move (Figure 8-8).

Thumb Loop and Thumb Abduction Splint

Variations of the thumb abduction splint have been proposed by several authors.[8,15,39] The papers cited in the references include fabrication guidelines; the splint also is commercially available.

The thumb abduction splint is considered a semidynamic splint,[15] and the focus of positioning is on thumb and wrist alignment. The strapping material used in the fabrication of this splint positions the thumb in abduction and aligns the wrist in a position of slight radial wrist extension. The hand is placed in a position that enhances prehension, manipulation, and release of objects and provides the freedom of movement needed for bilateral coordination.[15]

Stern[39] states that another indication for use is during any activity involving effort, particularly when performing fine activities with the unaffected limb results in increased thumb adduction on the affected side. Therefore this splint has been suggested for both positioning and enhancement of functional performance.

Stern cautions that "For this splint to be of any value, the patients must be able to use the affected hand for grasp and release, their main problem being adduction of the thumb, which prevents sufficient opening of the hand to allow for palmar grasp." Patients with fixed adductor contracture are less likely to benefit.

Research evaluating the effectiveness of this splint in the adult population is lacking. Currie and Mendiola[8] evaluated the effectiveness of a variation of this type of splint on five children with "mild to moderate spastic hemiplegic cerebral palsy." These children exhibited a cortical thumb (adducted thumb) at rest, and their hand function was limited to a "raking" ulnar type of prehension pattern.

With the use of this splint, all five children's resting thumb patterns were enhanced, and their prehension patterns improved to a radial grasp, usually in a three jaw chuck or large cylindrical prehension pattern, depending on the size of the object being manipulated (Figure 8-9).

Hand-Based Thumb Abduction Splint

If the patient has controlled wrist movement in flexion and extension (not necessarily full wrist range of motion, but some isolated control) but continues to have flexor activity influencing the digits, a hand-based thumb abduction C-spacer splint may be useful during functional activities. The splint is custom fabricated from thermoplastic material. The thumb abduction splint positions the thumb in an enhanced prehension pattern for manipulation of objects during grasp and release activities (Figure 8-10).

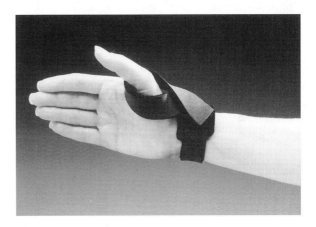

Figure 8-9 Thumb loop and thumb abduction splint. (Courtesy of Smith & Nephew Rolyan, Germantown, Wisconsin.)

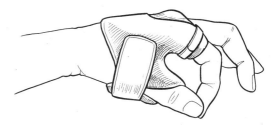

Figure 8-10 Hand-based thumb abduction splint to be used when wrist control returns; thumb requires abduction assistance for functional opposition activities.

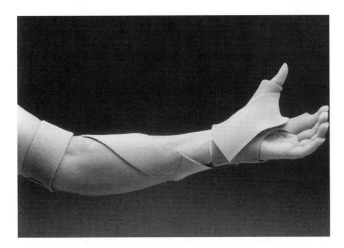

Figure 8-8 Tone and positioning (TAP) splint. (Courtesy Smith & Nephew Rolyan, Germantown, Wisc.)

MacKinnon Splint

Although the MacKinnon splint was developed for the pediatric population, it may be indicated at times for the adult population. The splint includes a dorsal-based forearm support that wraps three fourths of the distal half of the forearm, a dowel placed in the palm of the hand to provide pressure on the MP heads, and rubber tubing attaching the dowel to the dorsal forearm support; the fingers are left free to assume functional patterns.

The goal of this splint is to release the overactive finger flexors and adductor pollicis to gain balanced muscle action of the wrist. MacKinnon et al's[23] paper includes fabrication guidelines and observations of approximately 30 children who used the splint and gained improved hand awareness, increased use, and decreased spasticity when the splint was removed. Research on the effectiveness of this splint is not available, and it has not been documented for use with the adult patient recovering from CVA (Figure 8-11).

Submaximal Range Splint

The submaximal range splint was described by Peterson (as cited by Feldman[10]); its design is based on the clinical observation that muscles splinted on full stretch or maximal range of motion resulted in increased tightness.

The splint is fabricated in the fashion of a resting hand splint. The splint should position the distal extremity with the thumb in partial opposition to the index finger, the MP and PIP joints in 45° of flexion, with distal interphalangeal (DIP) joint extension, and the wrist in 10° to 20° of extension; the splint should provide pressure to the palmar arch. If the patient cannot achieve this ideal range, each joint should be positioned in 5° to 10° less than the available range.[10] Fabrication guidelines are the same as are those for a resting hand splint.

No research is available evaluating the effectiveness of this splint, but the precautionary statements about the resting hand splint are similar to those for this splint design (Figure 8-7).

Serpentine Splint

The serpentine splint must be custom fabricated from thermoplastic materials. It was originally designed for use with pediatric patients with cerebral palsy who had difficulty grasping objects. It is easily adapted to the adult with neurologic impairments. The serpentine splint provides sufficient thumb abduction support, positions the hand and wrist in a more optimal position for function, and allows "active wrist function in the child with moderately increased tone."[41] The designers of the splint feel that the serpentine splint inhibits the thumb-in-palm reflex by using the thumb abduction position.

The authors have used an adaptation of the serpentine splint with several patients after CVA, with positive outcomes. The serpentine splint can be used for patients with mild to moderate increased skeletal muscle activity (it is not recommended for the flaccid hand). This splint is never recommended for hands that exhibit severe increases in skeletal muscle activity for the reasons outlined earlier in this chapter.

The wrist is positioned in 20° to 30° of extension, the thumb is positioned in 30° to 40° of abduction, and the material continues two thirds of the length proximally up the forearm. The splint positions the hand in a more functional position for grasping exercises and activities.[41] It is worn during the day for activities and wrist support and removed at night. The serpentine splint requires maximal assistance for application and moderate assistance for removal. It is a practical alternative to more conventional static splints. Because it is an open splint, it is less confining; it also is lightweight and allows for air circulation, which results in decreased perspiration, decreased skin maceration, and reduced potential for skin breakdown. When fabricating this splint, the therapist places the roll in the palm, then wraps it around the ulnar aspect of the hand, forms it over the dorsum of the hand through the web space, brings the roll over the thenar eminence and under the base of the thumb, and continues wrapping the material two thirds of the way up the forearm. The seam made by rolling the splint material should face away from the skin to prevent skin irritation and breakdown (Figure 8-12).

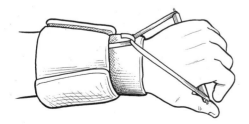

Figure 8-11   MacKinnon splint.

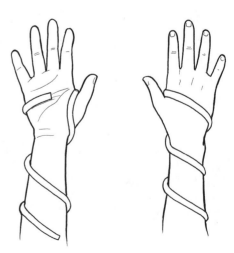

Figure 8-12   Serpentine splint.

Drop-Out Splint

The drop-out splint is a custom-fabricated splint designed to decrease elbow contractures that may be common in the patient after stroke. The splint is designed from thermoplastic material positioned volarly on the humerus, distal to the axilla; it extends into the palm of the hand proximal to the distal palmar crease. The splint is fabricated with the shoulder and humerus externally rotated and the forearm in as much supination as possible. The splint is customized with a gentle stretch to the contracted elbow joint (not to the point of discomfort) using the low-load prolonged-stretch principles in the Treatment of Joint Contractures section of this chapter. The splint is used during rest periods to maximize the low-load prolonged stretch to the elbow. The elbow contracture is measured with a goniometer before application of the splint and checked weekly to allow appropriate adjustments of the splint for increased extension as needed. As with all splints used in the patient who has had a stroke, but especially for splints using the low-load prolonged-stretching principles, the upper extremity must be monitored frequently for skin maceration and breakdown (Figure 8-13).

Belly Gutter Splint for PIP Joint Flexion Contractures

The belly gutter splint is a static PIP extension splint custom fabricated from thermoplastic material. Many PIP extension splints are commercially available; Joint Jack; LMB Wire-foam; and safety-pin splints, which apply two points of volar pressure to make a perpendicular pull on the involved segments, are but a few.[45] If the flexion contracture is greater than 35° these splints are not effective. Both dynamic extension splints and the belly gutter splint provide traction tension at a 90-degree angle to the phalanx. The belly gutter splint provides the 90-degree–angle pull by incorporating a convex belly in the middle of the gutter.[45] When fabricating and applying this splint, the therapist must place the Velcro strap directly under the PIP joint; the belly of the splint must be directly under the PIP joint axis for the splint to be effective. The authors have found this splint effective for flexion contractures of the PIP joint from approximately 15° of contracture to 35° of contrac-

ture. A PIP joint contracture of more than 35° requires dynamic splinting.[11] The belly gutter splint is used at the beginning of treatment for 1 hour on and 1 hour off. Gradually, as the contracture decreases the time may be extended to as much as 4 hours, but as always close monitoring of the splint is mandatory (Figure 8-14).

HandAssist Splint

The HandAssist splint, which is commercially available from MedAssist, is marketed for contracture management of the population in the chronic stages of stroke rehabilitation. The splint consists of an adjustable volar-based wrist support that is easily adjusted to achieve the desired range of extension. The palmar aspect of the splint is an air bladder that can be easily inflated or deflated, depending on the desired stretch and level of contracture. The splint is easily donned and comfortable (Figure 8-15).

Many of the splints described and researched in the available literature are for the most part based on neurophysiologic approaches to the rehabilitation of the patient who has had a stroke. Although a shift is occurring from these ap-

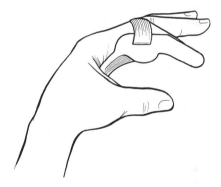

Figure 8-14 Belly gutter splint for PIP joint flexion contractures.

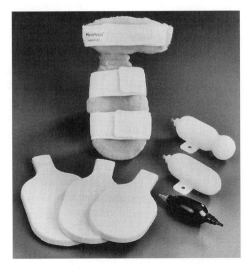

Figure 8-15 Handassist splint. (Courtesy MedAssist.)

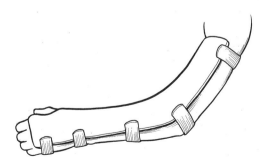

Figure 8-13 Drop-out splint.

proaches to a more current understanding of motor control, splinting interventions have not yet followed this trend.

The majority of splints described have not been validated through research. Many are supported solely by anecdotal evidence, and many are based on an outdated understanding of the nervous system.

Many issues must be considered when prescribing or designing a splint for use on persons after CVA. The following section exposes therapists to the complexity of issues to be considered during the splinting evaluation.

CONSIDERATIONS IN PRESCRIBING AND DESIGNING A SPLINT FOR THE DISTAL EXTREMITY AFTER STROKE

Spasticity

Many commonly used splints are applied in the hopes that they will to inhibit spasticity with an end result of improved function. As outlined in chapter 6, the cause-and-effect relationship between spasticity and function is being questioned.

The link between spasticity and contracture has been well documented; see Chapter 6. Therefore splinting patients who are experiencing distal spasticity may be indicated to prevent painful contractures and loss of tissue length. This differentiation is important if therapists are to analyze objectively the effectiveness of the splints provided.

Hummelsheim et al[16] have demonstrated that prolonged stretch resulted in "a significant reduction in the spastic hypertonus in elbow, hand and finger flexors" of the 15 patients they studied. Spasticity was measured by the Ashworth scale. The EMG recordings included in their study objectively demonstrated that late EMG potentials are reduced or disappear after sustained muscle stretch. The authors hypothesized that "the beneficial effect resulting from sustained muscle stretch is due to stretch receptor fatigue or adaptation to the new extended position. . . ."

Although this study was based on manual stretching techniques, the same principles may be applied to splinting. Therefore splinting may be used as an adjunct to interventions aimed at relaxing the distal extremity.

Feldman[10] recommends early splinting interventions for patients with spasticity; treatment should begin before the spasticity becomes severe. She states that "the longer tonal influences are left to bear on the joints, the greater the risk for contractures and other complications." Feldman also warns that patients with severe spasticity should not be considered for splinting programs. These patients are at risk for skin breakdown, edema, and circulatory impairment. Instead, Feldman recommends interventions with spasticity medication and nerve blocks for these patients.

Soft Tissue Shortening

Many of the wrists and hands that therapists evaluate are immobilized. This immobilization may be because of weakness, static splinting for prolonged periods, excessive skeletal muscle activity, or contracture. The deleterious effects of immobilization begin to occur soon after immobilization is initiated.

Consequences of prolonged positioning secondary to immobilization include anatomic, biochemical, and physiologic changes.[13] Specific changes include changes in the number of sarcomeres, changes in protein content, loss of muscle weight, changes in the amount of passive and active soft tissue tension, decreased aerobic function and Type I and II fiber atrophy.[13]

From their review of the literature, Gossman et al[13] concluded that "evidence from experimental studies and clinical observations clearly indicates that muscle is an extremely mutable (prone to change) tissue. Change is more pronounced when a muscle is shortened than when it is lengthened. The changes can be deleterious, but they are reversible, a condition that can be used in correcting movement dysfunction."

Halar and Bell[14] state that if mild contractures have formed, prolonged stretches for 30 minutes are effective. More severe contractures may require longer sustained stretch through splinting. They recommend application of heat before splinting to decrease the viscous properties of connective tissue and maximize the effects of stretching.

During the splinting evaluation the therapist must assess the differences between extrinsic and intrinsic tightness and joint contractures. Fess and Philips[11] suggest altering wrist posture to detect extrinsic soft tissue involvement. If extrinsic tightness is evident, changing the wrist posture from slight extension to flexion results in an increase in the range of motion of the digits (the tenodesis effect). In contrast, if range of motion limitations are secondary to joint pathology, an altered wrist position does not affect the range of motion (Figure 8-16).

Fess and Philips[11] suggest evaluating intrinsic tightness by holding the MP joint in extension and attempting to flex the PIP joint; full passive flexion of the PIP joint is absent if the intrinsics have become tight. With intrinsic tightness, however, full passive PIP flexion is possible with the MP joint in flexion (Figure 8-17).

Tubiana et al[42] suggest evaluating for shortening of the extrinsic flexors by evaluating extension (i.e., wrist and digits in full extension). If a patient can only assume full-digit extension with partial wrist flexion (tenodesis effect), a contracture of the extrinsic flexor tendons exists. Extrinsic tightness also can be tested by holding the MP joints in maximal extension and passively flexing the PIP joint and then placing the MP joint in flexion and flexing the PIP joint. If more PIP flexion occurs with the MP joint in extension rather than in flexion, extrinsic tendon tightness is present. If the motion of the PIP joint is unchanged regardless of the position of the MP joint, a PIP joint contracture is present[17] (see Figure 8-17).

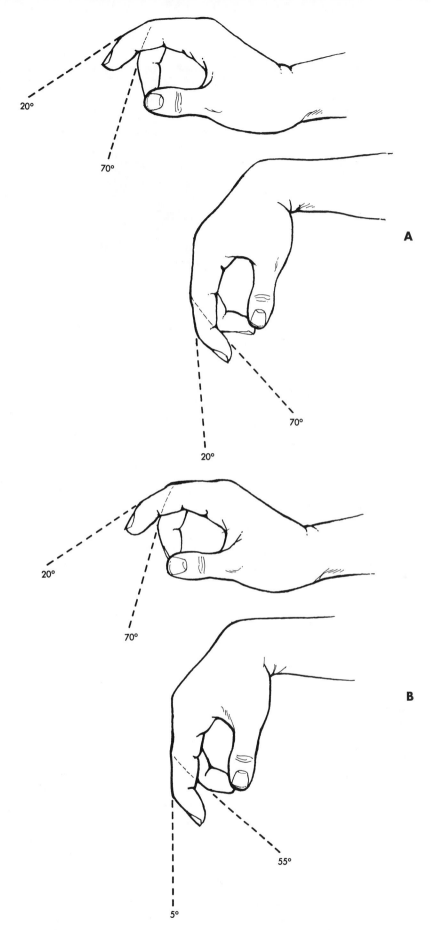

Figure 8-16 **A,** If stiffness is limited to the joint and periarticular structures, both the range and arc of motion are unaffected by altered wrist position. **B,** However, if extrinsic musculotendinous units are involved, the arc of motion remains constant, but range of motion measurements change as wrist posture is altered. (From Fess EE, Philips CA: *Hand splinting: principles and methods,* ed 2, St Louis, 1987, Mosby.)

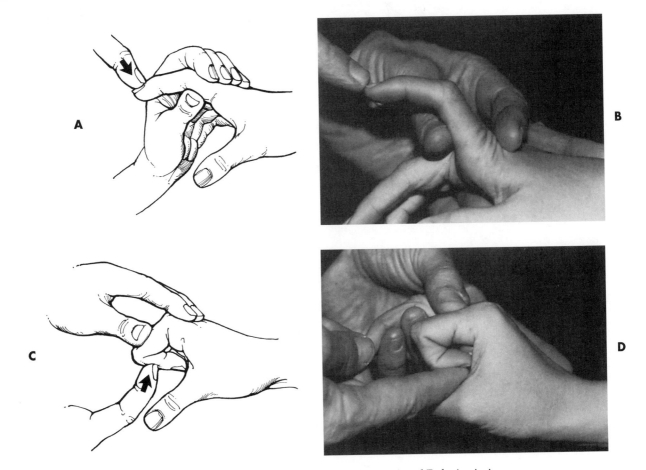

Figure 8-17   Intrinsic tightness and extrinsic tightness tests. In **A** and **B** the intrinsics are put on stretch by the examiner, who then passively flexes the PIP joint. The intrinsics are then relaxed by flexing the metacarpophalangeal joint, **C** and **D**. If the PIP joint can be passively flexed more with the MP joint in flexion than when it is in extension, tightness of the intrinsic muscles is evident. Conversely, in performing the same test, if the PIP joint can be passively flexed more with the MP joint in extension than when it is in flexion, tightness of the extrinsic muscles is evident. (**A** and **C** from Fess EE, Philips CA: *Hand splinting: principles and methods*, ed 2, St Louis, 1987, Mosby; **B** and **D** from Hunter JM, Mackin E, Callahan A: *Rehabilitation of the hand: surgery and therapy*, ed 4, St Louis, 1995, Mosby.)

Many patients also develop contracture of the extensor tendons. Therapists must determine whether the alteration of the position of the MP joint affects the amount of flexion obtained at the PIP joint. If shortening or adhesion of the extensor has occurred, the therapist is able to flex the PIP joint further with the MP joint extended than with it flexed.[42] This phenomenon occurs because extension relaxes the extensor system, whereas flexion builds up the passive tension.

Collateral ligament tightness of the PIP joint limits PIP joint motion regardless of the position of the MP joint.[17] The testing is performed by flexing the PIP joint with the MP joint extended and again with it flexed; if PIP joint motion is limited in both testing positions, the collateral ligaments of the PIP joint have shortened (Figure 8-18) and splinting of the PIP joint is indicated. A dynamic PIP extension splint is used if the contracture is greater than 35°; a static PIP extension splint is used if the contracture is less than 35°.[11] A combination of both splints is sometimes used; the dynamic splint is applied for the more severe contracture, and a static extension splint is worn after the contracture is reduced to less than 35°.

Loss of active flexion of the DIP joint may be caused by joint contracture or contracture of the oblique retinacular ligament.[17] The oblique retinacular ligament tightness test is performed by passively flexing the DIP joint with the PIP joint in extension and then repeating the test with the PIP joint in flexion. If more motion occurs when the PIP joint is flexed than when it is extended, a shortening or contracture of this ligament has occurred (Figure 8-19). If equal loss of flexion occurs with the PIP joint flexed or extended, a joint contracture is evident.[17] Contracture of the DIP joint with decreased DIP flexion can be treated with the use of a flexion strap with the MP, PIP, and DIP joints

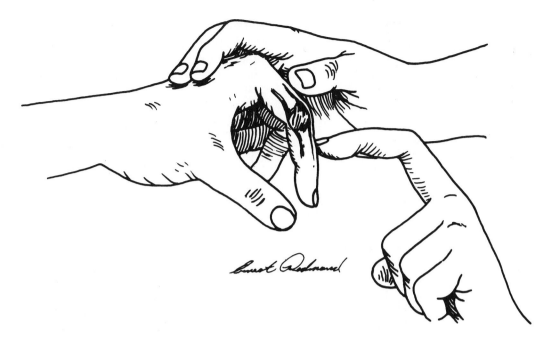

Figure 8-18 PIP joint contracture. Collateral ligament tightness limits proximal phalangeal joint motion, regardless of the position of the MP joint. (From Hunter JM, Mackin E, Callahan A: *Rehabilitation of the hand: surgery and therapy*, ed 4, St Louis, 1995, Mosby.)

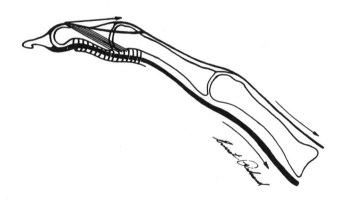

Figure 8-19 Oblique retinacular ligament. (Redrawn from Tubiana R: *The hand*, Philadelphia, 1981, W.B. Saunders.)

in as much flexion as possible. This strap can be fabricated from Velcro strapping and is commercially available (Figure 8-20). It can be used intermittently during the day for 1 hour on and 1 hour off.

Treatment of Joint Contractures with Low-Load Prolonged Stretch (LLPS)

Neuromuscular dysfunction is a common cause of physiologic joint restriction and contractures.[22] Splints are used to either maintain or lengthen soft tissues and maintain joint integrity. If a joint has become contracted, the joint capsule becomes stiff, the synovial fluid becomes thickened from nonmovement, and the ligaments around one side of the joint become shortened, whereas the ligaments on the other side become lax. Soft tissue involvement in contractures includes shortened tendons and skeletal muscle. High-load brief stretch (HLBS) manual therapy alone does

not achieve plastic elongation of tissues over time.[12] Low-load prolonged stretch (LLPS) involves holding the tissues in a moderately lengthened position for a significant amount of time; the tissue will grow, not stretch, to the new lengthened position.[22]

Current literature supports LLPS as the preferred method of lengthening shortened tissues.[22] The common clinical practice of stretching contractures manually with high brief-load periods for 1 to 2 minutes is contraindicated in the literature.[22] The elongation accomplished by manual stretch alone shortens when the force is relaxed.[12] Manual therapy prepares tissues but must be followed with splinting and activities to effect permanent changes.[12]

A study by Light et al[22] tested knee contractures using HLBS or LLPS on 11 geriatric patients. All subjects had bilateral knee contractures; HLBS was the treatment for one knee, and LLPS was the treatment for the other. The

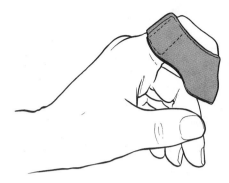

Figure 8-20   Flexion ("Buddy") strap.

LLPS in this study was accomplished by traction. LLPS produced a greater overall increase in passive range of motion than did the HLBS.

Splinting to provide an LLPS is a noninvasive, nonstressful, and ideally painless treatment.[22] The treatment for joint stiffness and contracture is stress, which involves intensity (amount of effort), duration (amount of time), and frequency (amount of repetition).[12] Although all these stress factors are important, duration is the most important for LLPS, the optimal time being 5 to 7 hours. This optimal duration usually must be built up slowly, beginning with 1 to 2 hours. As the joint contracture decreases, the splint must be readjusted regularly (usually weekly) to increase prolonged stretching. LLPS is the principle used in some of the splints mentioned earlier in this chapter, including the elbow drop-out splint, the belly gutter splint, and any dynamic splinting. As with all splinting, but especially in using LLPS splinting for patients with sensory impairments, therapists must monitor patients using these splints for skin breakdown.

Injury to the Extremity

Because of decreased motor control and perceptual dysfunction (e.g., body neglect, somatoagnosia), many patients are at risk for injuries to the already compromised extremity. Many times these patients assume malaligned upper extremity patterns for prolonged periods. A common example may be observed during bed mobility training. Patients assume sitting postures from side lying and end up bearing their weight through the dorsum of their hands with the wrist flexed. This posture puts patients at risk of developing traumatic synovitis, increased edema, and pain. The patient, depending on the level of awareness, may maintain this maladaptive posture during the next task (e.g., dressing) before noticing the problem, resulting in the potential for tissue damage.

Another commonly seen alignment problem that puts patients at risk for injury occurs if upper extremity positioning devices are ineffective. Many patients are prescribed half or full lap-trays to provide upper extremity support while they are seated in their wheelchairs. In many cases the supported extremity slides between the lap-board

and the patient's trunk, pinning the wrist in extreme flexion. Depending on patient and staff awareness, this position unfortunately may be maintained for prolonged periods. Injury also can lead to pain and swelling, which in turn may trigger the initial symptoms of shoulder-hand syndrome.

Biomechanical Alignment

The position a hand assumes at rest (the resting posture) has been documented by several authors. A summary of this posture is as follows:

- Forearm midway between pronation and supination[24]
- Wrist at 10° to 15° of extension[11]
- Thumb in slight extension and abduction with the MP and IP joints flexed approximately 15° to 20°
- Digits posture toward flexion, exhibiting greater composite flexion toward the ulnar side of the hand
- Second metacarpal aligned with the radius
- Palmar arches maintained (see following section)
- Hand exhibiting "dual obliquity"

The therapist must consider the concept of dual obliquity when evaluating the alignment of the hand. Because of a successive decrease in the length of the metacarpals from the radial to the ulnar side, objects held in the hand assume two oblique angles.[34] For example, if a pencil is held in the palm across the metacarpal heads (eraser toward the ulnar side) and the forearm is held in pronation resting on the table, the examiner can identify two oblique angles. The first angle is observed with the pencil point angled upward in relation to the wrist joint axis. The second oblique angle is observed on examination of height of each end of the pencil. The radial side is held higher than the ulnar side, i.e., the pencil is not parallel to the table (Figure 8-21).

The obliquity of the palmar transverse arch follows a line from "the second to the fifth metacarpal head and forms an angle of seventy-five degrees with the axis of the third ray."[42] Therefore from a biomechanical perspective the firm cone splint discussed earlier for a moderately relaxed hand should be placed with the narrow end in the ulnar side and the wide end on the radial side, following the normal obliquity.

Deviations from the resting posture must be noted; they assist in the design of the splint. Therapists must consider that patients may differ slightly from the normal resting posture because of heredity, habits, and job descriptions; examining the opposite hand is helpful in determining the "normal" resting posture for each patient.[21]

The distal extremity assumes several typical alignment deviations after stroke. These deviations and their consequences include the following:

1. Wrist flexion secondary to decreased skeletal muscle activity—This common posture (most often observed

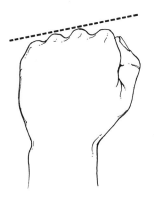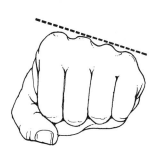

Figure 8-21 Dorsally, the consecutive metacarpal heads create an oblique angle to the longitudinal axis of the forearm. Distally, the fisted hand exhibits an ulnar metacarpal descent that creates an oblique angle in the transverse plane of the forearm. (From Fess EE, Philips CA: *Hand splinting: principles and methods*, ed 2, St Louis, 1987, Mosby.)

in the flaccid stage) produces a variety of pathologic processes. A hand positioned in wrist flexion results in the following:
- Flattening of the palmar arches
- Passive extension of the fingers as a result of tenodesis action[11]
- Shortened collateral ligaments secondary to the extended digits
- Narrowing of the web space[11]
- Inability to perform the grasping function (flexor action of the thumb and digits reinforced by extension of the wrist)[42]
- Blockage of ulnar and radial deviation of the wrist when it is in flexion[19]
- Overstretching of the wrist extensors and dorsal ligaments[42]
- Shortening of the long flexors
- Tendency to develop an edema syndrome

2. Extreme ulnar deviation—The posture of ulnar deviation results in a variety of compounded problems. A wrist positioned in extreme ulnar deviation produces the following:
- Effective blockage of wrist extension[19]
- Shortening of the ulnar deviators and overstretching of the radial deviators
- Shifting of both the proximal and distal rows of carpal bones[42]

3. Wrist and digit flexion—This posture may occur secondary to excessive skeletal muscle activity and soft tissue shortening. This posture results in the following:
- Loss of normal tenodesis function (wrist extension with digit flexion and adduction, wrist flexion with digit extension and abduction)
- Shortening of the extrinsic flexors with resultant overstretching of the extensors
- Potential for skin maceration
- Painful contracture and deformity

Loss of Palmar Arches

A familiar alignment problem seen in patients after stroke is the loss of palmar arches, or the development of a "flat-

tened hand." The maintenance of the palmar arches is crucial for hand function.[4] Kapandji[19] outlines the arches of the hand as follows (Figure 8-22):

- Transverse arch—This structure consists of two arches. It includes the carpal arch, which corresponds to the concavity of the wrist and is continuous with the distal metacarpal arch formed by the metacarpal heads. The carpal arch is rigid, whereas the metacarpal arch is mobile and adaptable. The long axis of the transverse arch crosses the lunate, capitate (the "keystone" of the carpal arch[11]), and the third metacarpal bones. Boehme[4] states that the functional significance of this arch stems from its forming the hand into a gutter, bringing together the radial and ulnar borders of the hand. This arch can widen or narrow the surface area of the hand.
- Longitudinal arch—This arch includes the carpometacarpophalangeal arches. These arches are formed for each finger by the corresponding metacarpal bones and phalanges. Kapandji[19] notes that the arches are concave on the palmar surface; the "keystone" of each arch lies at the level of the MP joint. According to Boehme,[4] in its simplest form this arch supports a basic cylindrical grasp. If the arches are expanded, the hand is longer. This arch allows the palm to flatten and cup itself around objects.[11]
- Oblique arches—These arches are formed by the thumb during opposition with the other fingers. Kapandji[19] states that the most important of these arches is the one linking the thumb and index finger; the most extreme is the one linking the thumb and the fifth digit. These arches are obviously crucial in the opposition of the digits.

Patients lose their arches after stroke for a variety of reasons, including edema in the dorsum of the hand that biomechanically forces the metacarpals inferiorly, inactivity of the wrist and hand, prolonged and extreme wrist flexion (resulting in a flattening of the arches), and inappropriate support of the hand during weight-bearing activities.[4]

Figure 8-22 **A,** Side view of the longitudinal and transverse arches of the hand. The shaded areas show the fixed part of the skeleton. **B,** The thumb forms, along with the other digits, four oblique arches of opposition. The most useful and functionally important arch is between the thumb and index finger, used for precision grip. The farthest arch, between the thumb and little finger, ensures a locking mechanism on the ulnar side of the hand in power grips. (From Tubiana R, Thomine JM, Mackin E: *Examination of the hand and wrist*, St Louis, 1996, Mosby.)

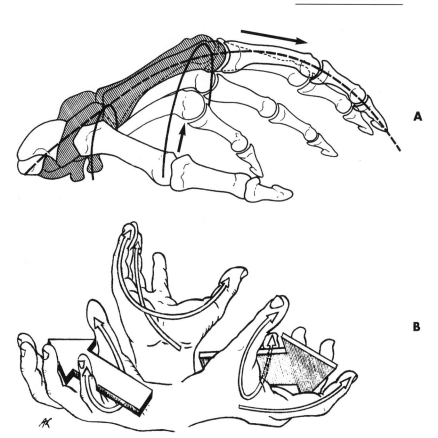

During evaluation of splinting, therapists should examine the arches of the hand and compare them with those of the unaffected hand. In a normal hand's dorsal surface at rest, the MP joints form an arch with the apex at the third metacarpal (i.e., the third metacarpal head is higher than the others) (Figure 8-22). Many patients present with a flattened arch (i.e., the MP joints lose their arches [flatten]), and in response, the proximal phalanges hyperextend. This posture puts the patient at risk for developing a permanent claw-hand deformity and effectively blocks opposition of the thumb (Figure 8-23).

In these cases, splinting may be indicated to give outside support to the arches through upward pressure on the palmar surface of the hand. To be effective and give full support to the metacarpals, the splint must conform to the arches and be contoured to the individual's hand. Commercially available splints are not effective for this type of intervention because they do not take into account the variability of arches.

Learned Nonuse

Current research (see chapter 6) has demonstrated the existence of a component of upper-extremity dysfunction resulting from a learned phenomenon of nonintegration of the hand into functional tasks. This process likely begins in the early stages after stroke, before any functional recovery has commenced. Patients learn to compensate with their unaffected sides, thereby repressing any return of function on the hemiplegic side.

Many CVA protocols call for splinting immediately after stroke. Some facilities have standing orders for splinting in their acute services. Current research indicates that early splinting in the early post stroke phase may be detrimental. The splint gives a message that an outside device is responsible for the maintenence and improvement of the affected hand. Because the hand is supported and aligned through outside means, the patient does not attend to the hand, stretch the wrist and hand, or attempt to integrate it into functional tasks. In other words, early splinting may predispose patients to a learned nonuse phenomenon. A sign that a patient is predisposed to learned nonuse is the observation that a patient, after cueing, can integrate functional return during a therapy session but does not integrate this new function outside the sessions. The therapist must balance interventions for contracture prevention with activities that encourage functional use of the hand, thereby negating the effects of learned nonuse. Splinting for contractures can be used at night instead of during the day to prevent learned nonuse behavior patterns.

THE DECISION-MAKING PROCESS

The therapist must evaluate all of the following areas when deciding whether to splint and choosing the type of splint

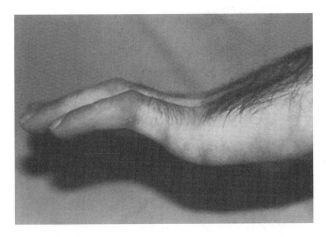

Figure 8-23 Flattening of the palmar arches resulting from hand paralysis. Hyperextension of the MP joints and flexion of the proximal and DIP joints occur because of an imbalance of the extrinsic flexor and extensor systems. (From Hunter JM, Mackin E, Callahan A: *Rehabilitation of the hand: surgery and therapy*, ed 4, St Louis, 1995, Mosby.)

to fabricate. This section is designed to help guide the therapist's clinical reasoning in making splinting decisions.

1. Evaluate cognitive and perceptual status—Does the patient attend to the extremity during the day (attending includes self-ranging, rubbing, positioning, and protecting)? Is the patient alert for the greater portion of the day?

   If the answer is yes, the patient may be able to maintain range of motion and alignment in the extremity without the use of splints; the therapist should consider not splinting.

   If the answer is no, neglect, decreased attention, somatoagnosia, and decreased alertness and arousal may place the patient at risk for contracture and malalignment; splinting may therefore be indicated.

2. Evaluate soft tissue tightness—Does the patient have full composite flexion and extension? Can the patient be ranged into a full intrinsic minus/intrinsic plus position? Does the patient have full and pain-free range of wrist motion, especially extension and radial deviation?

   If the answer is yes, the therapist should consider not splinting. Treatment should focus on teaching the patient and family techniques to maintain this range and prevent pain and contracture.

   If the answer is no, splinting may be indicated to improve or at least maintain soft tissue length. The splint should be designed to place the shortened soft tissues on prolonged stretch.

3. Evaluate bone and joint contracture—Splinting is necessary to ameliorate joint contracture and prevent further deformity.

4. Evaluate learned nonuse—Does the patient integrate the extremity into functional tasks in the clinic without carryover into nontherapy hours?

   If the answer is yes, the therapist should consider not splinting. In this situation the patient does have distal function; this function should not be impeded by splinting. The splint may in fact feed into the learned nonuse cycle.

5. Evaluate function—Does the patient exhibit distal motor control (including gross patterns) that can be integrated into activities of daily living (ADL) and instrumental activities of daily living (IADL)?

   If the answer is yes, the therapist should consider not splinting or should choose a splint that enhances the functional return (e.g., a basic wrist extension splint to provide a stable proximal segment for the digits to work from or a simple opponens splint to improve fine motor control).

   If the answer is no, splinting may be indicated, although the therapist must consider that splinting a hand without functional recovery may block the initial motor return (sometimes automatic reactions and protective responses) or the patient's initial attempts at function.

6. Evaluate potential for soft tissue injury—Is evidence of skin maceration and laceration in the palm of the hand and lateral aspect of the thumb from extreme flexion apparent?

   If the answer is yes, splinting must be seriously considered to prevent further damage and enhance the healing process; wrist extension splints with distal cones or palm guards are recommended.

   If the answer is no, the therapist should consider not splinting.

7. Evaluate biomechanical alignment—Are deviations from the standard resting position of the hand evident? Does realigning the hand result in increased relaxation?

   If the answer is yes, the therapist should consider splinting to improve resting alignment of the extremity to prevent shortening and overstretching of soft tissue.

   If the answer is no, the therapist should consider not splinting.

8. Evaluate sensation—Does the patient have sensory impairments?

   If the answer is yes, the therapist should consider the amount of cutaneous surface area that is covered by splinting. The splint may end up blocking the little sensory input the hand is receiving. A general goal for the involved extremity is to maximize sensory input. If sensation is impaired, extra precautions are necessary for careful, custom splint fabrication and diligent, ongoing monitoring of the skin condition by the therapist, patient, and family for any breakdown or maceration, which the patient may not detect. This is especially important if cognitive deficits are present.

9. Evaluate edema—Does the patient have distal edema?

   If the answer is yes, the therapist should consider whether a splint will support a flexed wrist with the goal of counteracting the dependent positioning of the hand, thereby decreasing or preventing further edema? Will the immobilization of the splint increase the edema by blocking the "pumping action" of muscles generated by active range of motion? Patients with edema tend to lose digit flexion, thereby keeping the collateral ligaments in a shortened position. Will the splint block digit flexion, thereby exacerbating this problem? Will the splint impinge on neuromuscular structures and further limit hemodynamic function?

10. Evaluate posturing—Does the patient posture in persistent flexion?

    If the answer is yes, the therapist should consider splinting to maintain stretch on soft tissues. Rechecking of biomechanical alignment is essential; proximal realignment may relax the hand.

    If the answer is no, the therapist should consider not splinting.

GENERAL SPLINTING GUIDELINES

1. Check for abnormal pressure and stress points, especially over bony prominences (e.g., ulnar styloid)
2. Decide during which activities and periods the patient will wear the splint. The splint must be evaluated or fabricated while the patient is in the most difficult posture and performing the most stressful activities if the effectiveness of the splint is to be evaluated. For example, fabricating a splint while the patient is seated and relaxed may result in a good fit with a relaxed hand. However, if the patient then leaves therapy to prepare a meal at home, the therapist may find the patient's hand "clawing" and flexing out of the splint. If the splint was fabricated with the patient standing and with the appropriate level of stretch, this phenomenon may not be a problem.
3. Splint for comfort. Pain and pressure responses may increase the patient's bias toward stereotypical posturing.
4. Patients need to experience full range of motion. Use positioning splints only as adjuncts to a comprehensive upper extremity program.
5. Monitor full range of motion. Many patients have been provided with resting hand splints to prevent flexion contractures only to end up with extension contractures, or "intrinsic lock."
6. Make wearing schedules practical to ensure patient compliance.

7. Therapists must have reasonable expectations for splints. An extremely tight hand may require several serial splints to achieve a desired position. Splints designed to provide correction at more than one joint can lead to added deformity if excessive skeletal muscle activity is present. For example, attempting to position both the wrist and digits into extension may create a clawing effect in the digits as a result of the amount of stretch at the wrist and digits.[43] A severely malaligned hand may respond best if the therapist only focuses on one particular aspect of the malalignment (proximal first). For example, counteracting the extreme ulnar deviation seen in this type of extremity may be the goal of the first splint, followed by neutral deviation with slight wrist extension for the next splint. The therapist must remember that with an extremely tight or contracted hand, all deformities cannot be addressed simultaneously; if simultaneous correction is attempted, compliance with splinting may be jeopardized because of the discomfort level and skin breakdown.
8. Educate patients about the realistic goals and expectations of the use of a splint. Many patients wear their splints for prolonged periods with the hope that the splint will "make their hand better." Most patients interpret "better" as a return in function. However, this may not be the case for all patients; therefore the patient should be aware of the reasons that the splint was prescribed. No splint should be worn continuously.

GENERAL FABRICATION GUIDELINES

Many splinting materials are commercially available today (Tables 8-1 and 8-2). They are basically thermoplastic materials, some with more rubber content base than others. The rubber content base materials tend to have increased conformability and drape compared with pure thermoplastic materials, but they may be more difficult to handle because of their draping quality.

Thermoplastic materials generally have a greater memory capacity than do the rubber-based thermoplastics. Memory indicates the capability of the material to return to its original shape after the reheating that occurs during fabrication of the splint. Some therapists prefer the thermoplastics because of the memory capacity. The thermoplastics are available in perforated and solids. Perforated materials are recommended to allow for breathability and decrease the chance of skin maceration (especially with patients with sympathetic nerve changes and sensory impairments). The therapist must take care when using maxiperforated thermoplastics to eliminate sharp edges after cutting the material. The edges must be heated with a heat gun and turned down to smooth the edging; the edges also may be covered with $\frac{1}{16}$-inch solid material, cut into 1-inch wide but long pieces, heated in water, and then applied to

Table 8-1

Splinting Materials: Rubber-Based Thermoplastics

RUBBER-BASED THERMOPLASTICS*	VENDORS
Orthoplast	Sammons/Preston, Smith & Nephew Rolyan
NCM Preferred	North Coast Medical
NCM Clinic D	North Coast Medical
NCM Spectrum	North Coast Medical
Kay Splint	Sammons/Preston
San Splint	Smith & Nephew Rolyan
Polyform/Polyflex	Smith & Nephew Rolyan
Synergy	Smith & Nephew Rolyan

*Most rubber-based thermoplastic materials are not perforated except for Polyform, San Splint, and Polyflex.

Table 8-2

Splinting Materials: Thermoplastics

THERMOPLASTIC MATERIALS	VENDORS
Aquaplast	Sammons/Preston, Smith & Nephew Rolyan
Orfit	North Coast Medical
Prism	North Coast Medical

the edging. A thin layer of moleskin also may be used to smooth the edges of perforated material.

The thermoplastic materials and rubber-based thermoplastics are available in various thicknesses ranging from ⅛ inch, 3⁄32 inch, ½ inch, and 1⁄16 inch; the most common width is ⅛ inch. Some of the splinting materials are available in a wide range of colors; these may help draw attention to the involved limb and prevent the splint from being lost in hospital bedding. Also, color may enhance compliance. Several vendors offer precut splint blanks and kits. These products can be cut to size for customization and to decrease the amount of splinting time required for fabrication. Prefabricated splints also are available for many splinting needs, but some may be difficult to customize. The authors do not recommend some of the commercially available spring wire splints for patients with sensory impairments because these splints may apply too much pressure that the patient will not be able to detect. Custom-fabricated splints are the splints of choice for patients with sensory impairments.

Velcro strapping materials are now available in multiple colors. Velfoam, a padded strapping material, is highly recommended for the patient with sensory impairments because it is a softer strapping material.

Splint padding does not compensate for a poorly fitted splint and increases the pressure within the splint. Splint padding is recommended to cushion fingers at the point of contact of the thermoplastic material in dynamic splints only. Splint padding is available under different trade names such as Contour Foam, Slo-Foam, Luxafoam, Terry Cushion, and Splintcushion, to name a few. Splint padding materials only increase the pressure of an ill-fitting splint. Splint padding materials used in this way may also be hot and uncomfortable for the patient; their use may increase the chance of skin maceration resulting from the increased perspiration that the padding may cause in a patient with increased sweating response.

Splinting the extremity of a patient with neurologic involvement is sometimes extremely difficult if severely increased skeletal muscle activity is evident in the upper extremity. Maintaining the desired alignment and molding the splinting material may be almost impossible. The assistance of another person for positioning is usually indicated for a proper fit. Pattern-making also may be difficult with this type of patient. The fabrication of a gross pattern on the unaffected hand and reversal of the pattern for transfer to the splinting material are helpful at times.

Allowances must be made for bony prominences by either cutting around or flaring the splinting material over the prominence. A helpful hint for flaring out the material is to place a spot of dark lipstick over the bony prominence (on the patient's skin); place the cooled, already formed splint on the patient; and remove the splint. The lipstick will now be on the splint in the exact spot at which the splint requires flaring.

During the use of thermoplastic materials in splinting, the placement of curve in the material increases the tensile strength of the material to approximately 20 times that of straight material. This is helpful to remember in the fabrication of dynamic outriggers from thermoplastic material or the creation of an additional roll in the material as a spine or support.

SPECIFIC FABRICATION GUIDELINES

Forearm Support

If the splint prescribed for a patient includes a forearm trough, basic splinting principles call for the trough to cover two thirds of the forearm. To compensate for the weight of the hand and the excess force created by increased distal flexor activity, the forearm trough should be two thirds of the length of the forearm to provide a sufficient lever.

Palmar Support

Many patients with neurologic involvement have flattened arches at the MCP joints, with resultant clawing of the digits. This malalignment is usually seen in patients with little or no skeletal muscle activity in the affected hand. In molding the splint into the palmar arch in these cases, the therapist can use the thumb to mold a letter T pattern over the palmar surface of the splint. The base of the T runs longitudinally through the center of the palm, whereas the top of the T runs across the metacarpal heads. The base of the T should connect to the top of the T at the third MP head. The T shape is molded into the palm to enhance the arch. To ensure sturdy arch support, the splint must progress distal to the distal palmar crease and does not need to clear the thenar eminence in a hand without movement. The patient should frequently be reevaluated for returning motor control, and the splint should be adjusted as needed. If the patient exhibits controlled digit flexion, the distal end of the splint needs to be rolled back proximal to the distal palmar crease so that returning function is not blocked. If the patient begins to exhibit thumb function, the palmar support surface of the splint must again be rolled back to clear the thenar eminence and therefore not block active movement.

After splint fabrication the palmar support section of the splint is evaluated by checking that the dual obliquity of the hand is maintained, the third metacarpal head is the apex of the arch formed by the metacarpal heads, and the hand is not "flattened" in the splint (Figures 8-24 and 8-25).

Wrist Support

When molding and evaluating the wrist component of a splint for the patient after stroke, the therapist must consider alignment:

- The third metacarpal should lie midway between the radius and ulna in a neutral deviated hand. Many hands with neurologic involvement have a tendency to assume a position of ulnar deviation. Splint modifications to the wrist component include raising the border of the splint that lies lateral to the fifth metacarpal. This modification effectively blocks the ulnar deviation (Figure 8-26).
- The wrist should be supported between 0 and 20° of extension. The final decision depends on which angle allows the maximal amount of function or (if the hand is not functional) which angle in this range decreases the usual abnormal flexor activity in the digits. (Many patients' digits relax if they are realigned proximally.) In some cases the splint may be fabricated in some degree of flexion. This may be required if contracture of the extrinsic flexors is evident and the goal is to systematically lengthen the flexors with serial splinting. In these cases, each subsequent splint should be molded with an increased stretch on the flexors. For example, the first splint may be molded in 20° of wrist flexion, the next in 10° of flexion, neutral wrist, and finally in some degree of extension. Therapists must remember that if the goal is to lengthen the extrinsic flexors, both wrist and digit support is required.

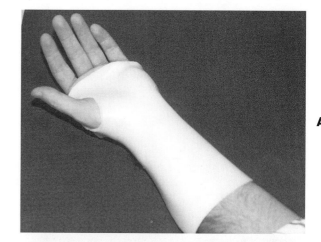
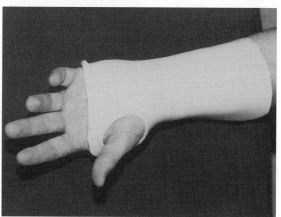

Figure 8-24 Variations on palmar support fabrication. **A,** Full palmar support (material progresses past distal palmar crease and gives thumb support over the first metacarpal). **B,** As function returns, distal and thenar aspects of the splint are rolled back to allow for joint excursion during functional tasks. Note the T shape molded into the palmar aspect of the splint.

- After molding the splint, the therapist should check that the hand is not in a position of medial or lateral rotation (neutral) compared with the forearm. Many patients who exhibit excessive skeletal muscle activity develop a tendency for the hand to rotate either medially or laterally in relation to the forearm. The hand should be positioned in the splint so that the fifth metacarpal is aligned with the ulna instead of lying inferior to the ulna (the hand is laterally rotated in relation to the forearm) or lying superior to the ulna (the hand is medially rotated in relation to the forearm).

Digit Support

A digit support platform should be used only as a last resort. A digit support platform must be included in the splint if the patient exhibits excessive flexor activity in the digits that cannot be otherwise controlled and if the pa-

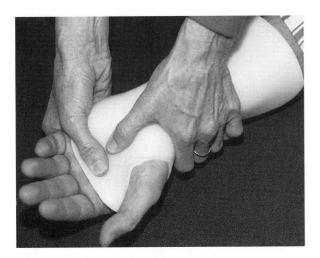

Figure 8-25 Molding the T support into the splint. The base of the T runs longitudinally through the palm, whereas the top of the T supports the metacarpal arch. The base of the T intersects the top of the T at the third metacarpal head. Palmar support is accurate if the arches of the hand are maintained and the third metacarpal head is superior to the metacarpal heads of digits two and four.

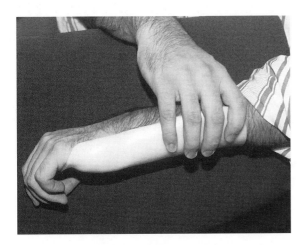

Figure 8-26 The lateral aspect of the splint is built up along the fifth metacarpal to effectively block ulnar deviation.

tient is being splinted for contracture management. If a digit platform is included, daytime use of the splint is discouraged.

If a patient exhibits excessive flexor activity, a forearm and wrist splint that enhances alignment should be tried at first. In many patients a proximal realignment of the joints and a prolonged state of accommodation of muscles to their resting length relaxes the hand. This phenomenon can be evaluated by therapists by manually realigning the joints with their hands and evaluating whether a relaxation response occurs.

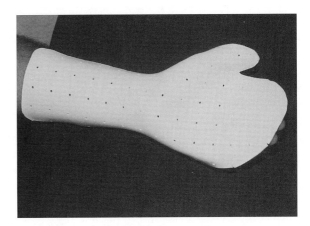

Figure 8-27 Full support provided to the distal extremity. This style of splint is only recommended if alternate attempts of proximal realignment do not relax the hand. This splint is recommended for night use only.

If a digit support platform is necessary, the digits should not be overstretched to the point that a "clawing" of the hand or a "bottoming out" of the metacarpals occurs. The therapist must ensure that the palmar arch remains intact when the digits are stretched onto the platform (Figure 8-27).

Thumb Support

In the nonfunctional hand the thumb should be supported in a position midway between palmar and radial abduction. This position can be maintained by the previously described palmar support, which also supports the first metacarpal; if the splint is rolled back to clear the thenar eminence, the thumb cannot be supported in this position (see Figure 8-24).

If the thumb is functional, the splinted position is dictated by evaluating the position of thumb that is the most effective at enhancing function with the thumb in opposition. Figure 8-28 describes the clinical reasoning process followed when deciding on the type and style of splint to fabricate.

SUMMARY

When designing or fabricating a splint for a patient after stroke, the therapist must consider each patient on an individual basis; no set of rules applies to all patients after CVA. No definitive answers or protocols are available. The reader is encouraged to consider the questions in the decision-making section of this chapter to guide clinical reasoning, because so many factors must be considered in treatment.

Any hand with a malalignment or deformity results in an overstretching of the soft tissues (muscles, ligaments) on one side of the joint and shortening of the soft tissue on the opposite side. All treatment, including splinting,

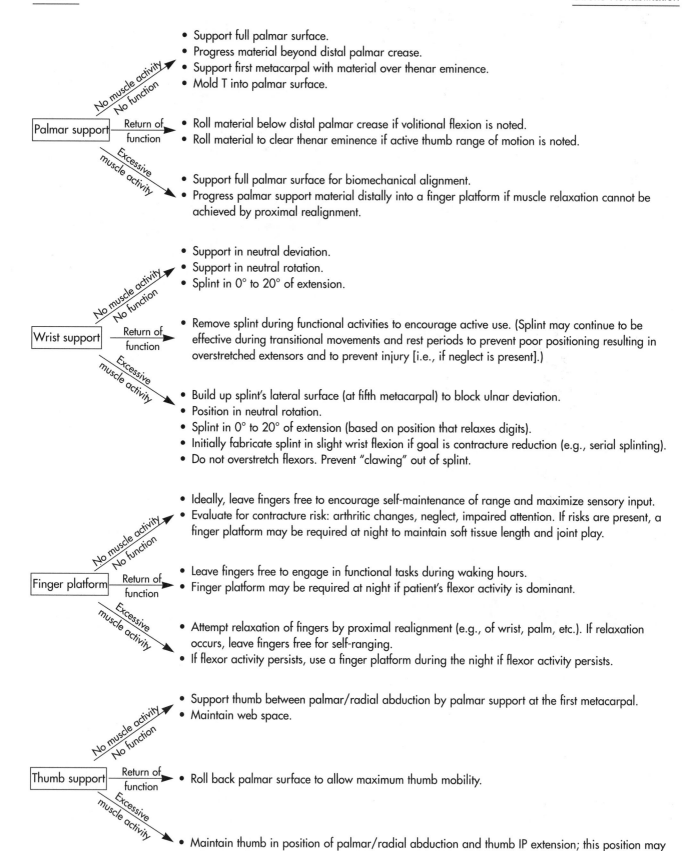

Palmar support

No muscle activity / No function
- Support full palmar surface.
- Progress material beyond distal palmar crease.
- Support first metacarpal with material over thenar eminence.
- Mold T into palmar surface.

Return of function
- Roll material below distal palmar crease if volitional flexion is noted.
- Roll material to clear thenar eminence if active thumb range of motion is noted.

Excessive muscle activity
- Support full palmar surface for biomechanical alignment.
- Progress palmar support material distally into a finger platform if muscle relaxation cannot be achieved by proximal realignment.

Wrist support

No muscle activity / No function
- Support in neutral deviation.
- Support in neutral rotation.
- Splint in 0° to 20° of extension.

Return of function
- Remove splint during functional activities to encourage active use. (Splint may continue to be effective during transitional movements and rest periods to prevent poor positioning resulting in overstretched extensors and to prevent injury [i.e., if neglect is present].)

Excessive muscle activity
- Build up splint's lateral surface (at fifth metacarpal) to block ulnar deviation.
- Position in neutral rotation.
- Splint in 0° to 20° of extension (based on position that relaxes digits).
- Initially fabricate splint in slight wrist flexion if goal is contracture reduction (e.g., serial splinting).
- Do not overstretch flexors. Prevent "clawing" out of splint.

Finger platform

No muscle activity / No function
- Ideally, leave fingers free to encourage self-maintenance of range and maximize sensory input.
- Evaluate for contracture risk: arthritic changes, neglect, impaired attention. If risks are present, a finger platform may be required at night to maintain soft tissue length and joint play.

Return of function
- Leave fingers free to engage in functional tasks during waking hours.
- Finger platform may be required at night if patient's flexor activity is dominant.

Excessive muscle activity
- Attempt relaxation of fingers by proximal realignment (e.g., of wrist, palm, etc.). If relaxation occurs, leave fingers free for self-ranging.
- If flexor activity persists, use a finger platform during the night if flexor activity persists.

Thumb support

No muscle activity / No function
- Support thumb between palmar/radial abduction by palmar support at the first metacarpal.
- Maintain web space.

Return of function
- Roll back palmar surface to allow maximum thumb mobility.

Excessive muscle activity
- Maintain thumb in position of palmar/radial abduction and thumb IP extension; this position may enhance relaxation.

Figure 8-28 Fabrication decisions: clinical reasoning. A volar-based forearm trough that supports two thirds of the forearm with sides parallel to the radius and ulna serves as the base splint in this decision-making process.

should be instituted after consideration of this phenomenon and should aim to preserve the length and balance of soft tissue on either side of the joint. This treatment prepares the hand for possible future integration into functional activities and prevents permanent deformity.

All splints applied to patients after CVA, especially patients with increased skeletal muscle activity and decreased sensation who are being treated with the principles of LLPS, must be continually monitored to assess for skin integrity by therapists, nursing staff, and families. This concept is particularly crucial for patients with cognitive and perceptual deficits. Factors in the monitoring of skin integrity include signs of skin discoloration, maceration, edema, and breakdown.

Splinting for patients after CVA that combines both the principles of biomechanical positioning and the neurophysiologic concepts of facilitation and inhibition may lead to the most favorable components of function.[44]

Realistic outcomes must be guiding forces in the decision-making process in the fabrication of splints for patients after stroke. Clinicians working with this population who use splinting as an adjunctive treatment should strive to gain a solid understanding of anatomy, biomechanics, and motor control theories.

Finally, therapists have a responsibility to not only stay current on research regarding this area of intervention, but also to add to the literature through research, from single subject case studies to qualitative trend analyses to large subject sample qualitative studies. Until more definitive and well-designed research studies are available concerning this treatment, the splinting controversy for patients after stroke will continue, and therapists may be providing patients with less than optimal care.

REVIEW QUESTIONS

1. What is the normal resting posture of the hand? What are the common malalignments observed after a stroke?
2. What precautions should be followed when splinting a patient after stroke?
3. What is the recommended rationale for splinting the patient after stroke?
4. How does the therapist differentiate among intrinsic tightness, extrinsic tightness, and joint contracture when evaluating for a splint?
5. What are the advantages of low-load prolonged stretch versus high-load brief stretch?

■ COTA Considerations ■

- Newly applied splint should be checked soon after initial application to ensure that no pressure areas have been created.

- When splinting patients with sensory loss, therapists must take precautions so that skin breakdown does not occur.
- Splinting should only be used as an adjunctive therapy intervention to a comprehensive upper extremity treatment plan.
- A variety of splinting options must be considered for patients after CVA.
- Therapists should continually check and recheck alignment of the distal extremity when molding and finalizing splints.

REFERENCES

1. Blashy MRM, Fuchs-Neeman RL: Orthokinetics: a new receptor facilitation method, *Am J Occup Ther* 13:226-234, 1959.
2. Bloch R, Evans MG: An inflatable splint for the spastic hand, *Arch Phys Med Rehabil* 58:179-180, 1977.
3. Bobath B: *Adult hemiplegia: evaluation and treatment*, ed 3, Oxford, 1990, Butterworth-Heineman.
4. Boehme R: *Improving upper body control: an approach to assessment and treatment of tonal dysfunction*, Tucson, 1988, Therapy Skill Builders.
5. Brennan J: Response to stretch of hypertonic muscle groups in hemiplegia, *Br Med J* 1:1504-1507, 1959.
6. Casey CA, Kratz EJ: Soft splinting with neoprene: the thumb abduction supinator splint, *Am J Occup Ther* 42(6):395-398, 1988.
7. Charait SE: A comparison of volar and dorsal splinting of the hemiplegic hand, *Am J Occup Ther* 22(4):319-321, 1968.
8. Currie DM, Mendiola A: Cortical thumb orthosis for children with spastic hemiplegic cerebral palsy, *Arch Phys Med Rehabil* 68:214-217, 1987.
9. Doubilet L, Polkow LS: Theory and design of a finger abduction splint for the spastic hand, *Am J Occup Ther* 21(5):320-322, 1977.
10. Feldman PA: Upper extremity casting and splinting. In Glenn MB, Whyte J, editors: *The practical management of spasticity in children and adults*, Philadelphia, 1990, Lea & Febiger.
11. Fess EE, Philips CA: *Hand splinting: principles and methods*, ed 2, St Louis, 1987, Mosby.
12. Flowers K: Orthopaedic assessment and mobilization of the upper extremity. *Scar Wars I & II*. Seminar conducted in New York City, 1992.
13. Gossman MR, Sahrman SA, Rose SJ: Review of length associated changes in muscles: experimental evidence and clinical implications, *Phys Ther* 62(12):1799-1808, 1982.
14. Halar EM, Bell KR: Contracture and other deleterious effects on immobility. In Delisa JA, editor: *Rehabilitation Medicine: principles and practice*, ed 2, Philadelphia, 1993, J.B. Lippincott.
15. Hill SG: Current trends in upper extremity splinting. In Boehme R, editor: *Improving upper body control: an approach to assessment and treatment of tonal dysfunction*, Tucson, 1988, Therapy Skill Builders.
16. Hummelsheim H et al: Influence of sustained stretch on late muscular responses to magnetic brain stimulation in patients with upper motor neuron lesions, *Scand J Rehabil Med* 26:3-9, 1994.
17. Hunter JM, Mackin E, Callahan A: *Rehabilitation of the hand: surgery and therapy*, ed 4, St Louis, 1995, Mosby.
18. Johnstone M: *Restoration of motor function in the stroke patient: a physiotherapist's approach*, New York, 1983, Churchill Livingstone.
19. Kapandji IA: *The physiology of the joints vol. 1: upper limb*, ed 5, New York, 1982, Churchill Livingstone.
20. Kaplan N: Effect of splinting on reflex inhibition and sensorimotor stimulation in treatment of spasticity, *Arch Phys Med Rehabil* 43:565-569, 1962.
21. Kiel JH: *Basic hand splinting: a pattern-designing approach*, Boston, 1983, Little, Brown.

22. Light K et al: Low-load prolonged stretch vs. high-load brief stretching in treating knee contractures, *Phys Ther* 64(3):330-333, 1984.

23. MacKinnon J, Sanderson E, Buchanan J: The Mackinnon splint—a functional hand splint, *Can J Occup Ther* 42(4):157-158, 1975.

24. Malick MH: *Manual on static hand splinting*, ed 5, Pittsburgh, 1985, Harmarvile Rehabilitation Center.

25. Mathiowetz V, Bolding DJ, Trombly CA: Immediate effects of positioning devices on the normal and spastic hand measured by electromyography, *Am J Occup Ther* 37(4):247-254, 1983.

26. McPherson JJ et al: A comparison of dorsal and volar resting hand splints in the reduction of hypertonus, *Am J Occup Ther* 36(10):664-670, 1982.

27. McPherson JJ: Objective evaluation of a splint designed to reduce hypertonicity, *Am J Occup Ther* 35(3):189-194, 1981.

28. Neeman RL, Neeman M: Efficacy of orthokinetic orthotics for post-stroke upper extremity hemiparetic motor dysfunction, *Int J Rehabil Res* 16:302-307, 1993.

29. Neeman RL, Neeman M: Orthokinetic orthoses: clinical efficacy study of orthokinetics treatment for a patient with upper extremity movement dysfunction in late post-acute CVA, *J Rehabil Res Dev* (Annual Supplement) 29:41-53, 1992.

30. Neeman RL, Neeman M: Rehabilitation of a post stroke patient with upper extremity hemiparetic movement dysfunction by orthokinetic orthoses, *J Hand Ther* 5:147-155, 1992.

31. Neeman RL, Liederhouse JJ, Neeman M: A multidisciplinary efficacy study on orthokinetics treatment of a patient with post-CVA hemiparesis and pain, *Can J Rehabil* 2:41-52, 1988.

32. Neuhaus BE et al: A survey of rationales for and against hand splinting in hemiplegia, *Am J Occup Ther* 35(2):83-90, 1981.

33. Nicholson DE: *The effects of pressure splint treatment on the motor function of the involved limb in patients with hemiplegia*, master's thesis, Chapel Hill, 1984, University of North Carolina.

34. Pedretti LW: Hand splinting. In Pedretti LW, Zoltan B, editors: *Occupational therapy: practice skills for physical dysfunction*, ed 3, St Louis, 1990, Mosby.

35. Peterson LT: *Neurological consideration in splinting spastic extremities*, unpublished paper.

36. Poole JL et al: The effectiveness of inflatable pressure splints on motor function in stroke patients, *Occup Ther J Res* 10(6):360-366, 1990.

37. Poole JL, Whitney SL: Inflatable pressure splints (airsplints) as adjunct treatment for individual with strokes, *Phys Occup Ther Geriatrics* 11(1):17-27, 1992.

38. Snook JH: Spasticity reduction splint, *Am J Occup Ther* 33:648-651, 1979.

39. Stern GR: Thumb abduction splint, *Physiotherapy* 66(10):352, 1980.

40. Stockmeyer S: An interpretation of the approach of Rood to the treatment of neuromuscular dysfunction, *Am J Phys Med* 46:900-961, 1967.

41. Thompson-Rangel T: The mystery of the serpentine splints, *Occupational Therapy Forum*, 4-6, September 20, 1991.

42. Tubiana R, Thomine JM, Mackin E: *Examination of the hand and wrist*, St Louis, 1996, Mosby.

43. Wilson D, Caldwell C: Central control insufficiency III. Disturbed motor control and sensation: a treatment approach emphasizing upper extremity orthoses, *Phys Ther* 58(3):313-320, 1978.

44. Woodson AM: Proposal for splinting the adult hemiplegic hand to promote function. In Cromwell FS, editor: *Hand rehabilitation in occupational therapy*, Redding, Calif, 1988, Hawthorne Press.

45. Wu SH: A belly gutter splint for proximal interphalangeal joint flexion contracture, *Am J Occup Ther* 45(9):839-843, 1991.

46. Zislis JM: Splinting of hand in a spastic hemiplegic patient, *Arch Phys Med Rehabil* 45:41-43, 1962.

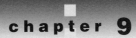

lauren joachim-grizzaffi

chapter 9

Casting Applications

key terms

casting

cerebrovascular accident

contracture

spasticity

hypertonia

reflexes

serial casting

inhibitory casting

heterotopic ossification

plaster

fiberglass

resting cast

holding cast

drop-out cast

bivalve cast

anteroposterior splint

chapter objectives

After completing this chapter, the reader will be able to accomplish the following:

1. List objectives of casting a patient who has survived a cerebrovascular accident.
2. List indications for casting a patient who has survived a cerebrovascular accident.
3. List precautions when casting.
4. List contraindications to casting.
5. Describe what to consider clinically when evaluating a patient for casting.
6. Compare and contrast plaster and fiberglass.
7. Compare and contrast various types of casts and their associated indications and pros and cons.
8. Develop an understanding of casting progression guidelines.
9. Describe cast application and removal procedures.
10. Describe fabrication of various casts including drop-out and bivalve casts.
11. Describe clinical issues relating to casting a patient who has survived a cerebrovascular accident.

Little documentation exists in the literature regarding the use of serial and inhibitory casting for patients who have had a cerebrovascular accident (CVA). Most of the literature published is developed for use with patients diagnosed with traumatic head injury, cerebral palsy, and quadriplegia.* Patients who have survived a CVA may be at risk for developing soft tissue contracture or severe spasticity. Casting may be necessary when traditional methods of treatment have failed and the patient is at risk for contracture because of severe spasticity. If not treated a variety of dysfunctions and problems may develop, such as functional limitations in self-care and instrumental activities of daily living (IADL); inability for caregivers to assist patients with bathing, hygiene, and dressing; and an unpleasant appearance, skin breakdown, or a negative perception of body image. Traditional therapeutic interventions include using passive range of motion (PROM) activities, generalized and localized inhibitory handling techniques, splinting, positional devices, myofascial release, acupressure, physical agent modalities, a tilt table, positioning, nerve blocks, and pharmacologic intervention.† Serial casting has been demonstrated to be effective in reducing spasticity as well as contractures.‡

Anesthetic and phenol nerve blocks, drugs, and topical anesthesia have been used for treating and diagnosing spasticity. Procaine or lidocaine hydrochloride anesthetic nerve blocks may be used before cast application to relax spastic muscles. Repeated use of nerve blocks may reduce spasticity enough to improve function. For example, an obturator nerve block may aid a patient who has a scissoring gait. Anesthetic nerve blocks can be used to differentiate spasticity from fixed contracture. In addition, they provide a preview of more permanent phenol nerve blocks and tendon-lengthening procedures.

Phenol nerve or phenol motor point injections enable further rehabilitation during recovery. Peripheral phenol nerve blocks may be used for severe spasticity because complete cessation of muscle activity occurs. An open peripheral nerve injection of nerves containing both motor and sensory branches should only inject the motor branches to prevent dysesthesia and loss of sensation after the nerve block. Phenol motor point injections may be performed at the bedside for patients with minimal spasticity that is interfering with function. The block lasts 1 to 2 months; repeat blocks may be performed. Spastic muscles are not completely relaxed as they are with peripheral nerve blocks.[12]

Drugs may benefit patients with spasticity resulting from a CVA. Medications more commonly used to treat spinal-cord injured patients with spasticity may be used in the stroke population. However, there is presently no known uniform treatment for this population. Drugs are used on each patient on an individual basis until, hopefully, a satisfactory effect is achieved. Side effects must be considered. Drugs most effective in reducing spasticity include baclofen, diazepam, dantrolene, chlorpromazine, clonidine, and progabide.[5,12] Baclofen (Lioresal) may be used orally or intrathecally. Baclofen is less sedating than diazepam and equally effective. The effects of baclofen on cerebral forms of spasticity are presently not clear. In the brain-injured population, it may interfere with attention and memory. It has been demonstrated to be safe for long-term use and has a low incidence of side effects. Oral diazepam (Valium) is generally not appropriate for patients with brain injuries because of its negative effects on attention and memory. Intellectual impairment and reduction in motor coordination are possible side effects, and physiologic addiction is possible. Withdrawal symptoms may appear if diazepam is tapered too quickly. Oral dantrolene (Dantrium) is the preferred drug for cerebral forms of spasticity such as spastic hemiplegia. It is less likely to cause lethargy or cognitive dysfunction than baclofen or diazepam. Dantrolene is likely to decrease clonus and muscle spasms from innocuous stimuli. It has also been suggested that dantrolene "weakens" muscles; however, motoric function is not affected by its effect on spasticity. Hepatotoxicity (liver toxicity) may occur in approximately 1% of the population. Oral chlorpromazine, oral and transdermal clonidine, and oral progabide may also be tried in an effort to decrease spasticity in cerebral forms of edema.[5] No spasticity-reducing drugs are given intravenously.

Topical anesthesia (20% benzocaine sprayed for 15 seconds) applied to the patient's skin is an additional treatment that has been used successfully to decrease hypertonicity resulting in increased active range of motion (AROM), PROM, and improved gait pattern.[28] An example of the use of this form of topical anesthesia is the "spray and stretch technique."

Casting can be done on upper and lower extremities. Tissues will shorten in a period of time if not lengthened on a regular basis. These tissues can lengthen if undergoing constant, prolonged stretching.[23] Through animal studies, Tabary et al[31] have demonstrated that changes in muscle fiber and sarcomere length and number occur with prolonged stretch. Although the same process is suggested to occur in humans, it has not been proven.

Serial casting is based on the biomechanics of muscle length. Casts are used with contracted muscles to provide prolonged stretch in a lengthened position to allow for changes in sarcomere distribution, increased muscle or tendon length, or both.[16] Multiple casts are applied to gradually increase range of motion (ROM) until full ROM is restored or maximum attainable range occurs. Inhibitory casting uses positioning to relax muscles and pressure to decrease excessive skeletal muscle activity.[16] This mecha-

---

*References 1, 3, 7, 9, 10, 16, 17, 19, 21, 23, 25, 29, 31, 32, 34, 36, 37.
†References 1, 8, 12, 16, 19, 23, 27.
‡References 1, 3, 16, 17, 19, 21, 23, 25, 31, 34, 36, 37.

nism remains unclear. Some rationales include neutral warmth and constant pressure, an increase in muscle or tendon length, and inhibition of Golgi tendon organs (GTOs), and muscle spindles.[1,4,23,30] Neutral warmth is a local inhibitory technique that causes a decrease in gamma motor neuron activity.[8] Continuous, slow stretching places the contracted muscle of the casted limb in a prolonged position at maximal tolerable length. Maintaining this position will cause cutaneous stretch receptors to rapidly adapt, thus causing inhibition by preventing additional stimuli from entering the system.[8,33] Continuous pressure is inhibitory; it activates the pacinian corpuscles which are rapidly adapting receptors. Pressure on a tendon insertion activates deep receptors by applying pressure across the longitudinal axis of a tendon.[33] Sometimes casting combines serial casts and inhibitive positioning.

When performing serial or inhibitory casting, the effects of long-term immobilization must be considered. In 1982, Booth[4] documented that when a muscle was immobilized in a shortened position the muscle atrophied. However, when the muscle was in a lengthened position the muscle enlarged. After weeks of immobilization, muscles composed of predominately slow-twitch fibers took on characteristics of fast-twitch muscles. Electromyographic (EMG) activity of immobilized limbs was reduced 5% to 15% when compared to controls. In addition, the resting membrane potential of immobilized limbs either did not change or decreased.

The effectiveness of prolonged stretch has been documented since as early as 1959,[6] in a study with 14 hemiplegic patients with spasticity for an average duration of 18 months since onset. The responses to stretch of 19 flexor muscle groups, 18 upper extremities, and 1 lower extremity were studied for 3 years. Each flexed limb was constantly stretched in extension with a polythene-polyurethane splint for an average of 3 months. When increased active extension was demonstrated and the flexor spasm terminated for at least 1 month, the splint was worn for shorter daily periods of time. The splint was removed twice daily for bathing. At that time, the patient was encouraged to actively move the limb. Most of the patients demonstrated decreased spasticity and increased AROM. A follow-up visit revealed that the gains were maintained with an increase in function. However, the length of the period before the follow up and the amount of increase in function were not specified. Those patients who did not improve in their functional abilities did at least demonstrate improved body appearance resulting from improved limb posture. The author of this study suggests the following time guideline for prolonged stretching that will abolish different degrees of spasticity with lasting effects: 12 weeks of constant stretching followed by 8 weeks of intermittent stretching for moderate spasm. This time should be adjusted for lesser and greater amounts of spasm.

In 1990, MacKay-Lyons[24] reported that low-load prolonged stretching with the Dynasplint successfully reduced elbow flexion contracture secondary to head trauma. A Dynasplint is a dynamic elbow splint that consists of two adjustable cuffs with medial and lateral struts hinged at the joint axis. By varying the tension of the springs housed in each of the distal struts, the amount of force applied across the joint can be altered. After a trial of the splint, the contracture decreased from −67° of elbow extension to −15° of elbow extension—a gain of 52°. ROM gains were still present at follow-up evaluations conducted 2 and 6 months after treatment. Average splint wear was 8 to 12 hours per day at a tension setting of 10. Positive outcomes included decreased flexion contracture, an increase in bilateral upper extremity use for activities of daily living (ADL), and the ability to ambulate short distances with a walker.

The use of serial and inhibitory casting for patients who have had a CVA has been documented in the literature.[1] The literature is inconsistent regarding which factors are necessary if casting will be used to decrease excessive muscle activity. It has been suggested but not demonstrated that the cast maintains the limb with excessive muscle activity in a reflex-inhibiting position. Reflex-inhibiting postures are defined by Trombly as positions that inhibit spasticity by passively elongating spastic muscles.[2] In addition, the roles of total even pressure and neutral warmth in reducing spasticity have been claimed and reported. It has been postulated that when the static position of the joint and muscle is combined with neutral warmth and constant pressure, it may cause thermal and rapidly adapting tactile receptors to turn off, thus reducing the influence on the excitability of interneurons, motor neurons, or both.[1] Barnard et al[1] reported the use of early cylindrical, short-leg plaster casts on an 11-year-old who sustained a closed-head injury and could not be treated with traditional therapies. Positive results were achieved—the patient's overall increased muscle activity decreased, and spontaneous movement of the left extremities and ankle ROM increased.

A 1994 study by Hill[17] compared casting to traditional treatment techniques, which included PROM activities, stretching, and splinting for severe brain-injury patients whose upper extremities had increased muscle activity. Fifteen subjects with brain injury were randomly assigned to receive one of two treatments: (1) 1 month of casting followed by one month of traditional therapy or (2) 1 month of traditional therapy followed by casting. The subjects were evaluated before intervention, after the first month of intervention, and after the second month of intervention for ROM, clinical indications of spasticity, and functional use. All but one patient's ROM improved with casting rather than with traditional therapy. Decreased spasticity when casted was seen in 11 of the 15 subjects. However, the decrease did not translate into improved function with either group.

In 1990, Yasukawa[34] casted a 15-month-old patient who was first seen with spastic hemiparesis. Initially, four short-arm serial casts were each used for 1 week. In the second phase, the unaffected extremity was casted to encourage active use of the involved extremity. In the third phase, a bivalved long-arm splint was used at night on the affected arm. Increased scapular stability and humeral flexion, use of the affected limb during transitions, and spontaneous use of the involved limb during bilateral tasks were reported after 1½ years.

Law et al[21] examined the use of a short-arm cast on 73 children with cerebral palsy. The children were divided into 4 treatment groups: (1) regular neurodevelopmental treatment (NDT), (2) regular NDT and a cast, (3) intensive NDT, and (4) intensive NDT and a cast. Quantitative differences were not found between the groups. However, quality of movement and wrist extension were found to be improved in casted groups.

King[19] discussed treatment of a 46-year-old patient who had suffered a subarachnoid hemorrhage and intraventricular bleeding secondary to aneurysm clipping. Traditional inhibitory techniques in conjunction with purposeful activity had been unsuccessful in reducing spasticity. A series of plaster drop-out casts were fabricated. A full circumferential portion enclosed the upper arm from axilla to the olecranon process; a volar forearm portion was added to prevent elbow flexion. The elbow was placed in maximum achievable extension. Ranging and bilateral upper extremity activities were implemented. Later a bivalved cast was worn for 12 hours at night for 2 weeks until the patient could actively and passively maintain range. PROM increased from −90° of elbow extension to −20° of elbow extension—a 70° gain. Once discharged from the inpatient rehabilitation unit, the patient was followed up biweekly for 4 months. The patient was monitored for an increase in independence with ADL and maintenance of active use of the impaired extremity with no return of spasticity. Specific gains regarding functional use were not reported. Gains were maintained and attributed to a reduction in elbow spasticity.

Smith and Harris[29] used casting to prevent an increase in elbow flexion contracture of a 5½-year-old girl with spastic quadriplegia. They initially observed a sharp decrease in elbow flexion contracture and then a slight increase.

Tona and Schneck[32] compared short-term upper extremity inhibitive casting with encased thermoplastic splinting on an 8½-year-old girl with upper extremity spasticity. Increased quality of movement, increased awareness and use of the casted extremity, and decreased spasticity and resistance to passive movement were noted but only lasted for 3 days.

Kaplan[18] examined the use of dorsal splinting on the surface opposite to the spastic muscles to provide prolonged stretching for hemiplegic upper limbs. A light splint consisting of three to four layers of plaster and one external layer of fiberglass impregnated with resin on the outside were used. Velcro straps held the splint in place. Patients wore the splint as long as it was tolerable. ROM and gross motor activity improved. The study did not report whether the patients were followed up.

Zachazewski and associates[37] described the use of short-leg inhibitory casts on a 25-year-old man who sustained a head injury in a motor vehicle accident. The patient had a positive support reaction in bilateral lower extremities, which was elicited during weight-bearing activities, transfers, and standing. Medications were not successful because of resulting drowsiness. Ice placed on the gastrocnemius and soleus muscles was also not effective. Bilateral lower-extremity inhibitory casts were fabricated and left in place for 4 weeks. When the casts were removed, the patient's gait had improved. The positive support reaction was decreased in the right lower extremity and absent in the left. Several days after cast removal the positive support reaction reappeared in the right lower extremity during ambulation. The casts were bivalved and used at night but were ineffective. A molded polypropylene "tone-inhibiting ankle foot orthosis" (AFO) was then fabricated for the right lower extremity. The patient's gait improved, and the positive scissoring was reduced enough to allow the patient to use a rolling walker to ambulate with supervision or minimal assistance. The authors of the study suggest that an inhibitory cast should be used to assess the patient for gains before fabricating a tone-inhibiting AFO because it is quicker, cheaper, and less complex to fabricate. In addition, casting may be needed to increase the patient's ROM and static stretching prior to fabrication of the tone-inhibiting AFO.

In summary, the serial casting has been demonstrated to be successful in increasing active and passive ROM, decreasing increased muscle activity, and improving function in some cases. If the therapist chooses this technique as an intervention, the goals must be clear (i.e., increasing function, improving cosmesis, improving hygiene), and the benefits must outweigh the risks.

CAUSES OF SOFT TISSUE CONTRACTURES

A patient who has had a CVA with resultant spasticity, cognitive and perceptual deficits (e.g., body neglect), hemiparesis, or hemiplegia is at risk for developing soft tissue contracture.[15] Tissues may shorten if not stretched over a period of time.[8] Traditional treatments to prevent soft tissue shortening include use of PROM activities, splinting, and inhibitory techniques.[1,23] A patient with a decreased level of alertness and poor attention, concentration, initiation, memory, or cooperation may not be able to volitionally perform the ROM activities necessary to maintain full joint range. This could potentially result in soft tissue contracture(s).[27] In addition, a patient with unilateral body neglect may not acknowledge the affected side. Therefore they usually cannot perform self-ROM activities. A patient with hemiparesis may not have the motor control to move the joint actively through full ROM, thus contributing to soft-tissue contracture. A patient with hemiplegia may also not be able to take the joint through full ROM as a result of pain or inability to effectively perform self-ROM. Patients who have suffered a CVA may develop spasticity to varying degrees. Patients with severe spasticity may develop reduced joint mobility as a result of ineffective treatment modalities to maintain joint ROM or reduce spasticity.

CASTING OBJECTIVES

1. Improve ROM.
2. Decrease influence of excessive skeletal muscle activity.
3. Decrease ineffective movement patterns.
4. Lengthen or maintain soft tissue contracture.
5. Decrease influence of pathologic reflexes by positioning limb(s) in inhibitory positions.
6. Obtain or maintain proper joint alignment.
7. Increase efficiency of available movement.
8. Increase functional use of an extremity.
9. Enable fit of a more definitive orthosis by improving ROM and positioning and decreasing spasticity.
10. Evaluate for "hidden" potential for motion.
11. Decrease joint posturing.

CASTING INDICATIONS

1. Spasticity[3,4,10,14,36]
2. Soft-tissue contracture[4,14]
3. Active and passive ROM limitations[3,4,10,14,16,22,36]
4. Pathologic reflexes
5. At least 10° limitation of ROM at a joint
6. Severe spasticity resulting in potential joint contracture or deformity that is not responding well to traditional medical or physical treatment
7. Demonstrated neurologic recovery when loss of ROM is a result of spasticity and not other factors, such as heterotopic ossification, healing fracture, or ligamentous injury[25]
8. A need for fit of a more definitive orthosis
9. A need to evaluate for "hidden" potential for motion

CASTING PRECAUTIONS

When casting a patient, observation of safety precautions is imperative.

1. Avoid poor casting technique, insufficient padding, or poor patient positioning, all of which may result in imperfect casting.[23]

2. Agitated patients are at risk for skin breakdown from cast abuse.[23] Fiberglass is generally not recommended because it splinters, leaving sharp edges.[3]
3. The therapist should use flat rather than flexed fingers and precise hand placement. Minimize indentations within the cast while the patient is being positioned during cast formation. Abnormal pressure points may cause skin breakdown.
4. Bony prominences such as the olecranon process, malleoli, and calcanei are common sites of skin breakdown. Bony prominences should be well padded.[3,23]
5. Cast cutters can abrade or cut the skin during cast removal. Have safety of the unit checked periodically.
6. Improper casting procedures can cause late-onset peripheral neuropathy resulting from nerve compression from the cast. Ulnar and peroneal nerves are most at risk for compressive neuropathy.[23]
7. Wrapping a limb too tightly in a cast can obstruct venous return and result in edema. Remove a cast that results in discoloration of toes or fingers of a casted limb for more than 20 to 30 minutes or when capillary refill is not observed from the outset. However, temporary skin discoloration during casting is not uncommon.[3,4,23,25] It may be associated with peripheral circulatory changes or in response to heat generated as the cast sets.
8. Do not initiate weight-bearing activities for 24 hours after cast application to promote hardening of casting material, prevent skin breakdown, prevent deformities of the interior plaster, and prevent indentations.[3,10,23,25]
9. Patients may not tolerate multiple casts well.[4] They can be heavy and limit function. In addition, they may interfere with homeostasis by elevating body temperature, and they limit limb access for monitoring vital signs or intravenous use.
10. Discomfort is expected within the first 24 hours after cast application. Analgesic medications usually alleviate this discomfort. Discomfort should not be severe.[4,9]
11. Edema can be caused by casting, which can result in decreased circulation because of cast compression of the vascular and lymphatic structures of the limb. Elevating the casted extremity can decrease the amount of occurrence of edema.[4,10]
12. Impaired sensation may place the patient at risk for skin breakdown.[10]
13. Dermatological conditions such as cellulitis, fungus growth, open wounds, and those caused by drug reactions must be considered when deciding whether to cast the patient. Skin maceration may occur if moisture builds up in the cast.

14. Patients with impaired communication abilities may not be able to express they are experiencing pain and discomfort.

15. Patients who have difficulty tolerating stress on related musculoskeletal areas may be prone to development of tendonitis or trigger points.

16. Perform a plaster sensitivity test before cast application if the patient has sensitive skin.

17. After cast application, check for (1) red areas, (2) pulse at points distal to cast, (3) pain, (4) temperature comparison of both extremities, (5) swelling, (6) discoloration of hand or foot and nail beds, and (7) dusky veins.

18. Check the patient's position before cast application.

19. Check whether the patient has a known allergy to a casting material.

20. Check whether the patient has adherent scar tissue.

21. The etiology of heterotopic ossification (HO) is not known. HO is the formation of bone in abnormal sites. The literature reports that HO can develop in patients who have had a CVA. HO most commonly develops in limbs with spasticity or those that have experienced trauma.[11] Clinical signs of HO include pain, decreasing ROM, and mildly swollen joints. Joints may be warm. The patient's alkaline phosphatase blood level will be elevated. Diagnosis is made by radiographs and bone scans. The role of PROM with HO remains controversial. Some authors report maintenance or increases in PROM with joint manipulation or judicious ROM.[12] Other authors report PROM or manipulation enhances the HO process.[12] Literature does not specifically document the role of PROM or joint manipulation for the patient who has survived a CVA. Generally, active and active assistive ROM may be used. When HO is present, it is controversial as to whether aggressive joint ROM or manipulation should be performed or if it worsens the situation.[13] Management of major HO may include aggressive joint manipulation while under general anesthesia. When the patient is under anesthesia, spasticity can be differentiated from bony ankylosis. Surgical excision has not always been successful.[12] Documentation regarding whether serial casting is contraindicated is inconsistent throughout the literature.[4,13] In cases of HO, stretch gently; change casts more frequently, range joints between cast changes to prevent solidification or fusion, and alternate bivalved casts between flexion and extension to prevent loss of ROM in either direction.

22. Plaster of Paris casts can burn a patient's skin. Lavalette and associates[20] found that skin could be burned under certain circumstances: (1) The water used to dip the casting material in is greater than 24° C. (2) The cast is greater than eight ply. (3) A pillow is used over the cast while setting and prevents dissipation of heat from the cast. (4) The casting material is not dipped in water for an adequate amount of time. Rapid, intense, localized heat may penetrate deep into the cast, which prevents dissipation of heat and places the patient at risk for being burned.

CASTING CONTRAINDICATIONS

The literature regarding contraindications to casting is inconsistent. Following is a list of contraindications that are most consistently found in the literature.*

1. Severe HO of the joint(s) may be enhanced[13] by casting.[23,25]

2. Fluctuating muscle activity may not be responsive to serial casting.

3. Skeletal muscle rigidity is not responsive to serial casting.[22,35] These limbs already resist passive stretch in both directions. Static positioning of a limb with a cast for 5 to 7 days may exacerbate the stiffness. An alternative may be to alternate bivalved casts in submaximal flexion and extension to reduce skeletal muscle rigidity and gradually increase joint ROM in both directions.[35]

4. Skin conditions (open wounds, abrasions, blisters, lacerations, skin graft) are contraindications.[3,16,23,25,26] Bivalving and windows may be options to open access to compromised skin in some circumstances.

5. Edema in the extremity may impair distal circulation, place the patient at risk for a compartmental syndrome, or have a tourniquet effect. A compartmental syndrome is a condition in which circulation to a structure such as a nerve or tendon is being constricted in an enclosed space. The structure may no longer be able to move freely in the compartment. The intracompartment pressure rises and circulation ceases. The tissues eventually necrose in the enclosed space.

6. Subluxation of the carpal bones or other orthopedic deformities that may require specialized interventions such as surgery are contraindications.

7. Impaired circulation indicated by pale skin color, low skin temperature, trophic changes, significant edema, and low distal pulse of the extremity to be casted may cause the casted limb to become cyanotic.[26] The patient may develop a compartmental syndrome.

8. Severe spasticity may cause microtears in the soft tissues resulting from improper fit, overstretching, and poor positioning.[7] Bleeding may result and cause a compartmental syndrome.

*References 3, 7, 16, 22, 25, 26, 34, 35.

9. Extreme wrist extension can cause carpal tunnel syndrome because pressure will be placed on the tunnel and magnify the symptoms. Circulatory problems may also cause cyanosis of the limb.

10. Uncontrolled hypertension may result because the cast causes an isometric contraction and may increase blood pressure.[26]

11. Lack of consent from patient, physician, or family is a contraindication to casting.[26]

12. Sensory or motor changes of the extremity to be casted may indicate circulatory problems, compartmental syndromes, or nerve impingement.[10,26]

13. Unstable fractures in the extremity to be casted are contraindications.[3,26] Do not serial cast until fractures are healed and stable because the patient may resist the cast and displace the fracture. It is possible to dislocate fragments or fixation.

14. Pathologic inflammatory conditions including arthritis of the joints proximal and distal to the casted joints and gout are contraindications.[26]

15. If limb access is required for an intravenous line or to monitor vital signs, casting is contraindicated.[3,23,25]

16. If patients are in danger of abusing themselves or getting injured, casting is contraindicated.[26]

17. Unstable intracranial pressure is a contraindication[3,14,23] because the cast is an isometric contraction and may increase intracranial pressure.

18. Diaphoresis, as well as the isometric effects of the cast, produce the potential for the skin to macerate under the cast.[23]

19. Contracture existing longer than 6 to 12 months.[3,4,23]

20. Poor compliance and/or attendance as an outpatient.

21. Internal fixation devices which limit ROM.

22. Metastatic disease secondary to risk of fracturing.

PRECASTING ASSESSMENT

When traditional methods for maintaining and improving range of motion or managing spasticity have failed and casting is being considered, it is advisable to do a precasting assessment. Initially, review the patient's hospital course and present medical status for potential contraindications to casting. Note baseline skin integrity, mental status, circulation, orthopedic conditions, course of rehabilitation therapy, and potential length of stay. Circulation may be evaluated by checking capillary refill. Pressure is applied and withdrawn from the fingertip or toe. The area touched should initially blanch (turn white) when pressure is applied and immediately return to its usual color when pressure is removed. If the patient is an outpatient, review compliance, the attendance record, and the support from caregivers. The risks and benefits of casting must be weighed. Cost, time, disposition, and goal of casting must be considered.

Initial Evaluation

The patient must be medically stable and without medical contraindications to casting (see the contraindications section of this chapter) if a casting program is to be initiated. Additionally, the patient and/or caregiver, as well as the physician, must consent to the casting program. Following is a list of initial evaluation considerations:

1. Skin integrity—Observe skin for open wounds; irritation; skin breakdown; edema; and excessively dry, moist, or sweaty skin. Is skin fragile or thin? If casting will be used despite skin irritation or breakdown, photograph skin before and after casting to compare skin integrity.[22] Consider using extra padding, T-foam, and drop-out casts. If skin is macerated, identify and manage the source of maceration before casting. Sources of maceration may include incontinence, vascular insufficiency, or sweating. Do not cast over an infection or wound. The wound would be enclosed and not have proper aeration and could not be accessed for wound care.

2. Sensation—Does the patient have absent or impaired proprioception; graphesthesia; two-point discrimination; or perception of sharp and dull, light touch, pressure?[22] If a patient's sensation perception is absent, function may be severely compromised. Therefore casting may not be appropriate unless the goal is to increase ROM.[4]

3. Circulation—Is blanching occurring? What are the color and temperature of nailbeds and extremities? Are pulses distal to the cast strong (e.g., radial for elbow and pedal for knee)? Is capillary refill good? Are trophic changes present?

4. Continence—Hygiene and cleanliness within the cast will be affected in an incontinent patient who requires lower extremity casting.

5. Joints—Assess active and passive ROM,[4] temperature, soft tissue restrictions, and end feel. End feel is the feeling at the completion of ranging a joint.[22] It may be empty, gradual, abrupt, nonyielding bony, or painful. When it is empty, nothing indicates an ending has been reached, but the therapist realizes that further pushing may cause damage. When end feel is gradual, it allows the therapist to feel a gradual tightening of soft tissues as end range is approached. When end feel is abrupt, end range is reached without any tapering. A bony end feels as if the therapist has hit one bone against another. A patient may complain of pain as the end of range is approached (a painful end feel). A local anesthetic nerve block may be used when it is necessary to differentiate spasticity from fixed contracture. Nerve blocks eliminate spasticity but do not affect muscle-tendon length. An anesthetic nerve block can be used to allow normal

joint position if the only cause of the deformity is spasticity.[4] Soft tissue contracture must be differentiated from joint contracture if the muscle crosses two joints. To evaluate for the type of contracture, flex the proximal joint and note the resultant position of the distal joints. Joint contracture will not be affected by change in position of the proximal joint. If the deformity is soft tissue contracture, a procaine nerve block will not correct the joint deformity. A hard end feel often indicates a bony block, which is usually not responsive to serial casting.[22] Do joints or soft tissues require mobilization before casting? What is the patient's active control, selective, or patterned movement?[4] What is patient's hand function?

6. Contracture—What is the duration of the contracture? Contractures of shorter duration tend to be more responsive to serial casting.[3,4,22]

7. Glenohumeral joint subluxation—If present, will the weight of the cast affect the proximal glenohumeral joint and pull the humerus into subluxation?

8. Position of scapula—What is the position of the scapula on the thorax (e.g., is there a subluxation)? Will the added weight of the cast adversely affect the position of the scapula on the thorax?

9. Effects on joints—In what way will the additional stress from the cast affect other joints proximal and distal to the cast?[22]

10. Joint stretching—Can one joint be stretched in isolation without other joints being stretched?[22]

11. Cast requirements—Will the cast require a plantigrade surface or wedge for ambulation or weight-bearing activities?

12. Muscle activity responsiveness—Does the patient respond to relaxation and handling techniques that optimize position for casting? Patients with muscle activity that is responsive to handling should benefit from casting. Rigid, unchanging skeletal muscle activity, probably will not be responsive. Are abnormal reflexes present that will affect casting?[22] For example, if an asymmetrical tonic neck reflex is present, will this affect application of the cast?

13. Mental status—Is the patient self-abusive or abusive to others? Is the patient combative? What is the patient's level of alertness? Can the patient communicate with others? Can the patient follow directions?[4] Are caregivers able to manage the patient with a cast?

14. Orthopedic considerations—Are fracture(s) present? HO may preclude casting.[4,22] Consider the option of using drop-out casts.

15. Sedatives—Will the patient require sedation and/or muscle relaxants before casting?

16. Goals—Will casting meet the patient's goals and result in gains in function? Will expected gains outweigh the cost and time required to cast the patient?[4]

17. Cast selection—Determine type of cast and type of material (plaster or fiberglass) required (Box 9-1).

CASTING MATERIALS

The following materials are needed for fabrication of casts. Materials should be gathered before initiating the casting process.

1. Plaster or fiberglass casting material: 2, 3, 4 and/or 6 inch, depending on the cast to be fabricated[3,9]

Box 9-1

Comparison of Plaster and Fiberglass Casting Materials

PLASTER
- Longer drying time[4] (approximately 24 hours)[9]
- Longer period before patient can bear weight (24 hours)
- More prone to indentations that may lead to areas of high compression and cause skin breakdown[4,14]
- Stronger[4]
- Heavier[4,16]
- Reinforceable[4]
- Easier to adjust[4]
- More difficult clean up after casting patient[4]
- More difficult to keep clean[4]
- More absorbent[4]
- Less expensive[10]
- Better when frequent cast changes are indicated
- More variability in setting time; can be varied according to the needs of the situation

FIBERGLASS
- Shorter drying time[4,14] (approximately 30 minutes)[14]
- Shorter period before patient can bear weight (20 to 30 minutes)[10]
- Higher risk of splintering[4,14]
- Harder[4]
- Lighter[4,10,16]
- More resilient[4]
- More soil resistant[10]
- Better when no further gains in range of motion are achieved[10] because final cast is usually a bivalved cast, which is usually made of fiberglass
- More adherence to skin or nonlubricated gloves[10]
- Less variability in setting time—must prevent a layer from hardening because subsequent layers will not bond well[10]
- More expensive[10]
- More durable[10]
- May be better for patients with neglect because bright-colored casts may assist with cueing strategies

2. Cast padding in the size corresponding to the casting material[3,4]
3. Stockinette: 3 inch for upper extremity casts, 4 inch for lower extremity casts[3]; on occasion, 2 inch for a small adult or adolescent
4. Bucket for water[3,4]
5. Water: warm if using plaster and cool if using fiberglass[3]
6. Cast spreader[3,4]
7. Cast-cutter scissors[4]
8. Cast saw[3,4]
9. Trimming knife[3]
10. Sticky-back foam padding
11. Plastic or rubber gloves
12. Sheets, newspaper, or plaster drapes to protect the patient, floor, etc.
13. Petroleum jelly, liquid soap, or lotion if working with fiberglass

COST

In 1990, Lehmkuhl et al[23] estimated the cost of materials for one serial cast to be $12 to $16 in addition to the $90 to $150 for the time of two staff members. If casting is being done in a hospital, the required materials for serial casting are often available through the orthopedics department, central supply, or on a mobile casting cart. Following is a list of supplies required for casting and their approximate prices.

Plaster cast material (box of 12 rolls)

2 inches x 3 yards = $17
3 inches x 3 yards = $21
4 inches x 4 yards = $30

Fiberglass casting tape: white (pack of 10) (Figure 9-1)
(Colored fiberglass casting tape is available for an additional cost.)

2 inches x 4 yards = $62
3 inches x 4 yards = $83

Stockinette (one box)

2 inches x 25 yards = $14
3 inches x 25 yards = $22
4 inches x 25 yards = $28
6 inches x 25 yards = $35

Acrylic cast padding (pack of 12)

2 inches x 4 yards = $17
3 inches x 4 yards = $29

Cotton cast padding (Figure 9-2)

3 inches x 4 yards = $16 (12 rolls)
4 inches x 4 yards = $24 (24 rolls)

Cast spreader (Figure 9-3)

$200.00

Cast cutter scissors (Figure 9-4)

$32

Bandage scissors (Figure 9-5)

$16

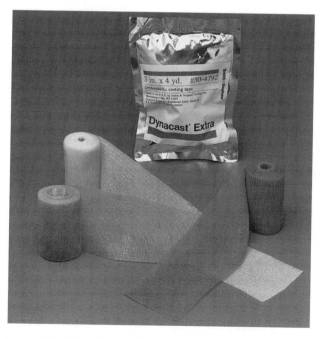

Figure 9-1 Fiberglass casting tape. (Courtesy Smith & Nephew Rolyan, Germantown, Wis.)

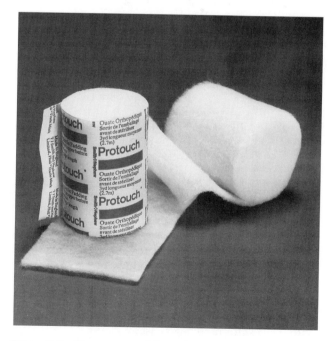

Figure 9-2 Cotton cast padding. (Courtesy Smith & Nephew Rolyan, Germantown, Wis.)

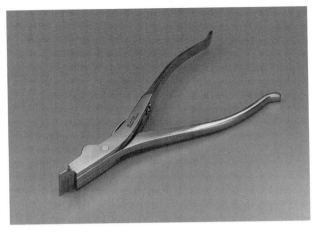

Figure 9-3   Cast spreader. (Courtesy Smith & Nephew Rolyan, Germantown, Wis.)

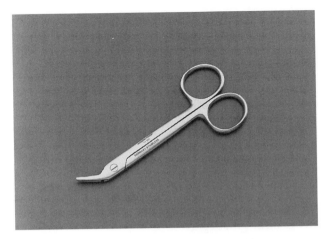

Figure 9-4   Cast scissors. (Courtesy Smith & Nephew Rolyan, Germantown, Wis.)

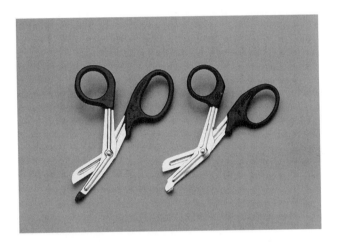

Figure 9-5   Bandage scissors. (Courtesy Smith & Nephew Rolyan, Germantown, Wis.)

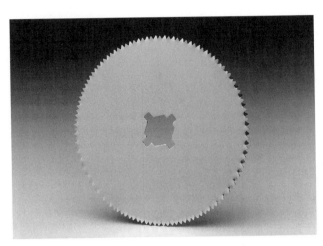

Figure 9-6   Saw blade. (Courtesy Smith & Nephew Rolyan, Germantown, Wis.)

Goggles

$14

Cast cutter (Figure 9-6)

$860

- Approximately 30 to 60 minutes of two staff members' time must be calculated into the cost for fabrication of each cast.[23]
- Approximately 30 continuous minutes for two staff members' time must be calculated into the cost for cast removal. In acute care settings, it may be helpful to arrange time with the treatment team to avoid interruptions.
- Approximately 60 to 90 minutes must be calculated into the cost for bivalving a cast.
- Two rolls of plaster are generally adequate for upper extremity casts.[3]

- Three to four rolls of plaster are needed for lower extremity casts.[3]
- Larger or stronger patients may require additional plaster.[3]

TYPES OF CASTS

Several types of serial casts are available. Each has its own implications for outcome (Table 9-1).

1. Resting cast—This is a cylindrical cast that is left on for 7 to 10 days. It is the initial cast in a casting program and is applied with the limb positioned at the end of easily attainable ROM.[3]
2. Drop-out cast—This cast consists of a series of cylindrical casts that have a portion of the cast cut out to allow for further range and stretching in the intended direction of stretch while preventing movement in the con-

Table 9-1

Comparison of Cast Types

CAST	PROS	CONS
Serial	Provides a constant prolonged stretch Provides an intimate fit Can help to maintain biomechanical alignment Ensures compliance	May interfere with ADL and mobility Does not allow access to a joint or extremity to monitor skin and provide other therapy (e.g., ROM, modalities, joint mobilization, weight bearing)
Bivalve	Allows access to joint and extremity to monitor skin Allows access to joint and extremity for other interventions Allows removal of cast for ADL and mobility May be used as a night or resting splint Allows quick removal of cast in emergencies	Impossible for cast to fit exactly together again once it is cut Can be difficult to maintain a wearing schedule Provides an intermittent stretch Has potential to pinch or cause soft tissue trauma
Drop-out	Gravity aids in stretching Allows enhanced active or passive movement in the desired direction while preventing further contracture Allows access to joint for mobilization, stretching, and soft tissue mobilization Allows AROM in desired range that may strengthen weak muscles opposing contracture Allows active movement that may increase patient's perception of movement via kinesthetic responses/stimulation if neglect is present	If cast is not precisely made and cut, is potential for movement within cast and subsequent skin breakdown and/or patient removal

tracted direction. Casts are changed weekly and reapplied, with the cast accommodating the limb in an improved position. An average of three to four drop-out casts are used to achieve maximally attainable ROM.

3. Holding cast—This cylindrical cast holds the limb in place for 7 to 10 days to maintain the newly acquired ROM; it is also known as a *final cast*.[3]

4. Bivalve cast—This type of cast is a holding cast that is cut lengthwise into two pieces (anterior and posterior), with the top portion comprising one third of the cast and the bottom portion comprising two thirds of the cast. The edges of the cast may be finished with padding or tape. The two pieces of the cast are held together around the extremity with straps. Patients are gradually weaned from wearing this cast as they become more active. If patients continue to have increased muscle activity, they continue to wear the bivalved cast at night.

Specific Cast Examples

- *Rigid circular elbow cast* (Figure 9-7): This rigid circular cast encloses the forearm and humerus and can be used to gradually increase elbow ROM in an elbow with contracture or increased muscle activity. In addition, it may be used for an elbow with fluctuating muscle activity because the cast can provide equalized pressure throughout the arm. A gradual increase in elbow ROM

is a result of the cast's stabilizing effect, which neutralizes abnormal muscle activity.[16,35]

- *Drop-out cast with humeral portion enclosed* (Figure 9-8): This type of cast is effective for treating severe elbow flexion contracture.[35]

- *Drop-out cast with forearm portion enclosed* (Figure 9-9): Enclosing the forearm increases elbow ROM while incorporating the wrist and forearm. This cast can be applied on a patient with skin breakdown in the humeral region.[35]

- *Long arm cast* (Figure 9-10): The long arm cast manages problems of the elbow, wrist, and forearm simultaneously. It can effectively control increased muscle activity in the forearm muscles.[16,35]

- *Reverse drop-out cast* (Figure 9-11): A reverse drop-out cast is used when increased muscle activity causes an elbow extension contracture that results in decreased elbow flexion ROM. It also puts weak biceps in a mechanically advantageous shortened position. The humerus is enclosed during fabrication. Casting application is most effective when the patient is in a supine or sidelying position, which allows gravity to assist the forearm into a position of elbow flexion.[16,35]

- *Elbow drop-out cast with wrist included* (Figure 9-12; see also Figure 9-11): This type of cast permits passive and active elbow extension while maintaining already-attained elbow extension ROM. The weight of the cast acts with gravity to provide a passive stretch when the

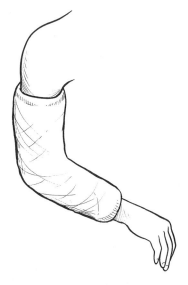

Figure 9-7   Rigid circular elbow cast.

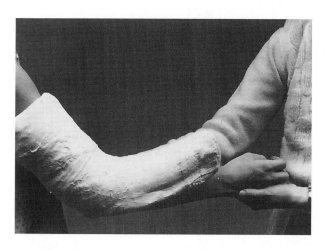

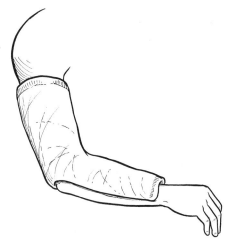

Figure 9-8   Drop-out cast with humeral portion enclosed. (From Hill J: Management of abnormal tone through casting and orthotics. In Kovich KM, Bermann DE, editors: *Head injury: a guide to functional outcomes in occupational therapy*, Gaithersburg, Md, 1988, Aspen.)

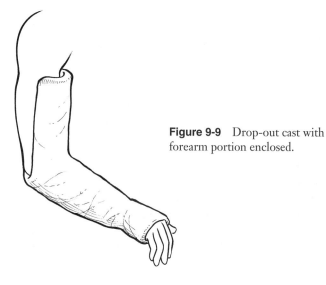

Figure 9-9   Drop-out cast with forearm portion enclosed.

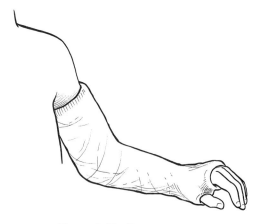

Figure 9-10   Long arm cast.

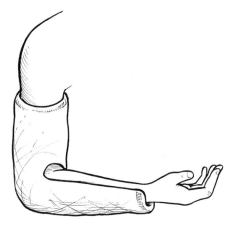

Figure 9-11 Reverse drop-out cast.

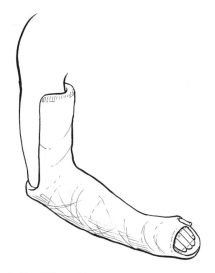

Figure 9-13 Elbow drop-out cast with hand included.

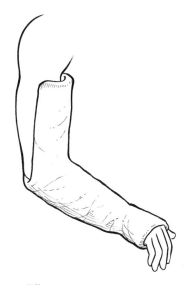

Figure 9-12 Elbow drop-out cast with wrist included.

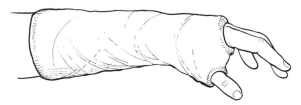

Figure 9-14 Wrist cast.

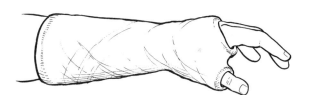

Figure 9-15 Short-arm cast with thumb post.

patient is seated or in an upright position. The wrist can be included. The forearm is casted in neutral.[3]

• *Elbow drop-out cast with hand included* (Figure 9-13): This drop-out cast is similar to the previously mentioned elbow drop-out cast with wrist included, except that it can include the hand. Its functions are the same.

• *Wrist cast* (Figure 9-14): A wrist cast is indicated when the wrist exhibits increased muscle activity, contractures, and general weakness. The problems may originate in the wrist only or in a combination of other joints. This cast facilitates functional movement by increasing wrist ROM, decreasing abnormal muscle activity, and isolating wrist movement from hand movement. It controls the wrist movements but leaves the digits free. This cast effectively influences distal hand function when the patient has active digit motion.[16,35]

• *Short arm cast with thumb post* (Figure 9-15): A wrist cast with the thumb enclosed manages the thumb-in-palm deformity caused by increased muscle activity of the thumb flexor and adductor. This deformity can decrease the effectiveness of hand functions such as grasp, pinch, and release. Thumb contracture or increased muscle activity may result in web-space shortening, joint subluxation, an unstable metacarpal phalangeal joint, or an overstretched extensor pollicis. A wrist cast with the thumb enclosed can enhance grasp or improve overall range and normalize muscle activity in the hand.[16,35]

• *Platform cast* (Figure 9-16): The platform cast is used when the patient has isolated muscle control but is still limited by increased flexor muscle activity that interferes with efficient and precise small muscle blend pat-

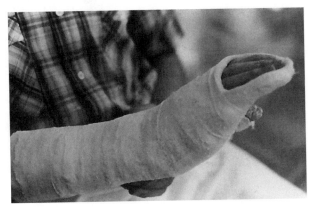

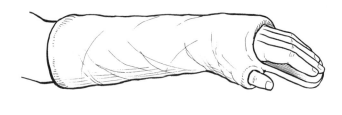

Figure 9-16 Platform cast. (From Hill J: *Management of abnormal tone through casting and orthotics.* In Kovich KM, Bermann DE, editors: *Head injury: a guide to functional outcomes in occupational therapy,* Gaithersburg, Md, 1988, Aspen.)

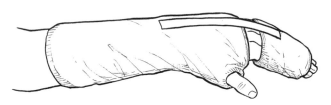

Figure 9-17 Finger shell.

terns. A platform cast can improve function with or without the thumb enclosed.[16,35]

- *Finger shell* (Figure 9-17): Severe wrist and digit contractures greatly impair function. Muscle activity is increased in the wrist and digit flexors as well as the intrinsics. A finger shell is attached to a wrist cast to slowly and gradually stretch the fingers into extension.[16,35]
- *Knee drop-out cast with anterior portion removed above the knee* (Figure 9-18): This type of cast is indicated for a knee flexion contracture. The anterior portion is removed to act as a knee flexion stop. Gravity can provide a prolonged stretch to tight flexors.[25]
- *Knee drop-out cast with anterior portion removed below the knee* (Figure 9-19): This knee drop-out cast has the same functions as the previously mentioned knee drop-out cast, except that the anterior portion removed is below instead of above the knee.[25]

CASTING PROGRESSION

Initially a resting cast is applied with the limb in submaximal range for 7 to 10 days.[3,4] Then a series of drop-out or positional casts are applied weekly in the improved position to increase ROM and decrease spasticity. PROM activities are performed between casts to stretch tissues and avoid reverse contractures.[3,4,16] ROM, sensation, and mo-

tor control should be reevaluated between cast changes to monitor improvements.[4,10,16] Skin integrity should also be checked.[4,16] This process is repeated until no further gains are obtained or full ROM is achieved.[4,10,22,26] Montgomery states that three to four cast changes are typically required to achieve a casting goal.[3] A final/holding cast is then applied for 1 to 2 weeks to maintain the maximum range that has been achieved.[10] The holding cast is then bivalved and converted to an anteroposterior splint.[4] The bivalve cast is used to maintain ROM and decrease spasticity. Initially the cast is worn at all times except during therapy sessions. The patient is gradually weaned from this splint until activity is increased.[3] Some patients cannot be fully weaned; for example, if a patient continues to have increased spasticity or weakness, the patient will wear the splint at night[3,4] (Table 9-2).

GUIDELINES FOR CAST APPLICATION

1. Obtain physician's orders.[16]
2. Perform the initial evaluation.
3. Pretreat the patient with sedatives if needed.[10,16,25]
4. Explain the procedure to the patient and what is expected of the patient.
5. Protect the floor with newspaper or plastic. Cover the mat, plinth, chair, etc. with plastic or sheets. Protect the patient's skin, face, and clothing with towels and sheets.[10]
6. Evaluate and document the patient's skin integrity, noting scars, open wounds, and discoloration.
7. If applicable, cut foam padding to size if the patient is at risk for skin breakdown over bony prominences. If fabricating a drop-out cast, cut straps.
8. Precut stockinette 4 to 6 inches longer than the length of the cast on each end so it can be rolled back over the ends of the cast.[10] This pads the ends of the cast and improves the final appearance.

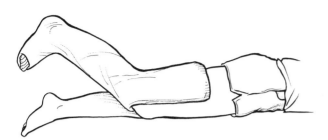

Figure 9-18 Knee drop-out cast with anterior portion removed above the knee.

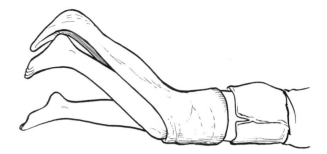

Figure 9-19 Knee drop-out cast with the anterior portion of cast removed below the knee.

Table 9-2

Purpose of and Wearing Times for Different Cast Types

TYPE OF CAST	GOAL	WEARING TIME
Resting cast positioned at end of easily obtainable range	To hold the extremity in a painless maximum range and decrease the influence of spasticity	7-10 days
Repeated series (often three to four) of serial or drop-out casts	To gradually increase the ROM of the joint and decrease the influence of spasticity	Weekly intervals with full PROM to immobilize joints between cast changes
Holding cast	To maintain the gained ROM and decrease the influence of spasticity	7-10 days
Anteroposterior splint (a holding cast bivalved and converted into a splint)	To maintain the gained ROM	Gradually decreased to night wear and discontinued when no longer needed

From Garland D, Doyle MM, Booth BJ: *Early management of spastic deformities*, Downey, Calif, 1979, Ranchos Los Amigos Medical Center, Adult Brain Injury Service.

9. Measure and record joint ROM.[10]
10. Mobilize the joint and soft tissue as needed.[26]
11. Fill the bucket with water.
12. Clean and dry the skin thoroughly.[10]
13. Apply the stockinette to the limb to be casted. Smooth out wrinkles to avoid skin breakdown.[3,4,10,16,25] Cut a slit for the thumb if necessary. A stockinette is not always required; however, a stockinette is needed for bivalved or anteroposterior casts to protect the cotton padding from fraying during frequent cast removal. The stockinette is easily replaceable if it becomes stained.[3]
14. Determine the cast length.
    Elbow or elbow and wrist cast
    The upper arm length should be 1 to 2 inches below the axilla and allow a sufficient lever arm.
    The distal end of an elbow cast should terminate just proximal to the ulnar styloid.
    A wrist cast should reach 1 to 1½ inches from the elbow joint and allow a sufficient lever arm. The distal end should terminate just proximal to the metacarpal phalangeal joints.

Knee or knee and ankle cast
A thigh-length cast should allow 3 to 4 inches from the groin and allow sufficient lever arm.
The distal end of a knee cast should be 3 inches above the malleoli or 1 to 2 inches below the fibular head.
The distal end of a cast incorporating the ankle should fully support the metatarsal heads.
If the patient is ambulatory or weight bearing, the plantar surface of the cast should include a wedge.
15. Open the casting materials: cotton padding, fiberglass or plaster rolls, and foam or felt padding. Fiberglass should be opened one package at a time and applied within 1 minute. Fiberglass will harden and not bond when left exposed to the air.[10]
16. The patient's extremity is casted in submaximal range (5° to 10° less than easily achievable range) initially and at end range with minimal stretching for subsequent casts.[10,16,23] Instruct helper in how and where to position the extremity to be casted.[10]
17. Apply one layer of cotton padding in a spiral fashion with ½ inch overlapping layers in a figure eight

around the elbow or knee. Avoid wrinkles to prevent pressure sores. The top and bottom ends should be cylindrical.[3,4,10,16,25]

18. Apply felt or foam padding to bony prominences.[3,4,10,16,25]

19. Add another two or three layers of cotton padding, and hold the felt or foam padding in place.[3,4,16,25] Apply padding 1 to 2 inches above and below the desired cast length to ensure a soft edge.

20. Don plastic gloves. Petroleum jelly, lotion, or liquid soap should be applied to gloves initially and throughout the procedure. Without it, gloves will be difficult to remove, and fiberglass may adhere to the patient's skin.[10] Gloves will protect the therapist's nailbeds if plaster is being used.

21. Apply plaster or fiberglass proximally to distally in a spiral fashion with the extremity positioned so that it has the correct amount of stretch.[4] Fiberglass should overlap itself by half a tape width.[10] Leave 1 inch of padding exposed (and do not cover it with plaster) to create soft cast edge. Keep the roll of material close to the limb to avoid pulling and decrease tension. If applying plaster, dip plaster roll in water while holding the end of the roll; dip it 5 or 6 times until it bubbles.[10] Crimp the end of the rolls to avoid wringing when removing excess water.[3] Removing too much water can cause the plaster to dry too rapidly before it bonds with the gauze. Additional water can be applied but only before the plaster dries. Avoid denting plaster to avoid pressure points. Fiberglass is submerged in cool water and gently squeezed 5 or 6 times, removed from the water, and applied immediately.[10] The assistant should stretch the joint without holding the cast by placing the hands proximal and distal to the cast.[10]

    After applying each roll (if using plaster), smooth the plaster material into the gauze. As layers are applied, rub the cast in circular motions to smooth the material.[4,10] If using fiberglass, applying petroleum jelly, liquid soap, or lotion to the top of the finished cast helps the material adhere to itself instead of the therapist.[10] Wrapping a wet Ace bandage around the cast can also shorten drying time and ensure a smooth cast.[4] The limb is held in position until the material is set or begins to harden.[3,4] Four to five layers of plaster or three to four layers of fiberglass casting material should be applied.[10]

22. While the cast is setting, insert one or two fingers between the stockinette and padding, and pull them out around the full circumference of cast at proximal and distal ends without applying a counterpressure with the thumbs. This ensures that the ends are not too tight, which may decrease the patient's circulation.[10]

23. Before applying the last layer of casting material, turn the ends of the stockinette back onto the cast to give a smooth, finished edge to the cast. Apply the last layer of casting material just below this edge.[10,16]

24. Allow the cast to set.

25. Write the patient's name, therapist's name, date of cast application, and anticipated date of cast removal on the cast with a permanent marker when it has dried.[16]

26. Draw lines on the cast in case emergency bivalving or removal is necessary.

27. Remove any plaster that may have dripped onto the patient's skin.[10]

28. Elevate the patient's casted extremity 10 to 20 cm above the patient's heart to prevent edema or decrease developing edema.

29. Check patient's circulation.

30. Communicate with medical staff, and post instructions above patient's bed and in nurses' cardex regarding wearing schedule, precautions, positioning, therapist's name and extension, and location of cast cutter for emergency cast removal in an "off hour."

FABRICATING A DROP-OUT CAST

Following is the procedure for converting a resting or holding cast into a drop-out cast:

1. If removing the posterior aspect of an upper arm cast, draw a line on the medial and lateral aspects of the cast. Connect the two lines with a horizontal line just distal to the olecranon process.

2. If removing the posterior aspect of a forearm cast, draw a line on the medial and lateral aspects of the cast. Connect the two lines with a horizontal line just proximal to the olecranon process.

3. If removing the anterior aspect of a lower leg cast, to increase knee extension, draw lines on the medial and lateral aspects of the cast. Connect the two lines with a horizontal line just proximal to the patella.

4. If removing the posterior aspect of a lower leg cast, to increase knee flexion, draw lines on the medial and lateral aspects of the cast. Connect the two lines with a horizontal line 2 to 3 inches proximal to the popliteal fossa.

GUIDELINES FOR CAST REMOVAL

1. Explain to the patient the way the cast cutter operates. Tell the patient that the cast cutter does not cut the skin. The blade oscillates back and forth. It can be touched to the skin very lightly while in motion without cutting.

2. Determine the line the cut will follow (which depends on the plan to bivalve the cast) according to

the mechanical force of pull and ability to clear bony prominences.

3. Drape the patient and surrounding area with sheets and newspaper.

4. Goggles should be put on the patient, the therapist, and the holder.

5. If a patient has pulmonary problems or a tracheostomy, consider using masks or careful draping to protect the patient from breathing in the dust from the cast as it is being cut.

6. Cut through the casting material. Cut with direct inward pressure in one place at a time. Do not lift the cast cutter until you feel the blade drop into the space that it has created. Do not move the cast saw proximally to distally along the length of the cast; searing can occur. Casts with severe angles will require two cuts.

7. Spread cast apart with the cast spreader.

8. Use bandage shears to cut through the padding and stockinette.

9. Completely separate and remove the cast.

10. Check the patient's skin for red areas, edema, or breakdown.

11. Record measurements and clinical observations.

12. Clean and dry the extremity. Moisturize the skin.[10]

FABRICATING A BIVALVE CAST

When the maximum achievable gain in ROM has been achieved, the cast may be bivalved and used to maintain gains.

1. The cast is usually fabricated from fiberglass but can be fabricated from plaster.[10]

2. Drape the patient and surrounding area with sheets and newspaper.

3. Cut the cast into anterior and posterior portions using the cast saw. (See #6 in the previous section for the correct technique.)

4. Bivalve the cast at the medial and lateral aspects of the forearm so that one third of cast is on top and two thirds is on the bottom. For a lower extremity splint, bivalve the cast at the medial and lateral aspects, slightly anterior to the medial and lateral malleolus so that one third of the cast is on top and two thirds is on the bottom. The blade cutter will not easily cut through the stockinette and padding, which should be taken into consideration. For example, do not double back the stockinette when bivalving.

5. Use the cast spreader to spread the cast apart. Use cast scissors to cut the padding and stockinette; discard them.

6. Realign the cast halves with cotton padding using same amount required for the original cast fabrication.

Extend the padding over the edges and sides of the shells. Do not cause ripples—the interior must be smooth. If necessary, rip the padding edges off to create a smooth surface. Replace the stockinette if it does not fit the splint.

7. Use adhesive tape or moleskin to secure the padding edges, which should be folded over the shells.

8. Cut the stockinette 4 to 6 inches longer than the length of each shell. Line each shell with a stockinette, and use adhesive tape to secure. NOTE: If too much underpadding is added, the cast angle will be reduced or shifted.

9. Secure bivalves on patient with Ace bandages or straps. Straps can be fabricated using 1- to 3-inch wide webbing and buckles that can be riveted, taped, glued, or sewn onto the stockinette. Webbing can also be attached using casting material (i.e., plaster, fiberglass).

CAST MONITORING

The patient, caregivers, and staff should monitor the cast every 2 hours[16,25,35] for the first 24 hours for the following:

1. Pain, discomfort

2. Edema

3. Sensory changes such as numbness, tingling, "pins and needles"

4. Circulatory changes such as coldness, changes in nailbed color

5. Increased or decreased movement inside the cast

6. Skin integrity including reddened or broken skin

7. Severe itching

8. Dents or cracks in or softening of the cast

CAST CARE

The patient can bathe in a tub or shower while wearing a cast but should avoid wetting the cast. The cast can be covered with a plastic bag or a commercially available cast cover. Tape the edges down to prevent the cast from getting wet. However, sponge bathing is preferred. Cover the cast when it is near water (e.g., when washing dishes).

CLINICAL ISSUES

Patients with diminished cognitive status may be casted if a caregiver assumes responsibility for safety. However, if the patient is acutely ill, medical needs and contraindications may preclude casting. For example, a patient may require the insertion of an intravenous line in the limb that needs to be casted. A cast can have a window around a line, which may be left open for Doppler ultrasound to check distal circulation. However, this is not optimal. In addition, poor skin integrity or fractures may preclude casting. Casting a cognitively impaired patient may allow the therapist to concentrate on improving the patient's positioning and motor function, so when the patient's cognitive status improves the patient can focus on performing functional tasks using maximum joint ROM and more normal movement patterns. In addition, casting can be used as an early intervention to work on a patient's cognitive status. For example, standing a patient with a lower extremity cast in a tilt table may improve the patient's level of alertness because of the maintenance of the upright position. The therapist can also focus on motor control of the pelvis, trunk, and shoulder girdle, which may result in improved abilities to move from sitting to standing, transfer, and position the wheelchair. Attempting to decrease excessive extension or flexion and enhance dissociated movements results in better positioning.

A patient may require multiple casts, which may affect the patient's nursing care and rehabilitation by other therapists. Alternate methods of positioning and nonverbal communication may need to be considered. The benefits of multiple-extremity casting for improved ROM or motor control must outweigh the risks, potential complications, and potential for improvement. The patient may not tolerate multiple casts well. Combining bivalve splints and casts may improve the patient's tolerance. Casts should be applied to the extremity in a way that severely limits ROM and spasticity. Bivalve splints can be applied to an extremity with minimal spasticity or ROM deficits and allow for increased function by easy removal.[36]

Casts should be changed as functional gains are achieved. For example, a long leg cast may interfere with sitting activities that are being used to encourage trunk control and trunk alignment. A long leg cast encourages a posterior pelvic tilt, kyphotic posture, and neck flexion—positions that do not lend themselves to developing effective postural control. A short leg cast with a removable splint for knee extension or a long leg cast with a hinged locking joint to permit knee flexion while sitting or extension to increase ROM may better suit the patient's functional status.[36]

Booth and associates[3] suggest that agitated patients' treatment is often directed at encouraging rather than restricting limb movement. Although serial casting inhibits movement, it is recommended because agitated patients' movements are random, and contractures can easily form. A cast also protects the limb from injury if the patient should become agitated. When choosing the casting material, several factors should be considered. Fiberglass dries quickly, which may be beneficial for patients who are agitated. The cast will less likely be dented,[3] and it is harder, lighter, and more resilient than plaster.[36] However, fiberglass can splinter if patients strike a hard object. Edges may be rough, and patients may be in danger of hurting themselves. Plaster, on the other hand, may be better for the ag-

itated or combative patient because additional layers may be added to increase the durability of the cast. However, increasing layers of plaster increases the overall weight of the cast. Regardless of the material selected, additional padding should be added to bony prominences to protect the patient from skin breakdown.

As motor control improves, the therapist must decide if the focus of treatment should be to continue to improve ROM or motor control. The goal is to have both ROM and motor control but not one at the expense of the other. If motor control is gained without sufficient range, the limb will not be functional. If ROM is gained at the expense of motor control, functional mobility will be difficult to maintain. The residual contracture, mental status, skin integrity, and severity of spasticity can aid in determining treatment priorities.[36] If the patient cannot follow directions and carry out an exercise program or incorporate gains into functional activities, casting should be discontinued. Casting may be discontinued on patients who can follow directions and actively use their contracted limb for functional tasks so that they can actively maintain the function of their contracted limb. A bivalve splint is recommended for easy access to the limb for therapy and to maintain ROM. A patient whose cognition is good but who has remaining severe contracture or spasticity, may need to stay in a cast for a longer period of time until a bivalve splint is indicated. However, if a drop-out cast is indicated, electrical stimulation can be used on the antagonist of the contracted muscle. Electrical stimulation of the antagonist of the contracted muscle combined with a drop-out cast can also be used if the joint is amenable to contracture management. Active participation of the patient is not required. Electrical stimulation may also facilitate motor control of the stimulated muscle.[36]

SUMMARY

Casting can be used effectively for patients who have suffered a CVA when traditional methods have failed to improve ROM and decrease spasticity. The goals of casting, type of casts, material to be used, time and cost of therapists, precautions, and contraindications must be carefully considered before initiating a casting program.

■

CASE STUDY

LP is a 72-year-old man who suffered a CVA that resulted in severe bilateral upper extremity spasticity in the elbow flexors. He was independent in ADL before admission. LP lived with his wife and daughter. Traditional methods of therapy had been unsuccessful during his brief time in the acute care service. LP had become dependent in all aspects of self-care. He was cognitively intact. There were no contraindications to a casting program. While on the rehabilitation unit, LP consented to being casted. He was casted with bilateral long arm casts that were left in place for 8 days. The spasticity reduced enough to allow the patient to perform hand activities, including self-feeding, shaving, and brushing his teeth. In addition, the spasticity decreased enough to allow traditional methods of therapy to be employed. LP was eventually discharged back to his previous living arrangement where he was again independent in all aspects of self-care.

■

CASE STUDY

SD is an 80-year-old female who suffered a CVA that resulted in soft tissue contracture of the elbow flexors to 90° of elbow flexion, severely increased skeletal muscle activity in the wrist and finger flexors, difficulty maintaining the web space secondary to the thumb posturing in flexion and adduction, and spasticity in the intrinsic muscles of the hand. SD did not have functional use of the extremity. She was globally aphasic and demonstrated ideational and motor apraxia. Sensation and skin integrity were intact. There were no contraindications to casting. SD was unable to consent to casting; however, her son consented. Initially, SD was fit with a long arm resting cast with full hand and thumb portions. The cast was left in place for 10 days. The spasticity in her wrist and hand reduced. She was then fit with a cylindrical elbow extension holding cast for 10 days to maintain maximum elbow extension. The cast was then bivalved into an anteroposterior cylinder splint and worn at night. The extremity did remain nonfunctional; however, SD was then able to be maintained with traditional therapies. The bivalved splint was worn at night.

■

REVIEW QUESTIONS

1. List five indications for serial casting.
2. List 10 precautions for serial casting.
3. List 10 contraindications to serial casting.
4. Describe the initial evaluation process for serial casting.
5. Describe the purpose of the following casts: resting, holding, anteroposterior/bivalved.
6. Compare and contrast plaster and fiberglass casting materials.
7. Describe the cast application procedure.
8. Describe the cast removal process.

■ COTA Considerations ■

- Casting provides slow, prolonged stretch for patients who are at risk for the development of contractures.
- Patients who have a decreased level of alertness, poor attention, poor concentration, decreased initiation, memory impairment, or poor cooperation are at greater risk for developing contractures.

- Casts are often applied in conjunction with the use of drugs that relax the skeletal muscles in the limb or after nerve-blocking procedures.
- Casts can provide support to a limb with muscle imbalance and provide a means of weight bearing, which can provide proprioceptive stimulation and allow redevelopment of muscle balance in the limb.
- If a patient who is wearing a cast complains of pain, swelling, or pinching from the cast or a change in sensation in the limb, the cast should be removed.

REFERENCES

1. Barnard P et al: Reduction of hypertonicity by early casting in a comatose head-injured individual: a case report, *Phys Ther* 64:1540, 1984.
2. Bentzel K: Remediating sensory impairment. In Trombly CA, editor: *Occupational therapy for physical dysfunction*, ed 4, Baltimore, 1995, Williams & Wilkins.
3. Booth BJ, Doyle M, Montgomery J: Serial casting for the management of spasticity in the head-injured adult, *Phys Ther* 63:1960.
4. Booth FW: Effect of limb immobilization on skeletal muscle, *Am Physiological Society*, pp. 1113-1118, 1982.
5. Braddom RL: Management of spasticity. In Buschbacher RM et al, *Physical medicine & rehabilitation*, Philadelphia, 1996, WB Saunders.
6. Brennan JB: Response to stretch of hypertonic muscle groups in hemiplegia, *Br Med J*, pp. 1504-1507, 1959.
7. Bronski B: Serial casting for the neurological patient, *Physical Disabilities Special Interest Section Newsletter* 18:4, 1995.
8. Cherry DB: Review of physical therapy alternatives for reducing muscle contracture, *Phys Ther* 60:877, 1980.
9. Davies PM: Overcoming limitation of movement, contracture and deformity. In *Starting again: early rehabilitation after traumatic brain injury or other severe brain lesion*, New York, 1994, Springer-Verlag.
10. Feldman PA: Upper extremity casting and splinting. In Glenn MB, Whyte J, editors: *The practical management of spasticity in children and adults*, Philadelphia, 1990, Lea & Febiger.
11. Garland DE, Blum CE, Waters RL: Periarticular heterotopic ossification in head-injured adults, *J Bone Joint Surg* 62-A(7):1143, 1980.
12. Garland DE, Keenan MAE: Orthopedic strategies in the management of the adult head-injured patient, *Phys Ther* 63:2004, 1983.
13. Garland DE, Razza BE, Waters RL: Forceful joint manipulation in head-injured adults with heterotopic ossification, *Clin Orthop Related Res* 169:133, 1982.
14. Giorgetti MM: Serial and inhibitory casting: implications for acute care physical therapy management, *Neurology Report* 17:18, 1993.
15. Grossman MR, Sahrmann SA, Rose SJ: Review of length-associated changes in muscle, *Phys Ther* 62:1799, 1982.
16. Hill J: Management of abnormal tone through casting and orthotics. In *Head injury: a guide to functional outcomes in occupational therapy*, Rockville, Md, 1988, Aspen.
17. Hill, J: The effects of casting on upper extremity motor disorders after brain injury, *Am J Occup Ther* 48:219, 1994.
18. Kaplan N: Effect of splinting on reflex inhibition and sensorimotor stimulation in treatment of spasticity, *Arch Phys Med Rehabil*, pp. 565-569, 1962.
19. King TI, II: Plaster splinting as a means of reducing elbow flexor spasticity: a case study, *Am J Occup Ther* 36:671, 1982.
20. Lavalette R, Pope MH, Dickstein H: Setting temperatures of plaster casts, *J Bone Joint Surg* 64-A(6):907-911, 1982.
21. Law M et al: Neurodevelopmental therapy and upper extremity inhibitive casting for children with cerebral palsy, *Develop Med Child Neurol* 33:379, 1991.

22. Leahy P: Precasting work sheet—An assessment tool: a clinical report, *Phys Ther* 68:72, 1988.
23. Lehmkuhl LD et al: Multimodality treatment of joint contractures in patients with severe brain injury: cost, effectiveness, and integration of therapies in the application of serial/inhibitive casts, *J Head Trauma Rehabil* 5:23, 1990.
24. MacKay-Lyons M: Low-load, prolonged stretch in treatment of elbow flexion contractures secondary to head trauma: a case report, *Phys Ther* 69:50, 1989.
25. Nash DL: Serial casting. In Lennard TA, editor: *Physiatric procedures in clinical practice*, Philadelphia, 1995, Hanley & Belfus.
26. Orest : Casting protocol for patients with neurological dysfunction, *PT Magazine*, pp. 51-55, 1993.
27. Ough JL et al: Treatment of spastic joint contractures in mentally disabled adults, *Orthop Clin North Am* 12:143, 1981.
28. Sabbahi MA, Powers WR: Topical anesthesia: A possible treatment method for spasticity, *Arch Phys Med Rehabil* 62:310, 1981.
29. Smith LH, Harris SR: Upper extremity inhibitive casting for a child with cerebral palsy, *Phys Occup Ther Pediatr* 5:71, 1985.
30. Stockmeyer S: An interpretation of the approach of Rood to the treatment of neuromuscular dysfunction, *Phy Med* 26:900, 1967.

31. Tabary JC et al: Physiological and structural changes in the cat's coleus muscle due to immobilization at different lengths by plaster casts, *J Physiol* 224:231, 1972.
32. Tona JL, Schneck CM: The efficacy of upper extremity inhibitive casting: a single-subject pilot study, *Am J Occup Ther* 47:901, 1993.
33. Umphred DA: Classification of treatment techniques based on primary input systems. In Umphred DA: *Neurological rehabilitation*, ed 3, St Louis, 1995, Mosby.
34. Yasukawa A: Upper-extremity casting: Adjunct treatment for the child with cerebral palsy. In Case-Smith J, Pehoski C, editors: *Development of hand skills in the child*, Rockville, Md, 1992, American Occupational Therapy Association.
35. Yasukawa A, Hill, J: Casting to improve upper extremity function. In Boehme R, editor: *Improving upper body control: An approach to assessment and treatment of tonal dysfunction*, Tuscon, Az, 1988, Therapy Skill Builders.
36. Zablotny C, Forte Andric M, Gowland C: Serial casting: clinical applications for the adult head-injured patient, *J Head Trauma Rehabil* 2:46, 1987.
37. Zachazewski JE, Eberle ED, Jefferies M: Effect of tone-inhibiting casts and orthoses on gait, *Phys Ther* 62:453, 1982.

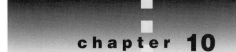

leslie a. kane
karen a. buckley

chapter **10**

Functional Mobility

key terms

mobility	scooting	upright function
bed mobility	transfers	transitional movements
trunk control	task-specific training	environmental strategies

chapter objectives

After completing this chapter, the reader will be able to accomplish the following:

1. Recognize the impact of performance component dysfunction on mobility tasks.
2. Analyze specific movement patterns observed during mobility tasks and common compensatory strategies.
3. Use a function-based approach to retraining mobility patterns.
4. Understand the impact of environmental changes on mobility tasks.

TERMINOLOGY

Many terms have been used in occupational therapy practice to describe an individual's ability to change the body's position in space and move within the environment. *Mobility* broadly refers to movements that result in a change of body position or location. The term *bed mobility* has been used interchangeably with *gross mobility* within the rehabilitation setting and traditionally has included such tasks as rolling to both sides, rolling to sidelying, moving from a sitting to a supine position and vice versa, and moving from sitting to standing. *Transfers* refer to movement from one surface to another such as from a bed to a wheelchair, from a wheelchair to a toilet, or from a wheelchair to a car, and involve varied methods of achievement.

OVERVIEW OF THE LITERATURE

Within the literature, numerous studies have carefully examined mobility functions of the adult in relation to gait and locomotion. Unfortunately, relatively few studies have examined functional mobility tasks. The analysis of the normal sit-to-stand sequence of movement has received attention and is reviewed later in this chapter.[18,75] Rising from bed has been examined in relation to age differences and the most common movement strategies selected.[30] This research demonstrates that age-related trends occur across the life span, but great variety remains evident in the selection of specific movement strategies. A limitation of this study is that the oldest age group examined was the 50- to 59-year-old group; thus information concerning older adults most at risk for cerebrovascular accident (CVA) was not included. A study of normal adult rolling patterns also has shown that adults exhibit great variability in the selection of movement patterns. In addition, the authors of this study have noted indications that a developmental sequence of movement patterns exists but is not inclusive of all individuals. Clearly many aspects of functional mobility still warrant further investigation.[82]

FUNCTIONAL MOBILITY: RELATIONSHIP TO PERFORMANCE AREAS

Occupational therapists have always approached functional mobility from the perspective that individual elements involved in changing the body's position were necessary to achieve competency in broad categories of human activity defined as *performance areas.* Improvement in activities of daily living, work and productive activities, and play and leisure activities has always been the ultimate goal of occupational therapy practice. The American Occupational Therapy Association (AOTA), in its 1994 Uniform Terminology, describes functional mobility as activities an individual performs in relation to the performance area of activities of daily living, including "moving from one position or place to another, such as in-bed mobility, wheelchair mobility, transfers (wheelchair, bed, car, tub, toilet, tub/shower, chair, floor), performing functional ambulation and transporting objects."[3]

In planning comprehensive treatment programs the occupational therapist should be mindful that functional mobility is not just a prerequisite to the performance of self-care tasks but also is integral to an individual's potential to return to work and productive activities or participate in favorite leisure activities. In practice the extent to which performance areas are addressed may be limited by time constraints imposed by the venue of treatment. Clinicians working within an acute-care setting often emphasize basic bed mobility tasks to prepare the patient for independence in grooming, bathing, and dressing activities. Within a rehabilitation setting, occupational therapists may have the opportunity to approach functional mobility more comprehensively in relation to more advanced tasks such as community mobility and tasks related to specific work and home-management requirements. The occupational therapist determines goals of treatment with the patient, contingent on imminent and future plans to resume responsibility for activities demanding advanced mobility.

Occupational therapy's task-related approach to intervention to improve functional mobility is consistent with present motor learning research emphasizing the important role environment plays in the organization of movement to solve motor problems.[8,32,33]

Performance components (sensorimotor, cognitive, psychosocial, and psychologic) have been used as the basis for assessing performance in the patient with hemiplegia. Each patient has different strengths, abilities, and deficits that have an impact on the performance of functional mobility. A patient may have strong neuromusculoskeletal abilities but demonstrate significant deficits in the ability to plan new motor acts in response to changes in the environment *(praxis).* Alternately a patient may have several problems affecting the neuromusculoskeletal system, including decreased alignment and postural stability, that interfere with the ability to roll efficiently toward the nonaffected side. Nevertheless, such a patient may demonstrate the ability to learn new strategies to accomplish tasks.

TRADITIONAL TREATMENT APPROACHES

Traditional treatment approaches emphasize the importance of sensation in the control of movement and functional mobility. Opinions differ concerning the specific use of sensory stimuli in intervention. Each treatment approach uses different techniques to enhance movement through the sensory system and alter intrinsic feedback through positioning and handling techniques. For example, sensory stimuli may be used to elicit reflexive patterns,[16] or positioning may be considered a method to gain reflex support for mobility.[83] Opposition to the use of reflexes is voiced by those who emphasize the importance of balance and equilibrium responses as the foundation for transitional movements.[10] Likewise, extrinsic sensory modalities may be applied to improve mobility and stability functions[77] and facilitate selective muscle activity.[26,77] Other therapists emphasize the importance of intrinsic sensory feedback to the relearning of mobility functions that integrate both sides of the body.[10,26]

Occupational therapists who have relied on these treatment approaches have been challenged to find an appropriate balance of techniques that can be combined readily with the task approach to treatment. This balance is necessary to achieve the primary goal of helping the patient regain as much independence in mobility as possible after stroke to permit the resumption of participation in desired performance areas.

INFLUENCE OF PERFORMANCE CONTEXTS ON FUNCTIONAL MOBILITY

Performance contexts are situations and factors influencing an individual's ability to become proficient in addressing mobility needs. Although always implied in practice, the emphasis on the importance of environmental features in planning comprehensive treatment programs is congruent to currently understood motor learning research and theory.

The understanding of performance contexts influences the selection of mobility interventions based on two primary factors: temporal aspects affecting the patient's life and the environment, including human and nonhuman aspects. Consideration of temporal aspects directs the therapist's attention to the "patient's age, phase of maturation, place in the life cycle, and the patient's current disability status."[3] When considering the age of an individual who has sustained a CVA and assessing expectations of the potential for functional mobility, the therapist must use caution. Many factors besides age contribute to the differences seen in the abilities older adults exhibit in functional mobility. The reader is encouraged to explore the literature examining the impact of aging on postural control and lifespan mobility.

Certainly the patient's stage in the life cycle more clearly guides assessment and interventions in the consideration of overall mobility needs. The young patient with hemiplegia who attends college has specific mobility needs. Sit-to-stand movements must be accomplished in changing environments and under varying conditions. For example, using public transportation, which may be moving or stationary; rising from a low seat at a football stadium; sitting down in a crowded and darkened movie theater; and getting into a truck all present different challenges. These mobility tasks are not unique to young persons, however. The retired person who enjoys traveling frequently and visiting family members also has special mobility needs.

The second major performance context, the environment, has always been an important aspect of occupational therapy interventions in relation to functional mobility. Environment determines a patient's function. The patient with hemiplegia may be able to roll to either side and come to a seated position on a mat or plinth within the clinical setting and engage in donning and doffing of upper extremity clothing. However, in bed within a home setting the patient may not be able to roll as efficiently or come to a seated position without some assistance. Grooming and dressing tasks may not be practicable because of changes in the height and firmness of the supporting surface. These occurrences and the reasons underlying the performance deficits are well represented in the current motor learning literature. The postural adjustments necessary to roll and come to a seated position to engage in self-care tasks can only be learned in the context of task performance[11,19] and in the expected environment.[32,33]

The treatment of a patient with hemiplegia often occurs on a continuum that directly influences the physical treatment environment. Many treatment environments impose constraints that limit the therapist's interventions. Ideally the relearning of motor skills and tasks should occur in the actual environment in which the task will be performed.[20,63]

Social and cultural variations also have an impact on the success of functional mobility interventions. Culturally derived boundaries of interaction must be considered[47] because the therapist must frequently work within an intimate distance during mobility retraining.[35] The physical environment in which interventions occur also affects the patient's willingness to participate actively. Some patients prefer treatment to occur in the privacy of their hospital rooms, whereas others are more comfortable with these "close encounters" occurring in the open space of a therapeutic gymnasium. The patient, family, significant individuals, and therapist all have perceptions and beliefs founded on their cultural conditionings. Similarities and differences of belief may occur in three areas influencing the success of functional mobility retraining: the perceived state of health and illness; the perceived relevance of therapeutic interventions; and the belief that functional mobility is relevant to resuming previous occupations.[49]

The therapist's ability to listen to personal needs and appreciate individual values helps ensure success.[49] The degree of independence a patient finds acceptable must be self-determined. The therapist must remember that compliance with home programs is influenced by cultural variations.[3,49,57]

FUNCTIONAL MOBILITY: THE OUTCOME OF MULTIPLE PROCESSES

Functional mobility requires the successful interaction of a number of systems. Carrying out skilled rolling, sitting, and standing does not depend solely on the integrity of the neuromusculoskeletal system. Occupational therapists must be mindful of the interdependence of various sensory, perceptual, and cognitive functions in the execution of these tasks and create evaluation tools that respect this relationship such as the Árnadóttir Occupational Therapy Neurobehavioral Evaluation (A-ONE) (see Chapter 13). This awareness ensures more appropriate treatment planning for the "total person" than do evaluations that look at motor behaviors in isolation. Occupational therapists' knowledge and expertise in task analysis render them uniquely qualified to evaluate and plan treatment to improve functional mobility skills while keeping all the patient's needs in mind.

Individual differences and variations in movement strategies may be related to factors such as the patient's build (short, tall, obese, thin) and history of activity before the CVA (i.e., the patient was a trained athlete, dancer, physically inactive, occasional exerciser, physical laborer). Additionally, each patient comes to a therapist with a history of customs and habits that influence movement.[26] A patient's psychologic state may indeed be reflected in movement (e.g., inhibitions or lack of them, reactive depression about the current situation). Pain before or after the stroke may affect movement patterns. These individual differences and their effects on functional mobility have been explored in the literature.[82] The occupational therapist must be cognizant of these factors and others in assessment and treatment planning.

Performance Component Impairments

Many sequelae associated with a CVA may produce difficulties in the carrying out of functional mobility tasks. The occupational therapist uses performance components as a structure for assessing impairments relevant to functional mobility. A review of components affected by CVA and their effects on performance of functional mobility skills is offered in the following sections.

Sensory Processing
Vision

Warren[84] presented a hierarchic model for understanding visual perceptual dysfunction in adults with brain injury. This model asserts that visual perceptual skill is comprised of lower and higher level skills interacting and subserving with each other. Lower-level skills such as visual fields, visual acuity, and oculomotor control form the foundation on which visual attention, scanning, pattern recognition, memory, and visual cognition can be developed and integrated.[84]

Visual field deficits are common after both CVA and traumatic brain injuries. The most common visual-field defect is a homonymous hemianopsia caused by involvement of the striate cortex or geniculocalcarine tract and usually congruent (the same for the two eyes). With or sometimes without cueing, patients can shift their eyes to compensate for such a defect. Hemianopsia often can coexist with visual inattention, but these are two distinct phenomena. According to Warren,[84] functional visual attention requires an efficient intrahemispherical and interhemispherical network for visual information processing to take place. An individual with visual inattention ignores objects in one visual field while attending to objects in the other field. Inattention usually occurs in patients with large right cerebral lesions involving the parietal and temporal lobes, supplied by posterior cerebral arteries (PCAs), or the parietal and frontal lobes, supplied by the middle cerebral arteries (MCAs).

Many patients with homonymous hemianopsia learn to compensate using gaze by turning the head a sufficient amount to bring the affected visual field into the unaffected one. With visual inattention, heightening the patient's awareness to the problem is instrumental to success in using compensatory strategies. Functional mobility skills can be significantly affected with visual inattention because the ability to scan the environment while moving is inconsistent at best. Decreased visual attention to one side may render transfers from bed to wheelchair difficult or even dangerous in cases in which awareness of the problem is poor (see Chapter 12).

Somesthetic Sensation

Disturbances of sensation are frequent in patients who have had acute strokes and are observed in 46% of 1000 consecutive patients,[13] usually in association with other neurologic deficits; in only 2% of those cases did the disturbances occur in isolation. The sensory involvement most commonly shows a face-arm-leg distribution (55.5%

of cases) and less commonly a face-arm (29%) or arm-leg (7%) distribution. Rarely only one of thee three areas is affected in isolation (arm 6%, face 2%, leg 0.5%).[13]

Diminished or absent somesthetic sensation resulting in hemisensory loss can account for difficulties with functional mobility tasks. Proprioceptive loss particularly can contribute to difficulties with purposeful movement, even if motor strength is relatively intact. Sensory loss in the affected extremities necessitates cognitive vigilance to that side during bed mobility and transfers of any kind. Additionally, decreased pain sensation is a risk factor for occurrences of self-injuries.

The use of peripheral feedback in the control of movement has long been debated. The research suggests that many gross motor activities involving the limbs may be achieved in the absence of somatosensory feedback. Researchers theorize that in the adult, many stored motor programs have been learned through a variety of experiences, giving the individual an extensive repertoire of movement possibilities.[50]

Pain can severely limit the extent to which a patient can work on functional mobility skill training. For example, many techniques in bed mobility and transfers require a pain-free arc of motion at the hemiplegic shoulder to be carried out easily. Addressing pain in this case may be the key to promoting function (see Chapter 6).

Perceptual Processing

Right-left disorientation (e.g., the patient gives the incorrect response to the command "show me your right hand") is usually associated with left hemisphere damage. In general these individuals have difficulty differentiating between the right and left halves of their bodies or the bodies of others.[44]

Disturbances of body image may cause an individual to fail to perceive stimuli on the left side, confuse body-positional and spatial relationships, misperceive left-sided stimulation as occurring on the right, and fail to realize that the extremities or other body organs are in some way compromised.[45]

Damage to the right hemisphere alters many aspects of visual-spatial and perceptual functioning. Disturbances can vary individually; however, typically these patients display difficulty with the analysis of geometric space, depth perception, distance, shape, orientation, position, perspective, and figure-ground recognition. The patient may misplace things; have difficulty with balance; stumble and bump into the walls and furniture; and become easily lost, confused, and disoriented while walking or driving. Attempting functional mobility skills training with these patients requires the therapist to be mindful that with each change of position patients undergo, the perception of position in relation to supporting surfaces and surfaces to which they are to move may be disrupted. These patients often misperceive the distance between themselves and the furniture toward which they are moving. Additionally these patients may experience fear when attempting to move; this may result in a "poverty of movement" since staying in one spot is less threatening (see Chapters 13 and 14).

Neuromusculoskeletal and Motor Components

Motor weakness is found in 80% to 90% of all patients after stroke.[13] Hemiparesis with uniform weakness of the hand, foot, shoulder, and hip is the most frequent motor-deficit profile, constituting at least two thirds of all cases.[55] Flaccidity may be evident early on; however, spasticity may develop in the acute phase as well. Limb flaccidity may be associated with retained reflexes; not infrequently reflexes remain normal or even increase. Although many authors have tried to find differences in frequency, severity, and profile of the hemiparesis in right- and left-sided lesions, the majority of such studies showed no significant differences.[55]

Patients after stroke typically experience changes in muscle tone, contralateral weakness (although ipsilateral weakness also is sometimes evident), and poor endurance. Left unattended over time, muscle stiffness and learned nonuse[79] are likely to occur. An extensive review of the causes of weakness in hemiplegia appears in the occupational therapy literature.[15] Although further study is clearly needed in this area, this review substantiates the notion that far too much emphasis has been placed on the role of spasticity in producing the inability to activate affected muscles. An increasing body of knowledge points to alterations in the physiology of motor units, particularly regarding changes in firing rates and muscle-fiber atrophy, and the contribution of other factors results in mechanical restraint of agonist muscles by their antagonists.[15] Early intervention aimed at avoiding contractures and facilitating activation of the more involved side is crucial even if consensus on the most effective means of management is lacking.

Many motor assessments used in the past emphasized the patient's limitations rather than the patient's abilities and created an emphasis on the quality of movement rather than on the actual movement accomplished by the patient. The inability to perform movements correctly can result from other neurobehavioral sequelae related to the stroke, not only from hemiparesis. Patients with motor neglect show a lack of initiation moving their limbs even in the presence of preserved strength, and patients with motor impersistence are unable to maintain voluntary action. Apraxia has been a challenging sequela to treat and is defined as a disorder of skilled, purposeful movement in the absence of impaired motor functioning and comprehension (see Chapter 14).[4]

Apraxic abnormalities are usually associated with left hemisphere damage, in particular injuries involving the left frontal and inferior parietal lobes.[44] Currently the shift in emphasis to appropriate task analysis is influencing occupational therapists in their assessments and broadening these assessments to include perceptual, cognitive, and behavioral features of the task.

Difficulties with postural control become evident for a variety of reasons after stroke. Shumway-Cook and Woollacott[76] view "postural control as the ability to control the body's position in space for the dual purposes of stability and orientation." They define postural stability as "the ability to maintain the position of the body (specifically the center of mass) within the specific boundaries of space, referred to as stability limits."[76] They further explain postural orientation:

Stability limits are boundaries of an area of space in which the body can maintain its position without changing the base of support. Postural orientation is defined as the ability to maintain an appropriate relationship between the body segments and between the body and the environment for a task.

Multiple sensory systems, including the vestibular, somatosensory, and visual systems, allow the individual to receive reference cues about gravity, the supporting surface, and the relationship of the body to objects in the environment, respectively. Disruption to any of these systems can occur after a stroke and must be accounted for in the evaluation process (see Chapter 5).[76]

Cognitive Integration

Arousal and Attention

Disorders of arousal and confusional states, not infrequently in combination, are the most common disorders of consciousness in patients who have suffered acute strokes. Arousal refers to the general state of readiness of an individual to process sensory information and organize a response.[28] Arousal undergoes slow fluctuations throughout the day (tonic arousal) and is influenced by factors such as sleep, food intake, and endogenous neural and endocrine circadian rhythms.[85] Rapid fluctuations in arousal (phasic arousal) occur in response to the presentation of challenging cognitive and physical tasks and signals indicating that an event requiring a response is about to occur (warning signals).[85]

The patient's level of arousal has an impact on readiness to participate in treatment and must be factored into the evaluation of performance of mobility skills. This necessity requires treatment planning in and of itself. The occupational therapist in the acute care or rehabilitation setting may have ample skills to monitor the patient's arousal through 24-hour nursing reports. In the home care setting, family members and other caretakers need to be educated about arousal and its fluctuation.

The neural structures mediating arousal are the reticular activating system (RAS), which has fibers of noradrenergic, dopaminergic, cholinergic, and serotonergic types[65]; hypothalamus; limbic system; and cerebral cortex. The neurotransmitter fibers of the RAS have a broad distribution to the cortex, and the RAS receives direct and indirect feedback from the cortical regions to which it projects. Large areas of the cortex are alerted during arousal; however, other parts of the cortex must be inhibited to allow for selective orientation and attention to specific stimuli. The RAS is able to alert the cortex, but cortical processing also is able to increase activity in the RAS.[65]

The right hemisphere appears to be dominant for tonic arousal and has greater noradrenergic and serotonergic content than does the left.[64] Right hemisphere lesions produce significant slowing of reaction time, particularly in unwarned tasks. Phasic arousal appears to be less significantly impaired by brain damage, including right hemisphere injury.

Selective attention can be thought of as the way and the direction in which the energy supplied by arousal is channeled. It refers to the ability to select and focus on one type of information to the exclusion of others. From a survival perspective the role of location in selective attention is formidable in accurately detecting food and predators. Posner[64] suggests that spatial selective attention can be divided into three sets of operations: disengagement of attention from its current location, movement of attention to a new location, and engagement of attention onto a new stimulus.

Many forms of neuropathology can impair spatial selective attention. Lesions in the cerebral hemispheres (particularly the right) can produce transient or long-lasting unilateral inattention. *Unilateral neglect* or *inattention* has been defined as a failure to orient to, respond to, or report stimuli presented on the side contralateral to the cerebral lesion in patients who do not have primary sensory or motor deficits; it may become manifest in a variety of ways with varying degrees of specific sensory, motor, and visual components.[43]

The impact of attention on evaluation and treatment is profound. Attention affects the ability to learn and remember. Disorders of attention manifest in a variety of ways and may include distractibility, impulsivity, hypersensitivity to stimuli, and decreased attention span, to name a few. A distractible patient, for example, may cue into external stimuli (i.e., anything in the environment) or internal stimuli (i.e., the patient's own thoughts, hunger, pain) and consequently "tune out" the interventions the therapist is attempting with them. Therapists may initially have to work with such patients in a distraction-free environment, if possible. In the patient's hospital room, bed mobility training can be begun with the curtain pulled around the bed to screen out potential distractions.

Most if not all assessments of functional mobility fail to take this most important cognitive ability into account in assessing the ability to perform functional mobility skills. If the patient's attention to task is poor, learning cannot take place. In fact, attention can be thought of as the prerequisite on which learning occurs.

Awareness

Awareness of disability is crucial in both treatment planning and outcome. Awareness is a distinct phenomenon from denial (which is characterized by overrationalization), and the two should not be confused in clinical situations. A significant proportion of brain-injured adults have demonstrated a lack of awareness of their deficits; this varies across domains and does not correlate with severity of brain injury.[38]

A model of awareness has been developed to aid the therapist's evaluation of the patient.[21] This model is hierarchic and describes different levels of awareness in the following order[21]:

1. Intellectual awareness
2. Emergent awareness
3. Anticipatory awareness

Patients tend to fall into one of these three categories, and one goal in therapy becomes helping the patient progress through these levels. The rehabilitation process only proves useful if the patient understands that a problem exists.

Although a greater tendency exists for patients to acknowledge deficits in motor areas, facilitating recognition of deficits in the cognitive and behavioral realms is far more difficult. Impulsivity (action not conditioned by reasoning), for example, which is exemplary of attention disorder, is not typically acknowledged as a problem by patients in the safe performance of functional mobility tasks. The ramifications of this in planning for a safe environment on discharge after hospitalization are obvious.

Memory and Learning

Learning can be defined as the acquisition of information and skills, and memory is the retention and storage of that knowledge. Learning can occur in the absence of overt behavior, but its occurrence can only be inferred from changes in behavior. Short-term memory (also referred to as *working memory*) describes the conscious retention and manipulation of information for recent, brief periods. *Declarative memory* refers to long-term memory amenable to conscious retrieval.[89] Declarative memory includes the learning of facts and experiences that can be reported verbally. Procedural, or nondeclarative, memory comprises a number of functions expressed in motor, perceptual, and cognitive skills and habits.[89] These skills and habits cannot be expressed verbally and are connected with Pavlovian conditioning. A special form of nondeclarative memory is priming, the preparation of a cognitive process by a previous task. Nondeclarative memory is typically spared in patients with amnesia because the memory people have of motor tasks is separate from the memories they have of other events in life.

Disruption of the underlying mechanisms subserving memory function occur frequently after CVAs. Declarative memory skill relies on the hippocampi, whereas the basal ganglia play a major role in procedural memory skills. The cerebellum probably plays a role in Pavlovian conditioning. To evaluate memory function, the therapist must assess whether the individual is taking in information efficiently by noting attention, association, organization, and other cognitive skills.

How much is understood about the way learning takes place? Studies on the neurobiology of learning after brain injury suggest that both functional reorganization and plasticity possibly play roles in the recovery of information-processing capabilities.[59] Understanding a patient's strengths and exploiting them are important in the learning process in occupational therapy. Teaching strategies should be geared to the patient's learning strengths (see Chapter 2).[59]

Many efforts at greater understanding are being made by researchers in motor learning. Recent research by Parasher and Gentile addresses the efficacy of "show" versus "tell" in providing instructions to the learner.[61] They emphasize that two types of instructions—visuospatial and visuowritten—involve different processing and working memory systems. Visuospatial instructions are associated with right hemispheric functions. Visuowritten instructions involve interhemispheric transfer from the left to right hemispheres to produce visual representations of desired action goals. Parasher and Gentile determined that elderly persons have "greater difficulty than the young with the interhemispheric transfer or recoding of speech-based input required to derive a central representation of the action-goal."[61] That is, showing the elderly learner the way to perform the task is better than verbally describing it. As more therapists involve themselves directly in research of this kind, occupational therapists may begin to elucidate differences in learning capabilities across the life span in the presence of a disability and hence be able to teach skills more effectively.

Executive Functions

Executive functions include the many skills used in problem-solving, including problem recognition, goal formulation, planning and organization, initiation, and self-regulation and monitoring. If a person is to engage in independent, purposeful, and self-serving behavior, intact executive functioning is essential. The frontal lobes are inextricably linked with executive functions. Patients with frontal lobe lesions have difficulties with (among other things) initiating behavior, switching from one strategy to another, using mistakes to alter performance, and dealing with distractions.

In functional mobility training, difficulties with executive functions may manifest as difficulties with problem-solving in novel situations. For example, the strategy employed to learn to roll on a mat is not applicable in a bed, in which sheets and pillows are present and the surface is often softer. A new strategy must be learned in this situation, which could prove difficult for patients with impaired executive functions.

Language and Communication

The left hemisphere is responsible for propositional language (conveying meaning through actual word order, word choice, and specific combinations of words and phrases into sentences). *Aphasia* is defined as the loss of language abilities (which may be on a continuum of mild to severe) caused by brain injury, usually to the dominant left hemisphere. It can affect the individual's auditory comprehension, verbal expression, repetition, naming, oral reading, reading comprehension, and written expression.[48] Aphasia must be addressed in therapy for functional mobility skills, and, depending on whether the patient has expressive or receptive impairments or both, a unique plan of action is needed to ensure success in treatment.

The right hemisphere is responsible for affective language (prosody, or melody of speech, and the conveying of meaning through emotional tone via changes in stress, tempo, rhythm, duration, and intonation of speech sounds). The right hemisphere also is said to process pragmatic language. Pragmatics refers to a rule system that delineates the appropriate use of language according to situational contexts and constraints. In other words, pragmatics involves the meaning conveyed by the words themselves through the use of gesture, body language, facial expression, and other nonverbal means.[62] With brain injury to the right hemisphere, deficits in communication can occur; however, they are frequently more subtle than those noted with dominant left hemisphere involvement. With right-sided brain injury, patients exhibit flattened affects. Their speech, though fluent, is characterized by aprosodia, verbosity, and tangentiality. Additionally, these patients may be unable to discern prosody or nonverbal cues in the communication attempts of others. This can have an enormous impact on the therapist-patient relationship, and attempts at training such patients in functional mobility skills may prove difficult unless the therapist understands that communication deficits are present. Only then can the therapist devise an individualized treatment plan with these specific problems in mind.

Psychologic Components

Psychiatric sequelae associated with CVA must be appreciated to facilitate the rehabilitation process (see Chapter 3). Cerebral ischemia is associated with two types of depressive disorders. One type is depression meeting *DSM-IV* symptom criteria for major depression. The other type is minor depression meeting *DSM-IV* symptom criteria for dysthymic depression (excluding the 2-year duration criterion). An association between the location of left-side anterior lesions and major depression among patients with acute stroke has been reported by three different groups of investigators.[5,37,67] Patients with depression in the rehabilitation setting are challenges for staff members and require supportive psychotherapeutic interventions. Additionally, they may benefit from psychopharmacologic treatment. Professionals working with these patients must recognize the signs of depression early because depression can have a significant impact on the patient's ability to participate in the rehabilitation process, concentrate during therapy sessions, and learn new skills.

In *Descartes' Error: Emotion, Reason and the Human Brain*, Damasio, a renowned neurologist, argues persuasively if not controversially that an inextricable link exists between cognition and emotion.[23] Damasio's thesis suggests for the work of occupational therapists a truth they have perhaps known implicitly for years: a person cannot be separated into apportioned packages of cognitive characteristics distinct from emotional and physical characteristics. The whole being, who is more than the sum total of biopsychosocial factors that interplay and are interdependent on each other, must be considered.

STRATEGIES FOR SPECIFIC IMPAIRMENTS

Language Impairments

Different types of strategies may be employed when approaching the patient with communication difficulties sustained as a result of damage to the right and left hemispheres. The therapist should consider the following guidelines when working with patients with left-hemisphere involvement resulting in aphasia[62]:

1. Avoid speaking in a loud voice. Although the temptation is great, no hearing loss has occurred, and loud speech often makes the patient feel like a child.
2. Give the patient ample time to respond so the patient has time to process the response for which the therapist is asking.
3. Observe the patient for signs of fatigue or anxiety; do not pressure the patient.
4. Encourage expression of thoughts or ideas through whatever means the patient has available (e.g., posturing, gesturing).
5. If comprehension is a problem, ask simple, short questions and deemphasize spoken interaction; use gesture, facial expression, and pantomime to provide the patient with clues as to the response desired.
6. For the patient with comprehension problems, cueing through the tactile medium is most beneficial. For example, if rolling is the desired activity, ensure that hand placement "tells" the patient the response needed.

Pragmatic Impairments

Therapists should consider the following guidelines when working with patients with right-hemisphere involvement[62]:

1. Minimize distractions because an attention deficit may be present and interfering in treatment.
2. Have the patient demonstrate the ability to do an activity rather than rely on a report of the way the activity is accomplished. Demonstration is crucial because patients with right-sided lesions have a tendency to minimize their deficits or simply not recognize them.
3. Ensure that the patient is focused on the task at hand.
4. Go through sequences with the patient, having the patient repeat the correct order in which to carry out the task. If the goal is sit-to-stand, have the patient describe with the therapist the necessary steps (i.e., come to the edge of the bed, bring the feet back, lean forward).
5. Provide feedback on statements irrelevant to the situation. Patients with right-sided lesions are verbose at times and may complicate simple directions in the process.
6. Try to promote awareness of facial gestures as communication. This awareness is important because patients have a tendency not only to be devoid of facial expression but also unable to perceive the expressions of others.
7. Increase awareness of the patient's current situation (e.g., the reason the patient requires assistance with bed mobility and transfers).
8. Help the patient relearn the rules of turn-taking in conversation.

Apraxia

Apraxia is a disorder of skilled movement in the absence of impaired motor functioning or paralysis.[36] The left hemisphere appears to be superior to the right in the control of certain types of complex, sequenced motor acts; if damage is sustained to the left hemisphere, the patient's ability to acquire and perform tasks involving skilled movements may be impaired. Many forms of apraxia have been identified; as with many of the other disturbances discussed, they may be attributable to a number of causes or anatomic lesions. The forms of apraxia, caused largely by damage to the left frontal and inferior parietal lobes, include ideational, ideomotor, and buccal-facial apraxia. Damage to the right cerebral hemisphere may cause dressing apraxia.

Affolter has developed a treatment technique of nonverbal guiding to stimulate and facilitate the patient's perceptual systems, thereby influencing cognitive systems. The therapist manually guides the patient in an activity, allowing exploration of objects and supporting surfaces in the process. This form of manual guidance is a "hand-over-hand" approach, with the therapist maintaining light but direct contact with the patient's extremities as the patient goes through the motions of carrying out a functional activity. The goal of this therapeutic approach is not the output of the movement pattern but rather the problem-solving process believed to be taking place.[14]

Heavy emphasis on the tactile-kinesthetic (TK) approach, that is, the tactile-kinesthetic exploration of the environment by the patient with facilitation from the therapist, is the defining feature of this technique; it is additionally a nonverbal technique, making it useful for the patient with apraxia. Affolter contends that the patient with apraxia is dealing with a perceptual deficit and needs to be treated with a functional approach.[14] The therapist can use this approach to assist the patient if motor movement breaks down; the therapist provides the intervention without the use of words, except perhaps after the movement in the form of feedback to the patient on performance. Thus the TK approach may be useful with patients with aphasia as well (see Chapter 14).[14]

The TK approach emphasizes the use of meaningful activities in the appropriate environmental context. In this approach the singular use of therapy equipment such as the mat table is meaningless because the patient needs to learn to roll and sit up from a bed and must learn sit-to-stand from a variety of surfaces such as a bed, chair, wheelchair, couch, toilet, and tub. Mistakes are needed for learning to take place. Patients need to learn to adapt to different situations and modify movement and strategy accordingly. Gradually the patient must take control over the personal movement repertoire for any carryover to take place.

Unilateral Inattention

Unilateral inattention is seen most commonly with right-hemisphere lesions and may exist with or without hemianopsia. Patients with unilateral inattention have symptoms that vary in specific sensory modality involvement and severity. A thorough assessment of sensory, motor, and visual manifestations should be made; particular attention should be placed on assessing the patient's level of awareness of the problem. Often these patients experience a lack of recognition of the left side of the body; this may make efforts at training in functional mobility tasks difficult because the ability to attempt to incorporate both sides of the body into the activity is neither automatic nor easy to facilitate by the therapist.

In her extensive work on the cognitive remediation of these patients, Toglia[80] describes specific treatment strategies that primarily focus on the need to heighten the patient's awareness of the problem. She recommends consistent use of self-monitoring strategies and error detection by the patient in the cognitive remediation process.[80] Modification of the environment also may be necessary; for example, a patient particularly susceptible to environmental distractions may need to begin functional mobility training in a low-stimulus environment and gradually build to a higher-stimulus environment in therapy (see Chapter 14).

Attentional Deficits

Depending on the nature of the patient's attention problem the therapist may choose to focus on increasing sustained attention, shifting attention, and sustaining attention in the presence of auditory and visual distractors. Initially therapy may have to take place in a minimally distracting environment, but gradually the patient needs to develop tolerance to stimuli in the environment.

FUNCTIONAL MOBILITY TASKS

Functional mobility tasks occur throughout the daily routine under varying circumstances within changeable environments. Each task requires the individual to stabilize the body in space or exhibit dynamic postural control. Das and McCollum identified three major requirements for locomotion that can be applied to all functional mobility tasks[24]:

1. Progression or movement in a desired direction
2. The ability to stabilize the body against the forces of gravity
3. The ability to make changes in movement in relation to specific tasks within different environments.

This view of functional mobility is congruent to a systems approach for analyzing and explaining normal movement, an approach that emphasizes the interaction of the individual, task, and environment.[76]

ACTIVITIES IN THE SUPINE POSITION
Bridging
Analysis of Movement

In the functional mobility task of bridging, the back and hip extensors support the body against the forces of gravity. The arch formed when the upper back and feet are in contact with the supporting surface is maintained by the activation of muscles located on the underside of the arch. Use of the arms or legs increases the demands placed on the trunk musculature. When an arm or leg is raised (as in attempts to dress), the muscles located above the arch (the oblique abdominal muscles) must become active to support the limb.[25]

Selected Problems

The mobility task of bridging is a challenge for patients with hemiplegia because of loss of activity in the extensors as well as the abdominal muscles. Combining this problem with early return of extensor activity results in ineffective and inefficient movement patterns.

Supine characteristics indicating decreased abdominal activity include the following:

- Upward and outward drawing of the ribcage (that is, the affected side rides higher in the cavity because the abdominals do not tether the ribcage downward)
- Shortening of the neck resulting from unopposed elevation of the shoulder girdle
- Hypotonic appearance of the abdomen
- Shift of the umbilicus to the nonaffected side
- Reduced proximal stability with an impact on the lower extremities

Primitive extensor activity for all movements further diminishes flexor control because of reciprocal inhibition.[25]

Treatment Strategies

Bridging is an important position that the patient should be instructed to assume early in the intervention process. It is a mobility function necessary for the use of a bedpan, reduction of pressure on the buttocks, and movement within the bed (bed scooting).[42] In addition, the position of the low back and hips approximates the alignment required for the normal stance position.[42,78] Movement within this position can further simulate the movement required of the pelvis and lower extremities during ambulation, specifically forward motion of the pelvis, lateral and rotational pelvic shift, and advanced movement combinations of hip extension with knee flexion.[25]

The patient with hemiplegia may experience difficulty in assuming the crooklying position and forming a bridge because of a variety of underlying causes. The lack of selective muscle activity on the affected side, caused by the use of mass patterns, prevents the patient from combining the necessary hip components of flexion and adduction.[10] Patient attempts to place the affected leg usually result in a mass pattern of movement characterized by hip flexion and external rotation and supination of the foot. The patient's inability to stabilize the pelvis while attempting this movement results in increased extension of the lumbar spine combined with forced extension of the nonaffected side into the supporting surface. Another possible reason for the increase in the extension of the lumbar spine is tightness of the hip flexors,[78] although this is unlikely in the early stages after CVA unless the patient exhibited tightness before sustaining the stroke.

The patient can be assisted to assume the crooklying position by the therapist. The patient is encouraged to assist with active flexion of the unaffected leg; the therapist may be required to assist and hold the required crooklying position. Active flexion on the affected leg helps position the pelvis forward and may promote active holding of the affected leg in a flexed position.[42] The therapist may provide downward pressure on the flexed knee of the affected side to ensure appropriate foot placement.[10]

Active bridging can be used to improve selective exten-

sion of the hip and abdominal muscle activity. As the patient lifts the buttocks from the supporting surface, the therapist should make sure the patient does not use excessive extensor activity, which is characterized by extension of the hips, overarching of the back, and pushing of the head into the supporting surface. To improve selective movement, the patient is encouraged to initiate the movement by actively tilting the pelvis up. The therapist may need to prepare the patient for this movement (Figure 10-1). After the pelvis is tilted forward, the patient lifts the buttocks off the surface while holding the pelvis level. The therapist may assist this movement by placing one hand under the hemiplegic hip and one hand on the abdominals. If the feet are positioned close to the body, the therapist may also guide the femoral condyles forward toward the feet while applying downward pressure (Figure 10-2).

After the patient can maintain this position, the next step is to lift the unaffected foot off the surface while maintaining the pelvis level. The therapist should observe any asymmetries or rotation of the pelvis. The patient must not be permitted to drop the unaffected side to gain more stability. This task is difficult for the patient with hemiplegia because it places demands on the oblique abdominal muscles.[20,26,78] Bridging can be graded according to the patient's ability to control movements selectively. Placement of the feet further away from the buttocks requires a greater degree of selective activity to maintain knee flexion with hip extension.[26] Alternate lifting of the feet off the supporting surface while maintaining the level of the pelvis requires increased muscular activity and greater coordination (Figures 10-3 and 10-4).[78]

Bridging can be used to move up in bed and don pants while in a supine position. Caregivers should be instructed

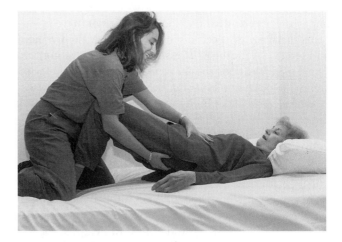

Figure 10-1 In bridging, increased extensor activity that results in arching of the back should be avoided. To facilitate selective movement of the pelvis, the therapist stimulates the gluteal region while facilitating the lower abdominals. This sequence may first be applied to the unaffected side, then to the hemiplegic side.

in the appropriate techniques to ensure that these movements are transferred into the patient's daily life routine. The occupational therapist can incorporate these movement strategies while training the patient in self-care activities.

Rolling

Analysis of Movement

Rolling is an important part of bed mobility and an essential part of many other tasks.[66] Research has demonstrated that normal adults use a variety of movement strategies to roll from supine to prone.[66]

One of the most common movement strategies used by young adults in rolling from supine to prone includes a lift-and-reach arm pattern. Movement of the head and trunk is initiated by the shoulder girdle; a unilateral lift of the leg also occurs. Rotation of the spine, which results in dissociation of the shoulder and pelvic girdles, is not observed

(Figure 10-5).[66] This rotation was once assumed to be a prerequisite to attaining the ability to roll in a normal pattern of movement.[10]

The most important finding of this study is that normal adults have a repertoire of movements available to them, unlike patients after stroke, who are limited to stereotypical patterns of movement.[22] The environmental conditions of

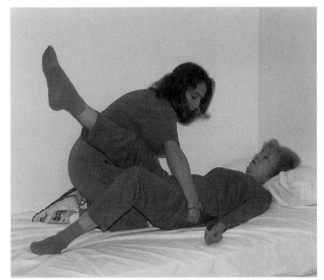

Figure 10-3 Lifting a leg off the supporting surface places increased demands on the abdominal muscles because the pelvis must be held up. The patient is asked to lift the unaffected foot off the bed so that all the patient's weight is placed on the affected side. The patient must maintain the pelvis in a level position. This patient is experiencing difficulty maintaining the optimal pelvic position (left hemiplegia).

A

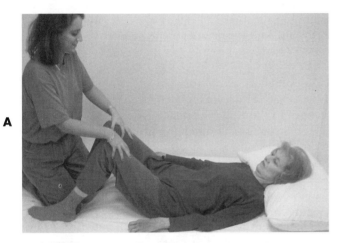

B

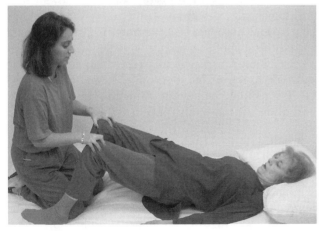

Figure 10-2 **A,** As the patient gains selective control over the pelvis, the therapist can provide downward pressure through the knees and guide the femoral condyles forward toward the feet. **B,** The patient is asked to lift the buttocks off the bed. Physical assistance can be diminished as the patient gains control.

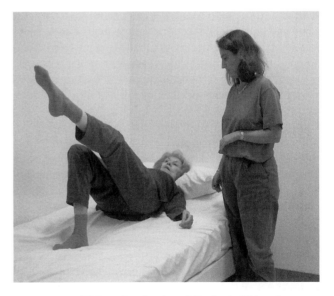

Figure 10-4 This patient has less difficulty in lifting the hemiplegic side (left hemiplegia).

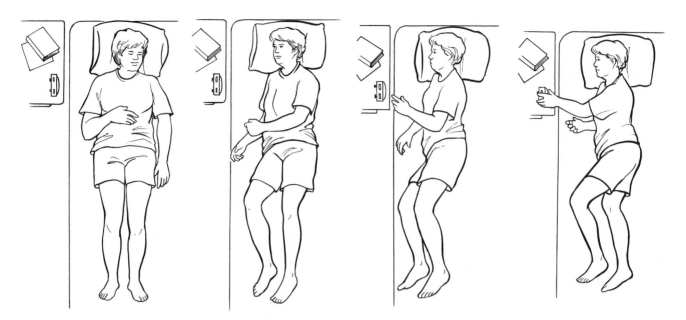

Figure 10-5 Research has determined that a common form of rolling observed in adults is initiated by a lift and reach above shoulder level; the shoulder girdle leads the movement, and a unilateral lift of the lower extremity follows. Many subjects also use a unilateral push of the lower extremity. A great variety of patterns is observed because of individual differences in build, strength, and the support surface.

this study were limited to rolling on an exercise mat, and the subjects were asked to roll "as fast as you can." Thus the variety of patterns observed may relate to the temporal demands and implied goal of the task. The strategies used to roll for speed may differ significantly from the strategies used to target a particular object in the environment. Therapists who work with patients with hemiplegia must consider the rolling surface (environment), the goal of changing the body's position while supine, and future mobility goals such as attaining supine-to-sit. Thus therapists must determine movement sequences most suitable to ensuring safety and maintaining essential components of movement that are nevertheless necessary for subsequent skills. Rotation of the spine during rolling it just one strategy that may be useful in providing a greater variety of movement possibilities for the patient with hemiplegia.[20,25,26]

Rolling to the Hemiplegic Side: Selected Problems and Treatment Strategies

The patient with hemiplegia frequently rolls over using an extensor pattern to initiate the movement sequence because of lack of flexor control of the trunk and the early return of extensor activity. The patient relies on the unaffected side to push against the supporting surface, resulting in an arching of the axial spine as the body is thrust forward in the direction of the roll.

Davies[25] suggests that rolling activities can be used to facilitate active flexion of the trunk and thus achieve subsequent improvement in active control of the trunk musculature. The need exists to balance the concentric and eccentric contractions of the trunk muscles in proportion to

the change in force exerted by gravity as the patient changes position.

The hemiplegic arm requires protection before rolling to the affected side is practiced. The therapist can provide this protection by prepositioning the arm, assisting the patient in bringing the shoulder and arm forward, and giving physical support to the hemiplegic arm while standing on the affected side.

The patient is encouraged to lift the unaffected arm and leg up and forward across the body; this movement is consistent with the pattern identified by Richter et al.[66] This movement should occur without the patient pushing against the supporting surface with the unaffected foot (Figure 10-6). The patient may repeat this movement by returning to the supine position. Either a part of or the whole leg should be held in abduction and slowly lowered to the surface as the patient returns to the supine position.

As the patient gains control of this movement sequence, the next step is to lift the head from the surface to assist with initiation of movement. As the patient turns, the head is rotated toward the direction of the movement. Throughout the sequence, physical assistance should be decreased as changes in the patient's ability to control movement occur.

Rolling to the Unaffected Side: Selected Problems and Treatment Strategies

Rolling to the unaffected side may be more difficult for the patient with hemiplegia. The movement is frequently initiated by an extensor pattern that includes extension of

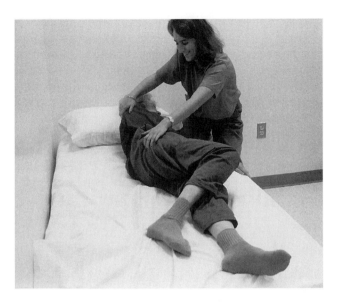

Figure 10-6 Rolling toward the hemiplegic side (left hemiplegia) is accomplished by lifting the unaffected leg over the hemiplegic side without pushing off the bed surface. The therapist assists with movement of the shoulder and pelvic girdles.

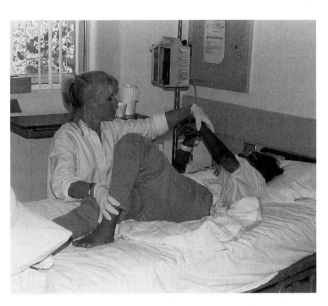

Figure 10-8 Early in the rehabilitation process the patient with left hemiplegia is instructed to clasp the hands to assist in bringing the shoulder forward; the hemiplegic leg is positioned in hip and knee flexion by the therapist to avoid an extensor pattern.

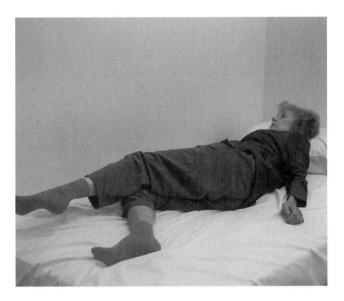

Figure 10-7 Rolling toward the unaffected side. The patient should avoid using the back extensors to bring the lower extremity forward while neglecting the hemiplegic arm (left hemiplegia).

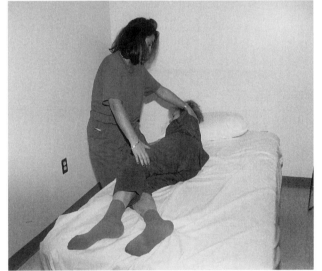

Figure 10-9 Sensory cues can be decreased as the patient gains control of the movement. The therapist is facilitating knee flexion and protraction of the shoulder (left hemiplegia).

the head, neck, and back. The patient relies on extension of the back to bring the hemiplegic leg over the trunk in a pattern of extension that may be viewed as an inefficient compensatory strategy. The affected arm may be left behind as the patient rolls (Figure 10-7).[26]

When teaching patients to roll to the unaffected side, the therapist's goals are to decrease maladaptive compensatory strategies contributing to inefficient movement and enhance more effective and efficient patterns of move-

ment. The patient may be instructed to clasp the hands together (Figure 10-8) and bring the hemiplegic arm up and forward while the therapist attempts to facilitate the movement of the pelvis and lower extremity. The therapist supports the affected leg while assisting with anterior movement of the pelvis (Figure 10-9).

Repetition of this sequence may assist with learning. The patient is encouraged to lift the affected leg off the supporting surface and lower it slowly after returning to the supine position. This strategy is used to assist the patient in maintaining a slight degree of hip and knee flexion, which decreases reliance on the extensor compensatory pattern. An alternative method is to flex both legs to roll.[10,26]

Supine-to-Sit

Analysis of Movement

The transitional movement from supine-to-sit may be achieved through a variety of movement strategies. Adults have a tendency to use a momentum strategy to achieve the goal (Figure 10-10). Their movements are smooth and

efficient as they "bound" out of bed, off the couch, or out of a chair. A momentum strategy requires forces within the trunk to be generated and transferred to the lower extremities to initiate the rolling sequence. Trunk muscles must contract concentrically to initiate and propel the movement; eccentric muscle contractions provide control. The reciprocal shortening and lengthening of muscle contractions provide maintained stability.

Many older adults demonstrate a tendency to use a force-control strategy (Figure 10-11). Here the individual transfers forces from one body part to another as gradu-

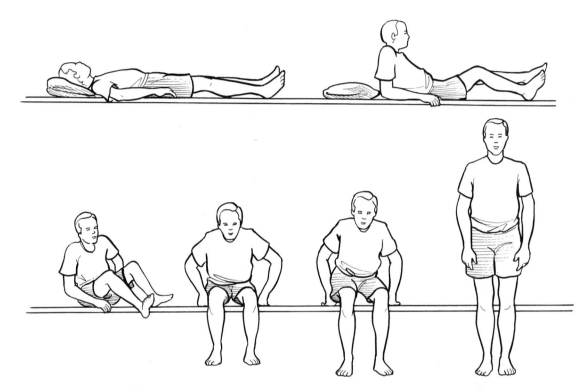

Figure 10-10   The most common movement strategy used by adults to get out of bed relies on momentum. Strategies are extremely variable.

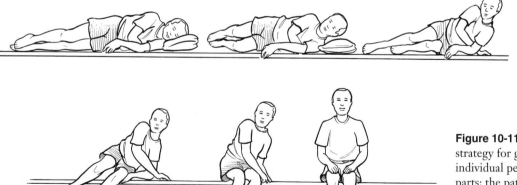

Figure 10-11   A force control strategy for getting out of bed has the individual performing the task in two parts: the patient moves from supine to sidelying, then pushes to a seated position. This strategy is useful for patients who exhibit reduced stability functions.

ated changes in position occur. Rolling to sidelying, then pushing up with the upper extremities, and swinging the lower extremities over the side of the bed is an example of this strategy. This method provides increased stability because concentric and eccentric forces are required in increments. Increased effort (force) must be used if momentum is lacking.[20,26,66,74]

A great variety of movement possibilities to achieve a supine-to-sit sequence remains. The described sequence is often used spontaneously by patients after CVA and by the therapists as a method of instruction.[20] This sequence is referred to as *sidelying-to-sit* for the remainder of this chapter.

Selected Problems

Movement from the sidelying to seated position becomes a challenge for the patient after CVA because of the combined effects of limited muscular activity and maladaptive compensatory strategies. Patients lack appropriate postural alignment and stability.[20,25] The lack of flexor control of the trunk and early return of extensor activity interfere with the patient's ability to grade concentric and eccentric muscle activity effectively relative to the changing forces of gravity.[25] If inadequate control of the trunk musculature is evident, the patient must rely on compensatory strategies that may include overuse of the unaffected arm or leg or exaggerated use of head movements. The patient uses these compensatory strategies instead of effective lateral movements of the neck and trunk. When sidelying the patient flexes the head forward instead of laterally; the unaffected arm is used to move the body away from the supporting surface. The forward movement of the head may be a compensatory strategy to shift the center of gravity forward. The patient may be unable to combine lateral flexion and extension of the trunk because of lack of selective muscle activity. Hooking of the unaffected leg under the affected leg to lift and lower the leg over the side of the bed is yet another compensatory strategy many patients are instructed to perform. This strategy prevents selective movement of the pelvis in an anterior and lateral direction.[20,25] The patient with hemiplegia experiences difficulty whether rising from the hemiplegic or the unaffected side because of the problems presented.

Additionally, while changing positions, the patient may not exhibit appropriate head-righting responses; this deficit requires the patient to flex the neck laterally while controlling eccentric muscle activity on the opposite side. Furthermore, the patient also may be unable to move or place the affected limbs appropriately in preparation for transitional movement, or the affected limbs may be neglected entirely.

Treatment Strategies

Many methods are suggested to retrain the patient in the supine-to-sit movement sequence. One method suggests that patients with hemiplegia be taught initially to roll toward the affected side to decrease the amount of ef-

fort required and reduce maladaptive strategies such as pulling and pushing to achieve the seated position.[20] Others suggest that the patient with hemiplegia be instructed to rise from both sides early in treatment to prevent associated reactions.[11,25,26] Another option is for the patient to start the movement sitting upright and learn to lie down first. This method may decrease the force gravity exerts on the trunk musculature as the patient first learns to control movement into gravity using eccentric muscle activity.[25] The physical environment and the patient's premorbid preferences for movement sequences also may influence the methods selected. Patients may benefit from learning more than one method to move more effectively in different environments.

Sidelying-to-Sit Toward the Affected Side

The therapist assists the patient in lifting the hemiplegic leg over the side of the bed; the head, neck, and upper thorax are brought forward, requiring the neck to flex laterally. Concurrently the nonaffected arm must be brought across the body and placed on the bed. The unaffected leg also must be lifted over the side of the bed as the patient pushes down with the hand. The movement of the unaffected leg as the patient simultaneously pushes with the hand adds a momentum strategy to this movement sequence; the weight of the leg assists the patient in attaining a seated posture. The therapist may be required to assist with bringing the unaffected shoulder forward over the body's base of support. The therapist's hand may be placed on the shoulder and pelvic girdle to give support and assist with movement of the unaffected leg (Figure 10-12). As the patient gains some control over this movement, the therapist may provide support to just the unaffected shoul-

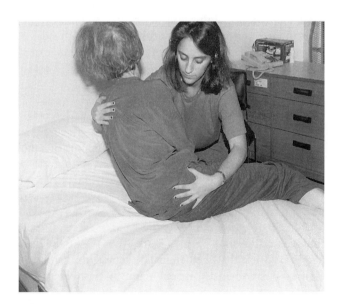

Figure 10-12 The therapist uses one arm around the patient's shoulders while the other hand provides downward pressure to the pelvis to assist with weight transfer in movement to a seated position (left hemiplegia).

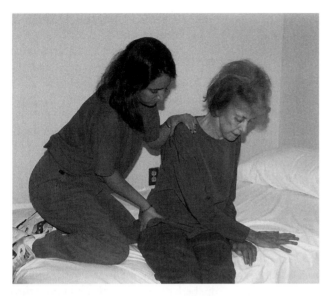

Figure 10-13   When the patient is able to control the trunk muscles actively, the therapist's assistance can be decreased. The therapist may facilitate lateral flexion of the head and trunk by providing downward pressure to the shoulder and pelvic girdles of the unaffected side.

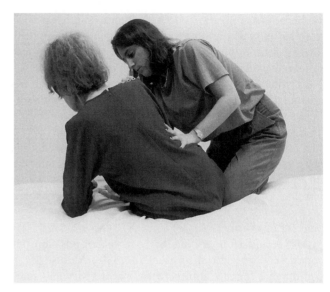

Figure 10-14   Propping of the affected upper extremity as the patient prepares to assume the seated position. The therapist is facilitating lateral flexion of the unaffected side while observing for appropriate head and trunk alignment on the affected side.

der and pelvis (Figure 10-13). Downward pressure on the shoulder facilitates lateral flexion of the trunk and appropriate head righting. To reverse this sequence, the patient may require assistance with lifting the hemiplegic leg onto the bed. Care should be directed toward maintaining the hemiplegic shoulder in a forward position as the patient turns and lowers the body to the bed surface.[25]

When assuming a sitting position from the affected side, the patient is active in the trunk, particularly as weight is borne on the affected upper extremity; therapists should be mindful of this. Furthermore, the therapist may have to facilitate movement of the trunk on both sides to promote the correct sequence of lateral flexion and extension responses (Figure 10-14).

Sidelying-to-Sit Toward the Unaffected Side

The sequence of movement in sidelying-to-sit toward the unaffected side remains the same as that in the previous example; however, the placement of the therapist's hands to assist movement changes. The patient should be instructed to lift the affected arm while lifting the unaffected leg over the side of the bed. The therapist assists with movement of the affected leg forward and over the edge of the bed as the patient lifts the head, neck, and upper thorax over the sound arm (Figure 10-15). The therapist needs to ensure that the hemiplegic shoulder remains in a forward position as the patient begins to push down with the unaffected side. A movement sequence that begins as a force-control strategy can with increased motor control of the head, neck, and trunk become a momentum strategy.

Patients demonstrating a lack of lateral flexion of the

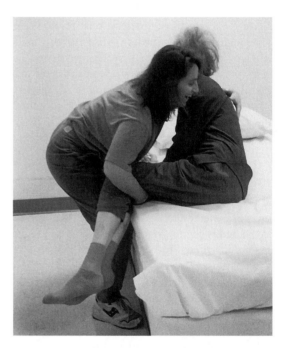

Figure 10-15   Rising from the unaffected side. For patients who require significant support the therapist places one hand on the scapula while assisting with movement of the legs.

neck require preparatory interventions. The patient should be positioned sidelying on the unaffected side with the head on the bed (Figure 10-16, *A*). The patient lifts the head with the therapist's assistance as needed (Figure 10-16, *B*). The patient is then requested to lower the head to the bed; this movement requires eccentric contraction of the lateral flexors. This maneuver is followed by active lift-

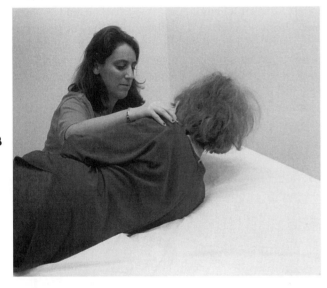

Figure 10-16 **A,** To encourage active control of the lateral neck muscles, the patient first learns to control eccentric contraction while lowering the head to the bed. **B,** This is followed by active lateral neck flexion while raising the head.

ing of the head, which requires concentric muscle contractions. The therapist should not permit the patient to rotate or flex forward while performing this task. A visual target such as an alarm clock, television, or family picture may assist in establishing this task-related goal.[20]

Additional interventions to promote lateral flexion and extension of the trunk, which are necessary to perform sidelying-to-sit, are described in the section on sitting.

ACTIVITIES IN SITTING

The ability to maintain a seated position and perform activities of daily living safely and efficiently is a goal many occupational therapists seek with their patients (see Chap-

ter 4). In the acute stages after CVA (if the patient is medically stable) the therapist should begin to work on control of sitting and standing with the patient as soon as possible to promote the ability to manage the upright position and increase overall visual input in functional positions.[20]

Analysis of Movement

For controlled movement in sitting the ability to bear and shift weight anteriorly, posteriorly, laterally, and in a rotary pattern must be present. This suggests that the concentric and eccentric abilities of the trunk flexors and extensors and the ability to activate these muscle groups selectively relative to the task demand must be present. For example, for controlled anterior weight shift through the pelvis the need for concentric contraction of the low back extensors and an associated eccentric contraction of the trunk flexors (abdominals) is evident. In a posterior weight shift through the pelvis, the need for concentric contraction of the trunk flexors and an associated eccentric contraction of the trunk extensors is evident. With lateral weight shift through the pelvis the trunk extensors and flexors work together concentrically (shortening) on the non–weight-bearing side and eccentrically (lengthening) on the weight-bearing side.[10] During trunk rotation the primary muscles involved are the oblique muscles.

Selected Problems

The trunk, often neglected in assessment, is crucial in postural control. The therapist must begin an assessment on functional capabilities in this area by close examination of the patient's ability to control movements in sitting. The neurodevelopmental treatment (NDT) perspective uses normal movement as a guiding principle in evaluation. Mohr[54] uses four areas of focus to assess normal trunk control:

1) Normal trunk control requires that any body part be able to dissociate (move separately from another body part); 2) An individual must experience movement and control at higher developmental levels against gravity prior to achieving full balance control at lower developmental levels; 3) Midline control is not complete without some ability to rotate, and; 4) Proper postural control of the trunk includes the need for normal range, dynamic stability and points of control.

Mohr contends that normal movement requires the upper trunk to be capable of dissociating from the lower trunk and the right side from the left side.[54] Indeed, this problem may be observed in patients with hemiplegia; as a result of this inability to dissociate within the trunk, voluntary movements are gross (one whole side moves to obtain a goal) and effortful. Additionally, this inability to dissociate precludes isolated limb function and hence a more normal reach and ambulation pattern.

A full appreciation of the normal ranges of motion within the spine is useful when comparing patients with hemiplegia and the patterns they use with the normal population. The therapist must be cognizant that these ranges decrease with age; ascertaining the baseline from which these patients were operating before the onset of hemiparesis is important. Mohr emphasizes the importance of establishing a patient's range of motion in spinal extension and flexion, lateral flexion, and rotation before treatment is implemented. This provides the therapist with information needed to decide whether interventions should include increasing ranges in these areas with the goal of promoting activation by the patient in these patterns for function. Davies[25] also recommends this approach. For example, passive mobilization of the lumbar spine for lateral flexion may be an important preparatory treatment to working on increased trunk control in activities requiring a lateral weight shift such as sidelying-to-sit. The therapist, having encouraged increased mobility in this plane, can progress to facilitation of the appropriate muscle contractions needed to hold and move into this position by placing the hand in the patient's axilla and assisting the side to lengthen while placing the other hand on the patient's opposite trunk to guide shortening on that side.

A deeper look at the location of movement and the way it is initiated is necessary before proceeding in evaluation. Mohr states the following[54]:

"Most gross mobility movements are initiated with the lower trunk and pelvis whereas movements involved in personal self-care involving reach are initiated in the upper extremity via the hand." Anterior and posterior movements of the trunk require a balanced flexion/extension response, and lateral flexion necessitates selected activation of flexors and extensors in combination with each other. Rotation, considered the most sophisticated movement pattern, requires flexion and extension responses in a more complex pattern between opposite sides of the trunk.

Davies indicates that the abdominal muscles tend to be neglected in treatment.[25] Appropriate recruitment of the abdominals is not possible because of the presence of hypotonicity in the trunk and changes in biomechanical alignment that keep the abdominals from working optimally.[25] Davies goes further and points out that a number of patients with hemiplegia from CVA appear to have a bilateral loss of abdominal muscle activity and tone. This seems to be a function of the attachment of the abdominal muscles through a central aponeurosis connected to the linea alba; each side depends on the other for skilled movement to take place. Davies maintains that as a result of the patient's loss of abdominal control and subsequent neglect of these muscles by clinicians, patients begin to use compensatory strategies to move. This is evidenced by overactivation of the back extensors when attempting to move (see Chapter 4).[25]

Treatment Strategies

As stated previously, controlled sitting requires the patient to have the ability to shift weight anteriorly, posteriorly, laterally, and in a rotary pattern. The therapist should

guide the patient to experience initiating trunk movements. Providing the patient with upper extremity support may be helpful initially to take the weight of the arm off the body. Use of tray table, therapy ball, or the shoulders of the therapist can help. The therapist may need to provide direct contact on the patient's pelvis to assist the patient to feel the origin of the movement. The therapist's hands around the patient's iliac crests may be sufficient to start, but occasionally the patient may need even more support from behind (in which case the therapist uses the body to support the patient) to maintain an upright position.

Teaching an anterior weight shift can be accomplished by facilitation of the low back extensors (Figure 10-17). Posterior weight shift is facilitated by direct contact to the trunk flexors (abdominals) (Figure 10-18). The therapist's contact should be direct but light enough that it provides the patient with the message to respond. Encouraging symmetry of the trunk while lending support is important to allow the trunk muscles to have a background of alignment from which to move efficiently. Controlled activation of the abdominals in this position is not simple, and patients have a tendency to slump into a posterior pelvic tilt instead of obtaining adequate abdominal contraction to achieve the weight shift.

Lateral flexion should be initiated next with the pelvis in a neutral position; too much extension literally blocks the ability to achieve a lateral weight shift. As mentioned

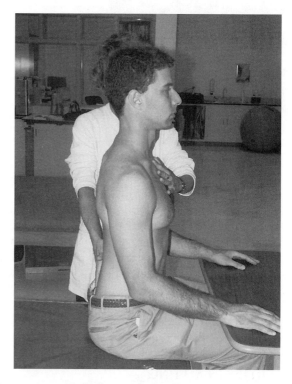

Figure 10-17 To facilitate anterior tilt of the pelvis, the therapist makes direct contact with the lumbar extensors with the right hand, encouraging concentric contraction of these muscles. Additionally, the therapist places the left hand on the sternum to promote elevation of the thorax.

previously, controlled lateral flexion requires the combined lengthening and shortening abilities of the trunk flexors and extensors working together. If patients are restricted in range into lateral flexion, mobilization of the lumbar spine should be performed by the therapist to prepare the patient to move (Figure 10-19). Patients may require a lot of direct contact initially to achieve lateral weight shift; the therapist may have to move the patient first by lifting one buttock and then the other off the supporting surface. The therapist should then "back off" and encourage weight shift with less contact. This is a useful activity to reestablish control of the midline because it requires moving to both sides and essentially moving back to the starting point with each attempt. With one hand under the patient's axilla and the other hand in the patient's opposite lateral trunk, the therapist can facilitate a weight shift first to one side and then to the other (Figure 10-20). Another way of achieving lateral weight shift is through facilitation of scapular depression (Figure 10-21). Controlling the weight shift to the affected side may be difficult at first, and the patient may have a tendency to "fall" to that side. The therapist should start in small ranges with this activity and gradually increase the range of weight shift slowly.[25] Patients may have difficulty trying to shorten the affected side to shift weight to the unaf-

fected side. This activity must be practiced and is often overlooked clinically.

Rotation, which takes place at the end ranges of lateral flexion, is a movement pattern that also is frequently overlooked in the clinic; nevertheless, for the purposes of function, it is a most important movement pattern of the trunk, requiring a sophisticated combination of selected muscle activity for successful accomplishment. Hand contacts here should promote forward and backward movement on a diagonal in the seated position first on one side and then on the other (Figures 10-22 and 10-23). The primary muscles involved are the obliques.

Restrictions of the trunk can occur rapidly after a CVA as the patient attempts to resist gravity and uses the compensatory movement patterns that are available. A shortening and splinting effect in certain muscle groups accompanies these movement strategies. These restrictions in turn affect the ability to move the upper extremity in an isolated manner, which by itself may develop restrictions.

Scooting

Analysis of Movement

Scooting, or "butt walking," involves the transfer of weight over first one buttock and then the other, creating overall movement of the body anteriorly in a seated posi-

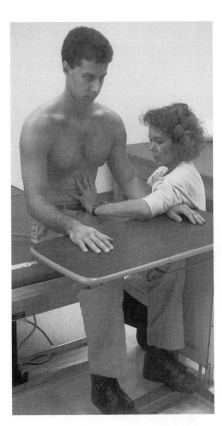

Figure 10-18 The therapist facilitates concentric contraction of the abdominal muscles through direct contact to these muscle bellies with the left hand, and the patient achieves a posterior tilt of the pelvis.

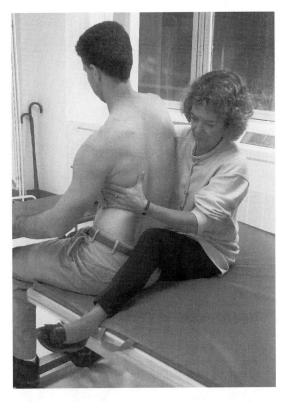

Figure 10-19 Mobilization of the lumbar spine into lateral flexion provides the patient with additional available range before the patient's active attempts to achieve and hold this position.

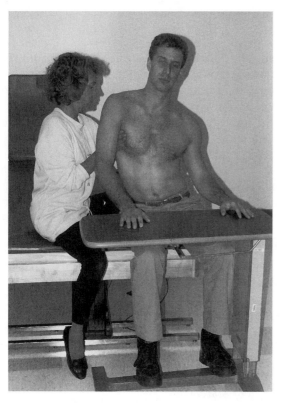

Figure 10-20   Lateral flexion, which occurs through activation of trunk extensors and flexors working together, can be facilitated with one hand under the patient's axilla and the other on the patient's lateral trunk, encouraging lengthening contractions on the weight-bearing side and shortening contractions on the non–weight-bearing side respectively.

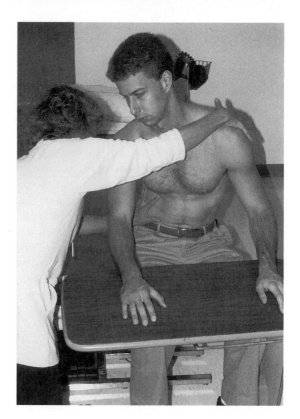

Figure 10-22   Trunk rotation can be facilitated through direct contact to the obliques with one hand while the other hand cues the opposite upper trunk with light pressure in a diagonal movement pattern.

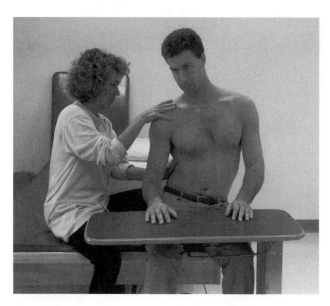

Figure 10-21   Light downward pressure on the shoulder encourages shortening of the trunk muscles on that side, thereby achieving lateral flexion of the trunk.

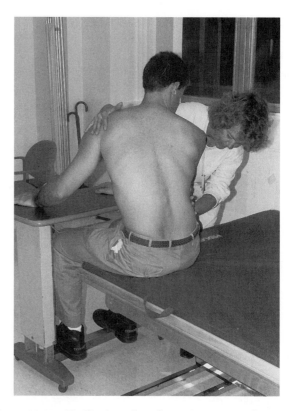

Figure 10-23   Facilitation of trunk rotation as viewed posteriorly.

tion.[11] Appropriate elongation of the trunk on the weight-bearing side and shortening on the non–weight-bearing side is required. This movement pattern is useful for a number of functional activities such as donning and doffing pants in a seated position. From a mobility perspective it allows the individual to approach the edge of a supporting surface to transfer.

Selected Problems

As indicated previously, problems with passive restriction in the trunk and the inability to activate trunk muscles selectively are of primary concern with this activity and may preclude the appropriate balance reactions needed for success and safety. The patient must have intact skin on the buttocks to practice scooting.

Treatment Strategies

Physical facilitation of scooting can be accomplished in a variety of ways, depending on the level of involvement of the individual. The desired movement pattern may be elicited through a series of contacts in which the therapist first facilitates a lateral weight shift and then places the hand on the patient's pelvis to stimulate forward advancing of the hip on the non–weight-bearing side.[11] The therapist then changes hands to facilitate forward movement of the opposite buttock (Figure 10-24). The pattern can be reversed to encourage weight shift backward onto the supporting surface. Patients requiring a less direct form of contact may "get the message" simply if the therapist provides some contact on the lateral aspects of their trunks that encourages rotary shift. Patients with more profound physical

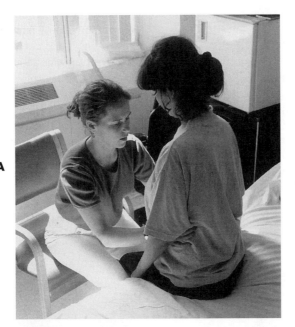

A

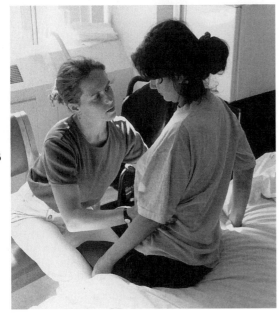

B

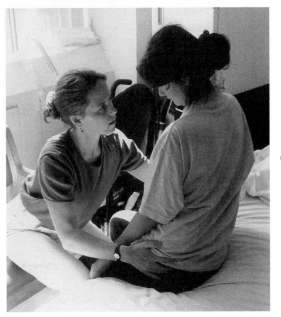

C

Figure 10-24 Scooting is an important skill for moving to the edge of a bed or seat and can be a useful movement pattern in activity of daily living tasks such as donning pants in a seated position. **A,** The patient begins in symmetric sitting. **B,** Scooting can be encouraged by first facilitating a lateral weight shift and then advancing the non–weight-bearing buttock to move anteriorly **(C).**

involvement may require added assistance by the therapist, particularly in advancing the buttock (Figure 10-25).

Transfers

Analysis of Movement

The ability to move from a given surface to an adjacent surface safely and efficiently is a primary goal in treatment for many of the patients with whom occupational therapists work. This maneuver requires enough forward flexion of the trunk over the feet to allow the individual to pivot about the feet and sit on the nearby surface.

Selected Problems

Patients with neglect who attempt to transfer often succeed in transporting only half the body onto the supporting surface. Additionally, the left foot may be neglected, and the patient may be oblivious to proper left foot placement before transferring.

Many patients require considerable help to maintain a flat foot on the floor. This may be because of unilateral inattention, poor sensation on the affected side, shortened trunk muscles resulting in asymmetric sitting, and shortening of the calf muscles on the affected side.

Treatment Strategies

Bobath[11] and Davies[26] describe the anterior weight shift that can be facilitated through contact on the patient's pelvis or scapulae. Carr and Shepherd[20] recognize the same forward weight shift and encourage patients to move the shoulders forward during active participation in transfers (Figure 10-26). All four therapists describe ways the therapist may use manual contact to the knee to draw the knee forward and encourage weight bearing on the hemiplegic side.

Patients have varying degrees of motor control for this activity. The therapist needs to create an environment in which the patient has enough guarding by the therapist to make training safe and enough "room" to try to make the transfer with as little assistance as possible. This is not always easy to do, and some patients inevitably require much assistance to transfer. However, the more the patient can be encouraged to do, the more the patient learns during the session. Consistent grading of the level of assistance a patient requires (i.e., minimal, moderate, maximal) is important in measuring progress and communicating to other staff members the amount of help required by the patient to carry out the task.

In the initial stages of transfer training a patient may require maximal assistance, and the therapist may need to clasp both hands around the pelvis to pivot the patient from one surface to another. As the patient gains greater strength and control over balance, this level of assistance may be reduced to a lighter hold around the pelvis and then the scapula.

Patients tend to be taught either stand-pivot or modified stand-pivot (squat pivot) transfers. Many therapists train stand-pivot transfers for the presumed benefits it affords in getting the patient into an upright position and putting full weight on the involved lower extremity. However, these transfers do not in any way resemble the maneuvers performed by normal subjects in moving from one

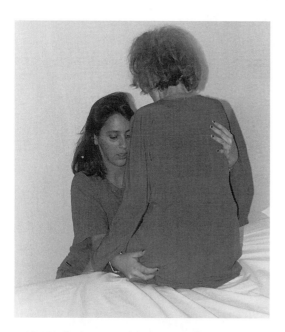

Figure 10-25 Patients requiring a more direct contact to scoot can be guided first by the therapist to advance the buttock.

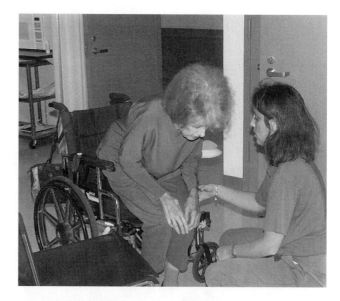

Figure 10-26 To teach a patient to perform a squat-pivot transfer, the therapist should encourage the appropriate amount of anterior weight shift by instructing the patient to move the shoulders forward.

surface to the other (i.e., coming to a full stand, turning and sitting down on an adjacent surface). As Shumway-Cook and Woollacott[76] point out, stand-pivot transfers may be more difficult because they do not allow the patient to use a momentum strategy; the need to come to a stand instead of pivoting blocks the benefits the momentum strategy provides.

Promoting weight shift onto the affected lower extremity is important during transfers and sit-to-stand activities. The therapist may position both knees around the patient's affected knee to facilitate forward weight shift onto the lower extremity and guard against buckling at the patient's knee. For patients requiring less cueing and guarding, the therapist may facilitate the knee by placing a hand on the patient's distal femur and gently pulling anteriorly and then down toward the floor as the patient takes weight on the leg.

The role of the arms in this training process has become somewhat controversial. Bobath[11] and Davies[26] support using clasped hands in front of the body to facilitate a forward weight shift, placing the arms on a stool, chair, or other supporting surface. However, a study by Carr and Gentile[18] examined the role of the upper extremities in sit-to-stand and determined that "fixing" the arms (by holding a rod as subjects in the study did) had a tendency to cause an increase in what was described as *extension force* (the force needed by the lower extremities to extend the body into an upright position) and a decrease in momentum of the body during sit-to-stand; this determination may have implications for transfers. The authors advocate that patients work on increasing strength in the lower extremities (particularly in extension) to enhance functioning in sit-to-stand. They contend that although patients tend to use the hands to push down on the armrests of a chair to stand or alternatively swing the arms forward to assist horizontal and vertical propulsion of the body mass, these strategies cannot be used in varying environmental conditions.[18]

Sit-to-Stand

Analysis of Movement

Sit-to-stand can be divided into different phases, depending on the description of the researcher (Figure 10-27). Shepherd and Gentile describe sit-to-stand using the terms *preextension phase*, a phase characterized by the beginning of the movement to the position in which the thighs are off the surface, and *extension phase*, the phase from the thighs-off position through the end of movement (full stand).[75] Shenkman[74] describes four phases in sit-to-stand (Figure 10-28). Phase I (Figure 10-29, *A*) is referred to as the *flexion momentum phase*; it is used to generate the initial momentum for rising. During this phase the center of mass (COM) is within the base of support (BOS), and eccentric contractions of the erector spinae are required to control forward motion of the trunk. Phase II (Figure 10-29, *B*) begins as the individual leaves the chair seat and ends at maximal ankle dorsiflexion. Forward momentum of the upper body is transferred to forward and upward momentum of the total body. The COM is now moving from within the BOS of the chair to the feet. It is by definition an unstable phase and requires coactivation of hip and knee extensors. Phase III (Figure 10-29, *C*) is an extension phase during which the body rises to its full upright position by extension of the hips and knees. The stability requirements are not as great as in Phase II because the COM is well within the BOS of the feet. Phase IV (Figure 10-29, *D*) is a stabilization phase in which complete extension of the hips and knees occurs. Regardless of the way researchers divide the task, an appreciation of the biomechanics of this movement pattern is crucial in training and understanding potential problems that occur in hemiplegia.

Selected Problems

As mentioned in the previous section, patients may have difficulty maintaining their feet flat on the floor because of

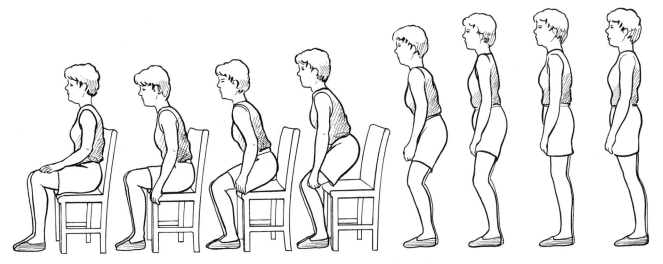

Figure 10-27 Sit-to-stand viewed laterally.

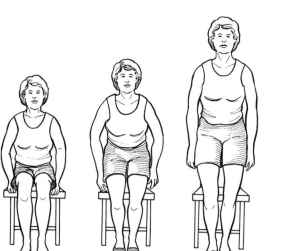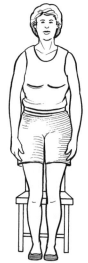

Figure 10-28 Sit-to-stand viewed anteriorly.

poor sensation, unilateral inattention, or shortening of the trunk and calf muscles.

Difficulties with spatial relations and praxis have been noted during transfer training, regardless of whether the therapist is training pivot transfers or sit-to-stand. Certain patients lean backward instead of forward while the therapist is attempting to transfer. These patients' actions are somewhat unpredictable and often run counter to those expected after instruction from the therapist.

As Arnadottir has noted, transfers also reveal problems with organizing and sequencing and conditions such as ideational apraxia. These problems may become evident when a patient attempting to rise from bed omits the appropriate steps of handling the bedclothes in preparation to transfer (see Chapter 13).[4]

Motor impersistence, a term first introduced by Fisher[29] to describe failure to persist at various tasks such as eye closure, breath holding, conjugate gaze, and tongue protrusion may explain some patients' inabilities to persevere with certain tasks such as transfers, sit-to-stand, and ambulation. These patients tend to collapse midway through the task, sometimes without warning, and reduced muscle strength, per se, does not appear to be the cause. Impersistence, in most studies, has been found to correlate more with right-hemisphere lesions than with left-hemisphere lesions.[29,46]

Treatment Strategies

Bobath[11] describes the need to begin training patients in sit-to-stand from a fairly high seat (Figure 10-30, *A*), progressing gradually to lower seats or a plinth (Figure 10-30, *B*). Other studies have substantiated her assertion such as the one concluding that high-surface chairs can significantly decrease the joint ranges of motion needed at the hip and knee, making rising from a higher chair much less stressful than rising from a lower chair.[17]

Stretching the arms forward also is recommended by

Bobath[11] and Davies[26] in practicing sit-to-stand. As mentioned previously, Carr and Gentile maintain that normal trunk flexion is accompanied by some arm flexion; fixing the arms in specific positions during the activity may actually prove detrimental to the normal movement pattern.[18] Encouraging weight bearing on the affected leg by pulling the knee forward also is emphasized. Bobath,[11] Davies,[26] and Carr and shepherd[19] all agree on the need to practice intermediate stages and sitting down by reversing the sequence.

Facilitation of the distal femur by the therapist to promote appropriate weight bearing on the affected lower extremity is recommended here as it is for transfer training. In Figure 10-31 (see p. 231) the therapist's handling provides a lot of stability for this patient. In Figure 10-32 (see p. 232) the therapist needs only to cue the patient through the distal femur to get the desired response.

Carr and Shepherd and Gentile have conducted studies clarifying the role of the trunk, arms, and feet in sit-to-stand.[18,75] Many implications can be drawn from these studies, including the importance of training patients to go from sit-to-stand by actively flexing the trunk, using momentum to swing the trunk forward, decreasing contracture of the calf muscles, and practicing from a higher-than-normal seat initially. Carr and Shepherd, through their extensive study of motor learning and control, have emphasized the importance of task-specific training, structured practice outside therapy sessions, correct feedback about performance, and a way to quantify and challenge performance.[19] A system for training sit-to-stand in which a gradual lowering of the seat occurs is considered beneficial because it provides a form of progressive resistive exercise that improves muscle strength and control in a task-specific activity.[18]

Because getting the feet back and under in sit-to-stand is so important, training patients to move to the edge of

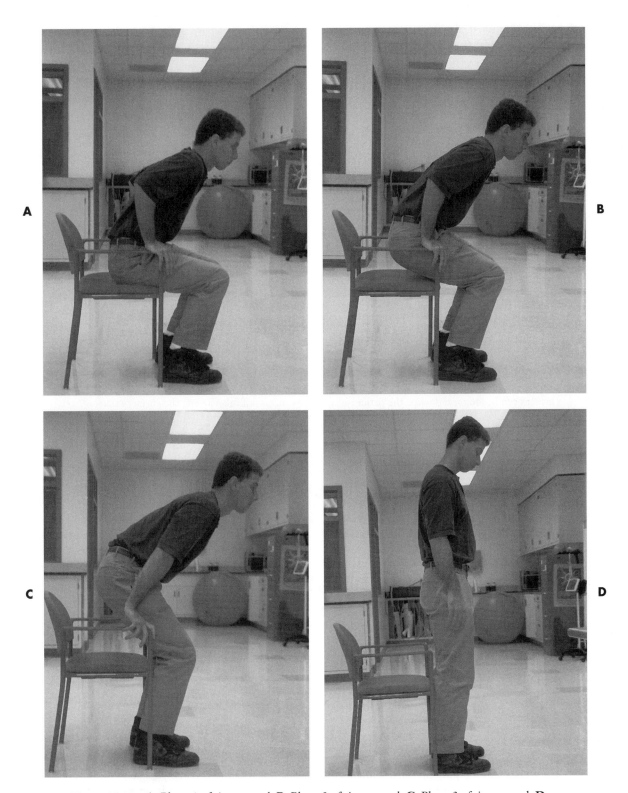

Figure 10-29 **A,** Phase 1 of sit-to-stand. **B,** Phase 2 of sit-to-stand. **C,** Phase 3 of sit-to-stand. **D,** Phase 4 of sit-to-stand.

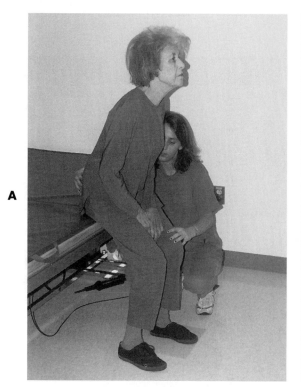
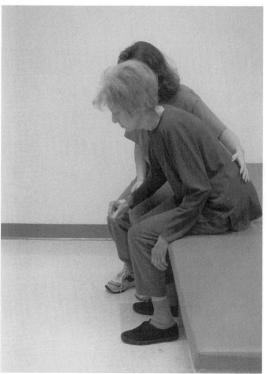

Figure 10-30 **A,** During the initial stages of learning, patients may find standing from a high surface easier. Among other things this provides the patient with a feeling of success. **B,** Lower surfaces can be attempted when the patient has become more skillful. Varying the surfaces that patients practice standing from is important to promote learning and enables the patient to cope with varying situations that arise in the "real world."

the supporting surface to allow for this is necessary. Afterward, forward flexion of the trunk to bring the COM over the BOS can occur. A patient who attempts to stand without doing this is set up for a tremendous struggle or failure (Figure 10-33).

Normal subjects frequently use a momentum strategy in mobility skills as a way to move with less energy requirements and hence with greater efficiency. It is frequently used in rising from bed, and no cessation of movement occurs. The momentum strategy can be used in a modified way with appropriate patients who have sustained CVA because it allows them to use the force generated by forward flexion to take them into an upright position. They then need adequate stability when their thighs are off the supporting surface to prevent them from falling forward. Momentum provides the patient with an efficient ability to move but by definition requires an ability to control for stability in its execution; patients with poor trunk control or marked cognitive impairments are not candidates for using such a strategy. When introducing the momentum strategy in therapy, the therapist must adequately guard the patient from falling.

ACTIVITIES IN STANDING

Analysis of Movement

The ability to stand is a goal many patients with hemiplegia want to achieve because the drive to be upright is very strong. Patients should be provided the opportunity to practice standing and shifting their centers of gravity in all directions and reaching for functional objects in the environment. The trunk responses needed for controlled sitting (i.e., selective lengthening and shortening depending on the requirements of the task) also are needed for controlled standing; however, these trunk responses are carried out over a much narrower base of support.

Selected Problems

Standing may prove challenging for patients with severe hemiplegia who have only one side of the body available to use for movement; moving with one half of the body is stressful work. The slow, laborious effort of standing and attempting to move in this position causes an increase in posturing and skeletal muscle activity. Movements are often lacking in spontaneity and must occur at a conscious level for the patient. Postural deviations noted in sitting in

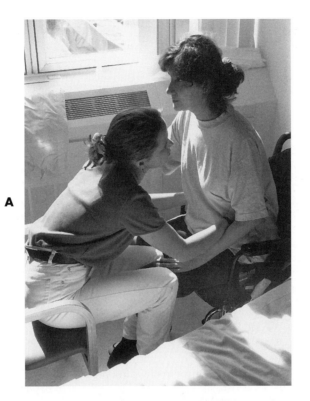

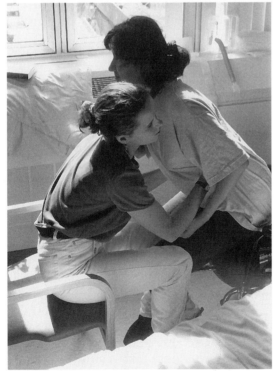

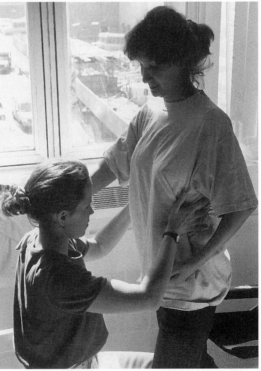

Figure 10-31 **A,** The therapist promotes weight bearing on the patient's affected lower extremity in sit-to-stand by placing the knees around the patient's affected knee, drawing the patient forward **(B),** and discouraging "buckling" when the patient achieves the standing position **(C).**

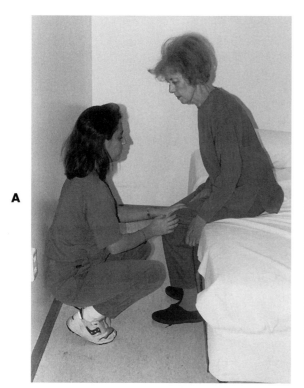
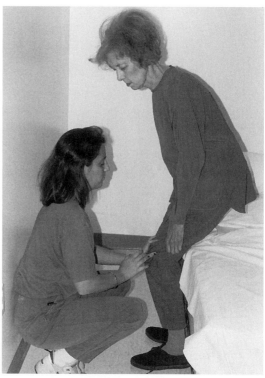

Figure 10-32 Patients with greater motor control may still require some facilitation to equalize the weight bearing between the lower extremities if they have a tendency to stand up using their unaffected side more than the other. **A,** The therapist places the hand on the distal femur of the affected lower extremity, draws the knee anteriorly, and then applies downward pressure as the patient comes to stand **(B).**

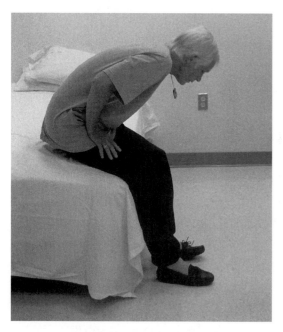

Figure 10-33 Foot placement is important in sit-to-stand. Note how far forward this individual's feet are as he attempts to stand.

these patients become even more exaggerated in standing. The patient who "fixes" the upper limb must stay upright while sitting because fixes even more in the struggle to stay upright on two feet.

Treatment Strategies

As stated previously, standing as early as possible if medical clearance is permitted is ideal for patients. Standing helps increase the patient's level of arousal and can be quite motivating. Bobath,[11] Davies,[26] and Carr and Shepherd[20] emphasize the need to help the patient stand so that body segments are properly aligned and weight is accepted through the affected lower extremity. For some patients, accomplishing this requires all of their attention and energy. Therefore the therapist should be mindful of the need (at least initially) to train the patient to stand and take weight on the affected lower extremity in a quiet, minimally distracting environment. This may be even more critical for patients with attention disorders manifesting as distractibility, impulsivity, and irritability with increased stimulation. As noted earlier, the need to incorporate competing stimuli into therapy gradually must be considered in treatment; otherwise the therapist cannot assert that functional balance has been achieved.

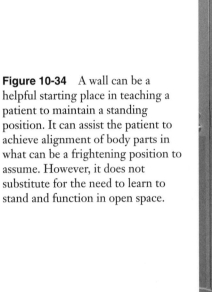
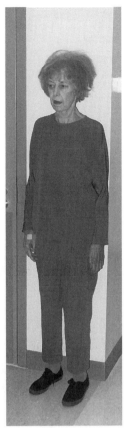

Figure 10-34 A wall can be a helpful starting place in teaching a patient to maintain a standing position. It can assist the patient to achieve alignment of body parts in what can be a frightening position to assume. However, it does not substitute for the need to learn to stand and function in open space.

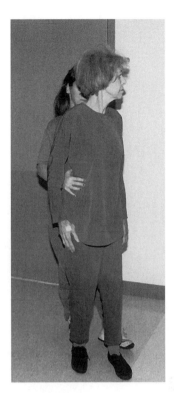

Figure 10-35 The therapist facilitates weight shifting in standing while encouraging the patient to scan the environment. Standing and looking around a room can prove challenging for patients in the initial stages of learning to stand.

Achieving weight shift in standing requires a substantial amount of cueing by the therapist, because patients often are fearful of standing on the affected leg because of reduced muscle strength, postural control, and sensation. Visual disturbances also may make standing a frightening activity for the patient.

Initially, the use of a wall (Figure 10-34) may be desirable to offer the patient substantial support; however, this should not be used to train functional reach in standing because postural muscle activity in the legs is reduced (with the help of the wall) when the patient makes an arm movement. A manually guided approach is useful to help the patient learn the desired end point of the movement pattern. Contact by the therapist directly on the pelvis (with one hand on each side) offers optimal control to guide the weight shift, and the therapist can gradually taper the amount of guidance required as the patient begins to activate more.

Free-standing balance should be attempted as soon as possible (see Chapter 5). Standing while simultaneously scanning the environment or having a conversation with the therapist is challenging and meaningful (Figure 10-35).

A progression to standing and reaching prepares the patient to be able to perform personal self-care and instrumental activities of daily living safely and efficiently in a standing position. Reaching in all directions in functional environments needs to be practiced (Figure 10-36). As Carr and Shepherd[20] have outlined, this should include reaching overhead, to the side, back, and down, progressing to unilateral and bilateral reaching to the floor. Recent research has demonstrated that the pattern of postural muscle activity in response to postural adjustments can be modified by training. This finding suggests the need for task-specific training to ensure the patient has a broad repertoire at hand when confronted with solving a movement problem in standing.

A commonly held view about asymmetric hemiparetic gait is that it may be subject to amelioration by balance training emphasizing weight bearing on the paretic lower extremity. However, a study by Winstein et al[87] in which hemiparetic subjects received specific balance training with a specially designed feedback device revealed that balance in standing may be improved but no carry-over into a more symmetric gait pattern occurs. This suggests that skill acquisition has a task-specific nature, and therapists cannot assume progress achieved in one skill area can be carried over or transferred to another. This finding calls into question many commonly held beliefs about the use of developmental progression to increase functional capabilities in upright positions. The effect of the environment

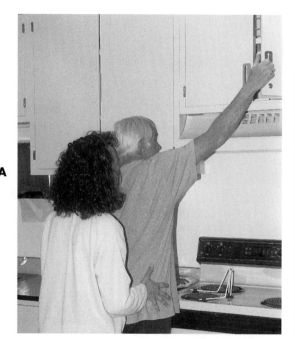

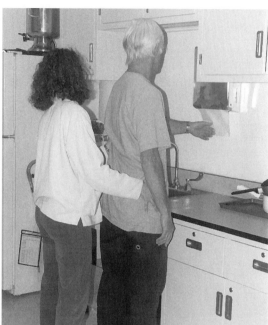

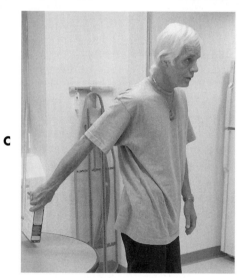

Figure 10-36 Training weight shifting and reaching in standing should occur within a functional context because task-specific training is most beneficial to the learner. Reaching up **(A)**, forward **(B)**, and backward **(C)**.

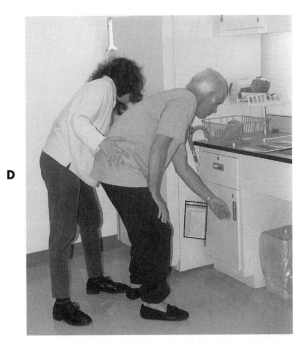 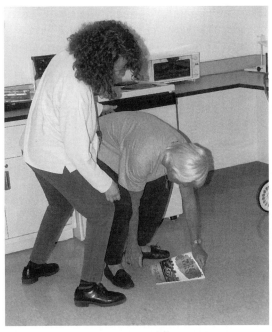

Figure 10-36, cont'd   Reaching down (**D**) and toward the floor (**E**). These patterns (**A** through **E**) are among the many patterns of movement that should be practiced within functional activities. Occupational therapists are uniquely qualified with their expertise in task analysis to train patients to perform basic and instrumental activities of daily living in standing.

on postural control has been explored increasingly in the motor learning literature, but research has typically been done on the able-bodied population. A study conducted by Abreu[1] examined the effect of environmental predictability on postural control after stroke. This study was conducted with subjects in a seated position; findings revealed that an unpredictable environmental model facilitated a more stable response from patients than the response seen with a predictable environment.[1] These findings challenge the assumption that therapy is best conducted in an undemanding environment. Abreu hypothesizes that the interaction between postural control systems and information processing systems is complex and requires significant exploration if therapists are to be successful in matching patients and tasks.[1]

Shumway-Cook and Woollacott[76] also note that although researchers have been painstakingly studying the biomechanical aspects of transfers, a paucity of information on the perceptual strategies used for these activities is available. Mulder et al[58] describe human beings as "biological problem-solving machines." They see no separation among motor, perceptual, and cognitive systems in the performance of movement problem solving. They describe the nervous system as a flexible, plastic, self-organizing entity. After injury the spontaneity under which it functions is lost. Mulder et al[58] carried out a series of experiments with amputees in which they studied balance by measuring postural sway. They note that these subjects, when given

the STROOP test while trying to maintain balance, displayed an increase in postural sway. They concluded that a dual-task world is the environment in which rehabilitation must take place, not the structured, unidimensional laboratory. Mulder et al[58] also assert that human movement studies should include more than isolated motor output and must examine the interaction between cognitive and sensory aspects of a task. Their conclusions have far-reaching implications for occupational therapists, whose primary role is to train patients in functional activities. Their dual-task paradigm[58] is a useful guide in standing activities because the patient is challenged to develop skill and not merely stand and think only of maintaining balance. This behavior is hardly functional and must be borne in mind as therapists label patients "independent" in these activities (see Chapter 5).

ADJUNCTIVE TECHNIQUES TO ENHANCE SKILL ACQUISITION

Feedback

Although encouragement of patients is important in the rehabilitation process and should not be eliminated, therapists must consider the relevance of feedback to the learning process and not confuse the two. Therapists are often too liberal in their use of feedback with patients, using the guiding principle of "more feedback is better" and that feedback facilitates learning.

In her review of this topic, Winstein[86] provides research findings indicating that less information feedback creates a better learning environment and probably forces the learner to develop problem-solving strategies. A great deal of research is being conducted on normal, healthy individuals in this area, and although the findings may prove applicable to the areas in which occupational therapists work, they have yet to be tested on patient populations who have sustained CVA and should be approached with some caution on the part of the therapist.

Gentile describes two kinds of augmented feedback an instructor can provide to learners[31]:

1. Knowledge of performance, defined as knowledge of information about movement
2. Knowledge of results, defined as knowledge of information about the performer-environment interaction

She goes on to suggest that the task's demands best dictate the most efficacious form of feedback. Activities that can be characterized according to the taxonomy of tasks as closed and consistent motion tasks require information about the movement to be transmitted from the instructor to the learner. For example, when training a patient in rolling over in bed or achieving sit-to-stand from a wheelchair, the provision of feedback about placement of the extremities and maintenance of alignment is useful. Tasks that can be categorized as open and variable motionless tasks according to the taxonomy of tasks by definition are subject to changing environmental conditions, and therefore feedback to the learner should focus on incorporation of environmental factors into the approach used and selection of movement strategy and pattern.[31] For example, standing up while on a bus requires anticipation of the bus's motion, movement of people in the immediate environment, and consideration of changing space constraints.

Many therapists videotape patients to provide information on performance and show and measure improvement in skill. This can prove useful, particularly with patients who may lack awareness about their performance.

Modeling

Recently some research in motor learning has been dedicated to the effects of modeling in teaching motor skill. However, the physical rehabilitation literature contains no published research studies examining the use of modeling and its effects on physically disabled adults during training in activities of daily living and mobility skills. Nevertheless, modeling is used frequently in rehabilitation settings to promote skill acquisition is self-care, transfers, walking, and wheelchair mobility. Therapists often use themselves and other patients as models. In addition, they use drawings, photographs, and videotapes to enhance motor performance. However, the most efficacious forms of modeling have yet to be explored with this population.

The viability of modeling as a topic for motor behavior researchers, however, has been well documented in the literature. Much of this research has been based on Bandura's social learning theory of modeling.[6] Bandura claims that modeling is not only a fundamental means of modifying existing behavior patterns but also is extremely important to the acquisition of new modes of behavior.[6] McCullagh et al[52] note that Bandura's original theory was actually designed for the acquisition and modification of social skills and behaviors, and motor learning researchers originally did not adopt this model, speculating that theories of motor skill acquisition would not be congruent with it. However, a shift in thinking in this area occurred in the 1980s, and many researchers are now examining the role visual demonstrations play in providing information to the observer before the action.[52] An integral component of Bandura's model is the concept of the formation of a cognitive representation by the observer viewing the model.[6] Understanding the nature of this cognitive representation is important in conceptualizing the way the modeling process aids or hinders the observer.

Research has shown that observers, even using nonhuman models, are capable of extrapolating accurate relative motion features needed to execute an action. Johansson[41] used point-light techniques in his research to demonstrate that observers differentiate human walking from wooden puppet walking. Scully and Newell[72] also carried out investigation using point-light models in which observers accurately perceived and judged the way gymnastic routines were executed. Accurate models, even point-light models, enhance response recognition in observers.[72] These studies support the importance of viewing the relative motion pattern of an action. Knowledge of the kinematics of an action is crucial in evaluating the way in which the movement is performed. Newell and Walter[60] have suggested in their study of modeling that in the initial stages of learning, the coordination function of a motor task is the strategy to be learned, that is, the kinematics of the action. The speed of the movement (scalar value) is learned in later stages with practice. This indicates that in the initial stages of learning, relative motion patterns must be provided in the demonstration.[60] These findings support the use of visual aids such as the therapist providing a movement pattern or videos of subjects practicing sit-to-stand, giving a gross kinematic view of the movement pattern to the patient. Therapists may infer from this that drawings and stick figures providing the correct angle of body parts in relation to one another may be useful.

The nature of the relationship between observer and model has long been considered an important variable in influencing the modeling process. In a study of the effects of attraction toward a model and the model's competence in adult imitative behavior, Baron[7] studied 48 subjects and manipulated attraction by varying the apparent degree of attitude similarity between subject and model. A high level of attraction toward the model facilitated imitation when the model was successful in performing the task but interfered with imitation when the model was unsuccessful.[7] Likewise, in a study by McCullagh et al,[52] similar findings were noted. She observed that subjects performed better after watching models they perceived to be similar to themselves than they did after watching models they perceived as dissimilar to themselves.[52]

These findings suggest that using a model similar to the patient in disability, gender, and age for teaching purposes may be a crucial variable in training success. Many rehabilitation centers have group activities aimed at teaching transfer skills with this in mind. Group members do not just support each other psychologically in the rehabilitation process, they provide optimal role models for a patient relearning basic self-care skills. Additionally, such models can provide feedback and suggestions during the learning process.

Mental Imagery

Mental imagery has been employed as a research treatment modality to enhance the rate of motor skill acquisition and improve skill accuracy. The literature to date suggests that imagery depicting successful task outcomes may be more effective in enhancing performance than imagery involving only mental rehearsal of motor activity.[88]

Studies by Meyers et al[53] confirmed the hypothesis most coaches have maintained: the effects on performance of mental activity can degrade or enhance performance. Occupational therapists should consider increasing the use of this clearly potent modality to improve their patients' performance in functional mobility tasks.

Manual Guidance

Manual guidance is a somewhat controversial subject because therapists often feel they cannot possibly begin to teach patients new movement skills without either helping them to "feel" the appropriate movement pattern or assisting the patient into the desired position. Too much handling encourages the patient not to be active and obviously runs counter to expectations desired in therapy. Selective use of hands-on support is obviously the more expedient approach to take, and therapists must become aware when their hands interfere with the active learning process that needs to take place for patients to develop skills.

EVALUATION TOOLS

Bobath[11] devised an evaluation tool for use with the adult hemiplegic patient that progressed from simple to more selective movement patterns with an emphasis on the quality of movement patterns executed by the patient. This assessment strictly looks at the quality of movement and balance reactions and does not address the way a patient carries out specific functional mobility activities. Rather it targets the places where movements may contribute to difficulty with the normal execution of mobility tasks. It is thorough in this regard but takes a long time to administer and is not standardized.

Currently the only standardized evaluation for mobility skills is Carr and Shepherd's Motor Assessment Scale for Stroke Patients (MAS). This test assesses eight areas:

1. Supine to sidelying
2. Supine to sitting over side of bed
3. Balanced sitting
4. Sitting to standing
5. Walking
6. Upper arm function
7. Hand movements
8. Advanced hand activities

The advantages of the MAS include the following:

1. It tests recovery specific for the patient recovering from CVA.
2. It takes less time to administer and infringes on little treatment time.
3. It is simple to administer and has objective and clear descriptions of criteria for rating patients.
4. It is sensitive to changes in patients' motor recovery status and therefore useful in describing patient progress over time.

The Functional Independence Measure (FIM) was developed by the Uniform Data System at the State University of New York (SUNY) at Buffalo as a standardized way for professionals to evaluate patient progress regarding levels of assistance needed to perform personal self-care, functional mobility, communication, cognition, and social interaction. Each area is graded on a one-to-seven scale, with a score of one indicating total dependence and seven complete independence. The areas of functional mobility covered in this test include transfers to bed, chair, and toilet and tub and locomotion and stairs. This test is used in rehabilitation centers across the United States and has been found to have good to excellent reliability.[33,34]

The Assessment of Motor and Process Skills (AMPS) is a standardized test created by occupational therapists that simultaneously evaluates motor and process skills to predict impact on the ability to perform instrumental activities of daily living. Such an evaluation tool, if developed for personal self-care and functional mobility skills, would prove invaluable for occupational therapists (see Chapter 15).

ANTICIPATING CHANGING ENVIRONMENTS

The ultimate goal of functional mobility retraining is to have the patient resume the roles and activities associated with the lifestyle before the CVA. This goal presumes that patients need to transfer reacquired mobility skills to environments unique to the individual lifestyle. The treatment setting presents a predictable environment in which the physical aspects of therapeutic equipment and furnishings remain unchanged from one treatment session to another. The patient's home environment also may be viewed as fairly predictable because of the patient's familiarity with the surroundings. The physical layout and home furnishings change little over time, even if home modifications are introduced. Nevertheless, therapists frequently observe problems as the patient attempts to make the transition from the treatment setting to the home environment. Unexpected problems occur within the closed home environment and community-based activities challenge the individual's ability to solve newly encountered problems. The occupational therapist is well qualified to address these dilemmas through task analysis of performance areas and careful consideration of the environmental contexts in which each task is performed.[68] The patient recovering from CVA is required to generalize and adapt mobility skills learned in the clinic setting to meet the changing environmental demands encountered on discharge. This generalization and adaptation occurs through the interaction among multiple systems: perceptual, cognitive, sensory, and motor. Earlier in this chapter, specific strategies for ameliorating performance component deficits influencing functional mobility were presented. These strategies should be incorporated throughout the intervention process as a means to attain generalization. (See Chapter 2 for a review of the issues associated with the learning process.)

Strategy Development

The research examining normal movement sequences has found great variety in the movement patterns used to perform each mobility task. A single pattern may be identified as occurring more frequently during rolling, although many subjects use alternative patterns that are equally effective. Similarly the methods described to retrain patients to roll over also vary. No single correct strategy is available to achieve this mobility task. Strategy development is more than learning to use a normal pattern of movement; it results from the patient's exploration of movement possibilities in relation to tasks occurring in different environments.[76] Thus the occupational therapist may use several methods of instruction while assisting the patient in learning movement limitations and determining future mobility potentials.[68,76] The two primary strategies for functional mobility include a force control strategy and a momentum strategy.[24] Early in the intervention process, patients may benefit from instruction in a force control strategy to prevent secondary impairments of fixations and resultant development of inappropriate compensatory strategies.[11,20,25,26] This method of instruction also is preferred for patients who do not have adequate stability of the trunk musculature because it may facilitate independent performance.[20] A momentum strategy or a combina-

tion of momentum and force control may be introduced if stability of the trunk is evident. Momentum is more efficient, requires less muscular activity, and approximates more normal-looking movement.

Not all patients are able to achieve a momentum strategy, but many patients may attempt to do so on their own in the home environment, particularly if it was their preferred method of movement before the CVA. Therapists need to anticipate this possibility and explore momentum as an alternative before discharge. Transition from a force control to a momentum strategy requires simple, concise instruction to move quickly without stopping the movement. The therapist may use manual cues at the shoulder girdle to ensure safety. Demonstration by the therapist also is helpful. The practice of momentum strategies also may prepare the patient to control movement during stressful life situations that occur unexpectedly and require quick transitional movements.

Practice Conditions

To prepare the patient to resume the previous lifestyle, the occupational therapist must carefully consider the conditions under which practice takes place. The goal of intervention is to maximize retention and transfer of acquired skills to everyday life situations the patient will encounter.[40] The therapist must increase the demands of the learning context during practice to prepare the patient to respond to unpredictable events. Chapter 2 presented an overview of factors the therapist considers when structuring the practice conditions in stroke rehabilitation. The following are considerations specific to functional mobility retraining.

Blocked and Random Practice

Blocked practice in functional mobility retraining is the rote practice of mobility functions in sequence. For example, the patient initially practices rolling to the unaffected side, then to the affected side, then to the seated position. Repetition of experiences and a degree of mastery must occur at each level before the patient proceeds to the next level of skill. This method of structuring practice may initially assist the patient in gaining proficiency during the practice session but is not effective in preparing the patient to engage in self-care tasks in which changes in the body's position occur randomly in response to task requirements. For example, the patient rolls to the left to reach for a brush on the table; it is just beyond reach. The patient rolls back to supine and assumes a bridge position, pushing upward in bed. The patient then rolls again and is able to grasp the brush. Random practice of mobility tasks improves learning, retention, and the ability to solve motor problems encountered in life situations.[73] Schmidt[70] recommends that randomized practice be incorporated throughout the intervention process. Mobility tasks should be interspersed with other tasks such as activity of daily living training in which transitional movements must be made in a natural context. The trial-and-error exploration of functional mobility in this context may initially prove difficult for the patient. Progress may be slow, and the therapist may be tempted to instruct the patient in a single movement strategy to speed progress. Varying the practice conditions increases the contextual interference, facilitating generalization as the patient relies on multiple processes and promoting the development of versatile motor strategies.[40,80]

Schmidt notes one exception in which a part-to-whole method of practice may be beneficial. Early in the intervention process, when the patient is acquiring foundational skills, practicing of component movements may be necessary. For example, the patient may initially need to gain control of lateral flexion of neck and trunk muscles before these movements can be incorporated into the sidelying-to-sit sequence. Schmidt suggests that as soon as patients are able to perform these component movements they should immediately be integrated into programs emphasizing random practice.[70] This method of practice can only be used with mobility functions that are readily divided into natural component parts.[71,86]

Varying the Practice Conditions for Specific Tasks

Chapter 2 introduced Gentile's taxonomy of motor tasks, which is useful for determining the most appropriate practice conditions for each mobility task. Objects, people, and the spatial temporal characteristics of each task all influence the motor strategies selected.[31,32] Sabari suggests that the occupational therapy process inherently considers the importance of the regulatory conditions to task performance. Occupational therapists frequently adapt and regulate the environment to facilitate mobility functions, as in adjusting the height of a bed in preparation for a transfer. Similarly, the amount of verbal cues and physical assistance is adjusted to foster independent performance and skill development. Sabari also directs attention to the crucial role occupational therapists assume as regulators throughout mobility retraining.[68]

Closed Tasks

Early in the treatment process, most functional mobility tasks may be considered closed, and the environmental features are easily regulated to improve performance. Rolling over and coming to a seated position in a hospital bed occurs on a stationary surface. The therapist can further regulate the environment by positioning pillows and bed linens appropriately, raising the bed guard rails, adjusting the height of the bed, limiting the number of people moving around the patient's bed, and positioning the body in a fairly static position to assist the patient if needed. Another important characteristic of a closed task is that movement is self-paced and no temporal constraints are placed.

The therapist's role as a regulator can be equated with the degree of assistance or handling provided. The therapist may initially give significant physical assistance and use a variety of adjunctive techniques to promote perceptual, cognitive, and sensory processing. As the patient regains control of movements in desired sequences, physical assistance and the amount of cueing is gradually reduced or eliminated.[68]

Variable Motionless Tasks

Bed mobility becomes a variable motionless task if the therapist is not present to regulate certain features of the environment. Patients preparing to get out of bed independently may find the pillows and bed linens in disarray, making movement difficult; the bed guard rails are lowered, the top of the bed remains slightly elevated, and the height of the bed may be too high. Simultaneously the patient may be receiving verbal encouragement to "hurry up." Without the therapist present to structure the environment, the patient may experience difficulty and may use compensatory strategies incompatible with the restoration of performance component deficits. The patient may hook the unaffected leg under the affected leg and use the hands to pull up to a seated position.

This comparison illustrates the way overstructuring the environment does not prepare the patient recovering from stroke to develop flexible motor strategies. The patient needs to have opportunities to process information and acquire the ability to solve future problems.[1,70] Abreu studied the effects of environmental regulation on postural control and found that unpredictable environments elicited improved control. These findings are contrary to beliefs occupational therapists have held concerning the grading of tasks from simple to complex and the structuring of environments from predictable to unpredictable.[2] Abreu postulates that the results of this study indicate both types of environments should be incorporated concurrently in the intervention process.[1] The therapist may regulate the environment but not on all trials. Perhaps the height of the bed is adjusted and the guard rails elevated on one trial, whereas the next session may require the patient to instruct the therapist verbally in the arrangement of the immediate surroundings in preparation for the mobility task.

Consistent Motion Tasks

During consistent motion tasks the pace of the environment remains the same and the environment moves. These tasks are associated with mechanical devices such as conveyor belts. Most functional mobility tasks do not meet this criterion.

Open Tasks

Many advanced mobility skills meet the criterion of an open task in which both the spatial and temporal parameters of movement are determined by events occurring in the environment. Open tasks require more precise timing of movement, and the patient is challenged to anticipate and react to unexpected events. Sit-to-stand on a moving train, plane, or bus are all examples of open tasks. Practice of these tasks should occur in the actual environment whenever possible.[39,68] Patients who are physically capable of attempting these advanced skills should be engaged in them while in the rehabilitation setting whenever possible.

Patients who do not have adequate foundational skills while hospitalized can benefit from interventions to improve future potential for the acquisition of advanced mobility skills. Patients need to be introduced to unpredictable environments in which they have the opportunity to explore movement strategies and develop problem-solving abilities. Early in the intervention process the therapist's handling techniques to prepare and assist the patient can be modulated using different degrees of tactile, proprioceptive, and kinesthetic input as the patient engages in functional mobility tasks. For example, as the patient learns to transfer, the therapist can vary the sensory cues and amount of assistance.[9] Responding to changes in sensory input may be helpful in the development of anticipatory postural adjustments (see Chapter 2).[76]

SUMMARY

The performance of functional mobility tasks should not occur in isolation, as in a gross mobility mat program. Practice of mobility skills while the patient is engaged in life tasks presents opportunities to solve unexpected problems that arise as the patient manipulates different objects and encounters changing support surfaces and changing temporal demands. The following are some suggestions for altering the regulatory features in the clinical environment.

Rolling

- Practice rolling on a narrow surface such as a sofa.
- Encourage abrupt change in direction, as in reversing the movement in midstream.
- Practice rolling under a heavy quilt.
- Try rolling with an object such as a newspaper in the hand.
- Attempt propping to sidelying to adjust pillows.
- Practice rolling in a darkened room.

Sidelying-to-Sit

- Attempt sidelying-to-sit with an immediate reach pattern.
- Practice sidelying-to-sit on a narrow surface.
- Try modifying the sequence to get out of a chaise lounge chair.
- Practice sidelying-to-sit on a soft surface such as a sofa.

Sit-to-Stand

- Use varying seat surfaces:
  Chair with arms
  Chair without arms
  Reclining chair with a significant seat depth
  Aluminum patio chair
  Side of the sofa
  Middle of the sofa
  Chair with wheels such as a desk chair
  Stool
  Swivel chair
  Dentist chair
  Chair in theater or stadium
- Incorporate varying standing surfaces:
  Different textures of carpet
  Linoleum
  Tile floor
  Grass
  Concrete
- Include varying speed of movement.
- Account for varying objects and pets in the environment.
- Incorporate changing lighting.
- Attempt holding various objects:
  Coat
  Briefcase
  Shopping bag
- Relearn turning right and left.

REVIEW QUESTIONS

1. What impact does the patient's place in the life cycle have on planning relevant treatment in functional mobility retraining?
2. What impact does damage to the right hemisphere have on functional mobility skills?
3. How does a lack of awareness of disability differ from denial and what are the implications of lack of awareness for functional mobility retraining?
4. How can the tactile-kinesthetic approach (such as the Affolter approach) be incorporated into treatment with a patient with apraxia?
5. What is the force control strategy?
6. What are the three major task requirements for locomotion that can be applied to all functional mobility tasks?
7. According to Mohr, what are the four areas of focus to assess in trunk control?
8. What three possible interventions can be used to maximize a patient's ability to achieve lateral trunk flexion?
9. What is the pusher syndrome?
10. What implications for treatment may be derived from the research done by Carr, Shepherd, and Gentile on sit-to-stand?
11. How can Mulder's dual-task paradigm be incorporated into occupational therapy interventions?
12. How can the therapist structure the practice of functional mobility tasks, considering the venue of care?

■ COTA Considerations ■

- Evaluate and treat mobility deficits in multiple settings using a variety of support surfaces (e.g., chair with arms, stool, recliner, couch, mat, bench).
- Note the way deficits in a variety of performance components can have an impact on a patient's ability to perform mobility tasks independently.
- Consider environmental adaptations that assist a patient in performing mobility tasks (grab bars, bed rails).
- Recognize the way the general population uses a variety of movement patterns during mobility tasks.
- Describe the way control of the trunk is crucial to efficient performance of mobility tasks.

REFERENCES

1. Abreu BC: The effect of environmental regulations on postural control after stroke, *Am J Occup Ther* 49:517, 1995.
2. Abreu BC, Toglia JP: Cognitive rehabilitation: a model for occupational therapy, *Am J Occup Ther* 45:439, 1987.
3. American Occupational Therapy Association: Uniform terminology for occupational therapy, *Am J Occup Ther* 48:1047, 1994.
4. Arnadottir G: Neurobehavioral deficits related to cortical dysfunction. In Arnadottir G, editor: *The brain and behavior: assessing cortical dysfunction through activities of daily living*, St Louis, 1990, Mosby.
5. Astrom M, Adolfsson R, Asplund K: Major depression in stroke patients: a 3-year longitudinal study, *Stroke* 24:976, 1993.
6. Bandura A: *Principles of behavior modification*, New York, 1969, Holt, Rinehart, and Winston.
7. Baron RA: Attraction toward the model and model's competence as determinants of adult imitative behavior, *J Pers Soc Psychol* 4:345, 1970.
8. Bernstein N: *The coordination and regulation of movement*, Elmsford, NY, 1967, Pergamon.
9. Bly L: What is the role of sensation in motor learning? What is the role of feedback and feedforward? *NDTA Network* 5:5, 1996.
10. Bobath B: *Adult hemiplegia: evaluation and treatment*, ed 2, London, 1978, Heineman.
11. Bobath B: *Adult hemiplegia: evaluation and treatment*, ed 3, Oxford, 1990, Butterworth-Heinemann.
12. Boehme R: *Myofascial release and its application to neurodevelopmental treatment*, Milwaukee, 1991, Boehme Workshops.
13. Bogousslavsky J, Van Melle G, Regli F: The Lausanne stroke registry: analysis of 1,000 consecutive stroke patients, *Stroke* 19:1083, 1988.
14. Bonfils KB: The Affolter approach to treatment: a perceptual-cognitive perspective of function. In Pedretti LW, editor: *Occupational therapy practice skills for physical dysfunction*, ed 4, St Louis, 1996, Mosby.
15. Bourbonnais D, Noven SV: Weakness in patients with hemiparesis, *Am J Occup Ther* 43:313, 1989.
16. Brunnstrom S: *Movement therapy in hemiplegia*, Philadelphia, 1970, Harper and Rowe.
17. Burdett RG et al: Biomechanical comparison of rising from two types of chairs, *Phys Ther* 65:1177, 1985.
18. Carr JH, Gentile AM: The effect of arm movements on the biomechanics of standing up, *Hum Move Sci* 13:175, 1994.
19. Carr JH, Shepherd RB: A motor learning model for rehabilitation. In Carr JH et al, editors: *Movement science: foundations for physical therapy in rehabilitation*, Rockville, Md, 1987, Aspen.
20. Carr JH, Shepherd RB: *A motor relearning programme for stroke*, Oxford, 1987, Butterworth-Heinemann.
21. Crosson C et al: Awareness and compensation in postacute head injury rehabilitation, *J Head Trauma Rehab* 4:46, 1989.
22. Crutchfield CA, Barnes MR, editors: *Motor control and motor learning in rehabilitation*, Atlanta, 1933, Stokesville.
23. Damasio AR: *Descartes' error: emotion, reason, and the human brain*, New York, 1994, GP Putnam's Sons.
24. Das P, McCollum G: Invariant structure in locomotion, *Neuroscience* 25:1023, 1988.
25. Davies PM: *Right in the middle: selective trunk activity in the treatment of adult hemiplegia*, New York, 1990, Springer-Verlag.
26. Davies PM: *Steps to follow: a guide to treatment of adult hemiplegia*, New York, 1985, Springer-Verlag.
27. Davis JZ: Neurodevelopmental treatment of adult hemiplegia: the Bobath approach. In Pedretti LW, editor: *Occupational therapy practice skills for physical dysfunction*, ed 4, St Louis, 1996, Mosby.
28. Edelbrock C, Raincurello MD: Childhood hyperactivity; an overview of rating scales and their applications, *Clin Psychol Rev* 5:429, 1985.
29. Fisher CM: Left hemiplegia and motor impersistence, *J Nerv Ment Dis* 123:201, 1956.
30. Ford-Smith CD, Van Sant AF: Age differences in movement patterns used to rise from a bed in the third through fifth decades of age, *Phys Ther* 73:305, 1992.
31. Gentile AM: Skill acquisition: action, movement and neuromotor processes. In Carr JH et al, editors: *Movement science: foundations for physical therapy in rehabilitation*, Rockville, Md, 1987, Aspen.
32. Gentile AM: A working model of skill acquisition with application to teaching, *Quest* 17:3, 1972.
33. Granger CV, Hamilton BB: The Uniform Data System for medical rehabilitation report of first admissions for 1990, *Am J Phys Med Rehab* 71:108, 1992.
34. Granger CV et al: Performance profiles of the Functional Independence Measure, *Am J Phys Med Rehab* 72:84, 1993.
35. Hall ET: *The hidden dimension*, New York, 1966, Doubleday.
36. Heilman KM: Neglect and related disorders. In Heilman KM, Valenstein E, editors: *Clinical neuropsychology*, New York, 1979, Oxford University.
37. Herrmann M, Bartles C, Wallesch CW: Depression in acute and chronic aphasias: symptoms, pathoanatomical-clinical correlations and functional implications, *J Neurosurg Psychiatry* 56:672, 1993.
38. Hibbard MR, Gordon WA: The comprehensive psychological assessment of individuals with stroke, *Neurorehab* 2:9, 1992.
39. Higgins JR, Spaeth RK: Relationship between consistency of movement and environmental condition, *Quest* 17:61, 1972.
40. Jarus T: Motor learning and occupational therapy: the organization of practice, *Am J Occup Ther* 48:810, 1994.
41. Johansson G: Spatiotemporal differentiation and integration in visual motor perception, *Psychol Res* 38:379, 1976.
42. Johnstone M: *Restoration of motor function in the stroke patient*, ed 2, New York, 1983, Churchill Livingstone.
43. Joseph R: Confabulation and elusional denial: frontal lobe and lateralized influences, *J Clin Psychol* 42:507, 1986.
44. Joseph R: Parietal lobes. In Joseph R, editor: *Neuropsychology, neuropsychiatry and behavioral neurology*, New York, 1990, Plenum.
45. Joseph R: The right brain. In Joseph R, editor: *Neuropsychology, neuropsychiatry and behavioral neurology*, New York, 1990, Plenum.
46. Joynt RL, Benton AL, Fogel ML: Behavioral and pathological correlates of motor impersistence, *Neurology* 12:876, 1964.
47. Krefting LH, Krefting D: Cultural influences on performance. In Christiansen C, Baum C, editors: *Occupational therapy: overcoming human performance deficits*, New Jersey, 1991, Slack.
48. Lapointe LL: Neurogenic disorders of communication. In Minifie FD, editor: *Introduction to communication sciences and disorders*, San Diego, 1994, Singular Publishing.
49. Levine RE: Culture: A factor influencing the outcomes of occupational therapy, *Occup Ther Health Care* 4:1, 3, 1987.

50. Marsden CD, Rothwell JC, Day BL: The use of peripheral feedback in the control of movement. In Evarts EV, Wise SP, Bousfield D, editors: *The motor system in neurology*, Amsterdam, 1985, Elsevier Biomedical.

51. Mathiowetz V, Bass Haugen J: Motor behavior research: implications for therapeutic approaches to central nervous system dysfunction, *Am J Occup Ther* 48:733, 1994.

52. McCullagh P, Weiss MR, Ross D: Modeling considerations in motor skill acquisition and performance: an integrated approach. In Pandolf KB, editor: *Exercise and sport sciences reviews*, Baltimore, 1979, Williams & Wilkins.

53. Meyers AW et al: Cognitive contributions to the development of gymnastics skills, *Cog Ther Res* 3:75, 1979.

54. Mohr J: Management of the trunk in adult hemiplegia: the Bobath concept, *Topics in neurology*, Lesson 1, 1990, APTA.

55. Mohr JP, et al: Hemiparesis profiles in acute stroke: the NCIDS stroke data bank, *Ann Neurol* 156, 1984.

56. Mosey AC: *Occupational therapy: configuration of a profession*, New York, 1981, Raven.

57. Mosey AC: *Psychosocial components of occupational therapy*, New York, 1986, Raven.

58. Mulder T, Pauwels J, Neinhaus B: Motor recovery following stroke: towards a disability-orientated assessment of motor dysfunctions. In Harrison AH, editor: *Physiotherapy in stroke management*, Edinburgh, 1995, Churchill Livingstone.

59. Neistadt ME: The neurobiology of learning: implications for treatment of adults with brain injury, *Am J Occup Ther* 48:421, 1993.

60. Newell KM, Walter CB: Kinematic and kinetic parameters as information feedback in motor skill acquisition, *J Hum Move Stud* 7:233, 1981.

61. Parasher RK, Gentile AM: Translating instructions into spatially-directed limb movements, *Abstracts Soc Neurosci* 21:422, 1995.

62. Pimental PA: Alterations in communication, *Nurs Clin North Am* 21:321, 1986.

63. Poole JI: Application of motor learning principles in occupational therapy, *Am J Occup Ther* 45:531, 1991.

64. Posner MI, Inhoff AW, Friedrich FJ: Isolating attentional systems: a cognitive-anatomical analysis, *Psychobiol* 15:107, 1987.

65. Rafal RD et al: Orienting of visual attention in progressive supranuclear palsy, *Brain* 111:267, 1988.

66. Richter RR, Van Sant AF, Newton RA: Description of adult rolling movements and hypothesis of developmental sequences, *Phys Ther* 69:63, 1989.

67. Robinson RG et al: Mood disorders in stroke patients: importance of location of lesion, *Brain* 107:81, 1984.

68. Sabari JS: Motor learning concepts applied to activity-based interventions with adults with hemiplegia, *Am J Occup Ther* 45:523, 1991.

69. Saunders JB, Inman VT, Eberhart HD: The major determinant in normal and pathological gait, *J Bone Joint Surg* 35:543, 1953.

70. Schmidt RA: Motor learning principles for physical therapy. In Lister MJ, editor: *Contemporary management of motor control problems*, Proceedings of the Second STEP Conference, Alexandria, Va, 1991, Foundation for Physical Therapy.

71. Schmidt RA: *Motor control and learning: a behavioral emphasis*, ed 2, Champaign, Il, 1988, Human Kinetics.

72. Scully DM, Newell KM: Observational learning and the acquisition of motor skills: toward a visual perception perspective, *J Hum Move Stud* 12:169, 1985.

73. Shea JB, Morgan RL: Contextual interference effects on the acquisition, retention, and transfer of a motor skill, *J Exp Psychol Learn Mem Cogn* 5:179, 1979.

74. Shenkman M et al: Whole-body movements during rising to standing from sitting, *Phys Ther* 70:638, 1990.

75. Shepherd RB, Gentile AM: Sit-to-stand: functional relationship between upper body and lower limb segments, *Hum Move Stud* 13:817, 1994.

76. Shumway-Cook A, Woollacott MH: *Motor control: theory and practical applications*, Baltimore, 1995, Williams & Wilkins.

77. Stockmeyer SA: An interpretation of the approach of Rood to the treatment of neuromuscular dysfunction, *Am J Phys Med* 46:900, 1967.

78. Sullivan PE, Markos PD, Minor MD: *An integrated approach to therapeutic exercise: theory and clinical application*, Reston, Va, 1982, Reston.

79. Taub E: Somatosensory deafferentation research with monkeys: implications for rehabilitation medicine. In Ince LP, editor: *Behavioral psychology in rehabilitation medicine: clinical implications*, Baltimore, 1980, Williams & Wilkins.

80. Toglia J: Generalization of treatment: a multicontext approach to cognitive perceptual impairment in adults with brain injury, *Am J Occup Ther* 45:505, 1991.

81. Twitchell T: The restoration of motor function following hemiplegia in man, *Brain* 74:443-480, 1951.

82. VanSant A: Life-span development in functional tasks, *Phys Ther* 70:788, 1990.

83. Voss DE, Ionka MK, Meyers BJ: *Proprioceptive neuromuscular facilitation*, ed 3, Philadelphia, 1985, Harper and Row.

84. Warren M: A hierarchical model for evaluation and treatment of visual perceptual dysfunction in adult acquired brain injury, part 1, *Am J Occup Ther* 47:42, 1993.

85. Weintraub S, Mesulum NM: Visual hemispatial inattention: Stimulus parameters and exploratory strategies, *J Neurol Neurosurg Psychiatry* 51:1481, 1988.

86. Winstein CJ: Knowledge of results and motor learning—implications for physical therapy, *Phys Ther* 71:140, 1991.

87. Winstein CJ et al: Standing balance training: effect on balance and locomotion in hemiparetic adults, *Arch Phys Med Rehab* 70:755, 1989.

88. Woolfolk RL et al: Effects of mental rehearsal of task motor activity and mental depiction of task outcome on motor skill performance, *J Sport Psychol* 7:191, 1985.

89. Zola-Morgan S, Squire LR: Neuroanatomy of memory, *Ann Rev Neurosci* 16:547, 1993.

sheila m. hayes

chapter **11**

Gait Awareness

key terms

gait analysis

"hemiplegic gaits"

cerebellar strokes

ipsilateral pushing

orthotic devices

assistive devices

gait patterns

proprioceptive deficits

visual deficits

neurobehavioral deficits

chapter objectives

After completing this chapter, the reader will be able to accomplish the following:

1. Understand normal gait components.
2. Identify common gait deviations after a cerebrovascular accident.
3. Understand the basics of gait retraining.
4. Identify and describe commonly used orthoses and assistive devices.

In the management of a cerebrovascular accident (CVA) patient, gait analysis and gait training have traditionally been the responsibility of physical therapists. Because of the interdisciplinary approach that is used in the rehabilitation of the CVA patient, much sharing of information regarding the patient's functional and mobility status occurs between team members. Occupational and physical therapists will often "cotreat" to enhance problem-solving regarding specific barriers to independence in activities of daily living (ADL).

Just as physical therapists have much to gain by familiarizing themselves with terminology and treatments used by occupational therapists (e.g., in the area of perceptual motor deficits), occupational therapists should find it beneficial to have a basic understanding of normal gait components, common gait deviations after a CVA, and gait re-

training. An integrated approach to treatment of the CVA patient necessitates a working knowledge of the other disciplines' terminology, evaluation techniques, and rationale for treatment.

Before gait analysis and retraining, a thorough evaluation must be performed by the physical therapist to examine such factors as range of motion (ROM), posture and bony alignment, strength, motor control, coordination, sensation and balance. Keeping in mind any deficits in these areas, the therapist is then ready to observe and analyze gait, and speculate on which of the deficits may be contributing to a specific gait deviation. Awareness of specific problem areas allows the therapist to address these issues with key treatment strategies and modalities.

Gait analysis is the objective documentation of gait.[46] It ranges in complexity from observational assessment to three-dimensional motion analysis and can include tools such as videotaping, dynamic electromyograms (EMGs), and force plates. Many physical therapists do not have access to highly technical evaluation equipment, although videotaping is now more commonly available. Observational gait analysis is used extensively by clinical physical therapists and in research and involves descriptions of the body and limbs as they move through the gait cycle. These assessments of movement patterns and joint displacements are called *kinematic analyses.*[41]

Observational gait analysis should take place in both the sagittal and frontal planes. The frontal or coronal view must include both anterior and posterior vantage points. Certain motions such as leg rotation and foot abduction and adduction take place in the transverse or horizontal plane, although the therapist usually is not in a position to observe motion specifically in this plane. In normal gait, most movement occurs in the sagittal plane, whereas in abnormal gait, many of the deviations are observed as compensations in the frontal (coronal) and transverse planes[46] (Figure 11-1).

TERMINOLOGY

To observe and analyze the gait of a person who has had a CVA, therapists must first be familiar with the components of the normal gait cycle and the terminology used to describe these components. A cycle begins when the heel of one foot touches the ground. It ends after the leg and body have advanced through space and time and the heel of that same foot hits the ground again.

The cycle includes a period when the leg is in contact with the ground, which is followed by a period when it is advancing through space. Thus the gait cycle of one leg can be divided into two phases: the stance phase (in which the leg is in contact with the ground) and the swing phase (in which the leg is off the ground). The stance phase makes up 60% of the gait cycle, and the swing phase makes up 40% (Figure 11-2). In a normal gait, the opposite leg is also going through a gait cycle simultaneously (i.e., has a stance phase and a swing phase). Each leg has two periods at the beginning and end of the stance when the opposite leg is also in contact with the ground. These are called the periods of *double support.* Together they account for 10% of the initial stance phase and 10% of the end of stance for both legs (see Figure 11-2).

The phases of swing and stance are further divided into substages. The language used to describe these subdivisions varies depending on whether the traditional terms are used or the terms developed at Rancho Los Amigos Medical Center in Los Angeles are used (Table 11-1). The terms are similar and physical therapists will often use a mixture of old and new terms unless the facility in which they work advocates strict adherence to one type of terminology. Most physical therapists are familiar with the Ran-

cho Los Amigos terminology because of the abundance of research, literature, and gait assessment forms that have been produced by the pathokinesiology service and physical therapy department at that facility.[47]

The Rancho Los Amigos definition of swing phase is divided into the substages of initial swing, midswing, and terminal swing. The stance phase is divided into initial contact, loading response, midstance, terminal stance, and preswing (Figure 11-3). Within these substages, the physical therapist observes the joint displacements and movements occurring at the trunk, pelvis, hip, knee, ankle, and toes. Figure 11-4 illustrates the phases of the gait cycle and

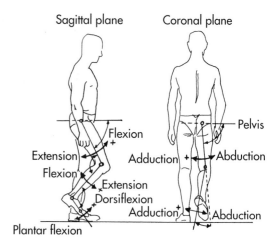

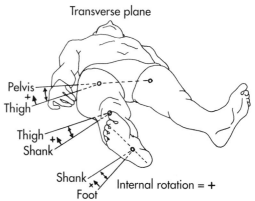

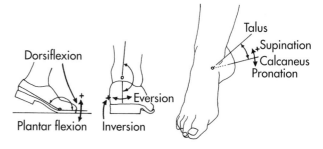

Figure 11-1 System of naming angular motion. (From Inman VT, Ralston HJ: *Human walking,* 1981, Williams & Wilkins.)

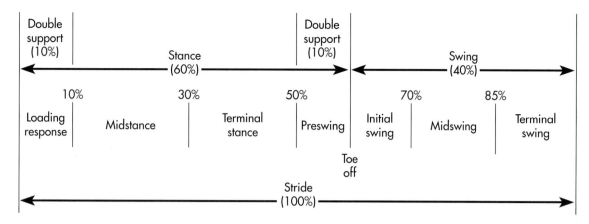

Figure 11-2   Phases of gait cycle and their proportions as percentages of gait cycle. (From Ounpuu S: *Evaluation and management of gait disorders*, 1995, Marcel Dekker.)

Table 11-1

Gait Terminology

TRADITIONAL	RANCHO LOS AMIGOS
Stance phase	
Heel strike: The beginning of the stance phase when the heel contacts the ground; the same as initial contact	*Initial contact:* The beginning of the stance phase when the heel or another part of the foot contacts the ground
Foot flat: Occurs immediately following heel strike when the sole of the foot contacts the floor; occurs during loading response	*Loading response:* The portion of the first double support period of the stance phase from initial contact until the contralateral extremity leaves the ground
Midstance: The point at which the body passes directly over the reference extremity	*Midstance:* The portion of the single limb support stance phase that begins when the contralateral extremity leaves the ground and ends when the body is directly over the supporting limb
Heel off: The point following midstance when the heel of the reference extremity leaves the ground; occurs prior to terminal stance	*Terminal stance:* The last portion of the single limb support stance phase that begins with heel rise and continues until contralateral extremity contacts the ground
Toe off: The point following heel off when only the toe of the reference extremity is in contact with the ground	*Preswing:* The portion of stance that begins the second double support period from the initial contact of the contralateral extremity to lift off of the reference extremity
Swing phase	
Acceleration: The portion of beginning swing from the moment the toe of the reference extremity leaves the ground to the point when the reference extremity is directly under the body	*Initial swing:* The portion of swing from the point when the reference extremity leaves the ground to maximum knee flexion of the same extremity
Midswing: Portion of the swing phase when the reference extremity passes directly below the body: extends from the end of acceleration to the beginning of deceleration	*Midswing:* The portion of the swing phase from maximum knee flexion of the reference extremity to a vertical tibial position
Deceleration: The swing portion of the swing phase when the reference extremity is decelerating in preparation for heel strike	*Terminal swing:* The portion of the swing phase from a vertical position of the tibia of the reference extremity to just before initial contact

O'Sullivan SB, Schmitz TJ, editors: *Physical rehabilitation assessment and treatment*, Philadelphia, 1994, FA Davis.

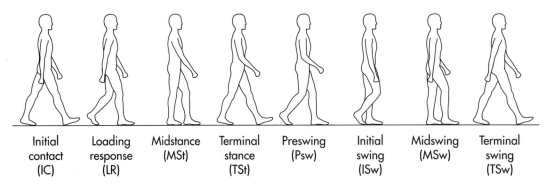

| Initial contact (IC) | Loading response (LR) | Midstance (MSt) | Terminal stance (TSt) | Preswing (Psw) | Initial swing (ISw) | Midswing (MSw) | Terminal swing (TSw) |

Figure 11-3 Phases of gait cycle shown with corresponding body position for sagittal plane motion. (From Ounpuu S: *Evaluation and management of gait disorders*, 1995, Marcel Dekker.)

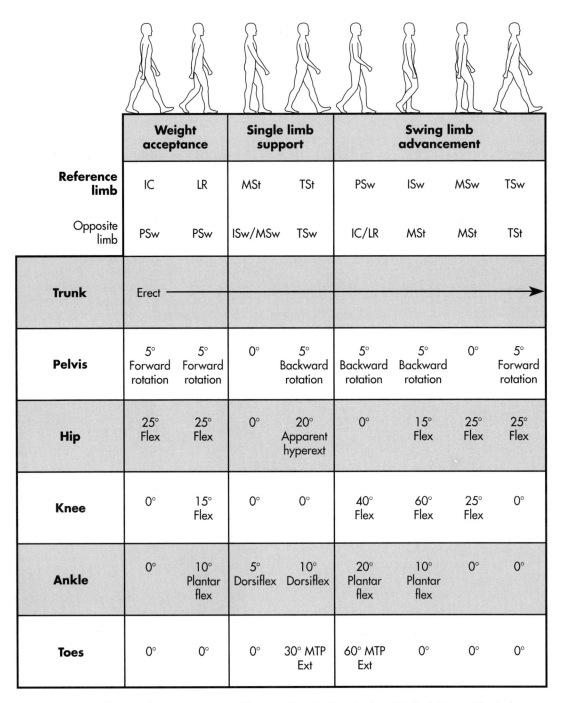

	Weight acceptance		**Single limb support**		**Swing limb advancement**			
Reference limb	IC	LR	MSt	TSt	PSw	ISw	MSw	TSw
Opposite limb	PSw	PSw	ISw/MSw	TSw	IC/LR	MSt	MSt	TSt
Trunk	Erect ————————————————————————————→							
Pelvis	5° Forward rotation	5° Forward rotation	0°	5° Backward rotation	5° Backward rotation	5° Backward rotation	0°	5° Forward rotation
Hip	25° Flex	25° Flex	0°	20° Apparent hyperext	0°	15° Flex	25° Flex	25° Flex
Knee	0°	15° Flex	0°	0°	40° Flex	60° Flex	25° Flex	0°
Ankle	0°	10° Plantar flex	5° Dorsiflex	10° Dorsiflex	20° Plantar flex	10° Plantar flex	0°	0°
Toes	0°	0°	0°	30° MTP Ext	60° MTP Ext	0°	0°	0°

Figure 11-4 Range of motion summary. (Courtesy Rancho Los Amigos Medical Center Physical Therapy Department and Pathokinesiology Laboratory, Downey, Calif.)

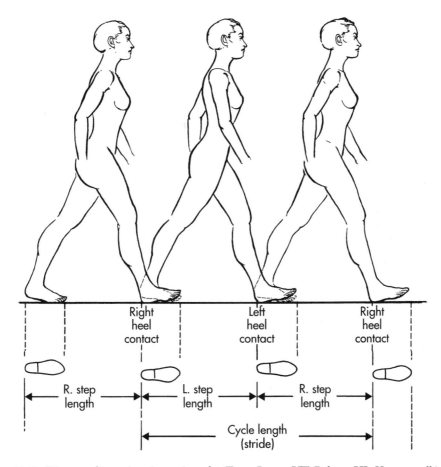

Figure 11-5 Distance dimensions in a gait cycle. (From Inman VT, Ralston HJ: *Human walking*, 1981, Williams & Wilkins.)

the corresponding normal joint displacements that occur as the body moves through the sagittal plane.

Other terms used in describing gait cycles are stride, step, cadence, and velocity. A stride is equal to a gait cycle (i.e., from heel strike of one leg to the next heel strike of the same leg). It can refer to distance (stride length) or time (stride time) in the gait cycle of one leg. A step is described as the distance (step length) or time (step time) from the heel strike of one leg to the heel strike of the opposite leg (Figure 11-5).

RELIABLE GAIT PARAMETERS

Cadence is the number of steps or strides per unit of time. Walking velocity equals speed—the distance walked divided by time. Because time-distance variables are the components of gait that can be most reliably measured, they can be utilized in assessing improvement in stroke patients.[25] For example, people who have had a CVA and have resulting hemiparesis typically walk with a slower than normal gait.[35] Routine recording of the cadence and velocity of these patients is an objective way of document-

ing change over time. It is a valid measure for showing improvement to physical therapists who do not have access to elaborate gait kinematic analysis systems.

Descriptive analyses of limb control are subjective and not easily quantified. Improvements in cadence and velocity can be an indication of functional improvement and limb recovery. A study by Harro and Giuliani[29] of hemiplegic patients showed positive correlations between high scores (greater than 90) on the motor portion of the Fugel Meyer Motor Assessment Scale and the ability to increase walking speeds.

Observational gait analysis is an acquired skill that requires much practice and repetition. The physical therapist must learn how to look at six different points on the body while simultaneously comparing the observed gait with normal gait parameters in three body planes. When first learning gait analysis, observing as many "normal" gaits as possible is useful. When first using observational gait analysis in the clinic, choosing patients who can tolerate walking for several minutes and developing a systematic approach to viewing trunk and limb excursions during the gait cycle is recommended.[47]

"HEMIPLEGIC GAITS"

The type of gait that a person has after a CVA depends on where the insult has occurred and which systems have been affected, such as motor, sensory, balance, coordination, perceptual, and visual systems. If a motor area in the cortex or a motor track has been involved, hemiplegia or hemiparesis is manifested in the contralateral limbs. Whether the arm or the leg is more impaired depends on the location of the infarction within these areas. Not all stroke patients are hemiplegic or hemiparetic, nor do all hemiparetic patients have the same degree of motor deficits. Unfortunately, the term *hemiplegic gait* is frequently applied to all individuals with hemiparesis, although many varieties and degrees of deficits exist.[25]

Individuals who have suffered ischemia in areas of the brain supplied by the anterior cerebral artery will usually have greater deficits in the leg, whereas those with ischemic lesions in areas supplied by the middle cerebral artery have greater arm involvement. Because middle cerebral artery infarctions are the most common type of CVA,[10] the deficits seen with these lesions are those most often associated with stroke patients and described by the generic term hemiplegic gait. Following are descriptions of gait deviations most often seen with hemiparesis at various joints and stages in the gait cycle.

During the stance phase of the hemiparetic leg, a patient may exhibit "foot flat" or even a "forefoot first" at the initial contact instead of a heel strike with adequate ankle dorsiflexion. The patient may exhibit both plantar flexion (forefoot first) and supination (in the frontal plane) at initial contact and then begin to weight bear precariously on the lateral border of the foot.[25,39,45]

During the loading response, while the patient is still in double limb support, weight is being "loaded," or accepted, onto the leg. Normally, 10° to 15° of knee flexion is needed to absorb the forces of momentum and body weight. The flexion may be absent, so instead the knee remains extended or even hyperextends (genu recurvatum) during midstance as the body moves forward. In this instance, no tibial advancement occurs over the foot because no dorsiflexion is occurring at the ankle (Figure 11-6).

Midstance begins the period of single limb support. In addition to knee hyperextension, trunk and hip flexion may also be observed as the body attempts to move its center of mass forward over a stiff knee. The problem may be compounded by pelvic retraction. Other patients may display the opposite scenario during midstance. There may be excessive knee flexion in the sagittal plane with concurrent excessive dorsiflexion and hip flexion.[2,39,45]

In the frontal plane, either excessive lateral trunk lean over the ipsilateral leg during midstance or a positive Trendelenburg's sign may be observed, both of which indicate weak hip abductors of the stance leg. A positive Trendelenburg's sign is present when excessive lateral displace-

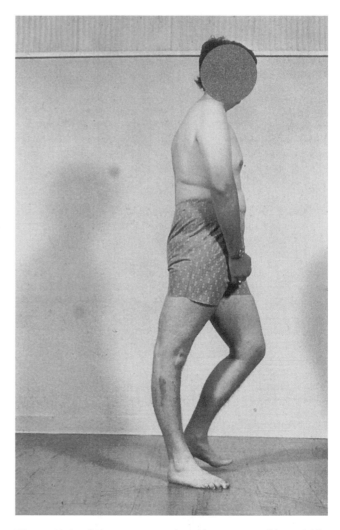

Figure 11-6 Genu recurvatum in midstance caused by a rigid plantar flexion contracture (greater than 15°). Tibia is prevented from advancing forward, driving the knee posteriorly into recurvatum, impeding progression, and reducing momentum. (From Adams J, Perry J: *Human walking*, 1994, Williams & Wilkins.)

ment of the pelvis occurs over the stance leg, with an excessive lowering of the pelvis on the contralateral swing leg.[41,46]

During the terminal stance phase, which is still a period of single limb support, the normal hip extension may be absent as well as the ability to transfer weight onto the forefoot in preparation for push-off. There may be continued excessive or diminished dorsiflexion at the ankle joint. Lack of heel rise can be observed combined with excessive dorsiflexion, and the contralateral leg makes initial contact early.[2,25,39,47]

In the preswing phase, the final stance stage and the second double support period, a lack of knee flexion (normally between 30° and 40°) is often observed, as is a lack of ankle joint plantar flexion at the end of preswing.[2,45,47]

Many of the deviations observed in the hemiparetic limb during stance can contribute to a decreased step length by the opposite leg. The body is not able to complete its normal excursion forward because of lack of movement, or ineffective movement, of the pelvis, hip, knee, or ankle of the hemiparetic limb. The opposite limb may "step to" instead of stepping past the paretic limb. Step length can also be reduced in the hemiparetic leg.

The swing phase of the paretic limb can sometimes be seen as a mass flexion movement instead of a series of sequential flexion movements.[25,35] More often it is characterized by a stiff-legged swing, with a decrease in hip flexion and in the velocity and amount of reciprocal knee flexion and extension. The velocity of the entire paretic limb is often decreased.[25] The decrease in hip flexion, plus lack of knee flexion and dorsiflexion, often results in circumduction to advance the stiff limb.* Circumduction is seen when the patient swings the leg through in a semicircle. It is most noticeable when looking at the patient in the frontal plane (Figure 11-7). The patient combines external rotation and abduction at the hip to lift the leg out to the side, then adducts and often internally rotates the leg to bring it back in.[41] In a normal gait pattern, no abduction, adduction, or external or internal rotation is observed in the frontal plane during the swing phase.[47]

The limited knee flexion in the preswing phase persists into the initial swing phase and often throughout the entire swing phase. The "toe drag" first seen in the initial swing phase may continue because of the decreased knee swing but may also be a consequence of decreased hip flexion and decreased ankle dorsiflexion. Compensatory hip hiking can be initiated at this stage to assist with clearing the toes as the leg advances.[2,25,39,45] Other compensations used to counteract toe drag are increased hip and knee flexion or vaulting by the opposite (stance) leg. During vaulting, the opposite leg rises up on the toes (causing excessive plantar flexion) for better clearance of the swing leg.[2]

In the midswing phase the pelvis may remain retracted instead of rotating forward to neutral. Hip hiking and leg circumduction may continue, especially if knee flexion and dorsiflexion remain limited. Dorsiflexion may be decreased or absent, with the ankle assuming a plantar-flexed ("footdrop") position. The foot may supinate during midswing because of an imbalance in ankle dorsiflexor muscle function[14,39,47] (Figure 11-7). Normally, both the anterior tibialis and long toe extensors dorsiflex the foot symmetrically. Some stroke patients have overactive anterior tibialis muscles and weak long toe extensors, causing the medially placed anterior tibialis tendon to pull the foot into supination.[14]

As the limb progresses toward the terminal swing phase, many patients are unable to extend the knee while simultaneously flexing the hip and ankle. Instead, knee exten-

*References 2, 25, 35, 41, 45, 47.

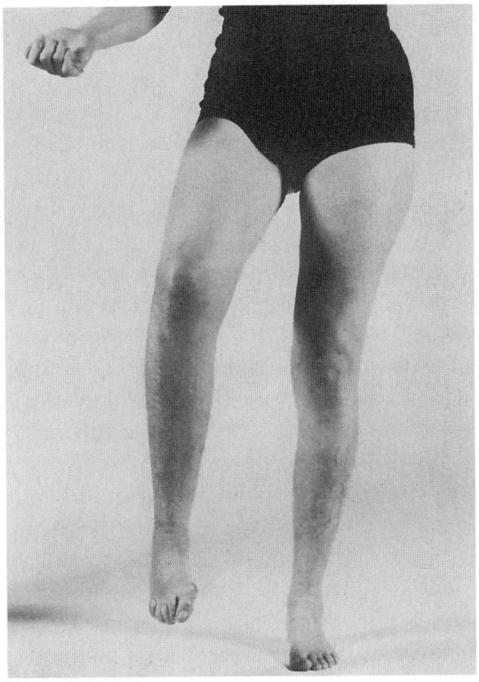

Figure 11-7 Supination of foot during swing phase resulting from uninhibited activity in the tibialis anterior. Circumduction of hip is also present during this swing phase. (From Davies P: *Steps to follow*, 1985, Springer-Verlag.)

sion is decreased, and they eventually make initial contact with the ground on a flexed knee.[39] The pelvis may still be retracted or may not have rotated forward past neutral. This, in addition to the decrease in knee extension, results in a decreased step length by the paretic leg. Other people may exhibit knee extension with plantar flexion during the terminal swing phase instead of the normal dorsiflexion seen in preparation for upcoming heel strike.[25,47] Others display adduction of the hip with knee extension that at times is so pronounced that the swing leg crosses in front of the stance foot. Patients literally end up tripping over themselves.

CAUSES OF GAIT DEVIATIONS

It cannot be overemphasized that the causes of observed gait deviations may vary from patient to patient. For example, a common deviation at initial contact is foot flat or forefoot first instead of heel strike. This aberrancy could be a result of weak dorsiflexor muscles,[16,17,36,38,47] abnormal activity of the plantar flexors,[2,35,36,47] a decreased ability to perform fast reciprocal movements,[25,31,36] a disruption in the central generation of preprogrammed muscle activation,[32] noncontractile soft tissue tightness in the plantar flexors,[2,13,16,47] or ankle joint pathology. Even when soft tissue tightness and joint contractures are ruled out, hypotheses vary and often conflict about the precipitating factor. This is especially true when the issue of voluntary versus reflex skeletal muscle activation is addressed. A number of recent papers and publications provide an abbreviated review of the literature on this topic.*

TREATMENT STRATEGIES

After a thorough evaluation and gait analysis the physical therapist needs to address identified deficits, such as decreased ROM and strength, with various modalities and therapeutic exercise. In addition, a variety of approaches are available to address the lack of movement and voluntary control deficits. Many are based on theories that advocate facilitation of normal movement and sensory stimulation of the patient by the therapist. In this context the patient is a somewhat passive recipient of the therapist's efforts. However, in the past 20 years, therapists have gradually shifted away from using the more traditional theoretical models underlying these therapeutic approaches to using the motor control perspective.[28] The motor control approach is also based on a theoretical model, but it does not advocate specific treatment techniques that are done by the therapist to the patient. In the motor control model the main task of the therapist is not to "facilitate" normal movement but to structure the environment in such a way that the patient will relearn to actively use the affected limbs functionally. The motor control relearning theory is based on research from a variety of fields: neurophysiology, muscle physiology, biomechanics, and psychology.[28] Patients are believed to learn by actively trying to solve problems. Therefore tasks should be structured to promote acquisition of the movements needed to solve specific motor control problems in a variety of situations (see Chapter 2).

The causes of disordered motor control most likely have many factors. Individual therapists have the responsibility to keep abreast of the latest research in this area as well as in the area of recovery of function after stroke. By doing so, gait training becomes an ever-changing and challenging task for the therapist and patient. As mentioned previously, not all stroke patients have a hemiplegic gait. Diverse manifestations can be seen, depending on which artery is occluded or has hemorrhaged and where the ischemic damage has occurred. Although this chapter focuses on deficits that impair gait, other deficits exist (and are noted). Recent publications provide comprehensive reviews of all the impairments that accompany specific stroke syndromes.[7,8,24,54] Even the list of abnormal gaits is too extensive to be covered completely in a single chapter. Therefore what follows are examples of abnormal gaits that are particularly challenging for the physical therapist to treat.

*References 13, 16, 20, 25, 29, 30, 31, 32, 36.

Cerebellar Strokes

A person who has an infarct in the cerebellum caused by occlusion or hemorrhage of a vertebral or a cerebellar artery may exhibit completely different gait deviations than a hemiparetic patient. The cerebellum is composed of three parts or lobes: the flocculonodular lobe, the anterior lobe, and the posterior lobe. The flocculonodular lobe is also called the *vestibulocerebellum* because most of its input is from the vestibular nuclei in the pons. The anterior lobe is also known as the *spinocerebellum* because most of its input is from the spinocerebellar tracts via both the inferior cerebellar peduncle and the superior cerebellar peduncle. The posterior lobe is also known as the *neocerebellum* and contains major portions of the cerebellar hemispheres. The hemispheres receive their major input from the cortex via the middle cerebellar peduncle.

In addition, the cerebellum can be divided longitudinally into functional zones perpendicular to the horizontal fissures dividing the lobes. The most medial structure is the vermis. Adjacent to the vermis, on either side, are the pars intermedia (intermediate sections) of the cerebellar hemispheres. Lateral to these are the bulk of the cerebellar hemispheres.

Gait is most influenced by the flocculonodular and anterior lobes. Consequently, lesions in these areas caused by ischemia or hemorrhage will lead to difficulty maintaining a proper stance and walking.[42] Damage to the flocculonodular lobe (vestibulocerebellum) will cause head and neck ataxia. Truncal tremor is often severe. A wide-based stance with the feet apart is usually used to increase stability. Any attempt to bring the feet together or walk with one foot directly in front of the other will cause loss of balance. Ataxia or dysmetria of the limbs is not common.

Damage to the anterior lobe, especially the medial aspect, will cause a disruption in the sensory input (via the spinocerebellar tracts) that is related to agonist-antagonist muscle activity. Lower limb ataxia or dysmetria is also present, but upper limb ataxia is usually absent. Lesions in a cerebellar hemisphere will result in ipsilateral limb dysmetria or hypotonia in addition to other deficits. Although the damage does not affect postural stability, the gait appears ataxic and staggering because of the limb dysmetria.[42]

The cerebellum is supplied by three main arteries, the posterior inferior cerebellar artery (PICA), the anterior inferior cerebellar artery (AICA), and the superior cerebellar artery (SCA). These arteries are part of the posterior circulation—the vertebrobasilar system. The PICA is a branch of the vertebral artery, whereas the AICA and SCA are branches of the basilar artery. The territories supplied by these arteries and their associated areas are described in detail in Chapter 1.[3,4] In general, they supply the areas of the cerebellum that their names imply in addition to parts of the brain stem. Some areas of vascularization in the cerebellum overlap because of the many free cortical anastomoses[3] (Figure 11-8). Although one artery may pre-

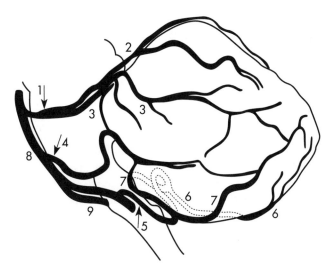

Figure 11-8 Lateral view of cerebellar arteries. *1,* Superior cerebellar artery (SCA); *2,* medial branch of SCA; *3,* lateral branch of SCA; *4,* anterior inferior cerebellar artery (AICA); *5,* posterior inferior cerebellar artery (PICA); *6,* medial branch of PICA; *7,* lateral branch of PICA; *8,* basilar artery; *9,* vertebral artery. (From Bogousslavsky J, Caplan L, editors: *Stroke syndromes,* Cambridge, 1995, Cambridge University Press.)

dominantly supply one particular lobe, this overlapping may result in additional blood coming from the distal branches of another artery. However, as a rule the SCA supplies the superior cerebellar peduncle, the AICA supplies the middle cerebellar peduncle, and the PICA supplies the inferior cerebellar peduncle.[3]

A cerebellar stroke resulting from occlusion of the PICA is usually referred to in the literature as a *lateral medullary syndrome* (Wallenberg's syndrome)[8,24,54] because it was believed that the PICA supplied the lateral medulla as well as parts of the cerebellum. Recently this term has been disputed based on evidence that the lateral medulla is less frequently supplied by the PICA than previously thought.[4] If the lateral medulla is spared, the cranial nerves VIII, IX, and X are not involved and Horner's syndrome does not develop. Regardless, a PICA territory infarct will damage the inferior cerebellar peduncle and cause ipsilateral limb ataxia and an ataxic gait. In addition, the patient tends to fall to the side of the lesion[4] and has difficulty shifting weight toward the contralateral leg.

It was reported in earlier texts that PICA infarcts are the most common,[8,54] but recent findings have shown that SCA infarcts occur as frequently.[3,4] SCA infarcts have several different clinical manifestations, but those that affect gait, such as cerebrovestibular signs, are among the most frequent, in addition to dysarthria. Limb dysmetria and gait ataxia as well as falling toward the side of the lesion (ipsilateral axial lateropulsion) are common symptoms.[4]

Gait retraining after a cerebellar stroke is focused on relearning the way to correct balance losses. Patients must first learn the point in space where their center of gravity

is optimally positioned over their base of support for stability. Then they must relearn the way to constantly readjust their center of gravity to align with their base of support. This task is most difficult during ambulation when the center of gravity is shifted anterior to the base of support as the body moves forward.[53]

Balance retraining should encourage active problem-solving by the patient (see Chapter 5). Being held upright by the therapist while walking will not promote functional independence. Likewise, assistive devices that require upper extremity weight bearing (e.g., walkers) may prevent loss of balance but do not promote functional improvement because they do not challenge the patient to relearn balance control.[5,9] The patient is merely stabilized externally and not required to utilize or integrate postural reflexes.

Activities that require active weight shifting and goal-oriented reaching are encouraged and practiced while the patient is standing (see Chapter 6). Progressively more challenging exercises and activities can be introduced as the patient becomes more adept.[5] Initially, some patients find it beneficial to walk along a high mat with their less affected side next to the mat. Having the stronger hip contact the mat as they step with the dysmetric limb provides a goal for weight shifting. Later, a cane is used only to prevent loss of balance or as a cue to shift weight to the less affected side—not as a maximal assistive device.

Ipsilateral Pushing

An unusual motor behavior sometimes displayed in the clinic by hemiplegic patients is ipsilateral pushing. The patients tend to push away from the unaffected side in any position. The syndrome was described by Davies in 1985 and called the *pusher syndrome.*[14] It is not a medically recognized syndrome, and the literature is scant on this subject. A study by Pedersen and associates[48] examined whether the syndrome was localized to a specific right parietal lobe lesion but no association was found. The same study also found no significant association between ipsilateral pushing and two perceptual deficits, hemineglect and anosognosia. Further research is needed to investigate the role of other deficits. For instance, Pedersen and associates suggested investigating the role of subcortical sensory pathways and relay stations and the effects of exaggerated sensory feedback from the affected side.[48] Damage to any area involved in processing sensory information can cause impairments when that input is needed to coordinate spatial movement.[6] In addition, occipital lobe ischemia can cause visual perceptual disorders[34] and needs to be studied for its effect on neurobehavior. The hippocampus is also believed to possibly play a role in spatial orientation,[6] and if it does the result of damage to that area needs to be examined.

The original description of the pusher syndrome was based solely on one clinician's observation. It was thought to be most often associated with left hemiplegia and perceptual deficits (especially left neglect), left visual field neglect with or without a homonymous hemianopsia, impaired body scheme and body image, and visuospatial deficits.[14]

Although research has not confirmed the existence of a pusher syndrome, ipsilateral pushing does exist. The cause may not be identifiable, but the behavior is still seen, as it was in as many as 10% of the 327 stroke patients in the Pedersen and associates study.[48] Gait training patients demonstrating ipsilateral pushing is a definite challenge, as is transfer training. During sit-to-stand activities, some patients will project themselves quickly out of a chair toward their hemiparetic side. If left unguarded, they will fall. Transferring toward the stronger side is extremely difficult because they are always pushing away from that side. Although easier, transfers toward the hemiparetic side are dangerous because of the lack of motor control on that side. Standing requires assistance to prevent falling to the weak side.

Walking with an assistive device, such as a cane in the stronger hand, is unproductive because these patients tend to use the cane to push themselves toward the hemiparetic leg. They appear unable to actively shift weight onto the strong leg. The more patients are supported (to prevent falling to the paretic side) the more they push into the helper.

Gait retraining is based on the same principles discussed in the ataxic gaits section. Patients must relearn the way to adjust their center of gravity over their base of support while standing. This implies a need for conscious awareness of loss of balance. Although Pedersen and associates[48] found no significant correlation between anosognosia and ipsilateral pushing, patients were questioned only about limb weakness and visual field deficits and not about balance deficits. Patient self-assessments of the location of their center of gravity in relation to their base of support has yet to be investigated. That these patients can relearn the way to balance themselves has been observed by this author and verified by the Pedersen study. Of interest is that data collected by Pedersen and associates demonstrated that patients with ipsilateral pushing had lower scores on the Barthel Index at discharge than those without ipsilateral pushing had on admission to the hospital. In addition, patients with ipsilateral pushing had significantly increased length of hospital stays and recovery periods. Relearning to maintain balance while walking is a formidable task indeed for those demonstrating ipsilateral pushing.

Trial and error are encouraged to promote active problem-solving. The degree of difficulty in relearning to maintain balance while walking is compounded by changes in sensation, strength, motor control, and normal feedback circuits secondary to the infarction. Visual goals and tactile goals can be most helpful. Having a patient walk around a high mat or table cues the patient where to weight shift to

avoid falling. The use of parallel bars is discouraged; a patient must learn to weight shift with the trunk to correct balance losses and not merely pull on a bar to remain upright. With improvement, the patient can advance to using a cane. Hands-on techniques used by the therapist to facilitate movement are discouraged. The patient will simply push into the hands of the therapist.

At times leg weakness will interfere with a "pusher's" ability to relearn postural control and weight shifting. Davies advocated splinting the hemiparetic knee in extension while having the patient work on active weight shifting during functional standing activities.[14] Splinting the knee this way reduces the amount of pushing by the patient while standing. Assumptions can be made that the added stability somehow reassures patients and allows them time to accurately assess whether they are balanced. Perhaps the degrees of freedom have been limited allowing patients to concentrate on one task—weight shifting—to achieve a functional goal without having to concern themselves with an unstable knee. At this time, only speculations can be made about what reduces the pushing tendency and why. Although treatment techniques were suggested for gait training patients demonstrating ipsilateral pushing, no controlled studies have been done to verify their efficacy and are based solely on this and other practitioners' clinical experiences.

Proprioceptive Deficits

Loss of sensation after a CVA can compound motor deficits. In particular, loss of proprioception can greatly impede motor recovery after stoke.[18] Proprioception is conveyed both to the cerebellum and to the cerebral cortex. Information about joint position and muscle activity is sent to both, but the information projected to the cerebellum is not recorded as conscious perception. It is used to ensure coordinated limb movements. In contrast, the information sent to the cortex can be perceived consciously and provides awareness of limb position and movement.[24]

Proprioceptive input from muscle spindles, joint receptors, and cutaneous touch receptors reaches the cerebellum through the inferior cerebellar peduncle via the ipsilateral dorsal spinocerebellar tracts. The same information reaches the somatosensory area of the cerebral cortex via the ipsilateral posterior columns of the spinal cord, which cross in the medulla and ascend in the medial lemniscus to the thalamus and then to the cortex.

Middle cerebral artery strokes can impair awareness of proprioception at the cortical level. Although all sensations can be affected, proprioception and two-point discrimination are usually more impaired than pain and temperature perception.[8] The deficits are manifested in the contralateral arm and leg. Cerebellar artery strokes will cause loss of the unconscious, rapid proprioceptive input required for the smooth, automatic movements of gait. A loss of sensory input regarding agonist-antagonist muscle activity causes a disruption in the continuous modulation of these muscles that is required for coordinated gait movements.

A study by Kusoffsky and associates[33] found that patients with proprioceptive loss after cortical stroke were able to regain a greater amount of function in the leg than the arm. One explanation for this was that gait is greatly dependent on centrally generated activation patterns that in turn are not dependent on peripheral sensory mechanisms.[33] These central pattern generators originate in the spinal cord and are controlled by locomotor centers in the brain stem. These centers are influenced by the cerebellum, the basal ganglia, and the cerebral cortex.[26] The physical therapist can take advantage of this phenomenon by emphasizing functional gait as much as possible.

Along with vestibular and visual input, proprioceptive information contributes to a patient's ability to maintain an upright stable position. Input from muscle spindles and joint receptors not only provide valuable information about the position of a limb in space but about the environment as well.[53] The ability to react to uneven surfaces or changes in ground texture depends on this input, and its impairment puts a patient at higher risk of falling. Coordinated limb movements may be decreased, and the person may be unable to judge the step length or limb joint excursions needed for maneuvering in the environment.

Vision can help to compensate for the proprioceptive loss.[24,44,53] As with other deficits, a problem-solving approach is encouraged by the physical therapist. The patient must learn to consciously use visual input, which was not necessary before. Occasionally mirrors are useful, although these aids should be evaluated individually for each patient. Mirrors can hinder as often as they help patients, especially those with visuospatial deficits.

The therapist's role is to provide a variety of settings in which the person can practice using visual cues. In addition, biofeedback can be used to provide auditory cues. One type of biofeedback unit is a limb load monitor that can signal a person when the foot contacts the ground. Standard biofeedback units can be used to provide information about the force of muscle contraction during strengthening exercises (see Chapter 6).

Visual Deficits

Visual impairments from strokes can also affect gait. The most common deficit in hemiplegic patients is homonymous hemianopsia,[34] which occurs when an infarction involves the optic radiation to one occipital cortex or as a result of damage to the visual cortex itself. A branch of the middle cerebral artery, the anterior choroidal artery, supplies most of the optic radiation, with some coverage by branches of the posterior cerebral artery. The visual cortex is supplied mainly by the posterior cerebral artery but is also supplied by some middle cerebral artery collaterals.[11,23] Homonymous hemianopsia can also be a result of an isolated occlusion of the calcarine branch of the posterior cerebral artery, but in this case no concurrent hemiplegia or hemisensory loss occurs.[24]

When homonymous hemianopsia is present, visual information about one half of a person's environment is missing. The temporal half of the visual field of one eye and the nasal half of the visual field of the other eye are absent. As mentioned previously, balance is maintained by an intricate communication network between the visual, vestibular, and proprioceptive systems. If vision is impaired, one aspect of this network is functioning abnormally. Balance is at risk if the patient does not learn to use other systems for feedback about the environment.

Self-awareness of the visual deficit is crucial for patients. They must test this new awareness in a variety of situations and environments to ensure safety on discharge from the hospital and maximize functional independence (see Chapter 12).

Neurobehavioral Deficits

Perceptual deficits such as left neglect or visual neglect are neurobehavioral deficits that can affect gait. These phenomena and their manifestations, causes, and clinical implications are discussed (see Chapters 13 and 14).[6,22,34] Ipsilateral pushing may also be classified as a neurobehavioral deficit.

Hemineglect and hemianopsia are separate entities that can often coexist. Likewise, neglect and sensory loss can develop together or independently. Communication between the occupational and physical therapists concerning a patient's perceptual status is critical in determining the best treatment approach to maximize function and ensure consistency of treatment interventions. Information obtained from formal testing by the occupational therapist can provide valuable insights for the physical therapist who is formulating the gait retraining program.

Orthotic Devices

An orthosis (from the Greek adjective *orthos*, meaning "straight") is an external device that improves a person's function when applied to a body part.[37] The more commonly used term for an orthosis is a *brace*. Orthoses are now named according to the joints they encompass. Short leg braces are known as *ankle-foot orthoses* (AFOs). A long leg brace is known as a *knee-ankle-foot orthosis* (KAFO) or a *hip-knee-ankle-foot orthosis* (HKAFO) if it contains a hip joint as well as a knee joint. The newer terminology is more descriptive and specific and avoids confusion.

Orthotic devices are prescribed by a physician and fabricated by an orthotist. The physical therapist provides input to the physician and orthotist about which temporary devices have been assessed in the clinic before a permanent orthosis is prescribed. The physical therapist is also responsible for gait training the individual with the orthotic device. Training includes donning and doffing instructions, skin inspections, and patient education as well as the actual gait training.

Orthotic devices are classified in four categories: stabilizing (supportive), functional (assistive), corrective, and protective. All orthoses are aimed at increasing function.

Stabilizing and functional orthoses are the two types most often used with CVA patients. Stabilizing orthoses are used to prevent unwanted motion such as plantar flexion at the ankle or knee buckling. Functional orthoses have an element that compensates for lost muscle strength by assisting with movement. Stabilizing orthoses are not intended as a way to correct a fixed deformity in an adult; they can only stabilize and accommodate a deformity. Corrective orthoses are used to correct or realign parts of a limb. They are used for infants and very young children to help correct flexible skeletal deformities. They should not be used to correct a fixed deformity in an adult. In such an instance, a stabilization orthosis can be used but only to support the fixed deformity. Protective orthoses protect a portion of a limb from weight-bearing forces (e.g., a limb with a fracture).[21]

The orthotist adheres to basic physical principles when fabricating an orthosis to control a weak joint. An orthosis that provides three points of pressure is the most common type.[52] One of the three forces is directed toward the joint itself, and the other two end forces are directed opposite to the main force (Figure 11-9). This principle is an important one for the occupational therapist to learn because of its relevance to adaptive shoe equipment. Figure 11-9, *B* illustrates the three points of pressure used with an AFO that is providing a dorsiflexion assist. Note that the main point of pressure is on the dorsum of the foot. The two counter pressures are at the posterior calf and the distal plantar surface of the foot. Elastic laces, often used to facilitate donning a shoe with stroke patients, eliminate the main point of pressure and result in loss of orthotic effectiveness. Therefore elastic laces should not be used with dorsiflexion-assist braces. Elastic laces should even be used cautiously with solid ankle AFOs that prevent dorsiflexion (see Figure 11-9, *A*) because the foot needs to be held

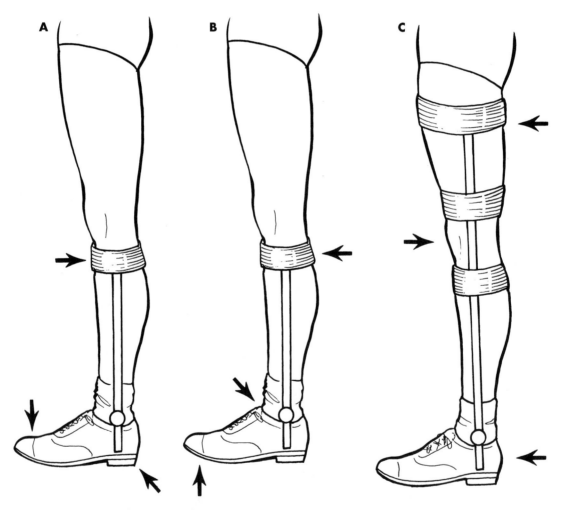

Figure 11-9 A, Three points of pressure of an AFO with dorsiflexion stop. **B,** Three points of pressure of a dorsiflexion assist AFO. **C,** Three points of pressure of a locked KAFO. (These illustrations are diagrammatic only.)

snuggly in the AFO and shoe. This is especially true if plantar flexion spasticity is present.

Another orthotic principle is the longer the lever arms, the less force that needs to be applied at the two ends and middle. Bony landmarks and superficial nerves need to be considered when implementing these principles.[51] The orthotic joint axis of motion should be aligned with the skeletal joint; otherwise, abnormal pressures can be applied in the wrong areas, such as under calf bands, with movement or positioning.[21,52]

Orthotic devices can be made of a variety of materials, the most common of which are metal and plastic. Plastic orthoses are in total contact with a limb and are worn inside the shoe. Metal orthoses are attached to a shoe and held in place on the limb with straps or bands.

The type of orthosis used most often with CVA patients is the AFO. The AFO can affect knee motion as well as ankle motion. If dorsiflexion is prevented at the ankle while standing, knee flexion or buckling is less likely to occur. If plantar flexion of the ankle is prevented while standing, knee hyperextension (recurvatum) is effectively blocked. Therefore using the heavier KAFO to control the knee in a stroke patient can usually be avoided.

Plastic orthoses are usually made from high-temperature thermoplastic materials such as polypropylene. They require high temperatures for molding and therefore are shaped over a model, such as a plaster cast impression of the patient's leg. They are more resistant to continued stress than the low-temperature thermoplastics used for upper limb orthoses.

The simplest and most commonly used plastic AFO is the posterior leaf splint or spring (PLS)[21] (Figure 11-10, A). It is used when the main gait deviation exhibited is "foot drop" during the swing phase. It functions as a dorsiflexion assist because of its flexibility. The plastic of the calf portion is displaced in stance and then springs back to a 90° angle during swing. The ankle joint is held at this 90° angle during swing. "Foot drop" and "toe drag" are avoided. However, it does not afford any mediolateral stability at the ankle joint. If this is of concern, then a more substantial orthosis can be tried.

A modified AFO or MAFO has a wide calf upright with lateral trimline borders that are just posterior to the malleoli (Figure 11-10, B). Usually the foot plate encompasses more of the lateral and medial borders of the foot. This results in more control of calcaneal and forefoot inversion and eversion. The increased width of the calf portion offers somewhat more resistance to plantar flexion in both swing and stance.

The most supportive AFO is the solid ankle AFO (Figure 11-10, C). The lateral trim lines extend even farther forward anterior to the malleoli. Because of its construction, the solid ankle AFO is designed to prevent ankle motion and foot motion in any plane. Dorsiflexion, plantar flexion, inversion, and eversion are controlled.

A variety of hinged plastic AFOs are now available to allow certain motions and block others. The ankle joint components are too numerous to mention, and newer components are continuously being designed. Different combinations of joints and stops can be used by the ortho-

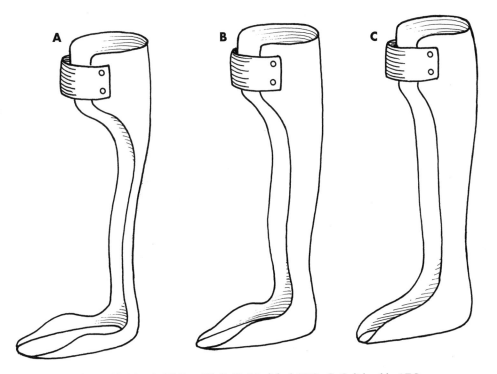

Figure 11-10   **A,** PLS or PLO. **B,** Modified AFO. **C,** Solid ankle AFO.

tist to allow, limit, or prevent movement. For example, the therapist may wish to allow dorsiflexion past neutral (90°) in stance to allow normal tibial advancement over the foot but block plantar flexion at neutral to prevent foot drop in swing and knee hyperextension in stance.

Another classification of plastic AFOs are referred to as *tone-inhibiting AFOs.* Most of these AFOs were initially designed for use with cerebral palsy children.[15] Several types have been designed more specifically for use with adult hemiplegics.[40] The common denominator is the flexibility allowed by these orthoses, in the foot as well as the ankle. In theory, this allows more normal weight-bearing contacts on the plantar surface of the foot throughout stance. This promotes normal mobility in the foot during stance, instead of it being held in one position. The foot-loading patterns obtained when using two different tone-inhibiting AFOs were documented in a study by Mueller et al.[40] Biomechanical alignment and foot stability were assessed, and one—the dynamic ankle-foot orthosis—was found to have had significant effects at the lateral forefoot with respect to force. The authors concluded that this effect may support the medial longitudinal arch of the foot and increase the stability of the forefoot as it is loaded. They theorized that this in turn may allow the forefoot to be loaded at a faster velocity. The effects of correct biomechanical alignment on muscle EMG activity were not investigated.

The tone-inhibiting effect attributed to these AFOs is based on hypotheses formulated on the basis of the effect of serial casting on spasticity and abnormal tone.[12,15] However, as the scientific literature readily attests, the evidence of a central inhibiting effect of prolonged stretch by inhibitive casting is inconclusive.[1,12,55] Changes in sarcomere number and connective tissue due to immobilization, positioning, and stretch can influence muscle contraction force.[1,13,27] In addition, muscle length can also influence the manifestation of hyperreflexia.[1,13] Perhaps it is these mechanical properties of muscle that are influenced by tone-inhibiting orthoses. By promoting better biomechanical alignment and normal muscle length, these AFOs may exert an effect on peripheral rather than central factors, that over time could otherwise augment stretch reflexes. Further research is needed, especially long-term, controlled studies, to investigate the many variables that influence motor control and muscle function. Until there is a more complete and universally accepted definition of tone and what contributes to normal and abnormal tone, the term *tone inhibiting* may need to be reconsidered.

Metal orthoses were the main type of orthotic devices used prior to the 1970s.[21] Metal AFOs are still used for certain stroke patients who cannot tolerate the total contact of a plastic AFO for whatever reason. The components usually consist of two metal uprights attached to an ankle joint. The metal is usually aluminum, but sometimes heavier steel is needed for control. The ankle joint is attached to a stirrup that is fastened beneath the heel of the shoe. The proximal ends of the upright are attached to a calf band.

The metal ankle joint is usually a single- or double-channel (chamber) type (Figure 11-11). Other types of ankle joints are described in detail elsewhere.[19,21,36] A single-channel ankle joint can assist dorsiflexion with a spring placed in the channel. Plantar flexion can also be limited to prevent genu recurvatum by placing a pin in the channel. A double-channel ankle joint can prevent dorsiflexion as well as plantar flexion by using pins in both channels. Small screws hold the pins in the chambers. The degree of dorsiflexion or plantar flexion (i.e., the ankle joint angle) can be determined by the degree to which the pins are driven into the channels by tightening the screws. Springs and pins can be used in combination to stop one movement and assist one another.

The metal uprights attached to the ankle joint and stirrup offer a certain amount of foot and ankle mediolateral control. However, if additional support is needed (e.g., to prevent severe foot inversion), a strap can be added that applies pressure to the lateral malleolus in a medial direction and is secured around the medial upright. Because it prevents varus positioning of the ankle, the strap is called a *varus correction strap.* Force can be applied in the opposite direction with a strap to prevent foot eversion and a valgus foot position. This strap is then called a *valgus correction strap.* A varus correction strap is more common.

The simplest type of metal AFO is the Veteran's Administration Prosthetic Center (VAPC) shoe clasp orthosis. It consists of a single narrow metal upright that attaches to the heel counter of a shoe with a metal clasp and a calf strap (Figure 11-12). It offers dorsiflexion assist only, with no mediolateral or plantar flexion control.

An AFO is the most appropriate orthosis to use with a hemiparetic patient.[39,49,56] Occasionally a KAFO with knee locks may be prescribed for a patient who requires additional knee control. However, the additional weight, prevention of normal knee joint excursions during swing, and increased energy cost greatly limit the potential for functional ambulation.[39,49,56] In addition, donning and doffing a KAFO are difficult for hemiplegic patients (see Figure 11-9, *C*).[56]

A KAFO combines the features of an AFO with a knee joint and (in the case of a metal orthosis) metal uprights that extend proximally up the thigh. Thigh bands secure the KAFO on the the upper leg. The simplest knee joint is a hinge, and the most common locks to maintain knee extension are drop ring locks.[21] The thigh component of plastic KAFOs is usually made of the same thermoplastic material as the AFO component. Metal and plastic combinations can also be utilized.[19,21,36]

As previously mentioned, KAFOs are seldom used for hemiparetic patients. Occasionally a preexisting knee joint deformity or ligamentous laxity is exacerbated by walking because of the now weak muscular support. In such in-

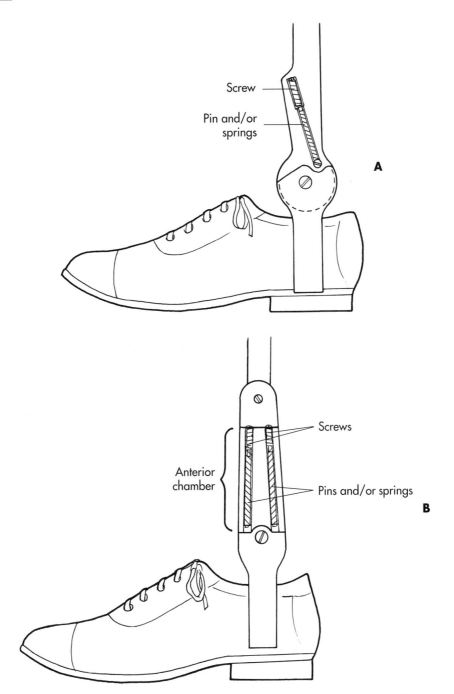

Figure 11-11 **A,** Single channel (chamber) metal ankle joint. **B,** Double channel (chamber) metal ankle joint.

stances, there may be no alternative to using a KAFO to allow minimal household ambulation. KAFOs are also sometimes used as initial training devices to enhance stability. They should be utilized only as temporary measures and not as long-term orthotic devices.[39,49,56]

The physical therapist, especially in the outpatient or home therapy setting, has the responsibility of reevaluating the orthotic device on an ongoing basis. In this era of decreased length of hospital stays, patients are sometimes prescribed an orthotic device while still in the early stages of recovery. As motor control improves, the orthotic device may need to be modified or discontinued to allow more active patient movement.

ASSISTIVE DEVICES

The assistive devices most commonly used with stroke patients are canes, walkers, and occasionally two crutches. A

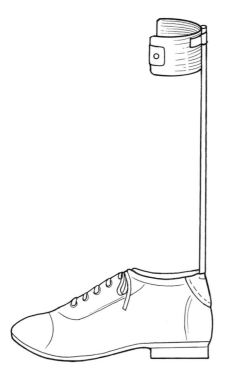

Figure 11-12 Veterans Administration Prosthetic Center orthosis for dorsiflexion assist.

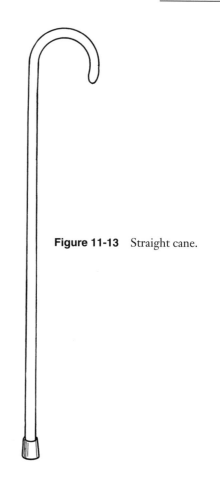

Figure 11-13 Straight cane.

cane may be used by hemiparetic patients whose balance is minimally impaired and who have functional strength in the opposite upper extremity. Two crutches or a walker require at least some functional use of both upper extremities. Both provide more external stability, with the walker providing more stability than the crutches. The main function of a cane is to increase the base of support and thereby improve balance.[50] The base of support is increased by providing another contact with the floor. Canes also decrease the need for abductor muscle tension to stabilize the pelvis in stance on the paretic side.[43,50] This in turn helps to prevent dropping of the contralateral pelvis (a positive Trendelenburg sign) in stance when the cane is used in the hand opposite the hemiparetic leg. Using the opposite hand also helps simulate the reciprocal arm and leg movements of a normal gait.

A variety of canes are on the market, ranging from a simple, wooden, straight cane to a tripod "walk cane" (also called a *hemiwalker*). At a level in between these two canes are the narrow- and wide-based quadruped canes (quad canes) (Figures 11-13 to 11-16). Widening the base of support provides more stability. Physical therapists may begin training with a fairly wide-based cane because of hemiparesis and impaired balance. They should advance patients as quickly as possible to the least amount of assistance required to ensure a safe, stable gait. Patients are often inadvertently kept on a maximally wide base of support cane when it is no longer needed. This prevents the patient from maximizing functional ambulation for two

reasons: (1) normal weight shifting to the hemiparetic leg is limited, and (2) cadence is slower than it is with a smaller device[50] or no device. The key word is *safety*. Maximum use of the involved leg should be encouraged as well as normal trunk and pelvic movement provided that patient safety is not compromised.

Two crutches are occasionally used—axillary or (more often) forearm (Lofstrand) crutches (Figure 11-17). Certain cerebellar stroke patients or others who have impaired balance but functional use of both arms and hands may be trained with these devices. These patients require the extra postural support afforded by the second crutch but have enough motor control to be able to advance the crutches reciprocally.

Walkers may be utilized for training stroke patients who have functional use of both arms and hands but have need of greater outside support than that afforded by two crutches. Occasionally a walker may be utilized to allow functional use of a hemiparetic arm even though balance is sufficient with a cane. In this case, gait training with a cane should also be practiced to promote optimum postural control as well. If the patients have sufficient control of the paretic arm, walkers may also be used when it is necessary for them to transport objects around the house (e.g., in the kitchen).

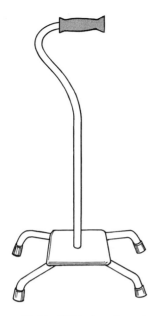

Figure 11-14   Wide-based quad cane.

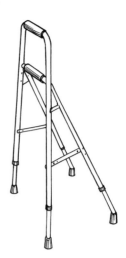

Figure 11-16   Hemiwalker or walk cane.

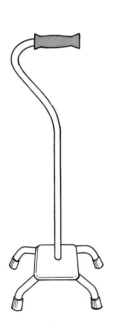

Figure 11-15   Narrow-based quad cane.

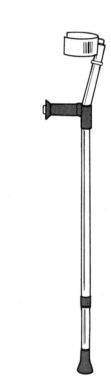

Figure 11-17   Lofstrand crutch.

Standard walkers are the most stable assistive devices because they provide four points of contact with the ground. The base of support is greatly increased. A variety of walkers are available as well. In addition to standard walkers with four legs, rolling walkers with front wheels only, four wheels, and platform attachments are also available. Rolling walkers allow a more normal reciprocal gait, but care must be taken to prevent the walker from "run-ning away" with the patient. A stroke patient with insuffi-cient arm and hand strength to lift a walker may have enough of an ability to maintain a grip on the rolling walker and push it forward. Some walkers have pressure-sensitive brakes that prevent forward movement when weight is borne on the arms and hands.

As mentioned in the cerebellar stroke section, postural control is sometimes sacrificed for stability when a walker is used. The patient has no need to relearn balance and control if the walker provides needed support. As mentioned, safety is the ultimate concern. If safe, functional ambulation is not possible without a walker, then safe independent ambulation with a walker is the preferred choice.

The type of gait pattern that is taught to the stroke patient depends on a number of factors, including balance, strength, and coordination.[43,50] Cognitive and perceptual deficits including apraxias should also be considered.

Terminology for describing walking patterns was suggested by Smidt and Mommens.[51] *Point* refers to the number of contacts that are being made with the floor, including with feet and assistive devices, during the forward progression of the gait cycle (Figures 11-18 and 11-19). For example, a four-point contralateral gait indicates that two feet and two assistive devices (such as canes being advanced one at a time) are being used (Figure 11-19, *A*). The more contacts on the floor at any given moment, the more stable the person is while walking. In addition, the pattern can be called a

delayed pattern if the assistive device is advanced before the limbs. Delayed patterns provide more stability than moving a limb concurrently with an assistive device. Following are the most common gait patterns taught to stroke patients.

GAIT PATTERNS

Two-Point Contralateral Gait Pattern Using One Device

Hemiparetic patients with a nonfunctional arm are often taught a two-point contralateral gait pattern using one assistive device. A device, such as a cane, is held in the unaffected hand. The cane and the paretic leg are advanced together (one point), and then the unaffected leg is advanced alone (second point) (Figure 11-18, *B*). The cane may be advanced first and then the paretic limb followed by the unaffected limb for a more stable pattern. This pattern is a delayed contralateral two-point gait pattern (Figure 11-19, *B*). In Figures 11-18, *B* and 11-19, *B*, the right leg is the hemiparetic leg.

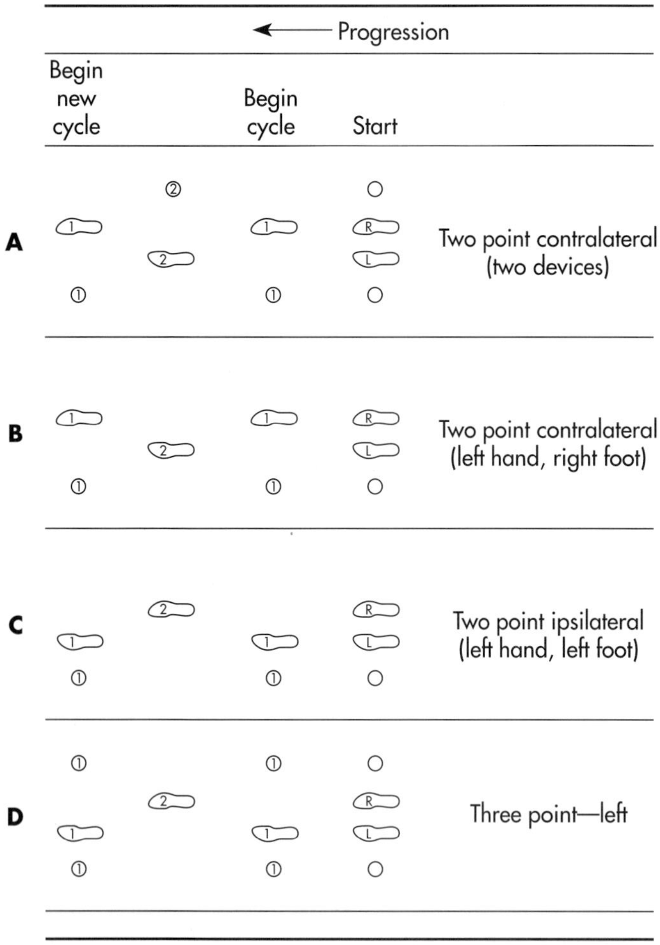

Figure 11-18 **A** to **D**, Diagrammatic view of assisted gaits. (From Smidt G, Mommens MA: Gait patterns, *Phys Ther* 60:553, 1980.)

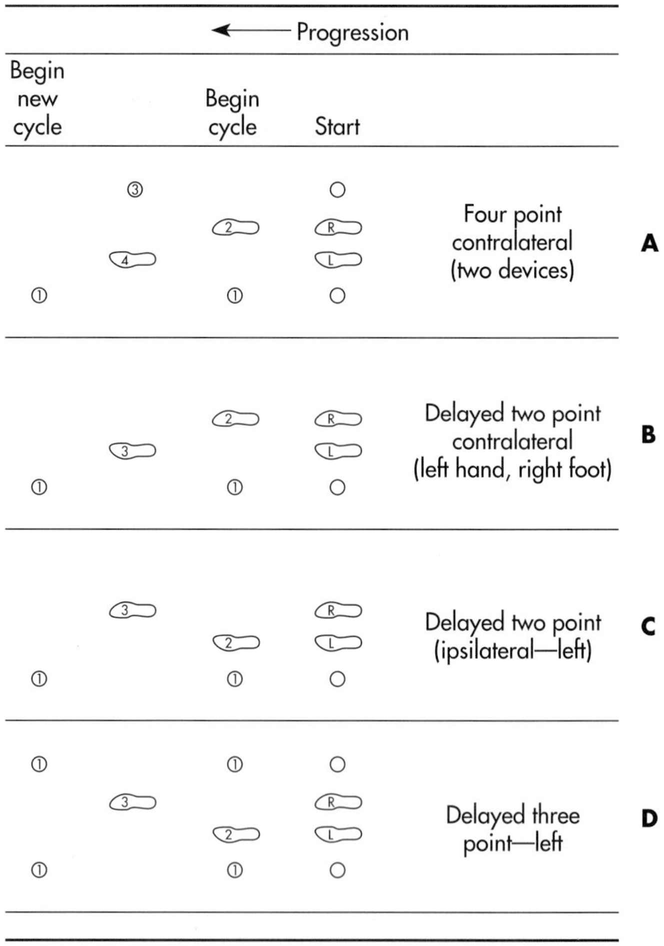

Figure 11-19 **A** to **D**, Diagrammatic view of assisted gaits. (From Smidt G, Mommens MA: Gait patterns, *Phys Ther* 60:553, 1980.)

Four-Point Contralateral Gait Pattern Using Two Devices

The devices used in a four-point contralateral gait pattern could be either canes or crutches. This type of gait may be chosen for stroke patients who have functional use of all four limbs but have impaired balance. They require bilateral support but are able to advance each device (two points) and each leg (two points) individually and reciprocally. Although this is a very stable gait pattern, it is not often used with hemiparetic patients. Sometimes a patient recovering from a cerebellar stroke will be taught this pattern to encourage coordinated reciprocal arm and leg movements as well as postural control.

Two-Point Contralateral Gait Pattern Using Two Devices

If the previously mentioned patients regained sufficient postural control, they might be advanced to using a two-point contralateral pattern (Figure 11-18, *A*). They still would be using two crutches or canes but would be moving one device and the opposite leg simultaneously (one point) followed by the other device and opposite leg (one point).

Five-Point Gait Pattern Using One Device

If patients have functional control of all four extremities but require greater trunk control, they may be trained with a walker. For example, certain patients who have had cerebellar strokes may never recover adequate postural stability to be able to use two canes. Walkers allow patients to utilize five points of contact: the walker's four legs and one of the patient's legs. If the walker is advanced simultaneously with one leg, the pattern is called a *five-point gait pattern* (Figure 11-20, *B*). If the walker is moved first and is followed by a leg, the pattern is called a *five-point delayed gait pattern* (Figure 11-20, *A*).

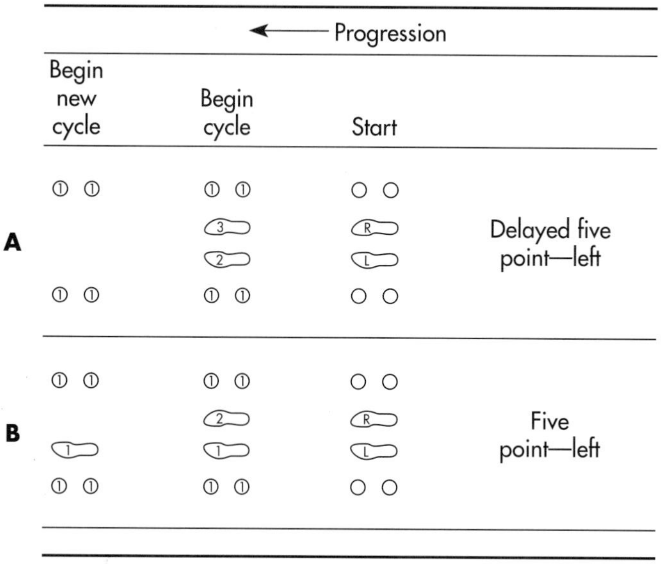

The previously mentioned patients may be trained with a rolling walker. This device may be chosen for two reasons: (1) because the walker is in constant contact with the floor while being advanced, maximum postural control is afforded; (2) because the walker is in constant motion, the patient is able to take equal step lengths and increase his speed. With the standard walker, the patient is forced to use a "step-to" type of gait pattern (walker is advanced, then the foot, then the other foot) that prevents a normal stride and limits velocity.[51] In making the decision to use a rolling walker, the physical therapist must also consider the patient's ability to control the continuous forward motion of the walker, as mentioned previously.

Three-Point Gait Pattern Using Two Devices

Three-point gait patterns are seldom used with stroke patients and are used more often with patients who have orthopedic conditions requiring weight relief on one leg (see Figures 11-18, *D* and 11-19, *D*).

GUARDING TECHNIQUES

The goal of gait training after stroke is to have the patient walk as efficiently, safely, and independently as possible. To promote optimum functional ambulation, it is important for the patient to experience postural instability to relearn the way to correct these imbalances.

With this in mind, it is important for the therapist to be as close to patients as necessary to prevent them from falling or injuring themselves and yet not inhibit them from learning the way to right themselves. Therapists must allow patients to take some risks without jeopardizing the patients' safety or their own safety. This is not an easy task, especially for new therapists. An ultimate horror for any therapist is having a patient fall. Obviously, until therapists are comfortable with patients and know how much if any outside support they need, it is better to guard too much than guard too little. Regardless, the goal should always be optimum function, and the therapist will need to reevaluate on an ongoing basis how much guarding is needed and in what type of setting and on what type of surface activities should be performed.

Hemiparetic patients walking with a cane are most often guarded on the weaker side. The therapist stands slightly posterior and lateral to the affected side.[50] The therapist is then in the best position to assist the patient. Should patients lose their balance or stumble, they may have difficulty preventing a fall to the weaker side because of decreased sensation and decreased strength and control of the paretic leg. The therapist can control patients with the hand closest to them at the hip or pelvis and can control patients' shoulder and trunk with the other hand if necessary.

Figure 11-20 **A** and **B**, Diagrammatic view of assisted gaits. (From Smidt G, Mommens MA: Gait patterns, *Phys Ther* 60:554, 1980.)

The use of gait belts or guarding belts varies from therapist to therapist and from institution to institution, but most facilities advocate their use in the initial stages of gait training and on stairs. The patient's safety is of the utmost concern. At times, a patient is uncontrollable without a gait belt. Other times, it can be a hindrance to patients relearning postural control if the therapist is inadvertently tugging on the belt with every step. Each patient must be evaluated individually. The size of the patient in comparison to the therapist may also need to be considered. The therapist should decide which anticipatory actions need to be taken to protect the patient from harm based on clinical assessment and sound judgment.

When guarding patients ascending stairs, the therapist is positioned posterior and to the weaker side. Patients should be trained using a railing at the stronger side. Initially they may be taught to ascend one step at a time, leading with the stronger leg. When patients are descending, the therapist stands in front of and lateral to the affected side so that assistance can be provided if patients' knees buckle on the weaker limb. Using the railing, patients step down one step at a time, leading with the paretic leg. Patients who regain functional strength of their paretic leg may be advanced to the step-over-step method with close guarding by the therapist. Ascending and descending stairs with only a cane or two canes is difficult and requires excellent balance. Some home environments may necessitate such training, but it should be undertaken with sufficient guarding, and the safety risks should be carefully weighed.

Guarding techniques need to be taught to family members as soon as possible during a patient's inpatient rehabilitation. Family participation in gait training provides the opportunity for practice and repetition of newly learned techniques.

CASE STUDY

Gait

This case study in no way reflects the patient's whole treatment program because emphasis is also placed on increasing strength and function in the trunk and left arm as well as in the leg. In addition, there are frequent sessions of cotreating by the occupational and physical therapists to enhance communication about specific treatment concerns (e.g., the subluxed shoulder) and functional goals.

HC is a 54-year-old male who was admitted to the emergency room of a university medical center with sudden onset of left-sided weakness. Two weeks earlier, he had undergone a mitral valve repair and a single coronary artery bypass with a left saphenous vein gaft. He had had an uneventful postoperative recovery course and was discharged to his home and prescribed a β-blocker.

On admission, the neurologic workup and results included

(1) a CT scan of the head showing early lucency in the right subcortical area; (2) noninvasive flow studies (on the second day) showing accelerated flow velocities in the right middle cerebral artery suggestive of stenosis and normal flows in the anterior cerebral arteries, posterior cerebral arteries, and basal artery; and (3) a transesophageal echocardiogram revealing trace mitral regurgitation, normal left ventricular function, and no intracardiac or aortic mass or thrombus.

The attending neurologist concluded that HC had suffered an infarct in the right corona radiata and putamen in the territory supplied by the lenticulostriate branches of the right middle cerebral artery. The cause of the infarct was most probably an embolus of cardiac origin that developed after the mitral valve repair. HC was prescribed anticoagulant medication and medically stabilized. Twelve days later he was transferred to the rehabilitation unit of the same medical center.

On admission to the rehabilitation unit, HC had symptoms of a pure motor syndrome with left upper extremity weakness that was greater than the left leg weakness, minimal left lower facial droop, and no sensory loss. He was alert and oriented and most cooperative although somewhat deconditioned because of the previous cardiac surgery.

Physical assessment revealed normal passive ROM of the left arm and leg, although both legs manifested tight hamstrings and could only perform a straight leg raise to barely 60°. A finger-width subluxation was present in the left shoulder. Strength testing revealed that the left arm was grossly 2-3/5 throughout. He was able to extend the left knee completely while sitting (3/5), but the hip flexors were weaker (2/5). He exhibited no isolated voluntary ankle movement, although dorsiflexion was two out of five with simultaneous flexion of the hip and knee, and plantar flexion was two out of five during simultaneous extension of these proximal joints. He did not at that time (or ever) exhibit any spasticity in the limbs during passive testing by the therapist, with the exception of mild, unsustained ankle clonus. He exhibited no ankle edema despite the leg weakness and previous vein graft for the coronary artery bypass graft surgery.

His gait was initially evaluated while he was walking around a high mat with his right side next to the mat, using his right arm and the mat to "unload" the left leg. During static standing, he required contact guarding and verbal cues to actively extend the left hip and knee. He had a tendency to bear most of his weight on the stronger right leg. When cued to stand with equal weight on both legs, he was unable to maintain an upright posture and would fall to the left because the knee would buckle. He required minimal assistance to maintain the hip and knee in extension when bearing weight symmetrically.

Initially he was able to take 10 steps around the mat with minimal assistance. His gait analysis was as follows: Uneven step lengths were observed; the left was greater although less controlled than the right. The shorter step with the right leg resulted in a "step-to" type of gait pattern—the right leg stepping to meet, instead of pass, the left leg. He exhibited a decrease in single-limb stance time on the left leg. His cadence was extremely slow—approximately 40 steps per minute.

During the left leg stance, the heel did not strike at initial contact; the foot was flat. The loading response resulted in excessive knee flexion that was greater than the normal 10° to 15°. To prevent buckling in midstance, the knee snapped back into hyperextension (genu recurvatum). Instead of bringing his body forward by allowing the tibia to advance over the foot (dorsiflexion), he kept the ankle angle fixed and flexed the hip and trunk over the foot. He did not push off at the end of stance. Instead he quickly took a short step with the right leg to unload the left one as soon as possible.

Because the resulting right leg position was next to the left leg instead of beyond it, the left leg was unable to assume the normal preswing position of hip extension and 40° knee flexion (see Figure 11-4). Instead both the left hip and knee were in full extension, and he was forced to initiate swing on the left from this position.

During the swing phase of the left leg, HC exhibited decreased hip and knee flexion and a foot drop because of the weak dorsiflexors. This resulted in his toes scraping the floor. He displayed mild lateral trunk flexion to the right in an attempt to first initiate swing from the previously mentioned abnormal preswing position and then to clear the toes throughout the swing phase.

HC was put on a program of active assistive ROM and strengthening exercises for the left arm and leg. Treatment of the leg emphasized functional strengthening in weight-bearing positions (e.g., sit-to-stand exercises for hip and knee strengthening).

During the initial stage of gait training, a posterior leaf splint orthosis was used to assist with dorsiflexion during the swing phase on the left side. This was chosen to encourage a more efficient swing phase and to discourage the patient from leaning to the right to clear the left leg during swing. Because of its flexibility, the posterior leaf splint did not restrict activity at the left ankle or knee during stance. Although the knee was unstable, HC was still in the early stages of recovery. It was not beneficial to sacrifice mobility for stability (i.e., block any ankle dorsiflexion and knee flexion in stance). Doing so would have forced him to move compensatorily because it is normal to dorsiflex up to 10° at the ankle during midstance and terminal stance. The therapist offered close supervison to contact guarding at the knee because of possible knee buckling resulting from excessive dorsiflexion. HC was taught to be aware of the difference between excessive knee flexion and recurvatum. He was soon able to correctly identify when he was in either of these abnormal positions even if he could not always prevent them.

HC quickly advanced from ambulation around the high mat to ambulation with a narrow-based quad cane and then a straight cane. He had the advantage of recovering much of his hip extension and abduction strength, which meant he did not require a large degree of outside support from an assistive device for these muscles.

Functional training included standing balance retraining in both single limb and double limb weight-bearing positions. Modified versions of activities that the patient had previously enjoyed (soccer) and a few new ones (golf putting and baseball) were introduced. Ambulation was practiced in a variety of environments and on both even and uneven terrains in preparation for discharge. Even getting through busy revolving doors was practiced.

After 6 weeks of inpatient rehabilitation, HC was evaluated for a permanent AFO. His left leg strength had improved enough to allow him to isolate dorsiflexion and plantar flexion in any position grossly in the 2/5 range, ankle inversion and eversion in the 2−/5 range, and toe flexion and extension in the 1+/5 range. His hip flexors improved minimally to two plus out of five, and knee extension also improved minimally to 3+/5.

During ambulation, he continued to manifest knee recurvatum in stance and did not push off at the end of stance because of weak plantar flexors. During swing, he continued to exhibit a foot drop and toe drag. The physiatrist, physical therapist, and orthotist performed a joint observational gait analysis. Because of the continued plantar flexor and dorsiflexor weakness during the swing and stance phases and less than normal knee extension strength, it was decided that HC required minimal knee control as well as ankle control from an AFO. In addition, the weak ankle invertors and evertors necessitated mediolateral control by an orthosis. Therefore a posterior leaf splint was deemed insufficient. However, because HC was continuing to progress and did not require maximum support at the knee, a solid ankle AFO was also inappropriate. The general consensus was that HC should be allowed to have as much movement at the ankle as possible without jeopardizing his safety to promote development of a normal gait pattern.

For this reason the team decided to order a hinged polypropylene AFO with free dorsiflexion at the ankle and a plantar flexion stop at 90°. The hinged ankle with free dorsiflexion allowed him to move the tibia normally over the foot (dorsiflexion) in midstance and terminal stance. The plantar flexion stop at 90° prevented foot drop in swing and recurvatum in stance. The orthosis improved his gait by allowing the normal joint excursions at the knee and ankle in stance while preventing abnormal movements in both stance and swing. The promotion of normal joint excursions at the ankle in stance allowed him to take equal step lengths with both legs.

On discharge to his home, HC was able to ambulate independently indoors with a straight cane and the hinged AFO, but required supervision outdoors. He was able to ascend and descend stairs step-over-step using a railing and ascend and descend curbs and ramps with the straight cane—all with distant supervision. He could independently perform simple home exercises for left leg and arm strengthening. He returned to work full-time as a university professor and continued with outpatient therapy three times a week for 6 months after discharge. He regained full functional use of the left upper extremity including finger function—albeit with decreased coordination—fine motor control, and strength. He also continued to receive occupational therapy for several months on an outpatient basis.

■

SUMMARY

The aim of this chapter was to familiarize the occupational therapist with processes used by physical therapists during gait evaluation and training of patients who have suffered a CVA. The most common type of gait disorders are those resulting from a middle cerebral artery infarction.

The application of orthotic devices is not an exact science. It is not accurate to assume that a particular abnormal gait always requires one specific type of orthotic device. Devices need to be evaluated on an individual trial basis. Use of a specific device or pattern requires individualized attention.

It is the belief of those well-versed and experienced in motor control research[13,25,28,30,57] that the trend in physical therapy is moving away from earlier theoretical models of treatment techniques and toward a motor control model. The emphasis is no longer on specific treatment techniques to "facilitate" movement but on active problem-solving by the patient to promote skilled movement and motor relearning. Treatment programs need to be based on specific motor control deficits, varied, meaningful to the patient, and must take place in a multitude of environments.

It can no longer be assumed that certain treatment techniques are effective. Effectiveness needs to be validated by research. Weinstein et al[57] examined the effect that balance-training and weight-shifting activities during standing have on the hemiplegic gait. Although patients who received training improved their standing symmetry significantly, it did not translate into improved weight shifting during ambulation. This study clearly demonstrates the hazards of assuming that transfer of training occurs from one functional task to another. For example, it would be convenient to assume that the techniques used to improve the standing balance of a patient with ipsilateral pushing will improve the ability to walk. However, there is no evidence to support this theory. Further research such as that of Weinstein et al[57] is imperative for therapists to validate the rationales for their treatment procedures for stroke patients. To do otherwise denies the patient the most beneficial treatment approach.

The case study was unusual because the patient exhibited no spasticity and had voluntary, isolated control of all muscles but had decreased strength. However, several authors questioned the role of spasticity in preventing normal movement[1,13,30] and pointed to weakness as the more limiting factor. It is well known that spasticity may increase the incidence of muscle contracture and thereby alter the biomechanical efficiency of a muscle.[1,13,16,27,30] In this respect, only the ankle joint was at risk and minimally so. The patient was a "model" patient for other reasons. He was not cognitively impaired, and he was very motivated to return to work. He was aware (although grudgingly at times) of the need for faithful adherence to a regular exercise program of repeated practice of newly learned motor skills.

Therapists should always be aware of the need for careful physical assessment, individualized treatment programs that are based on research findings, and ongoing reevaluation of the treatment program's effectiveness in promoting optimum function.

REVIEW QUESTIONS

1. What constitutes a gait cycle?
2. What are the phases and subphases of the gait cycle?
3. What are step, stride, and cadence?
4. What type of cerebral infarct is associated with the typical "hemiplegic gait"?
5. What are some of the variables that can cause a deviation from the normal joint excursions during a gait cycle?
6. In what way does the motor control model differ from the more traditional theoretical models underlying the different therapeutic techniques?
7. What are some of the manifestations of a posterior inferior cerebellar stroke?
8. What makes treatment of patients demonstrating ipsilateral pushing so challenging?
9. What helps compensate for proprioceptive loss after stroke?
10. What are the main differences between metal and plastic orthotic devices?
11. What orthotic device is most commonly used with stroke patients?
12. What assistive devices are used most commonly with stroke patients?
13. What determines the type of gait pattern that will be taught to a stroke patient?

■ COTA Considerations ■

- The gait cycle is made up of the stance phase, in which the leg is in contact with the ground, and the swing phase, in which the leg is off the ground.
- After a stroke, people walk slower. Physical therapists often measure cadence (the number of steps per unit of time) or the velocity (the distance walked in a given period of time) to document improvement.
- Trendelenburg's sign is present when there is excessive lateral displacement of the pelvis over the leg in the stance phase with excessive lowering of the pelvis over the contralateral leg in the swing phase.
- Circumduction is a semicircular movement of the involved hip—a compensatory strategy a person uses in place of hip flexion.
- Wallenberg's syndrome results in an ataxic gait and a loss of balance with falling toward the involved side.
- Engaging in weight shifting and reaching while in standing are encouraged for all persons with gait disturbances.

- Weight bearing on a leg that has a proprioceptive loss may help to restore leg function. Relying more on vision also helps to compensate for sensory loss.
- Stabilizing and functional orthoses are the most common types used by persons surviving a stroke. Stabilizing splints accommodate a deformity and prevent motion.

REFERENCES

1. Ada L, Canning C: Anticipating and avoiding muscle shortening. In Ada L, Canning C, editors: *Key issues in neurological physiotherapy*, Boston, 1990, Butterworth-Heinemann.
2. Adams JM, Perry J: Gait analysis: clinical application. In Rose J, Gamble JG, editors: *Human walking*, Baltimore, 1994, Williams & Wilkins.
3. Amarenco P: The spectrum of cerebellar infarcts, *Neurology*, 41:973, 1991.
4. Amarenco P: Cerebellar stroke syndromes. In Bogousslavsky J, Caplan L, editors: *Stroke syndromes*, Cambridge, 1995, Cambridge University Press.
5. Balliet R, et al: Retraining of functional gait through the reduction of upper extremity weight bearing in chronic cerebellar ataxia, *Int Rehabil Med* 8:25, 1987.
6. Bingman VP, Zucchi M: Spatial orientation. In Cohen H, editor: *Neuroscience for rehabilitation*, Philadelphia, 1993, JB Lippincott.
7. Bogousslavsky J, Caplan L, editors: *Stroke syndromes*, Cambridge, 1995, Cambridge University Press.
8. Branch EF: The neuropathology of stroke. In Duncan P, Badke MB, editors: *Stroke rehabilitation*, Chicago, 1987, Mosby.
9. Brandt T, Krafczyk S, Malsbenden I: Postural imbalance with head extension: improvement by training as a model for ataxia therapy, *Ann NY Acad Sci* 374:636, 1981.
10. Brust, JB: Cerebral circulation; stroke. In Kandel ER, Schwartz JH, editors: *Principles of neural science*, ed 3, New York, 1991, Elsevier.
11. Caplan LR: Visual perceptual abnormalities. In Bogousslavsky J, Caplan L, editors: *Stroke syndromes*, Cambridge, 1995, Cambridge University Press.
12. Carlson SJ: A neurophysiological analysis of inhibitive casting, *Phys Occup Ther Pedatr* 4:31, 1984.
13. Carr JH, Shepherd RB, Ada L: Spasticity: research findings and implications for intervention, *Physiother* 81:421, 1995.
14. Davies PM: *Steps to follow*, Berlin, 1985, Springer-Verlag.
15. Diamond M, Ottenbacher K: Effect of tone-inhibiting DAFO on stride characteristics of an adult with hemiparesis, *Phys Ther* 70:423, 1981.
16. Dietz V, Quintern J, Berger W: Electrophysiological studies of gait in spasticity and rigidity: evidence that altered mechanical properties of muscle contribute to hypertonia, *Brain* 104:431, 1981.
17. Dimitrijevic MR et al: Activation of paralyzed leg flexors and extensors during gait in patients after stroke, *Scand J Rehabil Med* 13:109, 1981.
18. Duncan PW, Badke MB: Determinants of abnormal motor control. In Duncan PW, Badke MB, editors: *Stroke rehabilitation*, Chicago, 1987, Mosby.
19. Edelstein J: Orthotic management and assessment. In O'Sullivan S, Schmitz TJ, editors: *Physical rehabilitation: assessment and treatment*, Philadelphia, 1994, FA Davis.
20. Engardt M et al: Dynamic muscle strength training in stroke patients: effect on knee extension torque, EMG activity, and motor function, *Arch Phys Med Rehabil* 76:419, 1995.
21. Faculty of Prosthetics and Orthotics, New York University School of Medicine and Post Graduate Medical School: *Lower limb orthotics*, New York, 1986, New York University School of Medicine and Post Graduate Medical School.
22. Ferro JM: Neurobehavioral aspects of deep hemispheric stroke. In Bogousslavsky J, Caplan L, editors: *Stroke syndrome*, Cambridge, 1995, Cambridge University Press.
23. Fox CR, Cohen H: The visual and vestibular systems: In Cohen H, editor: *Neuroscience for rehabilitation*, Philadelphia, 1993, JB Lippincott.
24. Gilman S, Newman SW: *Clinical neuroanatomy*, ed 8, Philadelphia, 1992, FA Davis.
25. Giuliani CA: Adult hemiplegic gait. In Smidt GL, editor: *Gait in rehabilitation*, New York, 1990, Churchill Livingstone.
26. Glatt SL, Koller WS: Gait apraxia. In Spivack BS, editor: *Evaluation and management of gait disorders*, New York, 1995, Marcel Dekker.
27. Goldspink G, Williams P: Muscle fiber and connective tissue changes associated with use and disuse. In Ada L, Canning C, editors: *Key issues in neurological physiotherapy*, Boston, 1990, Butterworth-Heinemann.
28. Gordon J: Assumptions underlying physical therapy intervention. In Carr JH, Shephard RB, editors: *Movement science foundations*, Rockville, Md, 1987, Aspen.
29. Harro CC, Giuliani CA: Kinematic and EMG analysis of hemiplegic gait patterns during free and fast walking speeds, *Neurol Report* 11:57, 1987.
30. Held JM: Recovery of function after brain damage: theoretical implications for therapeutic intervention. In Carr JH, Shepherd RB, editors: *Movement science foundations*, Rockville, Md, 1987, Aspen.
31. Knutsson E, Martensson A: Dynamic motor capacity in spastic paresis and its relation to prime mover dysfunction, spastic reflexes, and antagonist co-activation, *Scand J Rehabil Med* 12:93, 1980.
32. Knutsson E: Gait control in hemiparesis, *Scand J Rehabil Med* 13:101, 1981.
33. Kusoffsky A, Wadell I, Nilsson BY: The relationship between sensory impairment and motor recovery in patients with hemiplegia, *Scand J Rehabil Med* 14:27, 1982.
34. Lamm-Warburg C: Assessment and treatment planning strategies for perceptual deficits. In O'Sullivan S, Schmitz TJ, editors: *Physical rehabilitation: assessment and treatment*, Philadelphia, 1994, FA Davis.
35. Lehmann JF et al: Gait abnormalities in hemiplegia, *Arch Phys Med* 68:763, 1987.
36. Lehmann JH: Lower limb orthotics. In Redford JB, editor: *Orthotics etc*, ed 3, Baltimore, 1986, Williams & Wilkins.
37. Licht S: Preface, ed 1. In Redford JB, editor: *Orthotics etc*, ed 3, Baltimore, 1986, Williams & Wilkins.
38. McComas AJ et al: Functional changes in motor neurons of hemiparetic patients, *J Neurol Neurosurg Psychiatry* 36:183, 1973.
39. Montgomery J: Assessment and treatment of locomotor deficits in stroke. In Duncan PW, Badke MB, editors: *Stroke rehabilitation: recovery of motor control*, Chicago, 1987, Mosby.
40. Mueller K et al: Effect of two contemporary tone-inhibiting AFOs on foot-loading patterns in adult hemiplegics: a small group study, *Topics Stroke Rehabil* 1:1, 1995.
41. Norkin C: Gait analysis. In O'Sullivan S, Schmitz TJ, editors: *Physical rehabilitation: assessment and treatment*, Philadelphia, 1994, FA Davis.
42. Oestreich L, Troost BT: Cerebellar dysfunction and disorders of posture and gait. In Spivack BS, editor: *Evaluation and management of gait disorders*, New York, 1995, Marcel Dekker.
43. Olsson EC, Smidt GL: Assistive devices. In Smidt GL, editor: *Gait in rehabilitation*, New York, 1990, Churchill-Livingstone.
44. O'Sullivan SB: Motor control assessment. In O'Sullivan SB, Schmitz TJ, editors: *Physical rehabilitation: assessment and treatment*, Philadelphia, 1994, FA Davis.
45. O'Sullivan SB: Stroke. In O'Sullivan SB, Schmitz TJ, editors: *Physical rehabilitation: assessment and treatment*, Philadelphia, 1994, FA Davis.

46. Ounpuu S: Clinical gait analysis. In Spivack BS, editor: *Evaluation and management of gait disorders*, New York, 1995, Marcel Dekker.
47. Pathokinesiology Service and Physical Therapy Department: *Observational gait analysis handbook*, Downey, Calif, 1991, Professional Staff Association of Rancho Los Amigos Medical Center.
48. Pedersen PM, Wandell A, Jorgensen HS: Ipsilateral pushing in stroke: incidence, relation to neuropsychological symptoms, and impact on rehabilitation. The Copenhagen stroke study, *Arch Phys Med* 77:25, 1996.
49. Perry J, Hislop H, editors: *Principles of lower extremity bracing*, Washington, DC, 1977, American Physical Therapy Association.
50. Schmitz TJ: Preambulation and gait training. In O'Sullivan S, Schmitz TJ, editors: *Physical rehabilitation: assessment and treatment.*, Philadelphia, 1994, FA Davis.
51. Smidt GL, Mommens MA: System of reporting and comparing influence of ambulatory aids on gait, *Phys Ther* 60:551, 1980.
52. Smith E, Juvinall RC: Mechanics of orthotics. In Redford JB, editor: *Orthotics etc*, ed 3, Baltimore, 1986, Williams & Wilkins.
53. Tiderksaar R: Falls in older persons. In Spivack BS, editor: *Evaluation and management of gait disorders*, New York, 1995, Marcel Dekker.
54. Toole JF: *Cerebrovascular disorders*, ed 4, New York, 1990, Raven.
55. Walsh EG et al: Biodynamics of the ankle in spastic children—effect of chronic stretching on the calf musculature, *Exp Physiol* 75:423, 1990.
56. Walters RL, Garland DE, Montgomery J: Orthotic prescription for stroke and head injury. In Brunch WH et al, editors: *Atlas of orthotics*, ed 2, St Louis, 1985, Mosby.
57. Weinstein CJ et al: Balance training in hemiparetics, *Arch Phys Med* 70:755, 1989.

lorraine aloisio

chapter **12**

Visual Dysfunction

key terms

anatomy of the eye	saccades	stereopsis
accommodation	pursuits	functional optometry
visual pathways	vergence	visual screening
visual field	strabismus	visual perception
visual acuity	scanning	treatment

chapter objectives

After completing this chapter, the reader will be able to accomplish the following:

1. Present an overview of visual processing, including anatomy of the eye, neuronal processing, and pathophysiology in relation to stroke
2. Outline procedures for vision screening and visual perception evaluation
3. Outline treatment procedures as they pertain to functional abilities

Occupational therapy has made great strides in the screening and treatment of visual disorders in the past 2 decades. This chapter integrates the occupational therapy literature with various other disciplines. The goal of this chapter is to provide clinicians with a comprehensive evaluation and treatment framework for patients who experience visual dysfunction after stroke. A comprehensive understanding of the visual system and the way function is affected after an individual experiences a physical trauma (e.g., a cerebrovascular accident [CVA]) has been emphasized.

Acknowledgment: Special thanks to Dr. Joel H. Warshowsky for his vision.
Dedication: I wish to dedicate my effort in writing this chapter to my father, Fred R. Aloisio.

A TEAM APPROACH

The processing of visual information is a complex act that is usually screened and evaluated by one or more members of the rehabilitation team. These members may include the neurologist, psychologist, neuropsychologist, ophthalmologist, neuro-ophthalmologist, and occupational therapist. One highly important member often missing from this team is the rehabilitative optometrist, more commonly known as the *functional optometrist*. The functional optometrist works with the occupational therapist to assess and manage the functional aspects of vision. These aspects include but are not limited to the ability to use binocular vision, fixate, scan and locate objects, and use accommodation skills successfully.[9,12,14] The occupational therapist relies heavily on the results of the functional optometrist's assessment to provide appropriate treatment and enhance the patient's quality of life.

Many occupational therapists must go outside the rehabilitation program or clinic to use the services of the functional optometrist. Only a few rehabilitation facilities currently use a functional optometrist's services regularly.[19,30] With the high prevalence of visual system dysfunctions seen after stroke, a great need exists to have these professionals as part of the rehabilitation team. For example, an apparent deficit in a visual cognitive skill such as figure-ground (i.e., finding an article of clothing in a drawer) may actually be caused by refractive, binocular, accommodative, ocular motility, or pattern recognition problems. Therefore to help patients regain complex functions, treatment must start at the basic processing level and proceed through a hierarchy of skills, according to Hellerstein and Fishman.[13] Warren's hierarchy of visual perceptual skill development[28] is similar. This framework states that higher-level skills (visuocognition, visual memory, pattern recognition) evolve from the integration of lower-level skills (oculomotor control, visual fields, visual acuity) and are subsequently affected by disruption of lower-level skills.[28]

The functional optometrist's assessment, management, and collaboration with other team members is essential for the success of the individual. The functional optometrist's role does not replace the need for ophthalmologic and neuro-ophthalmologic intervention. If damage has occurred to ocular structures or to the ocular motor system, an ophthalmologist or neuro-ophthalmologist should be called to provide diagnostic and therapeutic care. Surgical or medical treatment may be necessary to minimize loss of sight. However, after the patient is stable, the functional aspects of vision must be evaluated and treated.[4,9,29]

ANATOMY OF THE EYE

The eye (Figure 12-1) includes the cornea, iris, lens, vitreous chamber, and retina.

Cornea

The cornea is the first structure light hits after it is reflected from an image.[6] Corneal tissue is completely transparent. Light is refracted, or bent, to a great degree by the cornea. Efferson[6] describes the refraction of light by discussing the way a stick placed into water appears bent at the point where it enters the water (Figure 12-2).

Damage to the cornea from abrasions, burns, congenital conditions, and disease-related processes can alter the spherical shape of the cornea and disturb the quality of the image that falls on the retina. In keratoconus the cornea slowly becomes steeper and more cone-shaped, distorting the image and causing reduced vision.[6,27]

Iris

Behind the cornea is the iris, the colored portion consisting of fibers that control the opening of the pupil, the dark circular opening in the center of the eye.[6] Constriction and dilation of the pupil control the amount of light entering the eye in a similar fashion to the way the f-stops on a camera change the size of the aperture to control the amount of light and depth of field.[6] In bright light the opening constricts, and in dim light conditions it dilates, allowing light in to stimulate the photoreceptor cells of the retina. This constriction and dilation are under autonomic nervous system (ANS) control with both sympathetic and parasympathetic components. Under sympathetic stimulation (fight or flight reactions) the pupils dilate, perhaps giving rise to the expression "eyes wide with fear." Under parasympathetic stimulation the pupils constrict.[6]

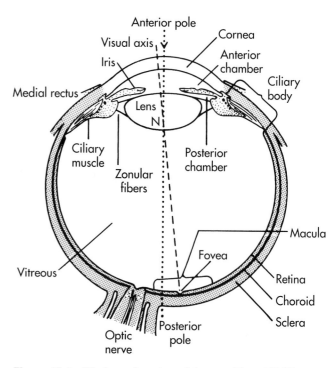

Figure 12-1 Horizontal section of the eye. (From Wolff E: *Anatomy of the eye and orbit*, ed 7, London, 1976, HK Lewis.)

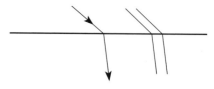

Figure 12-2 Refraction—the bending of light at the air-water interface. (From Umphred DA: *Neurological rehabilitation*, ed 3, St Louis, 1996, Mosby.)

Lens

Behind the iris is the lens. The lens is involved in focusing and accommodation. It is a biconvex, circular, semirigid, crystalline structure that focuses the image on the retina. The lens of the eye is analogous to the external optical lens system of a camera. A camera is focused by turning the lens to change the distance of the lens from the film, effectively increasing or decreasing the power of the lens and allowing near or distant objects to be seen more clearly.[6,8] The same effect (a change in the power of the lens) is achieved in the eye by the action of tiny ciliary muscles that act on suspensory ligaments, changing the thickness and curvature of the lens. A thicker lens with a greater curvature produces higher power and the ability to see clearly at near distances. A thinner lens and flatter curvature produce less optical power and the ability to see distant objects clearly (Figure 12-3). Accommodation is the process of lens thickening and thinning.[6,17]

Ideally, the lens brings an image into perfect focus so that it lands on the fovea, the area of central vision. If the focused image falls in front of the retina, however, a blurred circle falls on the fovea (Figure 12-4). In this case the lens is too thick and has too much optical power. This can be one of the causes of myopia (nearsightedness). One simple remedy is to place a negative (concave) lens externally in front of the eye in glasses to reduce the power of the internal lens and allow the image to fall directly on the fovea. A similar type of problem occurs in hyperopia (farsightedness), in which the image falls in the back of the retina. In presbyopia ("old eyes") the flexibility of the lens fibers decreases and the lens becomes more rigid. Accommodation becomes weaker until the image can no longer be focused on the retina. When this occurs, a positive lens may be worn externally to aid in vision.[6,19]

The lens also can be affected by cataracts, in which the general clarity of vision is impaired because of a loss of transparency in the crystalline lens. Incoming light tends to scatter inside the eye, causing glare problems.

Vitreous Chamber

The vitreous chamber, the space behind the lens, is filled with a gelatinous substance.[17]

Retina

The retina, located at the back of the eye, is the photosensitive layer that receives the pattern of light reflected from objects, similar to the film in a camera. Efferson's topography of the retina[6] (Figure 12-5) includes the optic disc, where the optic nerve exits and arteries and veins emerge. The optic disc also is called the *blind spot* because it con-

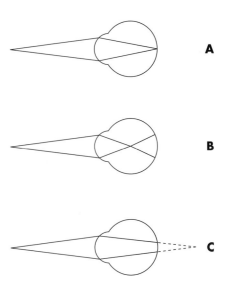

Figure 12-4 **A,** Perfect focusing as the lens brings the image directly onto the fovea. **B,** Focused image falling in front of retina with a blurred circle on fovea, producing myopia (nearsightedness). **C,** Focused image falling in back of retina producing hyperopia (farsightedness). (From Umphred DA: *Neurological rehabilitation*, ed 3, St Louis, 1996, Mosby.)

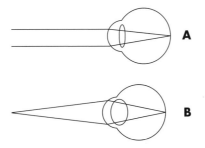

Figure 12-3 Focusing and accommodation. **A,** Thinner lens and flatter curvature produce less optical power and ability to see distant objects clearly. **B,** Thicker lens and greater curvature produce higher power and ability to see clearly at near point. (From Umphred DA: *Neurological rehabilitation*, ed 3, St Louis, 1996, Mosby.)

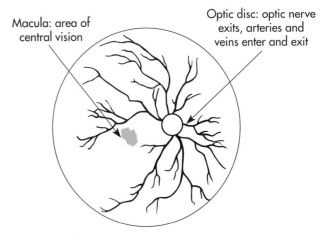

Figure 12-5 Retinal topography.

tains no photoreceptor cells. The macula is temporal to
the optic disc and contains the fovea, essential for central
vision. The surrounding retina is vital for peripheral vision
and defines a 180-degree half sphere.[6,17]

NEURONAL PROCESSING: VISUAL PATHWAYS

Retina

According to Kelly the visual fields are "the way in which
the visual world is projected onto the retina."[1,15] The left
and right hemivisual fields project to the temporal and
nasal hemiretinal fields. Figure 12-6 shows the visual pathways.[1] Based on the work of Mason and Kandel,[16] the visual field is the view seen by the two eyes without movement of the head. If the foveae of both eyes are fixed on a
single point in space, a left and right half of the visual field
can be defined.[16] The left half of the visual field projects
on the nasal retina of the left eye and the temporal retina

of the right eye. The right field projects on the nasal retina
of the right eye and the temporal retina of the left eye.
Light originating in the center of the visual field enters
both eyes; this area is called the *binocular zone*.[16] In either
half of the visual field a monocular zone also may be defined: light from the temporal portion of the hemifield
projects only onto the nasal hemiretina of the eye on the
same side because the nose blocks light from reaching the
opposite eye (Figure 12-7.)[16] This monocular portion of
the visual field also is called the *temporal crescent* because it
constitutes the crescent-shaped temporal extreme of each
visual field. Because no binocular overlap occurs in this region, vision is lost in the entire temporal crescent if this
region of the retina is severely damaged. Arnadottir[1] explains that fibers from the retina form the optic nerves on
each side. The optic nerves meet in the optic chiasma,
where fibers from the nasal hemiretina cross to the opposite side. The optic tract is continuous with the optic chiasma and carries fibers from the ipsilateral temporal

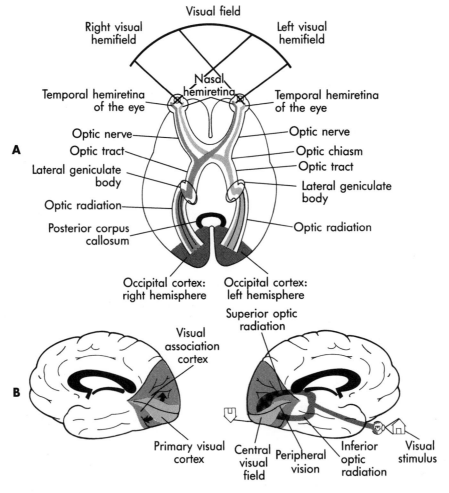

Figure 12-6 The visual pathways. **A,** Inferior view depicting flow of information from the visual
fields to the visual cortex. **B,** Medial view of components of the visual cortex and visual processing.
(From Árnadóttir G: *The brain and behavior: assessing cortical dysfunction through activities of daily living,*
St Louis, 1990, Mosby.)

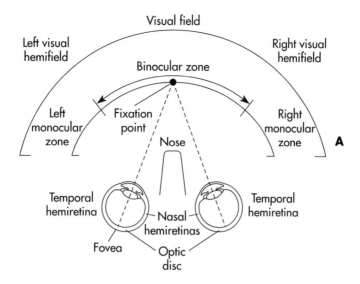

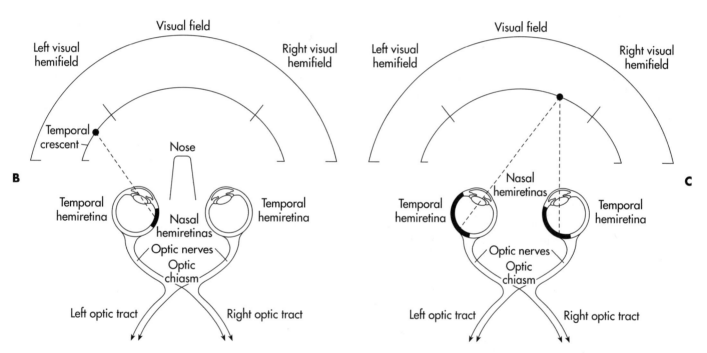

Figure 12-7 The visual field has both binocular and monocular zones. **A,** Light from the binocular zone strikes both eyes, whereas light from the monocular zone strikes only the eye on the same side. The hemiretinas are defined with respect to the fovea, the region in the center of the retina with the highest acuity. The optic disc, the region where the ganglion cell axons leave the retina, is free of photoreceptors and therefore creates a gap, or blind spot, in the visual field for each eye. **B,** Light from a monocular zone (temporal crescent) falls only on the ipsilateral nasal hemiretina and does not project on the contralateral retina because it is blocked by the nose. **C,** Each optic tract carries a complete representation of one half of the binocular zone in the visual field. Fibers from the nasal hemiretina of each eye cross to the opposite side at the optic chiasm, whereas fibers from the temporal hemiretina do not cross. In the illustration, light from the right half of the binocular zone falls on the left temporal hemiretina and right nasal hemiretina. Axons from these hemiretinas thus contain a complete representation of the right hemifield of vision. (From Mason C, Kandel ER: Central visual pathways. In Kanel ER, Schwartz TH, Tessel TM, editors: *Principles of neural science,* ed 3, Connecticut, 1991, Appleton and Lange.)

hemiretina (the inner visual field) and contralateral nasal hemiretina (the outer visual field) (Figure 12-6). The optic tract on each side projects to the lateral geniculate body of the thalamus. The optic radiation then carries visual information from the lateral geniculate body to the calcarine cortex in the occipital lobe. During the radiation, the fibers fan out from the upper part of the bundle carrying information from the lower visual field that runs posteriorly in the parietal lobe. The lower part of the bundle, with information from the upper visual field, loops around the temporal horn of the ventricles in the temporal lobe on its way to the visual cortex. A stimulus in the superior visual field is projected to the inferior retina, resulting in an inverted image (Figure 12-7).[1,16] Because of this inversion, information from the superior visual field is carried by the inferior optic radiation. The inverted image is then carried to the cortex. In the primary visual cortex around the calcarine fissure (Brodmann's area 17) the occipital pole is essential in vision from the central or middle visual field, whereas peripheral vision is facilitated by a more anterior part of the medial occipital cortex. The association areas (Brodmann's area 18 and 19) receive information from the primary visual cortex. They integrate this information with previous experiences and information from other sensory modalities and form visual memory traces.[13] The different processes can occur at the same time, a phenomenon termed *parallel processing*.[1,5,11]

Photoreceptors

Photoreceptors on the retina convert light energy falling on them into electrical impulses that can be analyzed by the brain. Cohen and Fox[5] state that the photoreceptor layer includes two classes of photoreceptors: rods and cones. Efferson[6] explains that the cone or rod shape is the dendrite of the cell. Variations in shape and slight variations in pigment give each cell different sensitivities. The rod cell has greater sensitivity to dim light but less sensitivity to color. The cone cell has greater sensitivity to color and high-intensity light but less to reduced-light conditions. The greatest concentration of cone cells occurs in the fovea and macula; the concentration of cone cells decreases and the concentration of rod cells increases with increased distance from the macula.[6]

Efferson[6] describes the phenomenon responsible for the high degree of neural representation in the foveal region that accounts for the tremendous conscious awareness of the central view, called *convergence*. The degree of convergence is greatest at the periphery of the retina; many photoreceptor cells synapse on each ganglion cell. This accounts for poor acuity but high light sensitivity. The closer to the macula, the smaller the degree of convergence; at the fovea, no convergence occurs. One photoreceptor cell synapses with one bipolar cell and one ganglion cell. The visual pathway begins a three-neuron chain exiting through the optic nerve; this chain consists of rods and

cones synapsing with bipolar and ganglion cells. This one-to-one correspondence between photoreceptor and ganglion cells in the fovea means that a significant degree of neural representation of the foveal image occurs in the brain.[6] This accounts for the individual's primary awareness of objects in the foveal field and secondary awareness of objects in the peripheral field. Conscious visual awareness of the environment is primarily influenced by objects in the foveal field. However, continuous information about the environment is flowing through the peripheral retina, usually subconsciously. Attention quickly shifts from foveal to nonfoveal stimulation if changes in light intensity and rapid movement are registered.[6] For example, when an individual is reading, the fovea is being used. If a familiar person enters the room, the peripheral field becomes stimulated and the individual becomes aware of the person's presence, clothing, ambulation pattern, scent, and possibly voice.

Five Neuronal Control Systems

Five separate movement systems maintain the fovea on a target, and each of these systems shares the same effector pathway, that is, the three bilateral groups of ocular motor neurons in the brain stem, according to Goldberg et al.[11] These systems include the following:

- Vestibulo-ocular movement uses vestibular input to hold images stably on the retina during brief or rapid head rotation. This movement stabilizes the eye as the head moves.
- Optokinetic movements use visual input to hold images stably on the retina during sustained or slow head rotation. These eye movements are used while driving in a car and reading street signs, recognizing people while walking down a hall, and window shopping.
- Saccadic eye movements keep the fovea on a visual target by keeping objects of interest on the fovea; these movements help the eye shift rapidly from target to target.[11] Saccadic movements resemble the quick phase of vestibular nystagmus. Accurate saccadic eye movements also can occur in response to sounds, tactile stimuli, memories of locations in space, and even verbal commands (e.g., look left).
- Smooth pursuit movements hold the image of a moving target on the fovea. The smooth pursuit system moves the eyes in space to keep a single target on the fovea by calculating the speed at which the target is moving and then moving the eyes accordingly. Smooth pursuit requires the individual to attend to an object and voluntarily pursue it, unlike optokinetic movements, which are involuntary.
- Vergence movements move the eyes in opposite directions so that the image is positioned on both foveae. When a person views a moving object, each eye moves differently to keep the image of the object aligned pre-

cisely on each fovea. If the object moves closer, the eyes must converge. If the object moves away, the eyes diverge.[11]

Eye Movement System

Six muscles attach to each eye: the superior rectus, inferior rectus, medial rectus, lateral rectus, superior oblique, and inferior oblique. The recti originate at the apex of the orbit and insert on the sclera (the outer coat of the eyeball) anterior to the equator of the eye. The obliques approach the eye from the anteromedial aspect and insert posterior to the equator (Figure 12-8).[11]

The medial rectus adducts and rotates the eyes inward, whereas the lateral rectus abducts and rotates the eyes outward. The superior rectus uses elevation and intorsion to move the eyes upward; it is assisted by the inferior rectus, which uses depression and extorsion to move the eyes downward. The superior oblique uses depression and intorsion to rotate the eye downward and outward, whereas the inferior oblique uses elevation and extorsion to rotate the eye upward and outward.[6-8]

In coordinated eye movement a muscle of one eye is paired with a muscle of the opposite eye to produce movement in the six cardinal directions of gaze. These paired primary muscles are termed *yoke muscles*. In any conjugate movement (both eyes moving the same amount in the same direction) the yoke muscles receive equal innerva-

tion.[27] To follow a moving target upward and to the left, the left eye moves upward and away from the nose and the right eye moves upward and toward the nose. This demonstrates that each pair of muscles in one eye has a functional complement in the other orbit that can rotate the eye in the same place but the opposite direction.[11]

Extraocular muscles are innervated by three groups of motor neurons whose cell bodies form nuclei in the brain stem. The lateral rectus is innervated by the motor neurons of the nervus abducens (cranial nerve VI) in the pons. The medial inferior and superior recti and the inferior oblique muscles are innervated by the ocular motor neurons that form the nervus oculomotorius (cranial nerve III) in the midbrain. The superior oblique muscle is innervated by the nervus trochlearis (cranial nerve IV) in the midbrain. Cranial nerve III is located at the level of the superior colliculus, whereas cranial nerve IV is located at the level of the inferior colliculus; both are located in the midbrain.[7,11,24]

PATHOPHYSIOLOGY REGARDING CVA

Individuals who sustain brain damage (CVA, traumatic head injury, tumor) often exhibit visual system dysfunctions, which may occur within the primary visual pathway (sensory or motor), associative visual pathway (perceptual), or within both pathways.[2] Dysfunction in the visual path-

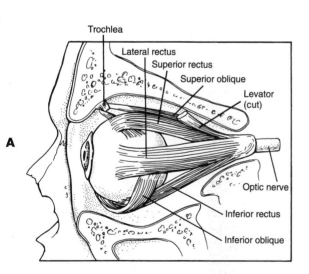

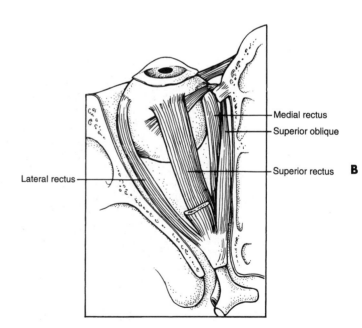

Figure 12-8 The origins and insertions of the extraocular muscles. **A,** Lateral view with orbital wall cut away. The recti insert in front of the equator of the globe and contraction rotates the cornea toward the insertion. The obliques insert behind the equator, and contraction rotates the cornea away from the insertion. The superior oblique muscle passes through a pulley of bone, the trochlea, before it inserts. **B,** Superior view with roof of orbit cut away. (From Goldberg ME, Eggers HM, Gouras P: Ocular motor system. In Kandell ER, Schwartz TH, Tessel TM, editors: *Principles of neural science,* ed 3, Connecticut, 1991, Appleton and Lange.)

ways lead to primary visual deficits, including decreases in near and distant acuity; accommodation; visual fields; oculomotor range of motion; convergence; quality of saccadic, pursuit, fixation, and functional scanning; color perception; stereopsis; symptoms of central blindness; and strabismus.[2,24] At times the terminology may be somewhat confusing. Bouska[3] refers to the above skills as *primary visual skills*, Hellerstein[12] refers to them as the *basic processing level*, Warren[28] describes them as the *lower level skills* in her hierarchic framework, and Scheiman[20] calls them *visual information processing skills*. Whatever the term, they are the most basic and functional visual skills necessary for the development and management of all visual perception and visual motor activities, and they must be intact to receive, process, interpret, and respond appropriately to input from the environment (Table 12-1).

Occupational therapists must be aware of the primary functional visual skills and the ways deficits in one or more of these areas have an impact on the quality of life of patients with whom they work. A comprehensive understanding of the visual system is necessary because the occupational therapist is often in the best position to observe functional vision problems, administer visual screening appraisals, and observe functional skills. The functional optometrist is the most qualified professional to assess and rehabilitate visual efficiency and the visual perceptual system. Vision, the dominant sense for gathering information, should be evaluated by a functional optometrist who has extensive experience in vision rehabilitation and functional vision care. Consultation with a functional optometrist by the rehabilitation team is crucial so that all health care providers have a good understanding of the patient's visual

Table 12-1

Visual Skills and Their Associated Functions and Resulting Dysfunctions After CVA

VISUAL SKILL	VISUAL FUNCTION	VISUAL AND PERCEPTUAL DYSFUNCTIONS
Visual acuity	Clarity of vision at near point and distance; 20/20 refraction	Vision blurred in one or both eyes consistently or inconsistently; visual fatigue; task incompletion
Accommodation	Process of focusing whereby the lens changes curvature so that various viewing distances remain clear	Blurred vision; inattention; poor concentration; eyestrain; visual fatigue
Visual fields	The peripheral area of vision up, down, in, and out when both eyes are positioned straight forward	Inability to read or starting to read in the middle of the page; ignoring of food on one half of the plate; difficulty orienting to stimuli in specific areas of space
Oculomotor range of motion; fixation; saccades and pursuits	Ability of both eyes to move within the six cardinal positions of gaze (right, left, inferior, superior, inferior oblique, superior oblique); maintenance of gaze for 10 seconds; small precise eye jumps; following a moving stimulus	Excessive head movement; frequent loss of place; skipping of lines; poor attention span; slow copying; difficulty when driving, reading, writing; difficulty tracking in all planes
Vergence	The ability to bring the eyes together smoothly and automatically along the midline to observe objects singly at near distance (convergence) or to move the eyes outward for single vision of distant objects (divergence)	Difficulty focusing; decreased depth perception; difficulty and confusion in interpreting space; decreased eye-hand coordination in self-care and hygiene; difficulty in driving, sports, communication, and ambulation
Strabismus	Deviation of one eye or one eye at a time from the object of regard, where the eye not in use is turned	Esotropia (inward turn); exotropia (outward turn); hyperopia (upward turn); hypopia (downward turn); double vision or suppression; decreased eye-hand coordination during mobility tasks; overreaching or underreaching; difficulty with reading and near tasks
Functional scanning	Ability to read or write from left to right precisely and smoothly without errors	Omitting letters, words, numbers; losing place when returning to next line; exaggerated head movement; using finger as pointer; abnormal working distance
Color perception	Ability to perceive colors	Muddy or impure color; color may fade out; difficulty finding items by color
Stereopsis	Depth perception and its relationship to spatial judgment	Problematic binocular system; deficits in three-dimensional perception; decreased spatial judgment especially in fine motor areas

deficits and functional results. Treatment strategies can then be established using a multidisciplinary approach. Improved visual processing often helps speed progress in other rehabilitative areas, including occupational therapy, speech therapy, therapeutic recreation, and physical therapy.[12]

Functional Visual Skills

The following sections describe primary functional visual skills; Table 12-1 lists the skill, function, and dysfunction associated with each.

Visual Acuity

Clarity of vision, or visual acuity, is essential in each eye at both near and far points.[8] Near vision acuity is the ability to see, inspect, identify, and understand objects clearly at near distances, within an arm's length. Distance acuity is the ability to see, inspect, identify, and understand objects clearly at a distance.[18] Refraction is the process used to evaluate the optical system of the eye. Refraction is used to determine whether an individual suffers from myopia (nearsightedness), hyperopia (farsightedness), and/or astigmatism (the lens is not spherical but oval and causes light rays to focus at two different points). Refraction also is used to determine whether an individual will benefit from glasses and the appropriate prescription.[8,19] If visual acuity is decreased for either near or distance tasks, vision is blurry and visual fatigue or eyestrain may be present. Corrective lenses focus the angle of light through the lens so the angle of reflection of the light on the retina is equal to the refraction and the environment is focused.

Accommodation

Accommodation is the ability to change the focus of the eye so that objects at different distances can be seen clearly.[18] The normal human visual system is physiologically focused for objects at distances of 20 feet and greater. If an object is brought closer than 20 feet, a focusing adjustment must be made or the object appears blurred. The accommodative system of the human eye works so well that most people are totally unaware that they even have a focusing system.[20] When an individual reads the mail and then looks up at the clock on the wall to determine the time, the accommodative system is used. If accommodative disorders are diagnosed, one or more of the following may be present: discomfort and eyestrain for all visual tasks, blurred vision, inattention during occupational therapy sessions, poor concentration, visual fatigue, rubbing eyes, or difficulty with activities of daily living (ADL) that require sustained close work.

Visual Fields

The visual fields extend approximately 65° upward, 75° downward, 60° inward, and 95° outward when the eye is in the straight forward position. The total field of vision is approximately 180°.[17] Visual fields are essential areas of the visual system that allow the individual to orient effectively to stimuli in specific areas of space. They are used when driving, walking, reading, eating, and in all daily living skills. Inferior field loss causes difficulty with mobility, including poor balance, tendency to trail behind others when walking, walking next to walls and touching them for balance, trouble seeing steps or curbs, shortened and uncertain stride while walking, and trouble identifying visual landmarks. Superior field deficit causes difficulty in seeing signs, reading and writing; misreading of words, poor accuracy, slow reading rate, inability to follow lines of text, and inaccurate check writing are additional difficulties.[1,9,19]

Oculomotor Range of Motion

Oculomotor range of motion is the ability to move the eyes in the six cardinal positions of gaze (right, left, inferior, superior, superior oblique, inferior oblique) using smooth and even motion without stress. For the eyes to move within these quadrants, three areas must be intact: fixation stability, saccadic function, and pursuit function. Fixation is the ability to locate and inspect a series of stationary objects with both eyes quickly and accurately. Most individuals are able to sustain precise fixation with no observable movement of the eyes for 10 seconds.[19] Saccadic functions include eye movements enabling the individual to redirect the line of sight rapidly so that the point of interest stimulates the fovea. Saccadic function consists of a jump from one fixation point to the next with a slight pause to process the information (as in reading). Pursuit function is the ability to follow a moving object such as a ball in flight or moving vehicle in traffic smoothly and accurately with both eyes. Difficulty with fixation results in off-task behavior and may give the impression that the person is inattentive or impulsive. Saccadic dysfunction usually manifests itself through undershooting of the target of interest; at times, overshooting of the target may be observed. Pursuit dysfunction is a condition in which the individual is unable to follow a moving target accurately. Pursuit problems play a significant role in ADL such as driving and sports and any other activities in which the individual or the object of regard is moving.[27]

Vergence

Vergence includes convergence and divergence. It is the ability to bring the eyes together smoothly and automatically to observe objects singly at near distance (convergence), or to move the eyes outward for single vision of distant objects (divergence). Vergence is reflexively associated with accommodation and divergence with relaxation of accommodation. The function of this reflex is to allow near or far objects to be single and clear. Problems in vergence can occur if the eye movement system is out of coordination with accommodation or damage to cranial nerves III, IV, or VI has occurred. Problems can be slight, with merely a tendency for the eyes to converge in or out too far, or they can be greater in magnitude. Tendencies to underconverge or overconverge are called *phorias* and are not visible to the observer. Some phorias may worsen to the extent that binocularity (the ability of both eyes to act as a single unit to obtain a three-dimensional scene viewed with depth and meaning) breaks down, at which point the individual displays strabismus. Vergence ability is needed for singular binocular vision and is basic to all activities. At near distances an individual may have difficulty finding objects; eye-hand coordination may be decreased, affecting self-care and hygiene tasks; and reading may be difficult. Distance tasks that may be affected include driving, sports, movies, communication, and frequently walking.[6]

Strabismus

Strabismus, or tropia, is a visible turn of one eye that may be constant, intermittent, or alternating between eyes. It may result in double vision; long-term strabismus may suppress or turn off the vision in the wandering eye.[6] Suppression is a neurologic function that is an adaptation to the intolerable situation of double images. It is only exhibited in long-term strabismus because apparently the brain cannot learn to suppress past the time of peak plasticity (until approximately 7 years).

The developing brain must choose which eye has the visual direction by using motor and tactile inputs. The other foveal image is then neurologically suppressed. The peripheral vision in the suppressing eye is still normal, and the eye is not by any means blind.[6,22] In strabismus one eye may turn outward (exotropia), inward (esotropia), upward (hypertropia), or downward (hypotropia). These are the most common forms of strabismus. Strabismus may be intermittent, occurring occasionally and alternating—switching use to the right or left eye or suppressing just the right eye or left eye. Strabismus may be constant (the same eye is always in or out) or comitant (the amount of turn is always the same regardless of whether the person is looking up, down, right, left, or straight ahead). Newly acquired strabismus (from stroke or head injury) is usually noncomitant; eye turn changes depend on the direction in which the eyes are looking. Any strabismic disorder may result in an inability to judge distance, underreaching or overreaching for objects, covering or closure of one eye, double vision, head tilt or turn, "spaced-out" appearance, difficulty reading, and avoidance of near tasks.

Functional Scanning

Functional scanning refers to the ability to scan a page of print from left to right without skipping letters, words, or lines. This should be accomplished with precise and smooth eye saccades. Functional scanning also relates to writing tasks and the ability to maintain print appropriately on each line. Problems with functional scanning re-

sult in poor speed and numerous errors, losing of place on a line of print, incorrect stating of letters or words while reading, inability to read or write from left to right, skipping around the page, and using the finger as a pointer.[2]

Color Perception

Color perception may be impaired in individuals who experience right hemisphere or bilateral lesions.[22] This symptom is different from color agnosia in which the patient is unable to name colors correctly as a result of an inability to interpret sensory information. Individuals with defective color perception may see colors as "muddy" or "impure" in hue, or the color of a small target may fade into the background, decreasing the ability to differentiate it from the background. Total loss of ability to discern color (achromatopsia) is rare but can occur.[3]

Stereopsis and Depth Perception

Stereopsis is binocular visual perception of three-dimensional space or depth. Depth perception is used during all activities involving spatial judgments, in particular fine motor and eye-hand coordination tasks in which judgment of relative depth is required (threading a needle, placing toothpaste on a toothbrush, hammering). Walking over curbs and up and down stairs requires depth perception.

Cortical Blindness

Cortical blindness refers to a marked decrease in visual acuity with severe blurring that is uncorrectable by lenses. It can be a total or almost total loss of vision resulting from bilateral cerebral destruction of the visual projection cortex (area 17). Deficits include blurred vision and decrease in acuity.

Age-Related Changes

Although CVAs affect many age groups, a much higher incidence occurs among elderly persons. The most common condition affecting the vision of elderly persons is cataracts. General clarity of vision is impaired because of a loss of transparency of the crystalline lens of the eye. The lens slowly loses its ability to prevent oxidation, and liquidation of the outer layer begins. The normally soluble proteins adhere, causing light to scatter; vision slowly declines.[6,7]

Age-related macular degeneration is the leading cause of blindness in the western world. Loss of central vision occurs from fluid that leaks from the deeper layers of the retina, pushing the retina up and detaching it from the nourishing layer. New vessel growth, hemorrhage, and atrophy further destroy central vision. All near-point ADL (reading, sewing, cooking) are affected, and safety is compromised.[6]

In arteriosclerosis, vision may or may not be affected. Hardening of the retinal arteries may occur, eventually leading to ischemia in the areas of the retina dying from oxygen deprivation. Hypertension is usually accompanied by arteriosclerosis. Retinal bleeding and edema may occur, which can affect central vision if the macula is involved.

Diabetes can affect the lens. In the "sugar cataract," sorbitol collects within the lens, causing an osmotic gradient of fluid into the lens, which leads to disruption of the lens matrix and loss of transparency. As the fluid increases and decreases within the lens, the person's vision also fluctuates, depending on the sugar level. Retinal effects include microvascular damage and microaneurysms. Central vision may be reduced because of retinal ischemia. Ischemia leads to the growth of new vessels that are very weak and frequently leak and cause hemorrhage. The hemorrhage attracts fibrotic development which puts traction on the retina, pulling it off and leading to retinal detachment and blindness.[6] (Laser treatment may prevent retinal detachment.)

Glaucoma is caused by an increase in intraocular pressure. This pressure interferes with the flow of blood and nutrients at the optic disc. Severe glaucoma can cause field loss and eventually complete blindness.

The occupational therapist should obtain the patient's visual history. Visual impairments may have existed previously and may not be a result of a stroke; previous impairments may have a greater impact with newly acquired deficits.

EVALUATION: VISION SCREENING

Much discussion is currently taking place regarding visual acuity and whether occupational therapists should screen for it. As long as a comprehensive understanding of vision and correct screening procedures are administered, screening can be performed. However, all the visual assessment tools used by occupational therapists are used for screening only. Visual acuity skills must be addressed before any other visual determination is made. The patient being screened is then referred for a comprehensive visual evaluation by an experienced functional optometrist.

Before screening, the head, neck, trunk, and pelvis should be aligned appropriately to the midline orientation. If the patient being screened wears glasses, they should be used during the screening. If the patient states they do not improve vision, the screening should be performed with glasses on and then with glasses off.

The occupational therapist should observe the patient during screening. Head position, eye alignment, eye-head dissociation, excessive head movement, and the use of the upper extremities to stabilize the head should be noted.

The following is a description of vision screening processes, which should be administered in a well-illuminated room free of glare and reflection[3,6,21]:

1. Distance Visual Acuity
   Equipment: Distance acuity chart (Snellen chart), occluder or eye patch, 20 ft measure
   Setup: Fixate distance acuity chart on a well-lighted wall at patient's eye level 20 ft away.
   Procedure: Cover the patient's left eye with occluder or patch. Ask the patient to identify letters on the 20/40 line. If the patient appears confused by the lines and letters, cover all other lines on the chart and expose only the line being used. If necessary, expose only one letter at a time. If the patient continues to have problems, attempt to test visual acuity using the Lea Symbols Test.[30] Continue until the individual misses more than 50% of the letters on a line. Cover the patient's right eye with occluder or patch and repeat the steps. Record acuity as last line in which the individual can successfully identify more than 50% of the letters.
   Functional implications: If visual acuity is poorer than 20/40 or if a two-line difference or more is evident between the two eyes, a referral is necessary and corrective lenses may need to be prescribed.[30]

2. Ocular Mobility
   Equipment: Penlight
   Setup: Have patient sit facing therapist. Penlight should be approximately 12 inches from the eyes. Do not shine the light directly into the eyes; instead direct the light so that it is pointing slightly above eye level at the brow.
   Procedure: Ask the patient to follow the penlight and move it in a large H pattern to the extremes of gaze. Then move the penlight in a large O pattern. Allow the patient to fixate on the light for 10 seconds before moving it.
   Functional implications: Observation of pursuits should be smooth and precise without anticipating responses. Note visual fatigue or stress and whether the patient reports diplopia (double vision). Observe whether the patient looks away, loses the target, or squints or blinks excessively. Inability to attend to visual tasks, difficulty reading or completing writing tasks, and problems with spatial orientation during walking may be displayed.[15]

3. Near Point of Convergence
   Equipment: Penlight and ruler
   Setup: Practice this procedure on a partner to determine when the penlight is positioned at 2, 4, and 6 inches from an individual's eyes.
   Procedure: Slowly move the penlight toward the patient at eye level and between the eyes, making sure not to shine the light in the eyes. Ask the patient to keep the eyes on the light and state when two lights are seen. After this occurs, move the light another inch or two closer and then begin to move it away from the patient.

Ask the patient to state when one light only is seen. Watch the eyes carefully and observe whether they stop working together as a team—one eye may drift outward. Record the distance at which the patient reports double vision and the recovery to single vision.

Functional implications: Double vision should occur within 2 to 4 inches of the eyes. A recovery to single vision should occur within 4 to 6 inches. A patient with a binocular vision problem may not report double vision because the eye that turns out is suppressed. Thus all eye movements should be observed before screening.

4. Stereopsis

Equipment: Viewer-free random dot test

Setup: Individual's head position should be vertical. If any head tilt occurs, it negates this screening.

Procedure: Hold the viewer-free random dot test 16 inches from the patient's eyes and ask the patient to describe what is seen. A patient with stereopsis should report seeing a square box in the upper left, an E on the upper right, a circle on the lower left, and a blank box on the lower right. Give the patient about 20 to 30 seconds to observe targets. If the patient has difficulty, try tilting the target slightly to the left or right.

Functional implications: The patient should be able to identify all three symbols correctly. A patient with constant strabismus is unable to identify any of the shapes. Patients with less severe strabismus or phoria may have normal responses. Some patients may report double vision on this task, which suggests that strabismus is present.

5. Accommodation

Equipment: Isolated letters and occluder or eye patch

Setup: Make a target by photocopying the near visual acuity chart, cutting out the 20/30 targets, and taping them to a tongue depressor. Place one target on each side of the tongue depressor so that you have two screening targets.

Procedure: Patch the left eye. Hold the tongue depressor with the 20/30 target about 1 inch in front of the right eye. The patient should be unable to identify the stimulus on the tongue depressor at this distance. Slowly move the target away and ask the patient to report as soon as the target is identifiable. Using a ruler, measure and record the distance at which the patient is able to identify the stimulus. Divide 40 by the measurement to determine the amplitude of accommodation. If the patient is able to identify the target at 8 in, divide 40 by 8, which equals 5 diopters. To compare the patient's amplitude of accommodation to the expected amplitude for

the patient's age, use the following formula: expected amplitude = 18 − one-third the patient's age.[19] The following are examples of the way to use this equation:

A 9-year-old child: Expected amplitude = 18 − [1/3 (9)]
                      Expected amplitude = 18 − 3 = 15 diopters

A 45-year-old adult: Expected amplitude = 18 − [1/3 (45)]
                      Expected amplitude = 18 − 15 = 3 diopters

Functional implications: The amplitude of accommodation should be 2 diopters of the expected finding for the patient to pass the screening test. Observe all eye movements. Problems include blurred vision, poor concentration, inattention, visual fatigue, and eyestrain.

6. Saccades

Equipment: Two fixators with red and green targets and scanning chart

Setup: Have the patient keep the head erect and vertical.

Procedure: Hold two tongue depressors (one with a red target and one with a green target) 16 inches from the patient's face and about 4 inches from the midline. Give the patient the following instructions: "When I say red, look at the red target. When I say green, look at the green target. Do not look until I tell you." Have the patient look from one target to the other five round trips or a total of 10 fixations. Determine whether the patient can maintain attention to complete five round trips (ability). Score 1 to 5. Observe accuracy using one eye movement or multiple eye movements. Score 1 to 5. Observe head and body movement and assign a score of 1 to 5.

Functional implications: Adults without visual impairment should receive a perfect score.[3] Any score less than that denotes problems with saccadic function; the patient requires further evaluation. Poor saccades result in poor concentration and attention and difficulty reading and writing.

7. Visual Field

Equipment: Occluder or eye patch, black dowels with white pins on the ends or a wiggling finger

Setup: Make sure the patient is seated facing the examiner.

Procedure:

1. One-examiner presentation—The patient holds the occluder over the left eye. Wiggle a finger out to the side and ask the patient to say "now" when the movement of the wiggling finger is

first detected. The patient should look at your nose the entire time and ignore any arm movement. Begin with the hand slightly behind the patient about 16 inches away from the head. Slowly bring the hand forward while wiggling a finger. Continue randomly testing different sections of the visual field in 45° intervals around the visual field. Proceed to the left eye, asking the patient to occlude the right eye. If using the dowel technique, slowly bring it in from the side until the patient reports seeing the small pin at the end of the dowel.

2. Two-examiner presentation—Examiner one stands behind the seated patient and examiner two sits facing the patient about 30 inches in front so that the face of the examiner and patient are at the same level.[10]

Test each eye individually, being careful to patch the other eye. Examiner two closes one eye and instructs the patient to "fixate and keep looking at my open eye. Examiner one will be showing you one or more fingers very quickly. Don't try to look at the fingers. Keep looking at my open eye and when you see a finger or fingers, tell me how many you see."[10]

Examiner one presents one or two fingers randomly for a 1-second duration to each quadrant of the visual field of the patient's unpatched eye. The fingers in the upper quadrant point down, and those in the lower quadrant point up. The fingers are presented 18 inches from the patient and at approximately 20° from the line of fixation.[10]

3. Two-examiner left-right field simultaneous presentation—No patch is used during this screening. The patient looks at examiner one while examiner two stimulates both hemifields simultaneously. This screening looks for visuospatial hemi-imperception (VSHI), which is usually referred to as *extinction, hemi-inattention,* or *unilateral spatial neglect.* When both hemifields are stimulated simultaneously, all or part of one hemifield is less responsive to stimulation; the patient responds to single stimuli and not to the affected side when both sides are stimulated.[10]

Functional implications: Visual field impairments have significant implications for the safe performance of many functional activities, including driving and mobility. Visually guided movement through space becomes impaired, as does efficient eye movement. Reading and near activities can be affected if central field loss is present.[6] Persons with visuospatial hemi-imperception leave out parts of the text when reading or fail to

perceive traffic to the left when driving or crossing the street.[10]

NOTE: These confrontation fields are considered a gross test as compared with a visual field perimeter test. Many patients cannot perform the perimeter test because it requires a higher cognitive level. These test are not usually performed by occupational therapists. Observations are important and give the occupational therapist much information about the way in which patients move about the environment and the way they move their bodies and use spatial orientation.[6]

VISUAL PERCEPTUAL EVALUATIONS

Tsurumi and Todd[26] state that much of the research on visual perception evaluation has been done using representations rather than real objects and real space. Visual perception testing uses two-dimensional representations of inverted forms as the stimulus material. They suggest that these two-dimensional figures, although useful measures of certain cognitive analysis skills, should not be correlated with the ability to perceive the three-dimensional world of objects and space.

Occupational therapists obtain more helpful information using more functional assessments. These assessments usually are in the form of checklists and observations of patients within the clinic or home setting.

Hemianopsia

Hemianopsia (Figure 12-9) is a visual field defect that results in loss of vision on the contralateral half of the visual field. This defect can be evaluated using confrontation testing, as described previously. Patients with pure hemianopsias are aware of their visual losses and spontaneously learn to compensate by moving their eyes (foveae) toward their lost visual fields to expand their visual spaces to gather information right and left of midline.

Unilateral Visual Inattention

Unilateral visual inattention is a condition in which a patient with normal sensory and motor systems fails to orient toward, respond to, or report stimuli on the side contralateral to the cerebral lesion. Efferson[6] states that this condition has been documented in patients who demonstrate no accompanying visual field defects or limb sensory or motor losses. It is usually not seen alone but is associated with accompanying sensory and motor defects such as hemianopsia, decreased tactile proprioceptive and stereognostic perception, and paresis or upper limb paralysis. LeDoux and Smylie (as cited by Efferson[6]) report that inattention is a hemisphere defect. They described a patient shown bilateral hemispheric visual perceptual slides who made visuospatial errors in left space. The pa-

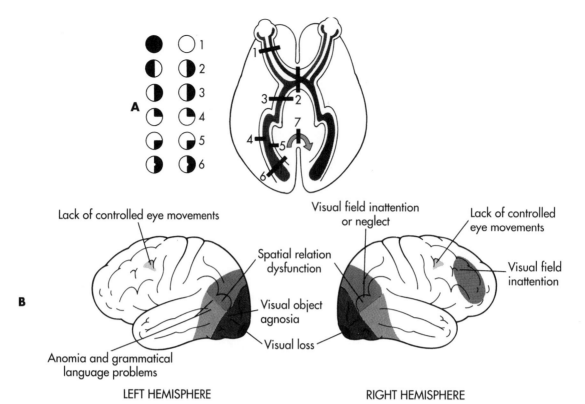

Figure 12-9 Visual processing deficits. **A,** The visual pathway viewed from the base of the brain (inferior view). The dark bars indicate lesions at different sites in the pathway. The numbers refer to visual-field disturbances according to location of the lesion: *1,* lesion of the optic nerve, leading to blindness in the corresponding eye; *2,* lesion of the optic chiasma, leading to bilateral temporal field defect; *3,* lesion of the optic tract, resulting in complete loss of visual field on the contralateral half of the visual field, or homonymous hemianopsia; *4,* lesion of the optic tract in the temporal lobe, resulting in loss of vision in the upper quadrant of the contralateral visual field in both eyes; *5,* lesion of the optic track in the parietal lobe, resulting in loss of vision in the lower quadrant of the contralateral visual field in both eyes; *6,* lesion in the occipital cortex, leading to visual loss in the contralateral visual hemifield with macular sparing; *7,* lesion in the posterior corpus callosum, resulting in a disrupted route, causing pure word blindness, or alexia without agraphia. **B,** Lesion sites that can produce visuospatial relation problems, or anomia and grammatical language problems related to spatial relations. Unilateral visual neglect is related to dysfunction of the inferior parietal lobe, cingulate gyrus, and dorsolateral frontal lobe, especially on the right side. (From Árnadóttir G: *The brain and behavior: assessing cortical dysfunction through activities of daily living,* St Louis, 1990, Mosby.)

tient suffered from a right-sided lesion. When the same slides were directed only to the right visual field (left hemisphere), performance improved. Efferson hypothesized that the deficient hemisphere failed to receive or orient toward incoming information, whereas the intact receiving hemisphere remains oblivious and goes about its own business. Efferson suggests assessing using confrontation testing. If visual field loss is ruled out, then the stimuli should be applied using auditory, tactile, and visual modalities. The patient's eyes, neck, head, and trunk position should be assessed at rest and during activities. Persistent deviation toward the side of the lesion may indicate inattention. Unilateral visual inattention may be ruled out if the patient is capable of tracking visual targets

from ipsilateral to contralateral space, maintaining fixation, and fixating on visual targets both right and left of midline on command. Very slow searching or failure to search may be considered inattention. Asymmetries in performance should be noted and carefully observed during functional activities such as eating, filling out a form, reading, dressing and maneuvering through the environment. The occupational therapist should note unawareness regarding doorways and hallways and turns made only in one direction (see Chapters 13 and 14).

Cancellation, crossing out, line bisection, and drawing and copying tasks may aid in indicating patient's functional ability. Toglia[25] developed a unilateral inattention functional rating scale, including shaving both sides of the face, combing both sides of the hair, and eating from both sides of the tray.

Cortical Blindness

Cortical blindness and variations of it should be assessed by a vision specialist or functional optometrist. Cortical blindness is a total or almost total loss of vision resulting from bilateral cerebral destruction of the visual projection cortex (area 17).

Color Imperception

Color imperception may be measured by using Ishihara's color plates or color-sorting or color-matching tasks. Patients with defective color perception have difficulty with some visual perceptual tasks because contextual cues related to color and shading are unavailable to them.[6]

Visual Agnosia

Visual agnosia is defined by Efferson[6] as a failure to recognize visual stimuli (objects, faces, letters) even though visual sensory processing, language, and general intellectual functions are preserved at sufficiently high levels. Three types of agnosia exist: visual, tactile, and auditory. Agnosia is tested by placing common objects in front of the patient and asking the patient to name them. Normal responses include the name of the item and its described or functional use. Abnormal responses are confabulatory and perseverative. Anomia must be ruled out before evaluation. A person with visual agnosia is able to name the object if another sensory modality (e.g., tactile) is used to obtain information about the object.

Spatial Relations

Spatial relations are discussed in Chapters 13 and 14 of this text but are mentioned here briefly. All visuospatial disabilities involve some problem with the apprehension of the spatial relationships between and within objects.[27] These problems include an inability to localize objects in space, estimate their size, and judge their distance and impaired memory for the location of objects and places. Further difficulties include the inability to trace a path or follow a route from one place to another and problems with reading and counting. Assessments to judge spatial relations include the following:

- Touching a number of targets in all parts of the visual field while fixating on a central point
- Determining which objects are closest, farthest, and in the middle
- Describing the position of objects in the patient's room from memory
- Describing a floor plan of the room arrangement in the patient's house.

Reading and counting may be assessed by asking the patient to read and observing performance and documenting errors. Pages of scanning materials (letters and numbers) often give additional information on spatial planning during reading. The size and density of the print should be controlled.

TREATMENT CONSIDERATIONS

Patients with visual field losses who are evaluated by a functional optometrist may be prescribed prism systems or yoked prisms to expand their viewing fields. They also may use oculomotor techniques emphasizing calisthenics, pursuit, saccades, and scanning techniques.

The occupational therapist should encourage the use of appropriate glasses or prisms during treatment sessions and use awareness techniques to help the patient understand the way visual defects interfere with various activities. The occupational therapist should emphasize conscious attention to detail while teaching organized scanning techniques for the deficient field. Increased speed and accuracy of eye movement during recognition tasks are essential aspects of therapy. Walking or another movement modality is necessary to integrate vision, movement, and perception. Planning routes verbally and visually assists the patient in thinking about and "going into" the deficit area. Use of markers when reading may be helpful. An L-shaped marker assists the patient in going over to that area before beginning to read each line.[10,13]

Treatment for unilateral visual inattention includes various techniques (see Chapter 14). Again, increasing the patient's cognitive awareness of inattention is a primary factor. The patient should be aware of the nature of the field loss and the way it affects vision. The patient with normal visual fields but with visual extinction should be treated the same as is the patient with an actual field loss; the visual experience is similar. Performance examples in the environment should be provided to demonstrate the biased view.

Visual scanning and awareness of the way eye and eye-head movements may be used to compensate should be emphasized. Training should then continue to the next level in which larger and quicker pursuits and saccades are made with longer fixations into unattended space. Training may be accomplished with interesting targets held by the therapist (small colored lights, bright objects of interest to the patient, pictures of family or friends taped to pencils). Pursuit and tracking of the target from attended to unattended space should be stressed first. Use of saccades in unattended space comes next. Initially, eye-head movements are acceptable, but eventually eye movements should dissociate from head movements. The visual field remains the same if the head moves into the unattended space but the eyes remain on a target in the attended space. Daily right-left scanning should be done independently and move farther into the unattended space each day.[6,17,28]

As treatment progresses, increased awareness and scanning abilities should be incorporated in increasingly complex visual perceptual and visuomotor tasks. However, inattention often increases with task complexity; the therapist must monitor the patient and tasks carefully. Useful tasks for assessment include the following:

- Surveying a room repetitively
- Using scanning techniques to observe and name objects
- Moving toward and touching objects right and left of midline
- Assembling objects from pieces on the floor and table
- Completing an obstacle course
- Bringing a chart back to the therapist who left it on a counter

Scanning should always be stressed, especially during functional activities—dressing, shaving, and moving through the environment. The patient must learn to monitor the influence of inattention on functional performance and heed the admonition that "When something doesn't make sense, look into the unattended space and it usually will."[6] Using markers when reading, slowing the pace by reading aloud, and following text using a finger as a pointer are helpful adaptations.

Patients cannot feed or dress themselves unless they have been taught to scan and locate objects in the affected field. Computer use may be difficult, especially if the patient did not use one before the impairment. If the patient did use a computer before the impairment, acuity and glare factors and scanning and pursuit abilities should be screened and evaluated. Scanning and depth perception are not intact in patients wearing eye patches. Some patients may suffer from vestibular disorders and depend more on their visual skills to compensate for balance reactions (see Chapter 5).

Efferson[6] reports that no reliable studies are available regarding treatment of cortical blindness, color imperception, and visual agnosia. She instead presents Bouska's[3] and other clinicians' principles. If cortical blindness or simultanagnosia is suspected, the therapist must first attempt to increase the patient's knowledge of foveal and peripheral vision—where the patient is fixating. A small headlamp under subdued lighting may be used to teach the patient to position the eyes in midline of the head. The patient is asked to move the light (and thus the head and eyes) to locate fairly large, bright stimuli placed on a plain background. As acuity and localization skills improve, stimuli and background become smaller and more complex (e.g., from a box to a paper clip). The patient should accurately point to and manipulate targets after locating them with the light or keep the light on the target while moving the target with one hand. With color imperception, treatment should involve materials and tasks employing sharp color contrasts with minimal detail and progress to less contrast (more hues) with more detail.[1]

The treatment of patients with agnosia should progress according to the abilities that return in spontaneous recovery from agnosia. Common objects should be used in treatment. Presentations should occur in front of the patient, not off to either side. Tactile input with or without visual input should be encouraged and can be used as a compensatory mechanisms; however, tactile input may not be helpful in every case.

Color and facial agnosia may be treated by continually drilling the patient regarding two or three personally important names or colors. The patient may be helped to pick out or memorize cues for associating names with faces.

Efferson points out that treatment for visuospatial deficits should follow basic developmental considerations and progress from simple to more complex tasks. (If the evaluation suggests disorders in body scheme, tactile or vestibular input, or right-left discrimination, these areas should be dealt with first.)

Patients who do not know their location in space must internalize spatial understanding before they can make judgments regarding the space around them. Gross motor spatial training should encourage movement in all planes wherever possible. Patients should look at or fixate on a target and move their bodies near it by rolling, crawling, or walking. Auditory stimuli should be used, including alternative sounds and playing music, and should be constantly presented to the patient. Patients should be able to state where the stimulus is, point to it, and move toward it. Vision should be occluded before movement activity but made available during movement. The next level after this training segment incorporates retrieving items from the occupational therapy kitchen. The therapist can ask the patient to retrieve items from "behind you in the drawer on the right," "the table next to you," or "the bottom cabinet below your waist." Patients also can place items in various positions within a room. They should then stand in the middle of the room, close their eyes and try to visualize, verbalize, and point to where the objects are in relation to themselves from memory. Having located them, the patients should then walk through the area and pick up each item they put down in sequence. Functional carryover should always be used (e.g., having patients remember through visualization where they put their glasses in the living room before they begin searching) (Box 12-1).[6]

Perceptual Retraining with Computers

Numerous computer programs have been developed for rehabilitation of brain damage sequelae such as impaired cognition, attention, sequencing, memory, and perception. Because the computer is a highly visual medium it has become an obvious tool for treatment of visual perceptual dysfunction. Treatment with computers has been termed *computer-assisted therapy*. No large or conclusive treatment

Box 12-1

Suggested Functional Activities to Treat Visual System Dysfunction After CVA

The following functional activities address visual fixation, scanning, and saccades. Some activities also address accommodation, eye-hand coordination, and figure-ground skills. Postural control and upper extremity performance play primary roles in these activities.

A vestibular component may be added as required by placing items behind patients so they must rotate to retrieve them or by placing items lower than the patient so a change in head position must occur. During activities the patient should always maintain as much visual fixation as possible, especially if using vestibular responses.

1. Sorting activities are necessary adjuncts to ADL and are performed every day. The more meaningful the task is to an individual, the greater the result in completion.
   a. Sorting of items on the shelf in a medicine cabinet—Sequence can be written by the therapist or demonstrated.
   b. Sorting of silverware from caddies or dishwasher bin into silverware receptacle in a drawer—If this task is too difficult, the therapist can color code sets of spoons, forks, and butter knives and then remove one a time.
   c. Sorting of dinnerware by pattern, color, and size; removing it from the dishwasher, dish drainer, or table; and placing it on another surface—After sorting the patient may set the table or put the dinnerware away in high or low cabinet.
   d. Sorting of coins in a coin holder
   e. Sorting of laundry by color, pattern, or size as stated on labels—The patient may be asked to hang pants in one section of closet and sweaters in another. Pants and sweaters may be placed on hangers in a different manner, which addresses spatial orientation.
2. Placing toothpaste on a toothbrush or a gel cleanser on a small brush to clean jewelry, small vases, or bowls is a useful task. So too is placing mustard from squeeze containers onto small cheese and bread wedges (cut out from cookie cutters or cut with a knife following a straight path distinguished with food coloring or mustard).
3. The therapist may place colored spots on a large mirror; the patient then cleans the spots off of the mirror.
4. The therapist may use baking activities. The patient should then place ingredients in all quadrants, including high, low, and rotary positions.

Box 12-2

Computer Programs for Visual Perceptual Training

Optometric Extension Program
2912 S. Daimler Street
Santa Ana, CA
92705
(714) 250-8070

Bernell Corporation
750 Lincolnway East
P.O. Box 4637
South Bend, IN
46634
(800) 348-2225

Psychological Software Services Programs
Odie Bracey
Psychological Software Services
6555 Carollton Avenue
Indianapolis, IN
46229

Life Science Associates Programs
R. Gianutsos
Life Science Associates
1 Fenemore Road
Bayport, NY
11705
(Diagnosis and Training)

studies have yet defined the outcome of computer-assisted therapy compared with conventional therapy. Some reports indicate that computer-assisted therapy helps to motivate patients with poor attention and motivation. It provides perceptual variables (number, size, speed) and immediate feedback and is an automatic control for learning. Visual perceptual training with computers should be viewed as one part of select patients' treatment programs. Some patients, especially elderly patients, have no interest in working on or learning the computer and are not motivated to use it. The computer does not require perceptual, vestibular, and motor responses that are typically required for daily living activities. Low-vision aids are available for individuals suffering from macular degeneration, cataracts, diabetic retinopathy, glaucoma, detached retina, or retinitis pigmentosa. Low-vision aids include magnification and enhancement for most software programs. These aids are quite helpful when used with the appropriate population. Low-vision aids should not be suggested unless a primary visual assessment or at least a visual screening has been administered. Use should be justified and not just based on trial and error. Use of the computer should be limited to those who have previous knowledge of computers, who have a stated goal to return to using a computer for work or leisure, and who enjoy computer work (Box 12-2).

REVIEW QUESTIONS

1. What is the role of the functional optometrist in the evaluation and treatment of vision dysfunction after CVA?
2. Which deficits are considered primary visual deficits?
3. What are the norms for visual fields?
4. What are examples of age-related visual dysfunctions that may complicate the evaluation of a stroke patient?
5. For which patient population are computers a useful treatment modality?

■ COTA Considerations ■

- A team approach to rehabilitation of the visual system after stroke is crucial for positive functional outcomes.
- After a CVA, visual system dysfunction may occur within the primary visual pathway (sensory, motor) or associative visual pathway (perceptual).
- Intact visual fields are necessary for effective orientation to stimuli in specific areas of space. Visual field loss may result in: poor balance, falls, uncertain gait, difficulty locating items in space, and difficulty reading and writing.
- Visual acuity skills must be addressed before any other visual determination is made.
- Functional activities such as scanning activities can address a variety of skills, including visual fixation and saccades.

REFERENCES

1. Árnadóttir G: *The brain and behavior: assessing cortical function through activities of daily living*, St Louis, 1990, Mosby.
2. Bouska MJ, Gallaway M: Primary visual deficits in adults with brain damage: management in occupational therapy, *Occup Ther Prac* 3:1, 1991.
3. Bouska MJ, Kauffman NA, Marcus SE: Disorders of the visual perception system. In Umphred DA, editor: *Neurological rehabilitation*, St Louis, 1990, Mosby.
4. Cohen AH, Rein LD: The effect of head trauma on the visual system: the doctor of optometry as a member of the rehabilitative team, *J Am Optom Assoc* 63:530, 1992.
5. Cohen H, Fox CR: The visual and vestibular systems. In Cohen H, editor: *Neuroscience for rehabilitation*, 1993, JB Lippincott.
6. Efferson L: Disorders of vision and visual perceptual dysfunction. In Umphred DA, editor: *Neurological rehabilitation*, St Louis, 1996, Mosby.
7. Farber S: *Neurorehabilitation: a multisensory approach*, Philadelphia, 1992, WB Saunders.
8. Gianutsos R, Matheson P: The rehabilitation of visual perceptual disorders attributable to brain injury. In Meier M, Diller L, Benton A, editors: *Neuropsychological rehabilitation*, London, 1986, Churchill-Livingstone.
9. Gianutsos R, Ramsey G, Perlin RR: Rehabilitation optometric services for survivors of acquired brain injury, *Arch Phys Med Rehab* 69:573, 1988.
10. Gianutsos R, Suchoff IB: Visual fields after brain injury: management issues for the occupational therapist. In Scheiman M, editor: *Understanding and managing vision deficits: a guide for occupational therapists*, Thorofare, NJ, 1997, SLACK.
11. Goldberg ME, Eggers HM, Gouras P: Ocular motor system. In Kandel ER, Schwartz TH, Tessel TM, editors: *Principles of neural science*, ed 3, Norwalk, Conn, 1991, Appleton and Lange.
12. Hellerstein LF, Fishman B: Vision therapy and occupational therapy: an integrated approach, *J Behav Optom* 5:122, 1990.
13. Hellerstein LF, Fishman B: Visual rehabilitation for patients with brain injury. In Scheiman M, editor: *Understanding and managing vision deficits: a guide for occupational therapists*, Thorofare, NJ, 1997, SLACK.
14. Kalb L, Warshowsky TH: Occupational therapy and optometry: principles of diagnosis and collaborative treatment of learning disabilities in children, *Occup Ther Pract* 3:77, 1991.
15. Kelly DD: Sexual differentiation of the nervous system. In Kandel ER, Schwartz TH, editors: *Principles of neural science*, New York, 1985, Elsevier.
16. Mason C, Kandel ER: Central visual pathways. In Kandel ER, Schwartz TH, Tessel TM, editors: *Principles of neural science*, ed 3, Norwalk, Conn, 1991, Appleton and Lange.
17. Moses R, Hart W: *Adler's physiology of the eye: clinical application*, St Louis, 1987, Mosby.
18. Richards RG, Oppenheim GS: *Visual skill appraisal*, Novato, Ca, 1984, Academic Therapy.
19. Scheiman M: Optometric model of vision, part one. In Scheiman M, editor: *Understanding and managing vision deficits: a guide for occupational therapists*, Thorofare, NJ, 1997, SLACK.
20. Scheiman M: Optometric model of vision, part two. In Scheiman M, editor: *Understanding and managing vision deficits: a guide for occupational therapists*, Thorofare, NJ, 1997, SLACK.
21. Scheiman M: Screening for visual acuity, visual efficiency and visual information processing problems. In Scheiman M, editor: *Understanding and managing vision deficits: a guide for occupational therapists*, Thorofare, NJ, 1997, SLACK.
22. Scotti G, Spinnler H: Color imperception in unilateral hemisphere–damaged patients, *J Neurolog Neurosurg Psych* 33:22, 1970.
23. Suchoff IB: Occupational therapy and optometry—a developing relationship, *J Behav Optom* 2:170, 1991.
24. Toglia J: *Cognition and perception: principles and practice workshop*, New York, 1990.
25. Toglia J: Unilateral visual inattention: multi-dimensional components, *Occup Ther Pract* 3:18, 1991.
26. Tsurumi K, Todd V: Theory and guidelines for visual task analysis and synthesis. In Scheiman M, editor: *Understanding and managing vision deficits: a guide for occupational therapists*, Thorofare, NJ, 1997, SLACK.
27. Vaughan D, Asbury J: *General ophthalmology*, California, 1974, Lange Medical.
28. Warren M: A hierarchal model for evaluation and treatment of visual perceptual dysfunction in adult acquired brain injury, Part I and Part II, *Am J Occup Ther* 47:42, 1993.
29. Warshowsky TH: Principles of optometric rehabilitation, *Pract Optom* 4:4, 1993.
30. Zoltan B, Siev E, Freishtat B: The adult stroke patient: a manual for evaluation and treatment of perceptual and cognitive dysfunction, Thorofare, NJ, 1986, SLACK.

guðrún árnadóttir

chapter **13**

Impact of Neurobehavioral Deficits on Activities of Daily Living

key terms

activities of daily living (ADL)	performance areas	somatoagnosia
neurobehavior	performance contexts	gnosis
activity analysis	ideational apraxia	topographical disorientation
A-ONE	motor apraxia	perseveration
standardized assessment	spatial relations	agnosia
occupational performance	spatial neglect	aphasia
performance components	body neglect	praxis

chapter objectives

After completing this chapter, the reader will be able to accomplish the following:

1. Establish a relationship between neurobehavioral concepts and activity performance.
2. Apply the A-ONE theory and provide a structure for clinical observations of stroke patients.
3. Provide conceptual and operational definitions for neurobehavioral impairments and disability.
4. Relate the *Uniform Terminology for Occupational Therapy* to neurobehavioral concepts.
5. Provide examples of how strokes can cause different patterns of impairments affecting task performance.

Referrals to occupational therapy (OT) for clients who have had cerebrovascular accidents (CVAs) are usually made when the resulting impairments are suspected to affect activity performance. In the United States, 3 million people with varying degrees of neurologic impairment are reported to be stroke survivors.[52] When neurobehavioral impairments result from a CVA, they can affect the performance of daily activities. This chapter contains discussions on the impact of neurobehavioral deficits on activity performance. Topics such as occupational performance, neurobehavior, function of the cerebral cortex, dysfunction of performance tasks, patterns of performance components dysfunction or impairment resulting from different types of CVA, and usefulness of standardized assessment methods are discussed. However, before considering these issues, it might be useful to consider the following questions: "What are activities of daily living (ADL)?" "What is neurobehavior?" "What is neurobehavioral deficit?" "How is neurobehavior related to activity performance?", and "How is the impact of neurobehavioral deficits on activity performance measured?"

ACTIVITIES OF DAILY LIVING

ADL are defined by the U.S. Department of Health and Human Services[52] as basic daily activities such as eating, grooming, toileting and dressing. The *Uniform Terminology for Occupational Therapy—Third Edition*,[1] which is an official document of the American Occupational Therapy Association (AOTA), defines ADL as self-maintenance tasks. These include grooming, oral hygiene, bathing or showering, toilet hygiene, dressing, caring for personal devices, feeding and eating, adhering to a medication routine, maintaining health, socializing, functional communication, performing functional mobility tasks, mobilizing in the community, responding to emergencies, and using sexual expression. These ADL can be classified as one of three occupational performance areas according to the *Uniform Terminology*. The other two performance areas are work or productive activities and play or leisure activities. Two parameters in addition to performance areas are defined: performance components and performance context.

The performance areas previously listed are human activities that are typically part of daily life. These areas can be broken down to specific tasks. For example, the area of dressing includes tasks such as putting on a shirt, trousers, socks, and shoes and manipulating different types of fasteners. Functional elements, or the performance components, are the foundation of human performance. Fundamental abilities are required for successful performance of different tasks. The three main groups of performance components include a group of sensorimotor components, including aspects of sensory awareness, sensory processing, perceptual processing, and neuromusculoskeletal and motor abilities; a group of cognitive integration and cognitive components; and a group of psychosocial skills and psychologic components. Each of these groups can be subdivided into smaller units of components. For example, the group of cognitive integration and cognitive components can be subdivided into arousal, orientation, recognition, attention span, initiation of activity, memory, sequencing, categorization, concept formation, spatial operations, problem-solving, learning, and generalization. These subunits are required for task performance. The performance components of task performance are used in different combinations and to varying degrees depending on the particular task. Nelson[38] has noted that not all necessary

subunits are included in this classification by the AOTA. For example, emotional aspects and various components of language have been omitted.

The performance contexts include temporal and environmental aspects that influence the engagement of the individual in performance areas.[1,2] Because the occupational therapist views the individual as an occupational being,[16] the occupational therapist's center of attention is the parameter of performance areas that include different tasks. The performance components are subsequently viewed in relation to those tasks. In addition, the performance tasks or areas are viewed in a particular context of the person, be it the person's age, developmental stage, culture, health status, or physical environment. The performance context can therefore either provide environmental support or produce barriers. Figure 13-1 shows, among other frameworks, the three performance parameters and some of the important subcomponents. The World Health Organization[54] (WHO) has four levels (pathology, impairment, handicap, disability), three of which are parallel to the three levels of dysfunction in the model of occupational performance (performance component dysfunction, performance area/task dysfunction, and performance role dysfunction).[42] Dickoff et al[20] describe four levels of theory development (factor-isolating theories, factor-relating theories, situation-relating theories, situation producing theories). The theory behind the A-ONE[3] is a factor-relating theory, relating ADL tasks to performance components.

Trombly[47,48] includes roles in her hierarchy of performance levels. She divides what the *Uniform Terminology*[1] describes as *performance areas* into roles, tasks, and activities. According to Christiansen,[15] roles represent the highest level of the occupational performance hierarchy and role responsibilities define the nature of occupational performance. The roles change throughout life.

Dunn et al[21,22] emphasize the impact of context on activity performance; people are "embedded in their contexts."[22] People perform when they interact with their context to engage in a task. People are surrounded by tasks; performance range is the range of tasks that can be performed during the interaction between the people and their context. Such interaction also affects roles. Roles include groups of different tasks that overlap. Persons may have many roles, and some of the tasks in their different roles may overlap.

According to Trombly,[47] occupational therapists have several models to choose from when working with physically disabled clients. A *conceptual model* of practice is considered synonymous with a frame of reference.[47] One model is the occupational performance model described by Pedretti and Pasquinelli[40] based on the *Uniform Terminology*.[1] This model was identified as one of the three most frequently used models in occupational therapy by Nelson et al.[39] According to Yerxa,[56] a frame of reference is "a set of ideas, beliefs, and tools which guide practice, and which

WHO CLASSIFICATION	OCCUPATIONAL PERFORMANCE FRAME OF REFERENCE	STAGES OF THEORY DEVELOPMENT

WHO CLASSIFICATION

Handicap
Societal consequences of disease; occurs when performance of social roles is impaired and task disabilities are severe

Disability
Restricted performance of daily activities; concerned with integrated functioning of the entire person, such as problems with feeding; occurs when impairment is severe and affects actions that have some meaning for the person

Impairment
Loss of abnormality of anatomic, physiologic, cognitive, or emotional structure of function; refers to direct physiologic consequences of the underlying pathology or the external manifestations of a disease (such as lack of ROM or visuospatial impairment)

OCCUPATIONAL PERFORMANCE FRAME OF REFERENCE

Dysfunction of Roles
- Housewife
- Carpenter
- Student
- Office Clerk
- Preschooler

Dysfunction of Performance Tasks

ADL Area	Work Area	Leisure and Play Area
• Grooming: hairbrushing	• Typing	• Playing chess
• Feeding: drinking from glass	• Writing	• Jogging
• Transfers: sitting up in bed	• Hammering	• Skating
• Dressing: putting on shirt	• Sanding	• Knitting
• Communication: asking for glasses	• Sawing	• Drawing
	• Cooking	• Gardening
	• Frying	

Dysfunction of Performance Components

Sensorimotor Components	Cognitive Integrative and Cognitive Components	Psychosocial Skills and Psychologic Components
• Tactile	• Memory	• Values
• Vestibular	• Sequencing	• Interests
• Stereognosis	• Learning	• Self-concept
• Kinesthesia	• Problem solving	• Self-expression
• Body scheme	• Concept formation	• Role performance
• Spatial relations	• Attention span	• Social conduct
• Strength	• Level of arousal	• Time management
• Endurance		
• Praxis		
• Muscle tone		

STAGES OF THEORY DEVELOPMENT

Factor-Isolating Theories
Develop terminology and definitions; most primitive theory level

Factor-Relating Theories
Develop interrelations among factors (e.g., A-ONE theory relates neurologic factors to activity performance)

A-ONE THEORY addresses both levels

Situation-Relating Theories
Predict that one situation will produce another (e.g., Neurobehavioral impairment results in dysfunction of self-care performance)

Situation-Producing Theories
Specify goals as aims of activities and prescribe activities to reach the goals

Figure 13-1 Relationship between different classification systems.

enable the practitioner to 'name and frame' what is relevant to consider in working with patients."

In summary, *occupational performance* is the ability of an individual to accomplish the tasks required by the role of that individual. Examples of roles are homemaker, student, and employee. The roles of a preschooler and a retired worker show the relationship between developmental stages and roles. The previously mentioned tasks, being performed in different performance areas by individuals in various roles, reflect the core concept of occupational therapy—purposeful activity. These tasks are further influenced by the performance context. The foundation for occupational performance consists of the previously mentioned functional elements, called *performance compo-*

nents, which are behavioral patterns based on learning and developmental stages.[3,40]

NEUROBEHAVIOR

According to Llorens,[33] neurobehavioral theory is concerned with the way environmental stimuli are processed in the central nervous system (CNS) and how they affect behavioral and emotional responses (Figure 13-2). Llorens defines processing of stimuli as "the recognition, interpretation, storage, and retrieval of information to which meaning is attributed from past and present experience."[33] Task performance in daily activities is a result of behavioral responses. The mechanism of nervous-system processing and neurobehavior is a complex interaction of processing and response. The processing of different performance components occurs in the nervous system with the goal of influencing behavioral responses. Thus neurobehavior is the basis for task performance.[3] The behavioral responses can be motor or emotional.

Neurobehavioral theory is based on functional neuroanatomy and neurophysiology. The theory addresses such areas as stimulation of the sensory systems and processing the stimulation in the CNS in addition to the generation of behavioral responses to link brain processes to behavior and emotional responses.[33] Occupational therapists assess and treat behavior as it appears during the performance of various tasks. All tasks provide sensory stimuli, and the ADL represent a group of these tasks. Performance components may therefore be viewed as different stimuli received and processed by the CNS through different mechanisms, which work together to elicit neurobehavioral responses and task performance.[3] Neurobehavior includes the different types of pertinent performance components necessary for performing different aspects of daily activities.

The three parameters of occupational performance can all be conceptualized along a continuum of function and dysfunction.[42] According to Christiansen,[15] dysfunction occurs when a "person cannot perform roles to satisfaction, either because of deficits in abilities and skills due to disease or disability, the conflicting demands of multiple roles, or because of unclear role expectations." Limitations in performance components and tasks will limit the performance range, as will inadequate context that does not provide the needed resources to enable performance.[21,22]

NEUROBEHAVIORAL DEFICITS OR IMPAIRMENTS

A *neurobehavioral deficit* is defined by Árnadóttir[3] as a functional impairment of an individual manifested as defective skill performance resulting from a neurologic processing dysfunction that affects performance components such as affect, body scheme, cognition, emotion, gnosis, language, memory, motor movement, perception, personality, praxis, sensory awareness, spatial relations, and visuospatial skills.

The World Health Organization (WHO) classified four concepts in its disablement model for describing the con-

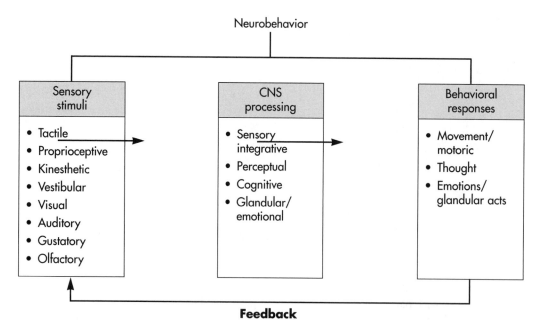

Figure 13-2   Elements of neurobehavior include different types of sensory stimuli. These stimuli are processed by different mechanisms in the CNS and result in different types of behavioral responses. Feedback from the responses affects new sensory stimuli. (Modified from Llorens LA: Activity analysis: agreement among factors in a sensory processing model, *Am J Occup Ther* 40:103, 1986.)

sequences of disease.[52,54] *Uniform Terminology*[1] organizes concepts related to occupational performance as mentioned previously; this classification is parallel with the WHO hierarchy according to Rogers and Holm[42] (see Figure 13-1). Townsend et al[46] recommend using the WHO International Classification of Impairments, Disabilities, and Handicaps (ICIDH) in occupational therapy (see Chapter 2).

According to Martini et al,[36] a proposed revision (PR) of the ICIDH has been suggested (ICIDH-PR). The ICIDH-PR considers a handicap the result of an interactive process between impairments, disabilities, or both, as well as social and environmental hindrances. This model is referred to as the *handicap creation model*, as opposed to the previous *disablement model*. The model differentiates between handicap situations that can be attributed to the environment rather than the individual. In this model, an impairment is a "structural organic anomaly or alteration."[36] Negative terms have been replaced by positive ones. Therefore, in the ICIDH-PR, impairment is defined in organic terms, disability is defined in relation to ability, and handicaps are defined in relation to obstacles to environmental factors and life habits, which in turn are related to activities and roles.

NEUROBEHAVIOR AND ACTIVITIES OF DAILY LIVING

The relationship between neurobehavior and ADL may be best described from a theoretical perspective. Yerxa[56] defines theory as a "set of related ideas that enable scientists to predict, control, explain, or gain a sense of understanding about phenomena." According to Reynolds,[41] theory development is an evolutionary process that starts with an idea and moves on to conceptualization. A classification system is needed in which *typology*, or a guiding set of ideas, must be developed. These concepts are the building blocks for the theory and must be defined, evaluated, and agreed on by the scientific community. The conceptualization eventually evolves into relational statements. A statement generated from a theory (on the basis of its typology) is selected for comparison with the results of empirical research designed to test the statement's correspondence with the theory.[41]

Dickoff et al[20] explain that theories used for practice disciplines are conceptual frameworks developed for a specific purpose. Four levels of theories could be viewed on a developmental continuum.[20] The first and most primitive level includes the factor isolating theories, which provide names for things (i.e., develop terminology). The second level is composed of factor-relating theories, which develop relationships among factors. The third level includes situation-relating theories, which make predictions about certain situations; as these theories predict that one situation will cause another, they may promote or inhibit con-

sequent situations. The fourth and most mature theory level includes the situation-producing, or prescriptive, theories. These theories specify goals as aims or activities and prescribe activities to reach the goals. The theory behind the Árnadóttir OT-ADL Neurobehavioral Evaluation (A-ONE)[3] explains how neurobehavior is related to ADL. This is a factor-relating theory, according to the conceptual framework described by Dickoff et al[20] because it relates factors from neurobehavioral performance components to ADL performance tasks. In the A-ONE theory, a relationship between different factors—the ability to perform daily activities, neurobehavioral impairments, and the CNS origin of the neurobehavioral dysfunction—is proposed. In other words, a relationship between daily activities and neuronal processing is proposed. Research studies that support these statements have been conducted.[3] Figure 13-1 lists the four steps of theory levels as described by Dickoff et al[20] and indicates which factors of the occupational performance framework the A-ONE theory relates. Following are several examples of relational statements from this theory.

The behaviors that are required for task performance are related to neuronal processing at the CNS level. Thus a relationship also exists between the defective behavioral responses of an individual with CNS damage during performance of ADL and the dysfunction of neuronal processing and performance components resulting from CNS dysfunction or structural damage.[3]

Performance of daily activities requires adequate function of specific parts of the nervous system. Consequently, impairment of certain components of the CNS may result in dysfunction of specific aspects of ADL. For example, a massive posteroinferior parietal lobe lesion in the left hemisphere may cause bilateral motor apraxia. This neurobehavioral impairment may make manipulation of objects difficult during functional activities such as combing hair, brushing teeth, or holding a spoon while eating. In contrast, a small precentral lesion in the primary motor area may cause muscle paralysis of the contralateral side but not apraxia. The paralysis would require that the patient perform some daily activities using one-handed techniques; performance of other activities might be impossible (Figure 13-3). Thus neurologic impairments that can be observed through the patient's engagement in daily activities indicate localization and the extent of neurologic damage. Therefore through analysis of ADL the integrity of CNS activity can be evaluated.[3]

Performance components needed to perform tasks can be used as sensory stimuli to elicit behavioral responses, allowing assessment of the neurobehavioral impairments that interfere with task performance of an individual with CNS damage. For example, a comb is a visual stimulus that results in task performance (i.e., the behavioral motor response of reaching out for the comb and combing the hair). A therapist instructing a patient to put on a shirt (an audi-

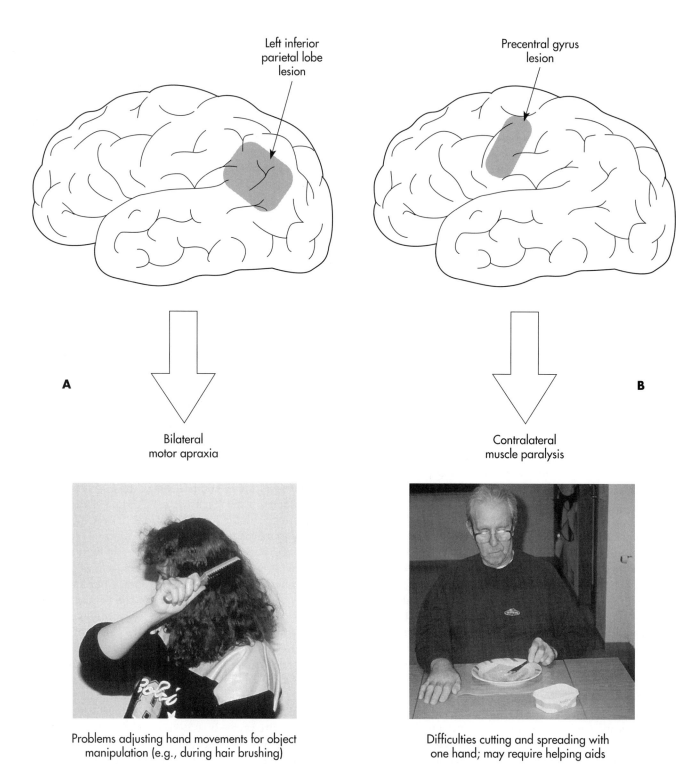

Left inferior
parietal lobe
lesion

Precentral gyrus
lesion

A

B

Bilateral
motor apraxia

Contralateral
muscle paralysis

Problems adjusting hand movements for object
manipulation (e.g., during hair brushing)

Difficulties cutting and spreading with
one hand; may require helping aids

Figure 13-3   Relational statements indicate that different neurologic impairments affect task performance differently and point to CNS localization of neurologic damage. **A,** Left posterior-inferior parietal lobe lesion causes bilateral motor apraxia, resulting in problems with adjustment of hand movements during hair brushing. **B,** Lesion in the precentral gyrus results in contralateral muscle paralysis manifested as difficulties with bilateral use of hands when buttering.

tory stimulus) can also evoke motor and cognitive behavioral responses such as turning the shirt and carrying out the necessary movements to put it on. Any behavioral response would be classified according to the previously mentioned activity analysis, which reveals dysfunction in performance components.[3] These theoretical statements indicate how neurobehavior and neurobehavioral impairments are related to ADL and task performance. The A-ONE theory will be used as a framework for the rest of this chapter.

MEASURING THE IMPACT OF NEUROBEHAVIORAL DEFICITS ON ACTIVITY PERFORMANCE

The impact of neurobehavioral deficits can be measured through observation of activity performance. Because neurobehavioral deficits often interfere with independence, therapists can benefit from detecting these impairments while observing ADL and gain an understanding of the factors affecting the patient's functional dependence. Subsequently, therapists could begin determining the most pertinent treatment for the neurobehavioral deficits that are causing the functional dependence.[3] A systematic evaluation of daily activities can be used as a structure for clinical reasoning that helps therapists detect neurobehavioral dysfunction or impaired neurologic performance components and assess functional independence in self-care activities. This method allows the therapist to analyze the nature or cause of a functional problem that requires occupational therapy intervention, so the analysis is made from the view of occupations.

Activity analysis is the process of examining activities in detail by breaking them into their components to understand and evaluate tasks. Performance components that are needed to perform specific skills or tasks are studied, as well as the effects impaired performance components will have on task performance.[3,33]

In the A-ONE, activity analysis is used to identify different performance components and possible manifestations of CNS dysfunction during ADL performance. During the instrument development of the A-ONE, activity analysis was used to determine which performance components are necessary for performance of particular tasks and how dysfunction of performance components is revealed by neurobehavioral responses during performance of specific activities.

An example might explain this process better. A meaningful task, such as eating, calls for a goal-directed, purposeful response. Various factors are involved, such as food and cutlery, as well as performance components, such as visuospatial-spatial relationships, muscle tone, and emotional state. Carrying out the behavior required to eat requires different performance components. When analyzed with the required performance components in mind, the quality

of the response reveals information not only about independence in ADL but also regarding performance component dysfunction—the problems that interfere with independence, such as misjudging distances when reaching out for a cup or not knowing how to use cutlery[3] (Figure 13-4).

Rogers and Holm[42] defined functional assessment as "the collection, analysis, and synthesis of data and the making of recommendations related to an individual's ability to perform work, self-care, recreation, and leisure tasks." Rogers and Holm[30] warn that complications may develop when functional assessment focuses on the level of performance components or role performance—a compilation of tasks—rather than on task performance. Complications include the failure to collect information and form hypotheses about task performance dysfunction and the failure to recognize functional problems that should be addressed by an occupational therapist.

Christiansen[14] acknowledged that "assessing function without regard to the patient's life tasks and roles has serious shortcomings" and that assessing occupational performance components such as ROM without regard to tasks and roles should be reconsidered.

Fisher and Short-DeGraf[23] agree with Christiansen's view. They propose an assessment method with which to obtain information through direct observations of meaningful task performance in natural environments. This method allows the therapist to directly assess the impact of "performance component deficits or occupational contexts on occupational performance." This direct assessment eliminates the need to infer relationships between different hierarchical levels.

Machiowetz[37] also supports this view. It is suggested that evaluation of occupational performance components should be secondary to assessment of performance areas and roles, which should be the main focus of evaluation.

According to Trombly,[51] assessment procedures should reflect the concept of occupational function. Trombly[49] identifies the need in therapy to develop standardized instruments that relate occupational performance components to task performance.

Árnadóttir[3] notes that cognitive perceptual tests uniquely designed for occupational therapy have not been available for therapists interested in evaluating neurobehavior. The items used appear to be borrowed from neuropsychology and neurology.

It is important for a profession's identity and autonomy to use evaluation tools based on its own concepts and theories. A profession should also have instruments developed according to the knowledge base of that profession to prevent its members from being misled and moved away from the profession's goals.[3] Árnadóttir developed and standardized the A-ONE[3] on the basis of the previously mentioned theoretical principles and viewpoints. Functional assessments may be nonstandardized observations or standardized evaluations.

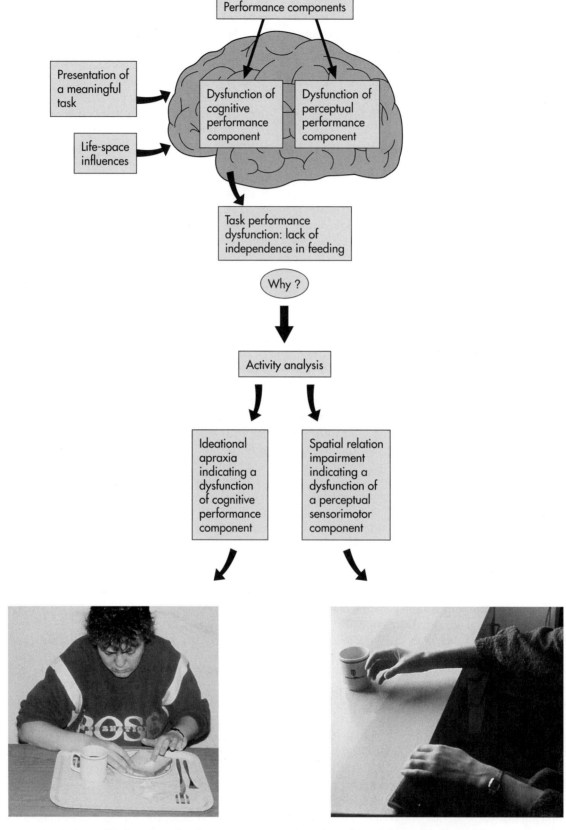

Figure 13-4 Dysfunction of performance components such as ideational apraxia and spatial relations impairment can be revealed by activity analysis during the observation of feeding performance. (Modified from Árnadóttir G: *The brain and behavior: assessing cortical dysfunction through activities of daily living,* St Louis, 1990, Mosby.)

FUNCTION OF THE CEREBRAL CORTEX: THE FOUNDATION OF TASK PERFORMANCE

Performance of daily activities is observed on a regular basis by occupational therapists working with CVA patients. With the use of activity analysis, it is possible to detect occupational performance components necessary for task performance and subsequently to detect the type and degree of severity of neurobehavioral impairments that interfere with activity performance. The performance components can then be related to functional areas of the brain responsible for different neurologic processing functions. The performance components are based on neurologic function, which takes place at different levels of the CNS. Several CNS areas may contribute to a particular type of neurologic processing, resulting in simultaneous or parallel processing at different locations, which contribute to processing of the same performance component. During activity performance, different types of processing may be taking place simultaneously. Neuronal processing in the brain varies in complexity. It is common to view three levels of functional complexity in the cortex based on Luria's[34] theories. These are commonly called *primary, secondary,* and *tertiary cortical zones* or *projection areas.*

Functional Localization for Processing Performance Components

Primary areas are concerned with direct processing of primary sensory and motor information. These areas include the primary somesthetic sensory cortex in the postcentral gyrus of the parietal lobe, the primary visual cortex around the calcarine fissure on the medial side of the occipital lobe, the primary auditory cortex in the superior temporal gyrus of the temporal lobe, and the primary motor cortex in the precentral gyrus of the frontal lobe. The cells in these areas respond mainly to information from a particular sense modality. Function in the primary areas is fairly symmetrical in both hemispheres; asymmetry increases in secondary and tertiary cortical areas.[3]

All cortical areas, other than the primary ones, are association areas, which (except for the motor association cortex) receive information from the primary areas and integrate it with information from other areas. The secondary association areas are adjacent to and connected with primary cortical areas. They are involved in more complex processing aspects of a single sensory or motor function. These areas include the visual association cortex surrounding the primary visual cortex in the occipital lobe, the auditory association cortex in the temporal lobe, the somatosensory association area in the superior parietal lobule, and the premotor cortex in the frontal lobe. The secondary association areas are connected with each other and with higher-order association areas, as well as with adjacent primary areas.[3]

The tertiary, or higher-order, association areas are involved in complex integration of information from many different cortical areas. Three such higher-order cortical association areas exist: the prefrontal cortex, the limbic cortex, and the parietotemporaloccipital cortex, on the border of the three posterior lobes. The dorsolateral prefrontal cortex is involved in complex motor functions, concept formation, abstraction, intelligence, judgment, attention, intention, sequencing, and timing and organization of activity steps and behavior as well as emotional processing. The limbic association cortex includes the orbitofrontal part of the prefrontal cortex, the temporal pole, and the parahippocampal gyrus on the medial aspects of the temporal lobes and the cingulate gyrus of the cortex. The limbic association cortex is concerned with memory as well as with motivation and emotional aspects of behavior. The parietotemporo-occipital cortex is involved with processing of complex sensory functions on the basis of information from two or more of the secondary association areas of the three posterior lobes. Figure 13-5 illustrates functional organization of the cerebral cortex. The secondary and tertiary association areas are connected, as are the different tertiary areas.[3] Although function can be related to different anatomic areas, it must be remembered that plasticity permits deviations from the usual localization sites under certain conditions such as injury or developmental abnormality.

To summarize, the frontal lobes are responsible for motor functions including motor speech, motor praxis, attention, cognition, emotions, intelligence, ideation, intention, judgment, motivation, working memory (i.e., sensorimotor components including neuromusculoskeletal and motor components), cognitive integration, cognitive components, and psychosocial skills and psychological components. The parietal lobes are concerned with the processing of somesthetic information as well as more complex sensory input from different sources, which thus includes sensorimotor components related to somesthetic sensation, sensory awareness and processing, perceptual components concerned with spatial relations, gnosis and body scheme, and the motor components of praxis. The occipital lobes process visual information (i.e., visual sensory and perceptual components, including visual recognition), and the temporal lobes process auditory information as well as long-term memory, emotion, and motivation (or as described in the AOTA Uniform Terminology classification,[1] sensorimotor, cognitive integration, and cognitive components). Table 13-1 summarizes the functions of the different cortical lobes of the brain and relates them to primary, secondary, and tertiary functional areas in these lobes. As indicated in the table, several functional areas in different lobes may contribute to a particular function. Therefore different cortical areas may be responsible for processing particular functions.

The cortex does not function in isolation. It communicates by various pathways with other CNS areas that also contribute to neuronal processing, including the thalamus, which contains nuclei that relay information to and from the cortex. The thalamus is involved in sensory, motor, emotional, memory, and complex mental func-

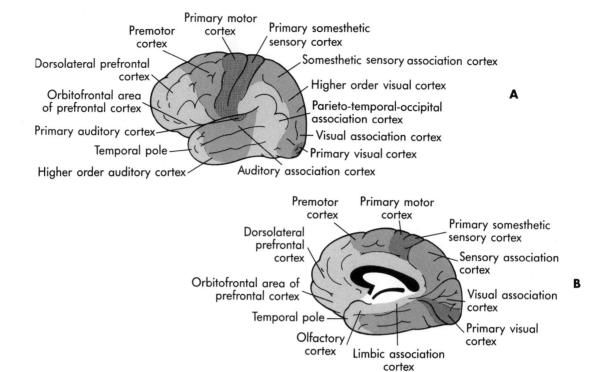

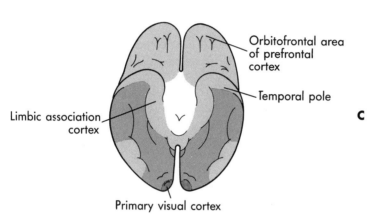

Figure 13-5 Functional organization of the cerebral cortex. **A,** Lateral surface. **B,** Medial surface. **C,** Inferior surface. The different shades refer to primary, secondary, and tertiary functional areas of the cortex. (From Árnadóttir G: *The brain and behavior: assessing cortical dysfunction through activities of daily living,* St Louis, 1990, Mosby.)

Table 13-1

Functions of the Cerebral Cortex

FUNCTIONAL AREA	ANATOMIC AREA	FUNCTION AND PERFORMANCE COMPONENTS
Frontal lobes		
Primary motor area	Precentral gyrus	Execution of movement
Secondary association area	Premotor cortex	Planning and programming of movement
		Sequencing, timing, and organization of movement
	Frontal eye field	Voluntary eye movements
	Broca's area in the left inferior frontal gyrus	Programming of motor speech
	Supplementary motor area	Intention of movement
Tertiary association area	Orbitofrontal and dorsolateral prefrontal cortex	Ideation
		Concept formation
		Abstract thought
		Intellectual functions
		Sequencing, timing, and organization of action and behavior
		Initiation and planning of action

Modified from Árnadóttir G: *The brain and behavior: assessing cortical dysfunction through activities of daily living,* St Louis, 1990, Mosby.

Table 13-1

Functions of the Cerebral Cortex—cont'd

FUNCTIONAL AREA	ANATOMIC AREA	FUNCTION AND PERFORMANCE COMPONENTS
Frontal lobes—cont'd		
Tertiary association area—cont'd		Judgment
		Insight
		Intention
		Attention
		Alertness
		Personality
		Working memory
		Emotion
Parietal lobes		
Primary somesthetic sensory area	Postcentral gyrus	Fine touch sensation, proprioception, kinesthesia
Secondary somesthetic sensory association area	Superior parietal lobule	Coordination, integration, and refinement of sensory input
		Tactile localization and discrimination
		Stereognosis
Tertiary association area	Inferior parietal lobule	*Gnosis:* recognition of received tactile, visual and auditory input
		Praxis: storage of programs or visuokinesthetic motor engrams necessary for motor sequences
		Body scheme: Postural model of body, body parts, and their relation to the environment
		Spatial relations: processing related to depth, distance, spatial concepts, position in space, and differentiation of foreground from background
Occipital Lobes		
Primary visual sensory area	Calcarine fissure	Visual reception (from the opposite visual field)
Visual association area	Brodmann's areas 18 and 19	Synthesis and integration of visual information
		Perception of visuospatial relationships
		Formation of visual memory traces
		Prepositional construction of language comprehension and speech
Temporal Lobes		
Primary auditory sensory area	Superior temporal gyrus	Auditory reception
Secondary association area	Superior and middle temporal gyri (Wernicke's area)	Language comprehension
		Sound modulation
		Perception of music
		Auditory memory
Tertiary association area	Temporal pole, parahippocampus	Long-term memory
		Learning of higher-order visual tasks and auditory patterns
		Emotion
		Motivation
		Personality
Limbic Lobes		
Tertiary association area	Orbitofrontal cortex in frontal lobe, temporal pole, and parahippocampus in the temporal lobe	Attention
		Motivation
		Emotions
		Long-term memory
	Cingulate gyrus in frontal and parietal lobes	

tions. The hypothalamus affects automatic functions, such as endocrine and emotional functions, and regulation of metabolism, temperature, and sleep. The basal ganglia and cerebellum affect coordination and tone of motor functions. The cerebellum is also involved in equilibrium. The brain stem houses fiber tracts that bring information to and from the cortex as well as different types of nuclei and the reticular formation. Reticular formation plays an important role in alertness and attention and contributes to cardiovascular and respiratory control.

Processing of Praxis

Although certain functions can be assigned to specific lobes, several CNS areas help process particular performance components.[3] Árnadóttir[3] constructed several different processing models indicating processing sites of different functions in the cortex. One example is the processing model for praxis. Praxis takes place in two steps: ideation, referring to concept formation related to an activity; and planning and programming of movement, which include timing and sequencing of movement components.[4] The result of praxis is motor execution. The ideation involved in praxis requires function of the frontal lobes (prefrontal and premotor areas) as well as of areas around the lateral tissue. The visuokinesthetic motor engrams or memory molecules for movement are stored in the left inferior part of the parietal lobe,[27] the left hemisphere in general being superior in storing routinely used codes.[26] Access to the left inferior parietal lobe is needed for either side of the body to move. Information goes from this area to the premotor area, which programs movement before the information is conveyed to the primary motor cortex in the left hemisphere (which controls execution of movements of the right side of the body). The premotor cortex on the left side connects with the premotor cortex of the right side by way of the anterior fibers of the corpus callosum and in turn relays the visuokinesthetic motor information to the right hemisphere. The right premotor cortex programs movements and instructs the adjacent primary motor cortex on the execution of movement of the left side of the body (Figure 13-6).

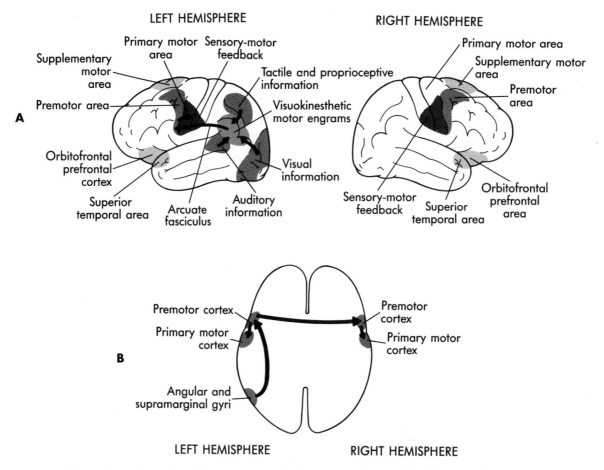

Figure 13-6 Processing of motor praxis. **A,** Active functional areas of the left and right hemispheres during praxis. **B,** Transverse view of the most commonly accepted sequential processing model of motor praxis.[27] (From Árnadóttir G: *The brain and behavior: assessing cortical dysfunction through activities of daily living,* St Louis, 1990, Mosby.)

Processing During Task Performance

Motor praxis (as described previously) is only one type of neurobehavioral performance component related to neurobehavior. The type of component and the degree of involvement depend on the task to be performed. As mentioned, several processing mechanisms may be simultaneously involved in the performance of a functional activity. This has been demonstrated by Árnadóttir through analysis of activity such as combing hair.[3] A person sitting in front of a mirror by a sink where the brush is located has three routes by which sensory information related to this particular task will reach the cortex. The person notes the brush visually, and this information travels through the visual pathway to the primary visual cortex where it is synthesized and further analyzed by the association areas. Memories and ideational processes are brought into play; as a result, the person gets the idea to want to brush the hair. Similarly, when the person is verbally instructed to brush the hair, this auditory input travels over the auditory pathway to the primary auditory area of cortex in the temporal lobe where it is processed by the association areas. Subsequently the input is compared with information in memory stores, yielding an idea based on the auditory information.

The third pathway is somesthetic. A person who grasps or is handed a brush receives tactile and proprioceptive information, which (after it reaches the primary sensory cortex in the parietal lobe) is analyzed by the association areas and integrated with prior experiences.

Information from all three pathways travels from the pertinent primary receptive areas to secondary and tertiary areas where further processing takes place. Attention processes, memory processes, emotions, and higher-order thought are brought into play. The sensory information is integrated with previous experiences, and responses are planned. A response may be emotional or motoric, resulting in different processing mechanisms depending on the nature of the response. Simultaneous processing of information takes place as information from the different secondary association areas is fed into the limbic system, the tertiary association areas in the prefrontal lobe, and the temporal pole, where higher cognitive functions including emotion and memory take place. Different fiber connections in a hemisphere, between hemispheres, and between the cortex and other CNS structures play important roles in this processing.

During processing, ideation, intent to perform an action, and preparation of a sequenced plan of action occur; all result in flow of information to the primary motor cortex and ultimately in the functional response of picking up the brush. This process requires praxis. The intention to perform an action is relayed to the frontal lobes and supplementary motor areas. From the lower left parietal lobe (which houses visuokinesthetic motor engrams), information travels to the left premotor cortex (which is responsible for planning and sequencing of movement) on its way

to the middle part of the primary motor cortex of the frontal lobe in the left hemisphere (which is responsible for movement performed by the right hand). A series of feedback movement interactions and readjustments follow. This series is based on continuous sensory information from the activity. During the complex process of performing "simple" activity, other responses (e.g., emotional and verbal) may be elicited. Such responses require function of processing areas different from the ones mentioned previously. Figure 13-7 illustrates some of the processing components that take place during the activity of brushing hair. The task performance that results from this kind of processing may reveal substantial information about function and subsequent dysfunction of the cerebral cortex.

DYSFUNCTION OF PERFORMANCE AREAS AS A RESULT OF CEREBROVASCULAR ACCIDENTS

CVAs may affect performance components. Dysfunction of performance components may subsequently interfere with primary ADL. Neurobehavioral impairments may be related to dysfunction of performance components, which have been classified into three groups according to the *Uniform Terminology for Occupational Therapy—Third Edition* outline.[1] These components are (1) sensorimotor, (2) cognitive integration and cognitive, and (3) psychosocial skills and psychological. There are two ways of defining terms. A concept is traditionally used for a general, abstract idea. Conceptual definitions are definitions of the concepts themselves, generalized and abstract. Conceptual definitions can be found in dictionaries. On the other hand, operational definitions refer to how particular concepts are measured and observed (e.g., test items with which particular concepts can be measured).

Conceptual Definitions of Terms

Frontal Lobe Dysfunction
The frontal lobes process sensorimotor components, including neuromusculoskeletal and motor components and cognitive integration and cognitive components. Dysfunction of the frontal lobes may affect sensorimotor components processed in the primary motor and premotor areas. Subsequently, a host of impairments including paralysis of the contralateral body side, muscle weakness, and spasticity may be observed. The distribution of impairments is related to lesion localization in the primary motor cortex. Dysarthria results if a lesion of the primary motor cortex is present above the lateral fissure. Dysarthria refers to weakness or altered neuronal control of the muscles responsible for speech production, or defective sensory feedback about the movements of those muscles.

If a lesion of the premotor cortex is present, apraxia and perseveration may be observed. Apraxia is a dysfunction of skilled purposeful movement that is caused neither by

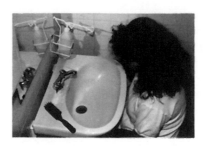

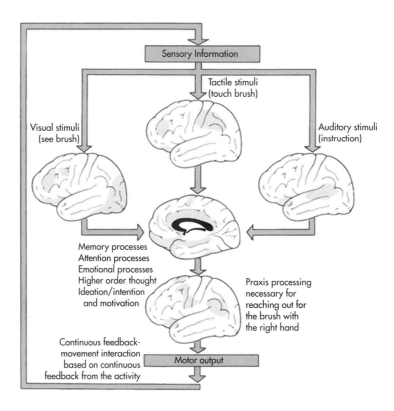

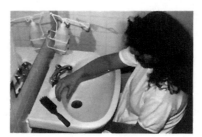

Figure 13-7   Different cortical areas involved in processing of various performance components during an ADL task. A person sitting by a sink preparing for grooming is asked to brush the hair. Note that three types of sensory stimulation can lead to performance. (From Árnadóttir G: *The brain and behavior: assessing cortical dysfunction through activities of daily living*, St Louis, 1990, Mosby.)

deficits in primary motor execution nor by comprehension problems.[27] Apraxia can be divided into ideational apraxia and motor or ideomotor apraxia. Ideational apraxia is conceptually defined as a breakdown of the knowledge of what is to be done to perform. This breakdown results from loss of the neuronal model, or a mental representation of the concept required for performance. It further refers to lack

of knowledge regarding object use or use of objects in relation to each other as well as lack of planning, sequencing and timing of activity steps.[4]

Motor apraxia is conceptually defined as a loss of access to kinesthetic memory patterns so that purposeful movement cannot be achieved because of defective planning and sequencing of movements, even though the idea and purpose of the task is understood. It is used by Árnadóttir[3] as a synonym for ideomotor apraxia as defined by Ayres.[4] Motor apraxia can result from a lesion in the inferior parietal lobe of the left hemisphere where the visuokinesthetic motor engrams or memory molecules for praxis are stored. It can occur as a lesion of the frontal lobe of either hemisphere where the premotor cortex is involved in planning and programming of movement of the contralateral body side. The movement is subsequently executed by the primary motor cortex of the corresponding hemisphere. Motor apraxia can also result from a lesion of the corpus callosum.[27] Thus a lesion in the left hemisphere, where the memory molecules for praxis are stored, can result in bilateral apraxia that may become apparent if the right side of the body is not paralyzed. If the right side is paralyzed, the motor apraxia may only show up in the left side of the body during movement. However, if the lesion is located in the anterior fibers of the corpus callosum or in the premotor area in the right frontal lobe, unilateral motor apraxia of the left body side may result, if that side is not paralyzed. Figure 13-8 shows lesion sites in motor apraxia caused by dis-

rupted processing of praxis. Motor apraxia can show up in fine movements and in gross movements and gait. Oral apraxia is a form of motor apraxia affecting speech and swallowing movements. Oral apraxia is defective planning and programming of movements of the oral musculature.

Perseveration can be divided into premotor perseveration and prefrontal perseveration as related to location of the lesion within the frontal lobes, according to Luria.[34] Perseveration has been defined as repeated movements or acts during functional performance as a result of difficulty in shifting from one response pattern to another. It refers to inertia or initiation or termination of performance.[18,35,45] Premotor perseveration is compulsive repetition of the same movement, whereas prefrontal perseveration is repetition of whole actions or action components. Prefrontal perseveration and ideational apraxia are both related to dysfunction of cognitive integration and cognitive components. Organization and sequencing of activity steps are related to ideation. Impaired organization and sequencing are the inability to organize thoughts with the activity steps properly sequenced. This impairment is a component of ideational apraxia, but it can occur separately as the first

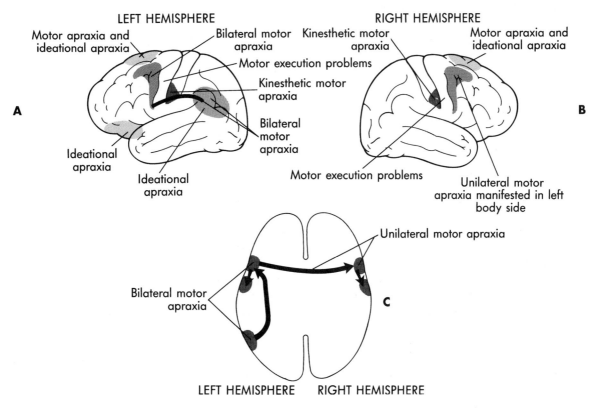

Figure 13-8 Disrupted processing of praxis. **A,** Lateral view of left hemisphere. **B,** Lateral view of right hemisphere. Lesion at praxic sites of left hemisphere, where kinesthetic motor engrams are stored, can produce bilateral motor apraxia, whereas lesion of the praxic sites in right hemisphere, or affecting anterior fibers of corpus callosum, can produce unilateral motor apraxia of left side of body. **C,** Transverse view of praxic areas, including association and commisural fibers believed to be involved in the process. (From Árnadóttir G: *The brain and behavior: assessing cortical dysfunction through activities of daily living*, St Louis, 1990, Mosby.)

indication of an impairment in a progressive disease process or as the remains of ideational problems such as when CVA improves. Perseverations can affect language as well as motor movements. Language perseveration is repetition of speech, including words and phonemes. The patient is unable to shift from one phoneme or word to another. Echolalia is a form of perseveration in which persons echo what they hear.

Dysfunction of Broca's motor speech area in the left hemisphere, resulting in expressive aphasia, is indicated by loss of speech production. Dysfunction of the supplementary motor cortex or cingulate gyrus[17]; disconnection of corpus callosum[9]; or disconnection of the supplementary motor cortex from the reticular activating system in the brain stem may result in mutism,[29] or impaired initiation of speech. The affected person does not speak, although speech function is present.

Other impairments related to dysfunction of cognitive integration and cognitive components accompanying dysfunction of the prefrontal cortex include impaired alertness, lack of attention, distraction, field dependency, memory problems, and disorientation. Impaired alertness is the basic arousal process in which an awake person cannot respond to any stimulus in the environment.[45] Lack of attention is the inability to attend to or focus on a specific stimulus and screen out irrelevant stimuli. The presence of other irrelevant environmental stimuli may result in distraction or diversion of attention. Field dependency comprises an attention component and a perseverative component. In field dependency, inadequate and irrelevant stereotypic actions are not inhibited, and these actions replace selective goal-directed actions corresponding to specific tasks. This behavior includes impulsiveness related to the elementary orienting reflex.[34] Lack of initiation, whereby a person cannot initiate performance of an activity despite the need to perform, may be present as may memory problems. Memory problems are related in particular to lack of registration and temporary storage of information received by the different memory modalities. This short-term memory has sometimes been referred to as working memory,[5] or the time needed to keep different aspects in mind while working on different memory tasks such as reasoning, comprehension, and learning.

Confabulations—unconscious fabrications of stories or excuses to fill memory gaps—may accompany impaired memory if a dysfunction of the frontal lobes is present. The confabulations may lie within the limits of reality; if they do not the falsehood is easily identified. Confabulations are also associated with poor judgment and lack of inhibitions.

Disorientation may accompany frontal lobe dysfunction. It is a specific memory problem involving the inability to give personal information regarding self, disability, hospital stay, or time of day despite intact language. Disoriented individuals understand the context of the situation but cannot remember details (e.g., date, name of hospital). Confusion is a more profound impairment than disorientation. It is a cognitive problem rather than just a memory problem. Confusion is the lack of ability to think clearly, which results in disturbed awareness and orientation with regard to time, place, and person. Interpretation of the external environment is impaired and responses may be slow. The affected person is severely disoriented and does not understand the context of the external environment.

Difficulties related to altered or reduced motivation, impaired judgment, lack of insight, and lack of abstractions or concrete thoughts may also result from dysfunction of cognitive integration and cognitive components processed by the prefrontal cortex. Lack of judgment is the inability to make realistic decisions based on environmental information. When judgment is impaired, the affected individual cannot make use of feedback from errors. Lack of judgment includes lack of safety considerations during performance, as well as socially unacceptable behavior. Lack of insight is related to lack of judgment, with specific reference to lack of insight into personal condition and disability and their effects on performance of daily life tasks. Lack of abstractions can result in concrete thinking, or inflexible thinking. The affected individual is unable to use internal speech to generalize information from situations. This style of thinking is the opposite of abstract thinking on a continuum of thinking.

Emotional and affective disturbances can also be related to frontal lobe dysfunction. These disturbances include depression, apathy, lability, euphoria, frustration, restlessness, irritability, and aggression. Depression has been conceptually defined as an affective disorder manifested as sadness, hopelessness, or loss of general interest in usual performance. It may be accompanied by loss of appetite, loss of energy, sleeping disorders, and feelings of worthlessness. Apathy comprises shallow affect, psychomotor slowing, blunted emotional response, lack of interest in the environment, and inaction. Lability is pathologic emotional instability appearing as alternating states of gaiety and sadness, including inappropriate crying. Euphoria is inappropriately elevated mood or a feeling of subjective well-being accompanied by self-confidence. Frustration is agitation and intolerance in behavior that may be manifested emotionally, verbally, or physically. Restlessness is uneasiness, impatience, and inability to relax. Aggression is defined as angry and destructive ideas or behaviors that are intended to be physically or emotionally injurious. Such behaviors are aimed at domination. Aggression may be manifested as hostility and attacking, destructive behavior. Irritability is excessive sensitivity to stimulation, manifested as quick excitability and displayed as annoyance, impatience, or anger. Table 13-2 includes definitions of impairments or dysfunction of performance components and relates these to different cerebral lobes.

Text continued on p. 307.

Table 13-2

Cortical Impairments as Related to Anatomic Location and Definitions of Terms*

IMPAIRMENT AND CORTICAL LOCATION	CONCEPTUAL DEFINITION	OPERATIONAL DEFINITION
Aggression		
Prefrontal cortex, hypothalamus, medial forebrain bundle	Angry, destructive ideas or behaviors intended to be physically or emotionally injurious and aimed at domination; may be manifested as hostility and attacking and destructive behavior	Shows hostility or aggression towards activity or people; may throw things at therapist when therapist tries to encourage performance
Impaired alertness		
Prefrontal cortex, particularly orbitofrontal area; reticular formation	A basic arousal process "in which the awake person is unable to respond to any stimulus in the environment"[45]	Is more or less unaware of what is going on in surrounding environment
Anomia		
Auditory association cortex on the lateral side of the left temporal lobe	Loss of the ability to name objects or retrieve names of people; fluent speech	Has difficulty finding names of objects
Anosognosia		
Right inferior parietal lobule; specific sensory thalamic nuclei, reticular formation, basal ganglia; prefrontal and premotor frontal lobe[44]	Denial or lack of awareness of a paretic extremity accompanied by lack of insight with regard to the paralysis; paralyzed extremities may be referred to as objects or perceived out of proportion to other body parts	Does not identify a paralyzed body part as own—may deny it completely as a separate object or recognize it and reject it (e.g., patient may complain about "somebody's" arm and not recognize it as own)
Apathy		
Prefrontal cortex; posterior internal capsule, basal ganglia[44]; medial forebrain bundle and reticular formation	Shallow affect, psychomotor slowing, blunted emotional responses, lack of interest in the environment and inaction	Has a lack of emotion or feeling during activity performance and communication; lack of interest in things that are generally found exciting; indifference during performance
Astereognosis		
Superior parietal lobule	Sometimes referred to as *tactile agnosia*; failure to recognize objects, forms, size and shape of objects by touch alone; includes failure of shape discrimination, texture, size, and weight. Refers to a failure of somesthetic recognition (tactile and proprioceptive), although somesthetic reception of tactile and proprioceptive stimuli is still intact	Needs to observe performance to accomplish dressing activity; unable to button shirt unless compensating by observing performance; if in doubt, should be checked by having patient recognize objects of different shapes, size and texture with eyes closed (e.g., coins, ring, pen)
Impaired attention		
Prefrontal cortex, thalamus, reticular formation	Inability to attend to or focus on a specific stimulus; possible distraction from presence of other irrelevant environmental stimuli; inability to screen out irrelevant stimuli	Does not continue an activity; does not attend to instruction or activity; does not attend to mistakes; may focus attention on irrelevant details and not on global environment

Courtesy G. Árnadóttir, Reykjavík, Iceland.
*Conceptual definitions of some common impairments seen in individuals with CVA and examples of operational definitions from the A-ONE instrument. Relation of impairments to dysfunctional CNS areas is simplified.

Continued

Table 13-2

Cortical Impairments as Related to Anatomic Location and Definitions of Terms—cont'd

IMPAIRMENT AND CORTICAL LOCATION	CONCEPTUAL DEFINITION	OPERATIONAL DEFINITION
Broca's aphasia/expressive aphasia		
Premotor area of left frontal lobe	Dysfunction of Broca's motor speech area, resulting in expressive aphasia indicated by a loss of speech production; used in the A-ONE as a synonym for expressive aphasia	Has total expressive aphasia or nonfluent speech; is unable to express self verbally
Concrete thinking (lack of abstract thinking)		
Prefrontal cortex	Inflexible thinking; cannot use internal speech to generalize from similarities among situations; opposite of abstract thinking on a linear continuum of thinking	Is unable to generalize from one situation to another; may ask what time it is while eating breakfast; cannot think of simple solutions that require some thought (e.g., calculations); unable to gain abstract meaning of proverbs
Confabulations		
Prefrontal cortex	Unconscious fabrication of stories or excuses to fill in memory gaps; may be within limits of reality or patient may not consider rules of reality and will then be easily identified; associated with lack of inhibitions and lack of judgment, as well as memory problems	Does not remember what happened during weekend and comes up with an explanation that does not have ground in reality
Confusion		
Prefrontal and diffuse dysfunction—bilateral; thalamus and reticular formation	Lack of ability to think clearly, resulting in disturbed awareness and orientation in regard to time, place, and person; impaired interpretation of external environment and slowed responses to verbal stimuli[19]; cognitive disturbance	Talks about past as present; talks out of context; is not oriented to time and place
Depression		
Left frontal lobe and left basal ganglia, right frontal and right parietal lobes[44]	Affective disorder manifested as sadness, hopelessness, or loss of general interest in usual performance; may be accompanied by loss of appetite, loss of energy, sleeping disorders, and feelings of worthlessness	Has sad affect or expression during activity performance
Disorientation		
Limbic system and limbic cortex in medial temporal lobe and prefrontal cortex	Inability to give personal information regarding self, disability, hospital stay, or time of day, without language problems; relates to specific memory problems	Has an inability to give exact information regarding date (day, month, year) and time of day; may not be able to name institution but knows context of situation (i.e., that current environment is an institution); may not be able to name therapist but knows that therapist belongs to staff
Distractibility		
Prefrontal cortex, reticular formation	Diversion of attention	Becomes distracted by environmental stimuli such as conversation in next room or somebody entering the room; (Note two components of field dependency—distraction and perseveration)

Table 13-2

Cortical Impairments as Related to Anatomic Location and Definitions of Terms—cont'd

IMPAIRMENT AND CORTICAL LOCATION	CONCEPTUAL DEFINITION	OPERATIONAL DEFINITION
Dysarthria		
Primary motor cortex in frontal lobe, primary sensory cortex in parietal lobe and cerebellum	Weakness or altered neuronal control of muscles responsible for speech production, or defective sensory feedback about movement of those muscles	Has problems with articulation of speech musculature; has slurred speech
Echolalia		
Prefrontal cortex	A form of perseveration; echoing back what is heard	Repeats what is heard: Patient asked, "Can you comb your hair?" Patient replies, "Can you comb your hair?"
Field dependency		
Prefrontal cortex	Uninhibited inadequate and irrelevant stereotypic actions that replace selective goal-directed actions corresponding to specific tasks; impulsiveness related to elementary orienting reflex[34]; field dependency thus has both a dysfunction of an attention component and perseverative component	Becomes distracted from particular task performance by specific stimuli (e.g., is washing hands, suddenly sees denture brush, and incorporates it into the hand-washing activity by scrubbing the hands with the denture brush)
Frustration		
Prefrontal cortex, hypothalamus	An appearance of agitation and intolerance in behavior that may be manifested emotionally, verbally, or physically	Becomes exited or intolerant when trying hard to perform or unable to perform (may be manifested emotionally, verbally, or physically)
Homonymous hemianopsia		
Primary visual cortex around calcarine fissure in either hemisphere	Loss of a visual hemifield contralateral to a cerebral lesion	Has visual field defect to visual field that is contralateral to a cerebral lesion; is aware of deficit and tries to compensate for it by using head movements to scan both visual fields
Ideational apraxia		
Prefrontal and premotor cortex in either hemisphere, left inferior parietal lobule and corpus callosum	A breakdown of knowledge of knowing what is to be done to perform—results from loss of a neuronal model or a mental representation about the concept required for performance; lack of knowledge regarding object use; also refers to sequencing of activity steps or use of objects in relation to each other; (NOTE: should rule out comprehension difficulties)	Does not know what to do with toothbrush, toothpaste, or shaving cream; uses tools inappropriately (e.g., smears the toothpaste on face); sequences activity steps incorrectly so that there are errors in end result of tasks (e.g., puts socks on top of shoes)
Impaired initiative		
Prefrontal cortex and supplementary motor cortex—predominantly right hemisphere	Inability to initiate performance of an activity when need to perform is present	Sits without initiating an activity; can describe activity performance but displays inertia in initiating it

Continued

Table 13-2

Cortical Impairments as Related to Anatomic Location and Definitions of Terms—cont'd

IMPAIRMENT AND CORTICAL LOCATION	CONCEPTUAL DEFINITION	OPERATIONAL DEFINITION
Decreased insight		
Prefrontal cortex	Insight—a discovery stage, with increasing awareness of the whole self; decreased insight—lack of insight into personal condition and disability	Does not have insight into disease or disability; does not make realistic statement regarding future plans; makes unrealistic comments regarding disability
Irritability		
Prefrontal cortex—particularly orbitofrontal cortex and hypothalamus	Excessive sensitivity to stimulation; includes quick excitability manifested as annoyance, impatience, or anger	Appears annoyed; may verbally indicate dislike or be physically agitated out of proportion to stimulus that evoked behavior
Jargon aphasia		
Left auditory association cortex in left temporal lobe	Language disorder manifested as fluent speech output that cannot be understood by others because the sequences necessary for intelligible speech phonemes are not available—results from a failure of comprehension because person receives no feedback about own speech performance	Has fluent but unintelligible speech
Impaired judgment		
Prefrontal cortex	Inability to make realistic decisions based on environmental information; unable to make use of feedback from own errors	Does not turn off water taps after washing; does not put brakes on wheelchair and makes unsafe transfers; goes to dining room without dressing or combing hair; does not care whether clothes are turned inside out or back to front, even when those facts have been pointed out
Lability		
Prefrontal cortex	Pathologic emotional instability; alternating states of gladness and sadness, including inappropriate crying	Has mood swings; cries or laughs inappropriately
Long-term memory loss		
Hippocampus of limbic system connected to parahippocampus of medial sides of temporal lobes by dentate gyrus; thalamus, corpus callosum	Lack of storage, consolidation and retention of information that has passed through working memory by way of different sensory networks in a permanent form, as well as the ability to retrieve this information	Demonstrates failure in retrieving information that was processed before onset of disability and information that should have been mobilized from working to long-term memory after disability occurred
Impaired motivation		
Prefrontal cortex—particularly orbitofrontal cortex, medial forebrain bundle, and hypothalamus	Lack of willingness to perform, with or without a perceived need	Does not initiate or continue an activity unless really accepting the need, although physical ability to perform is present (e.g., does not attempt to eat at mealtimes and may refuse to participate in activity); refuses to get up in morning or perform activities although physically able to perform and has previously been motivated to perform by same activities

Cortical Impairments as Related to Anatomic Location and Definitions of Terms—cont'd

IMPAIRMENT AND CORTICAL LOCATION	CONCEPTUAL DEFINITION	OPERATIONAL DEFINITION
Motor apraxia		
Premotor frontal cortex of either hemisphere, left inferior parietal lobe, corpus callosum, basal ganglia, and thalamus	Loss of access to kinesthetic memory patterns so that purposeful movement cannot be achieved because of defective planning and sequencing of movements, even though idea and the purpose of task is understood; used as a synonym for *ideomotor apraxia*	Has difficulties related to motor planning (e.g., cannot sequence and plan movements necessary to adjust grasp on a hairbrush when moving it from one side of head to other to turn the bristles toward hair)
Impaired motor function		
Primary motor cortex, anterior internal capsule, basal ganglia, thalamus, and cerebellum	Flaccidity, decreased strength, rigidity, spasticity, ataxia, athetosis, tremor	Has difficulty stabilizing objects such as containers that must be opened; has difficulty reaching unaffected axilla when washing; has difficulty dressing because of a paralyzed arm or inability to button because of tremor
Mutism		
Supplementary frontal cortex, cingulate gyrus, reticular formation	Impaired initiation of speech; lack of speech although speech function present	Does not attempt to speak or communicate
Impaired organization and sequencing		
Prefrontal cortex	Inability to organize thoughts with activity steps properly sequenced; (component of ideational apraxia but can occur separately as the first indication of impairment in a progressive disease process or last step of regressing ideational problems)	Has difficulties sequencing and timing steps of an activity; does not complete one activity step before starting another (e.g., does not take off glasses before taking off a T-shirt with a tight neck hole; puts on shoes before putting on the trousers; washes too quickly, resulting in poor performance)
Paraphasia		
Prefrontal cortex or left lateral temporal lobe	Expressive speech defect characterized by misuse or replacement of words or phonemes during active speech	Replaces words with incorrect similar or dissimilar words (e.g., may identify an apple as an orange because both are fruits)
Perseveration		
Premotor and/or prefrontal cortex	Repeated movements or acts during functional performance as a result of difficulty in shifting from one response pattern to another; refers inertia on initiation or termination of performance; *prefrontal* perseveration—repetition of whole actions or action components; *premotor* perseveration—compulsive repetition of the same movement	Repeats movements or acts and cannot stop them once initiated (e.g., attempts to put on shirt without any progress—may pull a long sleeve up arm past wrist [premotor perseveration]; moves comb toward mouth instead of hair after having brushed teeth [prefrontal perseveration])
Restlessness		
Prefrontal cortex	Uneasiness, impatience, inability to relax	May be impatient (e.g., cannot wait for therapist to start an activity); may have trouble staying in one place during activity

Continued

Table 13-2

Cortical Impairments as Related to Anatomic Location and Definitions of Terms—cont'd

IMPAIRMENT AND CORTICAL LOCATION	CONCEPTUAL DEFINITION	OPERATIONAL DEFINITION
Right-left discrimination impairment		
Right inferior parietal lobule; could also be left temporal or parietal lobe dysfunction	Inability to discriminate between right and left body sides or to apply the concepts of left and right to the external environment; includes an inability to understand and use concepts of left and right; comprises several factors, including a verbal component, a nonverbal component of tactile sensory discrimination and stimuli location, and spatial relations and visuospatial components[43,53]	Does not discriminate between left and right side of body on verbal command
Short-term memory loss		
Limbic system and limbic association cortex in orbitofrontal areas or temporal lobes	Lack of registration and temporary storing of information received by different sensory memory modalities, be it somatosensory, auditory or visual; refers to working memory in that a person must keep different aspects in mind while working on different memory tasks such as reasoning, comprehension, and learning; length of working or short-term memory dependent on nature of assignments	Does not remember instructions throughout evaluation; may have to be reminded to comb hair several times
Somatoagnosia		
Right inferior parietal lobule	Disorder of body scheme; diminished awareness of body structure and failure to recognize own body parts and their relationship to each other[43]; difficulty relating own body to objects in external environment	Puts legs into armholes or arms into legholes; brushes mirror image of teeth instead of own teeth or washes mirror image of face instead of own face
Somesthetic sensory loss		
Postcentral gyrus in either parietal lobes, posterior internal capsule, specific thalamic sensory nuclei	Loss of tactile sensation, proprioception, or kinesthesia	Has difficulty manipulating objects because of lack of sensation; is aware of sensory loss and tries to compensate (e.g., using visual clues)
Spatial relations impairment		
Usually right inferior parietal lobule	Difficulty relating objects to each other or to the self; synonymous with *visuospatial agnosia* when such difficulties are due to visuospatial impairment	Is unable to find armholes, legholes, or bottom of shirt; pulls sleeve in wrong direction; overestimates or underestimates distances when reaching for objects
Topographic disorientation		
Inferior parietal lobule or occipital association cortex	Difficulty finding way in space as a result of amnestic or agnostic problems; manifested as problems finding way in familiar surroundings or learning new routes	Does not know way to bedroom or bathroom

Table 13-2

Cortical Impairments as Related to Anatomic Location and Definitions of Terms—cont'd

IMPAIRMENT AND CORTICAL LOCATION	CONCEPTUAL DEFINITION	OPERATIONAL DEFINITION
Unilateral body neglect		
Inferior parietal lobule, right cingulate gyrus, prefrontal cortex, reticular formation, specific sensory thalamic nuclei, posterior internal capsule	Failure to report, respond, or orient to a unilateral stimulus presented to body side contralateral to a cerebral lesion; can be a result of defective sensory processing or attention deficit, resulting in ignorance or impaired use of extremities; (used as a synonym for unilateral body inattention); usually affects left side of body	Does not dress affected body side; does not pull shirt all the way down on affected side; gets shirt stuck on affected shoulder—does not try to correct it or does not realize what is wrong
Unilateral spatial neglect		
Inferior parietal lobule, right cingulate gyrus, prefrontal cortex, reticular formation, specific sensory thalamic nuclei, posterior internal capsule	Inattention to or neglect of visual stimuli presented in extrapersonal space of side contralateral to a cerebral lesion as a result of visual perceptual deficits or impaired attention[28]; it may occur independently of visual deficits or with hemianopsia[43]; (synonymous with unilateral visual neglect)	Does not account for objects in visual field on affected side—usually left side; when moving, runs into furniture, doorways, or walls located in affected visual field
Visual object agnosia		
Visual association cortex, left or bilateral and posterior corpus callosum	Inability to recognize, name, or demonstrate use of objects seen, resulting from distorted visual perception regardless of visual acuity[43,45]; can see and describe components of object but cannot recognize object itself	Does not identify objects in either visual field on verbal command but can if allowed to touch them; may not be able to recognize a razor but can describe it as a T shape; is not able to explain its use either, but recognizes it when allowed to touch it
Wernicke's aphasia/sensory aphasia/receptive aphasia		
Auditory association cortex in left lateral temporal lobe	Deficit in auditory comprehension of language; may affect semantic speech performance (manifested as paraphasia or nonsensical syllables because auditory feedback is impaired)[8,25]; impaired repetitions	Has difficulty comprehending spoken language; does not understand one- or two-word commands; does not perform according to verbal instruction; may have problems obtaining meaning from complex language (e.g., prepositions)

Parietal Lobe Dysfunction

The parietal lobes process somatosensory and complex sensory information from multimodal stimuli. When a dysfunction of the parietal lobes occurs, impairments related to different functional areas may develop if the sensorimotor component is affected. Dysfunction of the primary sensory cortex in the postcentral gyrus results in impaired sensory reception of somesthetic stimuli from the contralateral body side (i.e., tactile, proprioceptive, and kinesthetic information). If a dysfunction affects the superior parietal lobule, recognition of stimuli received in the postcentral gyrus is affected, resulting in tactile agnosia, or astereognosis. Astereognosis has been conceptually defined as a failure to recognize objects, as well as form, size, and shape of the objects, by touch alone. It includes failure to discriminate shapes, texture, size, and weight. Two-point discrimination and sharp-dull discrimination are also impaired.[3]

A dysfunction of the inferior parietal lobe, which processes information from the secondary association areas of all three posterior lobes may lead to impairments related to perceptual and motor processing of sensorimotor components. These impairments include motor and ideational apraxia, if the left inferior parietal lobe is involved, because the visuokinesthetic motor engrams are stored in this area. Spatial relations disorders may also be present. These disorders have been conceptually defined as difficulties in relating objects to each other or to the self. Such difficulties may include difficulties with foreground and background perception, depth and distance perception, perception of form constancy, perception of position in space, or constructional apraxia.[3]

Body scheme disorders and agnosias may be present. Body scheme disorders are perceptual deficits people have regarding their own postural model, including defective perception of body position, such as the relationship of body parts to each other.[43] Agnosia is an impaired ability to recognize the significance of and to differentiate among sensory stimuli. In the inferior parietal lobe, agnosia involves stimuli of more than one type of sensory input. Body scheme disorders and agnosia related to dysfunction of this area of cortex, usually the right hemisphere, include unilateral body neglect, somatoagnosia, left-right discrimination problems, and anosognosia (a person's denial of a paretic extremity as own).

Unilateral body neglect is the failure to report, respond, or orient to a unilateral stimulus presented to the body side contralateral to a cerebral lesion. This type of neglect can result from defective sensory processing or attention deficit, resulting in ignorance or impaired use of the extremities. The literature frequently refers to two terms: unilateral body neglect (often including paralysis); and unilateral body inattention. Use of the term "unilateral body neglect" carries a connotation of greater severity. Because the right hemisphere is superior in terms of attention and the left hemisphere cannot compensate for lack of attention to the left body side or visual field, unilateral body neglect and unilateral visual neglect usually occur toward the left side.[3,28]

Somatoagnosia, another disorder of body scheme, is defined as diminished awareness of body structure and the failure to recognize one's body parts and their relationship to each other.[43] Individuals with this disorder also have difficulty relating their bodies to objects in the external environment. This impairment usually results from a severe cortical dysfunction and is accompanied by ideational apraxia and spatial relation disorder.[3] Right-left discrimination impairment is the inability to discriminate between the right and left sides of the body or apply the concepts of left and right to the external environment. The impairment includes the inability to understand and use the concepts of the left and right. It comprises several factors, including a verbal component, a nonverbal component of tactile and sensory discrimination and stimuli location, and components of spatial relations and visuospatial components.[43,53] Dysfunction of other posterior lobes may also contribute to this impairment. Anosognosia is a person's denial of a paretic extremity, accompanied by lack of insight with regard to the paralysis. The paralyzed extremity may be referred to as an object or perceived as being out of proportion to other body parts.

Other perceptual impairments related to the inferior part of the parietal lobe include unilateral visual neglect,

topographical disorientation, and some forms of agraphia, alexia, and acalculia. Unilateral spatial neglect, also referred to as *unilateral visual neglect*, is defined as inattention to or neglect of visual stimuli presented in the extrapersonal space of the side contralateral to a cerebral lesion. This dysfunction results from visual perceptual deficits or impaired attention.[28] It may occur independently of visual deficits or with hemianopsia.[43] Unilateral visual neglect and unilateral visual inattention are sometimes treated as synonyms in the literature or as indicating different levels of severity.

Topographic disorientation results from amnestic or agnostic problems. The affected person has trouble finding the way in familiar surroundings or learning new routes.

Alexia is the inability to read or comprehend written language as a result of brain damage. It can be related to dysfunction of language, as well as to visual processes.[24,45]

Agraphia is an acquired writing disturbance.[45] According to Friedman et al,[24] it refers specifically to language errors, not to motor errors in letter formation or poor handwriting.

Acalculia is difficulty solving mathematic problems. It can be produced by spatial relation disorders, alexia, or number agraphia (impaired calculation).[32]

Occipital Lobe Dysfunction
The occipital lobe houses primary and secondary processing areas for visual information. The tertiary area for visual processing is located mainly in the inferior parietal lobe. If a dysfunction of the occipital lobe occurs, impairments are related to visual sensory components and perception of visual information. If there is a unilateral dysfunction of the primary visual cortex, located around the calcarine fissure on the medial side of the hemispheres, homonymous visual loss in the contralateral visual field—also referred to as *hemianopsia*—will result. Lesions of the association area cause visual agnosia. There are different types of visual agnosias, including visual object agnosia; visuospatial agnosia, which is a spatial relations disorder of visual origin; prosopagnosia; color agnosia; and associative visual agnosia.[3] Visual object agnosia is the inability of a patient to recognize, name, or demonstrate use of objects seen. It results from distorted visual perception, regardless of visual acuity.[43,45] The affected person can see and describe the components of the object but cannot recognize the object itself. Prosopagnosia is the inability to recognize familiar faces and color agnosia the inability to recognize colors. In patients with adequate visual perception, associative visual agnosia occurs when the visual cortex has been disconnected from the language areas of the temporal lobe. Clinically the object can be recognized and its use demonstrated, but it cannot be identified by name.

Temporal Lobe Dysfunction
The temporal lobes are involved with two types of processing: auditory and limbic. The lateral sides of the hemi-

spheres house primary and secondary processing sites for auditory stimuli and perception of such information. The tertiary processing area for these functions is located in the inferior part of the parietal lobe. A lesion of the primary auditory cortex in either hemisphere does not produce a readily detectable hearing impairment, although hearing acuity is affected, because reception from both ears is received bilaterally in the cortex.[6] A lesion of the auditory association cortex in the left temporal lobe results in Wernicke's aphasia, also termed receptive or sensory aphasia. This disorder has been defined as a deficit in the comprehension of language. Auditory feedback is affected; therefore semantic speech may be impaired, as well as repetitions.[8,25] Jargon aphasia may be associated with Wernicke's aphasia. It is a language disorder manifested in speech output that cannot be understood by others because the sequences necessary for intelligible speech phonemes are not available. Jargon aphasia results from a failure in comprehension; the affected person receives no feedback about the speech performance. A lesion of the auditory association cortex in the left hemisphere can also cause anomia because the memory stores for nouns are located in this area. Anomia is loss of the ability to name objects or retrieve names of people; the person does have fluent speech. Agraphia and acalculia may also be related to temporal lobe disorder. A lesion of the superior temporal gyrus of the right hemisphere results in a different type of auditory agnosia than the receptive aphasia of the left hemisphere. Comprehension of nonverbal sounds such as music is impaired, as well as of tonal sequences, timing of sounds, and sound modulation.[7,31]

Lesions of the limbic association cortex of the medial sides of the temporal lobes and temporal pole can cause disturbances of cognitive integration and cognitive components. These disturbances include impaired long-term memory and learning. Long-term memory disorder is lack of storage, consolidation, and retention of information that has passed through working memory by way of different sensory networks in a permanent form, as well as the ability to retrieve this information. Long-term memory is not modality specific. Emotional disorders may also be present. The right hemisphere has a dominant influence on reception and expression of emotions.[11] Table 13-2 relates defined impairments to dysfunction of different cortical and subcortical areas.

Operational Definitions of Concepts: Manifestation of Neurobehavioral Impairments During Task Performance

Operational definitions are how concepts are measured and observed. Following is a review based on Árnadóttir's[3] operational definitions of terms from the A-ONE regarding how neurobehavioral impairments can be detected during task performance in the areas of grooming and hygiene, dressing, functional mobility, eating, and functional

communication. Each of these performance areas comprises several tasks. For successful completion of each of the tasks, involvement of several performance components is necessary. Dysfunction of performance components resulting in the previously defined impairments is manifested differently during performance. The following examples indicate the impact of different impairments on task performance in the various performance areas (see Table 13-2 for conceptual and operational definitions of terms). Some impairments affect specific ADL areas. Other impairments are more pervasive and may appear in any performance area or may need to be addressed specifically. It must be kept in mind that behavior is flexible and neurobehavioral impairments are complex. Some have similar components—such as the impairments of unilateral body neglect and unilateral spatial neglect, which both include attention to stimuli—and may be manifested similarly. For others the anatomic neuronal networks lie close together. The following behavioral examples are guidelines for detecting impairments. However, they cannot be taken for granted without knowledge of neurobehavior, cortical function, activity analysis, and clinical reasoning because similar behaviors may be a result of different impairments at times. Thus the behavior of not washing one arm during the task of washing the upper part of the body may be caused by unilateral body neglect when it occurs in an individual with right hemisphere dysfunction. However, an individual with left hemisphere dysfunction may need assistance to wash the affected arm, partly because of motor paralysis, and may also need guidance to wash the other arm and body parts because of ideation problems and difficulty in organizing and sequencing the activity steps of the task. The patient may also have comprehension difficulties, which complicates the situation. The behavior of not washing an arm may therefore be a result of unilateral body neglect or ideational apraxia, depending on the situation. Therefore the following samples are to be used only as guidelines. Clinical reasoning and knowledge of neurobehavioral impairments and how the impairments group together in different diagnostic categories are crucial for effective differentiation and classification of impairments.

Hygiene and Grooming Performance Area

The performance area of grooming and hygiene comprises several tasks—for example, washing the face and body and bathing or showering; performing oral hygiene (including brushing teeth); combing hair; shaving; applying cosmetics, deodorants, or perfumes; performing toilet hygiene; and managing any aids or devices required for successful activity performance. These tasks may be affected by dysfunction of different performance components, resulting in various behavioral outcomes. Dysfunction of the sensorimotor components can result in paralysis, muscle weakness, and spasticity. Motor apraxia, perseverations, impaired tactile and proprioceptive sensation, astereognosis, or hemianopsia with a loss of a visual field or a loss of part of a visual field may be present.

Paralysis or muscle weakness may be manifested as difficulty in washing the affected arm or axilla (Figure 13-9, A). The individual may need to learn to use one-handed techniques to overcome the impairment. Adapted equipment may also be needed for the individual to reach body parts such as the back or, if balance is poor, the feet. Stabilizing objects may be a problem; the individual may need a nonslip pad under the soap. While brushing the teeth the person may have problems opening the tube of toothpaste and may need to learn to compensate by stabilizing it between the knees or teeth. The same applies to other containers and opening of lids. If the individual uses dentures, an adapted toothbrush or a suction brush for stabilization may be necessary (see Chapter 22).

Problems with tactile sensation, proprioception, or stereognosis affect object manipulation. An individual with such problems who does not suffer from inattention or neglect will be aware of the impairment and attempt to compensate for it (e.g., by using vision for sensory feedback).

Individuals with motor apraxia will have difficulty with motor planning; they may have difficulty adjusting the grasp of a razor when moving from one side of the face to another or when moving the razor to the chin. This requires sequencing and planning of fine finger and wrist movements so that the razor will be turned toward the face for effective use (see Figure 13-9, B). Similarly, motor apraxia may influence the ability to comb or brush the hair. The performance may be adequate on the side where the individual starts brushing but when moving the brush to the other side of the head or to the back, the individual will have difficulty adjusting the hand movements required to turn the brush toward the hair. Manipulating a toothbrush and other items may be similarly difficult and manifested as "clumsiness."

Premotor perseveration may be manifested as repetition of the movements of washing the face; the individual cannot stop the movements and take the washcloth to other body parts. Prefrontal perseveration is perseveration of whole acts. The affected individual, having completed one task such as brushing the teeth, begins another activity such as combing but perseverates a part of the previous action program. As a result, the individual approaches the mouth with the comb (see Figure 13-9, C)

If a part of a visual field is defective or hemianopsia is present, an individual may have to compensate by turning the head. If an individual only has this impairment and not neglect the individual will be aware of the problem and will be able to describe it, with insight into the dysfunction, and compensate for it.

If a dysfunction of the perceptual processing aspect of the sensorimotor component is present, a spatial relation disorder, difficulty with left-right discrimination, unilateral body inattention or neglect, unilateral visual inatten-

tion or neglect, anosognosia, or somatoagnosia may be expected. Spatial relation disorder may be manifested during hygiene and grooming tasks as difficulty in determining distances. An individual reaching for a toothbrush may overestimate or underestimate its distance. When the individual squeezes toothpaste onto the toothbrush, the paste may end up beside the brush (see Figure 13-9, D). When trying to stabilize objects, the individual may reach next to the object, resulting in ineffective performance. For example, an individual may reach with the washcloth into the space next to the water faucet instead of under the faucet. When manipulating objects such as dentures, the individual may have problems determining the top from the bottom part of the dentures, as well as front from back and left from right.

In unilateral body neglect, or inattention, the individual does not use the affected limb according to available control. For example, the individual may not use the arm for stability while attempting to open a bottle. An individual with unilateral body neglect may not wash the affected side but washes other body parts systematically. The same may apply to other tasks as well, such as shaving and combing, in that the individual only attends to one side of the face or hair. A man holding an aftershave bottle in the left hand while looking at his own face in the mirror and reaching with the right hand to the face may tilt the bottle without noticing it and spill the liquid (see Figure 13-9, E).

In unilateral spatial inattention or neglect, the individual may randomly locate all items in the affected visual field only when accidentally seeing them or may not notice an object at all in the affected visual field and does not systematically compensate for the impairment by rotating the head as required.

An individual with somatoagnosia cannot differentiate between the mirror image and self. An individual thus affected may attempt to wash the mirror image of the face instead of the actual face (see Figure 13-9, F). These individuals may not be able to differentiate between their own body parts and those of others. For example, an individual may grab another person's arm and attempt to use it to hold onto objects. Somatoagnosia is defined in the A-ONE as a severe dysfunction that is usually accompanied by ideational apraxia and often by spatial relation disorders.

Dysfunctions of cognitive integration and cognitive components with an impact on grooming and hygiene tasks include ideational apraxia, organization and sequencing problems related to activity steps, impaired judgment, decreased level of arousal, lack of attention, distraction, field dependency, impaired memory, and impaired intention. Ideational apraxia may appear during grooming and hygiene activities; an individual may not know what to do with the toothbrush, toothpaste, or shaving cream or may use these items inappropriately (e.g., smear toothpaste over the face or spray the shaving cream over the sink (see Figure 13-9, *G*). An individual with organization and sequencing difficulties only may have the general idea of how to perform but may have problems timing and sequencing activity steps. Such a patient may not complete one activity step before starting another or may perform activities too quickly as a result of problems in timing activity steps, resulting in a poor performance.

Lack of judgment may appear as an inability to make realistic decisions based on environmental information, providing that perception of those impulses is adequate. An individual so affected may leave the sink area without turning off the water taps or may leave the wash cloth in the sink, not noticing that the water level is increasing and threatening to overflow (see Figure 13-9, *H*).

Field dependency has both an attention component and a perseverative component. Individuals with this dysfunction may be distracted from performing a particular task by specific stimuli that they are compelled to act on or incorporate into the previous activity. For example, if an individual with field dependency sees a denture brush while washing the hands, the brush may be incorporated into the activity as the individual scrubs the hands with the denture brush.

An individual with short-term memory problems may not remember the sequence of activity steps or instructions throughout activity performance. The therapist may have to remind an individual several times to comb the hair, even though the individual does not have comprehension problems.

Lack of initiation may occur during performance of grooming and hygiene tasks; the individual may sit by the sink without performing, even after being asked to wash. With repeated instructions to begin, the individual may in-

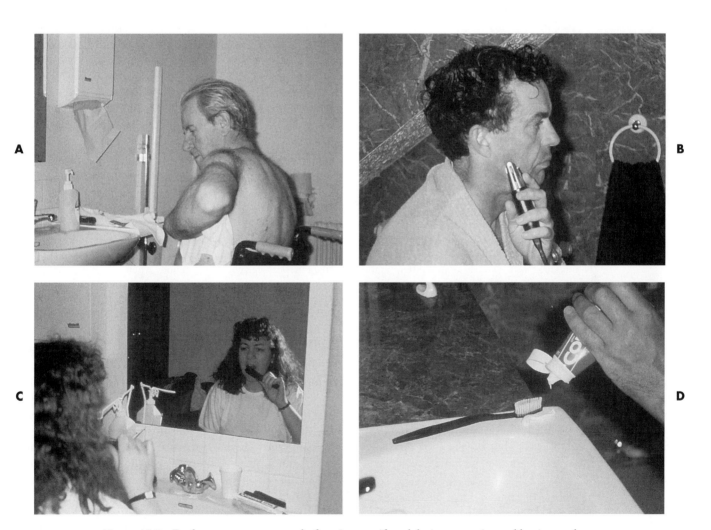

Figure 13-9 Performance component dysfunction manifested during grooming and hygiene tasks. **A,** Paralysis results in difficulty washing the affected axilla. **B,** Motor apraxia makes manipulation of razor difficult. **C,** Prefrontal perseveration—a part from the previous task of brushing the teeth is perseverated during combing, so that the comb is moved toward the mouth instead of the hair. **D,** Spatial relations impairment results in underestimation of distances when the individual attempts to place toothpaste on toothbrush.

Continued

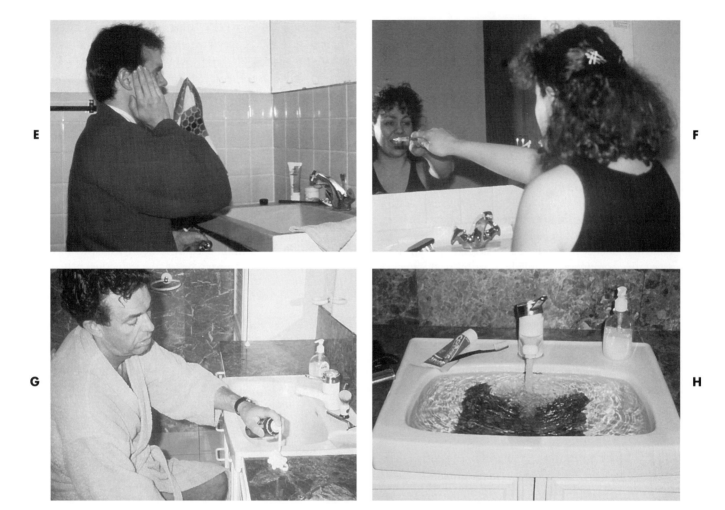

Figure 13-9, cont'd **E,** Unilateral body inattention during shaving. Aftershave lotion is spilled from a bottle held in left hand while individual is reaching with right hand to face and looking into mirror. **F,** Somatoagnosia. Woman cannot differentiate between a mirror image and her own body when brushing her teeth. **G,** Ideational apraxia. Man does not know what to do with shaving cream. **H,** Lack of judgment. Water has been left running with the washcloth in the sink, producing a safety hazard.

dicate that the activity is about to start, yet nothing happens. After several such incidents and if the therapist asks for a plan, the individual may state a detailed plan of action in which the water will be turned on, the washcloth will be picked up and put under the running water, soap will be put on the cloth, and washing will begin. The individual has a plan of action but cannot start the plan. This impairment may be associated with ideational problems as well.

Dressing Performance Area
The dressing performance includes the tasks of dressing the upper part of the body, including putting on items such as underwear, T-shirts, pullovers, sweaters, shirts, bras, cardigans, or dresses; putting on pants, socks, pantyhose, and shoes; and manipulating fasteners, such as zippers, buckles, laces, or Velcro. Following are some exam-

ples of the impact of neurobehavioral impairments on task performance in this area. Dysfunction of sensorimotor components affecting this performance area can result in paralysis of a body side. Individuals with one-sided paralysis must learn one-handed dressing techniques (Figure 13-10, *A*). Premotor perseveration may appear during dressing; the individual is unable to stop movements that have been initiated. For example, when the individual is placing an arm in a sleeve, the individual may keep pulling the arm into the sleeve until the end of the sleeve is up to the elbow or shoulder (see Figure 13-10, *B*).

Defective perceptual processing may result in spatial relation disorders such as difficulty figuring out the front and back, the inside and outside, and the top and bottom of an article of clothing. Although the individual knows that the shirt goes on the upper part of the body and is trying to get the arm through the sleeve, the arm may be

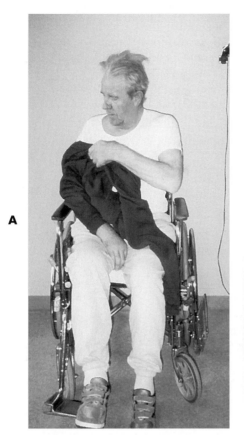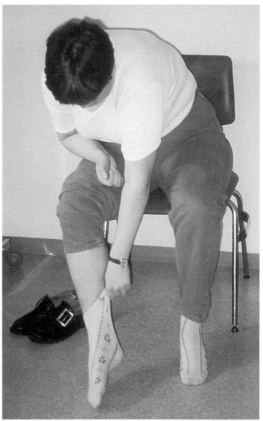

Figure 13-10 Performance component dysfunction manifested during dressing tasks. **A,** Paralysis requires use of one-handed dressing techniques. **B,** Premotor perseveration results in repetitions of movements so that leghole may be pulled up to knee; sock is pulled repeatedly, although it is already in place.   *Continued*

put through the neckhole instead of the sleeve or in the right sleeve instead of the left. An individual may place both legs in the same leghole (see Figure 13-10, *C*) or may not perceive that one of the legholes is turned inside out. Right-left disorientation can be related to visuospatial problems; for example, an individual may put the right shoe on the left foot. An individual with spatial relation disorder may pull the sleeve in the wrong direction when attempting to put on a shirt. The individual may be unable to tie shoelaces because of difficulty handling the spatial relations aspects of manipulating shoestrings. Velcro fastenings on shoes may be folded back on themselves instead of being passed through the D-loop before being folded backward. Somatoagnosia may manifest as a patients attempting to dress a therapist's arm instead of their own (see Figure 13-10, *D*) or when they attempt to place their legs into the armholes of a shirt. Thus they have problems with differentiating their own body from the therapist's body and relating objects to corresponding body parts. This is not only a spatial relation problem as described above, but also a defect in body image. An individual presenting with only a visuospatial problem cannot find the correct armhole but realizes that a shirt is related to the upper body.

This realization is not evident in individuals with somatoagnosia because of their body scheme dysfunction.

Unilateral body neglect may be severe, or less severe unilateral body inattention may be present. In severe cases an individual may not dress or undress the affected arm. The individual may even leave the arm in the armhole when undressing and attempt to hang the shirt on a clothes peg on the wall, not cognizant that the arm is still in the armhole (see Figure 13-10, *E*). However, the problem is not always this severe or apparent. At times the shirt may get stuck on an affected shoulder without the individual noticing it, or it may not be pulled properly down on the affected side. An individual with unilateral visual neglect or inattention may not put on clothes that are placed in the left visual field as they remain unnoticed.

Dysfunction of cognitive integration and cognitive components may be seen as field dependency, ideational problems, or impaired judgment. Field dependency is illustrated by an individual in the middle of the activity of putting on a sweater. Having placed both arms through the correct armholes and the neck through the neckhole, he or she is distracted by the sight of a comb. The activity of dressing is subsequently immediately discontinued as the individual grabs

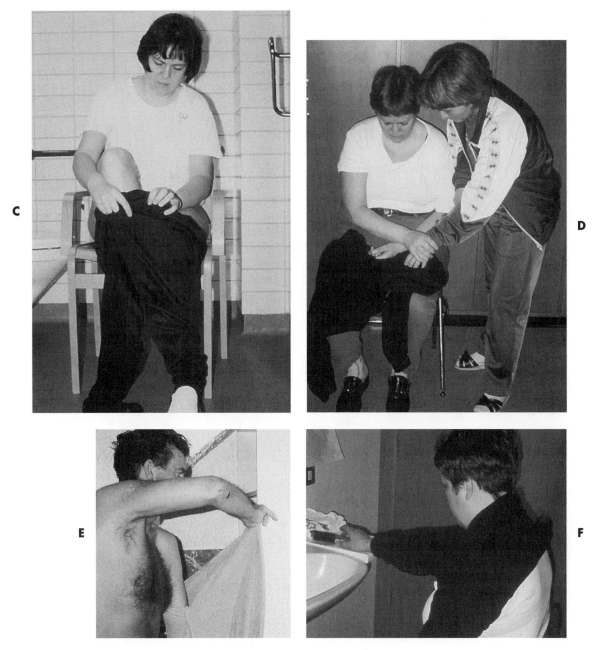

Figure 13-10, cont'd C, Spatial relations impairment, in which both legs are placed in same leghole. **D,** Somatoagnosia. Woman attempts to dress therapist's arm instead of her own. **E,** Unilateral body neglect. Man attempts to hang up his gown without having undressed his left arm. **F,** Field dependency. The sight of a comb distracts a woman in the middle of a dressing task. Dressing is discontinued and the woman begins combing.

the comb and starts combing his or her hair. After combing, the individual may or may not go back to the task of putting on the shirt. (Figure 13-10, *F*). A person might not know what to do with the clothes or how to put them on. A person with ideational apraxia may be able to perform certain activities automatically, such as putting on a sweater. Difficulty arises when the person realizes the t-shirt or undershirt hasn't been put on under the sweater. The individual may not be able to plan the necessary activity steps to correct the

mistake. The t-shirt may get tucked down the neckhole instead of the sweater being removed and the activity started over (see Figure 13-10, *G*). An individual with ideational apraxia may also attempt to put a sock on over a shoe. An individual who only has organization and sequencing problems might put shoes on before putting on trousers (see Figure 13-10, *H*). However, the general ideas of how to put the clothes on and where they fit are intact. Organization and sequencing problems may also appear when an individual

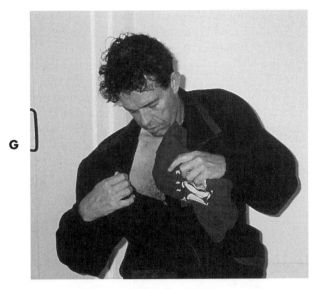
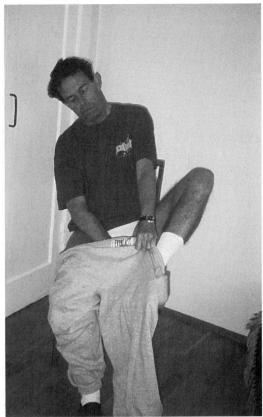

Figure 13-10, cont'd **G,** Ideational apraxia. Man knows that the t-shirt should go under the sweater but does not know how to accomplish the goal. **H,** Organization and sequencing impairment. Man puts on socks and shoes before trousers, resulting in difficulties donning trousers.

dresses the unaffected arm before the affected one and then runs into difficulty dressing the affected arm.

Impaired judgment may also be detected during dressing performance. An individual may be improperly dressed in the hallways or the dining area, indicating a lack of social judgment. Spatial relation disorder may also affect dressing performance. An affected individual may not be able to differentiate the front and the back of the clothes. Trousers may be put on with the front pockets and fastenings turned backward. Because these spatial relations deficits are of visual origin, the affected individual may not be able to identify the mistakes. However, when a therapist points out that the trousers are backwards, an individual with a lack of judgment might comment that it does not matter how the trousers are worn. A subject with intact judgment would attempt to make corrections, ask for assistance, or otherwise indicate a desire to have the performance corrected.

Functional Mobility Performance Area
The performance area of functional mobility includes the tasks of rolling over and sitting up in a bed, transferring to and from a bed, transferring to and from a chair, transferring to and from a toilet, transferring to and from a

bathtub or a shower, and moving from one room to another. The previously defined impairments or performance components dysfunction may interfere with the tasks of this performance area (see Chapter 10). Following are some examples of how these dysfunctions may be manifested.

If a dysfunction of the sensorimotor component, such as paralysis is present, it will affect strength and control of one body side and thus affect mobility and balance. An individual may therefore need assistance with transfers, require a wheelchair or walking aids, or require supervision or personal assistance for mobility (Figure 13-11, *A*). Individuals with premotor perseveration may not be able to stop the movements of wheeling a wheelchair; as a result, they continue wheeling and moving after the desired destination has been reached.

Dysfunctions of perceptual processing may result in spatial relation disorders in which the affected individual may misjudge distances. The individual may park a wheelchair too far from a bed or chair for a transfer. An individual with unilateral body neglect or inattention may not account for the affected body side when moving. Such an individual may hit furniture with the affected arm or walk into obstacles such as doorways. When transferring from the bed to a chair, an individual may only move the unaffected side to the chair, leaving the affected side in bed or off the chair (see Figure 13-11, *B*). An individual with severe neglect may also have the impairment of anosognosia. These individuals may deny that their affected arm or side is a part of themselves. The affected limb may be referred to as an object, or the individuals may claim that someone else's arm is lying in bed with them. One man with anosognosia was heard to comment that he was going to occupational therapy and that he would "need to bring the arm along," because the occupational therapist "always works on the arm." Unilateral spatial neglect or inattention refers to the phenomenon in which the individual does not account for visual stimuli from the affected visual field. The individual may walk or wheel into obstacles such as garbage cans, furniture, doorways, or other individuals (see Figure 13-11, *C*). Topographic disorientation, in which the person has visuospatial problems or memory problems with regard to spatial locations may also be present. The individual does not know the way to different, familiar lo-

cations such as the bathroom, dining room, bedroom or therapy department.

If a dysfunction of the cognitive integration and cognitive components is present, ideational apraxia or organization and sequencing problems may occur during transfers and mobility tasks. Individuals with ideational apraxia may not know how to get into bed. They may literally "throw" themselves into the bed. An individual may not know how to wheel a wheelchair, and repeatedly push down on the armrest (see Figure 13-11, *D*). (However, the therapist should rule out attention problems.) An individual with organization and sequencing problems may sit up in bed without taking off the blanket but will remove the blanket before standing up (see Figure 13-11, *E*). An individual with additional ideational apraxia may, on the other hand, sit up without lifting the blanket off and then attempt to stand up and walk away without moving the blanket, thus producing a safety hazard (see Figure 13-11, *F*). An individual with organization and sequencing problems only may not put on wheelchair brakes before trans-

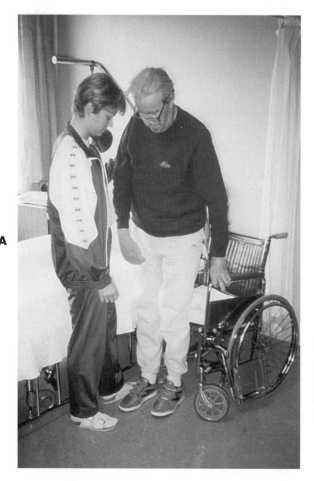

A

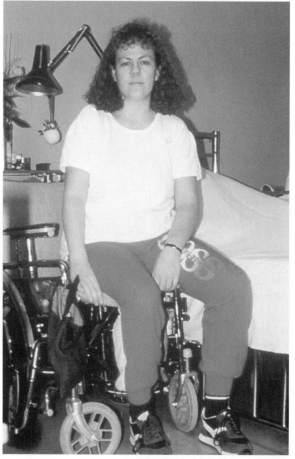

B

Figure 13-11 Performance component dysfunction manifested during functional mobility tasks. **A,** Paralysis affects strength and balance. Individuals require assistance when transferring from bed. A wheelchair is needed for mobility. **B,** Unilateral body neglect. Woman only moves intact body side over to wheelchair and leaves affected side in bed.

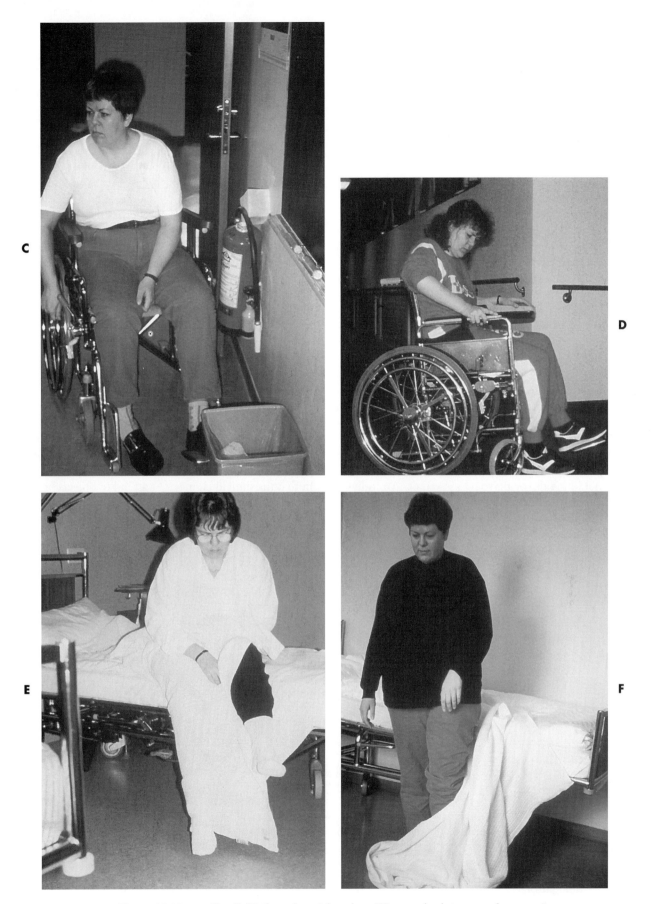

Figure 13-11, cont'd **C,** Unilateral spatial neglect. Woman wheels into a garbage can in a neglected left visual field. **D,** Ideational apraxia. Woman does not know how to propel wheelchair and pushes down on armrest instead of wheel. **E,** Organization and sequencing impairment. Woman does not lift off blanket before sitting up in bed. **F,** Organization and sequencing impairment and ideational apraxia. Woman attempts to walk away from bed without having moved blanket.

ferring or take them off before moving. This particular performance difficulty might occur when memory problems are present as well. If memory problems without impaired judgment are present, the results of the unsafe transfers (e.g., instability) may remind these individuals to lock the brakes.

Eating Performance Area

Dysfunction of eating performance may be affected by neurobehavioral impairments or dysfunction of the previously mentioned performance components. Chewing and swallowing, drinking from a glass or a cup, eating without utensils (only using the fingers), eating with a fork or a spoon, and using a knife to cut or spread may be affected. Many of these tasks are accomplished earlier in the developmental sequence than some of the tasks mentioned previously.

A dysfunction of the sensorimotor component may result in paralysis of one side of the body, resulting in poor sitting balance and use of only one arm. Tactile and proprioceptive sensation in the affected hand and arm may be impaired. All these impairments may affect eating tasks that require sitting balance and bilateral integration of the arms (e.g., stabilizing a slice of bread while buttering it or a slice of meat while cutting it, eating an egg, or peeling an orange). Because of the impairments, these eating tasks may require different performance techniques, helping aids, or personal assistance. An individual with motor apraxia may spill soup when moving the spoon from the bowl to the mouth—a task that requires much significant adjustment of fine finger and wrist

movements to keep the spoon level. Motor apraxia may result in "clumsy movements" when spreading butter, resulting in problems manipulating the knife (Figure 13-12, A). Premotor perseveration is demonstrated when an individual cannot stop the movements of bringing the spoon to the mouth from the bowl after having finished the soup. Another example is the continuation of chewing movements after the food has dissolved in the mouth. Prefrontal perseveration, or perseveration of actions rather than movements (a cognitive component), may manifest when an individual who has finished eating yogurt with a spoon reaches out for the spoon again to use it to get a sip of milk from a glass rather than drink directly from the glass (see Figure 13-12, B).

Dysfunction of perceptual processing affecting eating behavior may result in spatial relation disorders; an individual trying to stabilize a slice of bread to butter it may misjudge distance and grab the plate instead of the bread (see Figure 13-12, C). The individual may also overestimate or underestimate distances and reach beside the cup instead of grabbing the cup. Unilateral body neglect may occur during eating when the individual does not use the hand in a natural relation to its available function. Individuals may start eating bread using the left hand, "forget" that the bread is in the hand, and proceed to eat other items as the hand holding the bread slides off the table (see Figure 13-12, D). Unilateral spatial neglect may manifest in that the individual may not attend to objects or food in the affected visual field. For example, an individual may not notice a fork in the left visual field and attempts to solve the problem by grabbing the next person's fork lo-

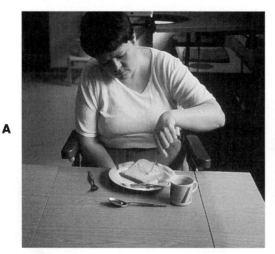

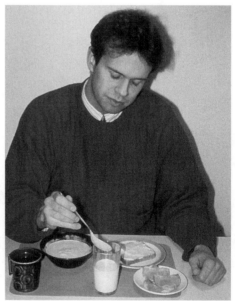

Figure 13-12 Performance component dysfunction manifested during feeding and eating tasks. **A,** Motor apraxia makes manipulation of knife difficult when buttering bread. **B,** Prefrontal perseveration. Man continues to move spoon toward glass instead of drinking from it, after having used the spoon to eat yogurt.

cated by a plate in the right visual field (see Figure 13-12, *E*). Individuals may not eat food located in the affected visual field although they enjoy that particular type of food.

Dysfunction of the cognitive integration and cognitive components may result in ideational apraxia in which the affected individual does not know which utensils to use or how to use them. The individual may simplify the activity by using the fingers to eat meat instead of a fork. Objects may also be misused. An individual may attempt to eat the soup with a knife. Activity steps may be left out of the sequence, resulting in defective performance. An affected individual may not take the shell off an egg before eating it or may not peel an orange before biting it. An individual may have the proper object in hand but may not know how to use it for the situation at hand: the individual may open a teabag, remove the tea leaves, and place them in the cup instead of placing the bag in the cup. Individuals may misuse objects: for example, they may sprinkle salt on the butter container (see Figure 13-12, *F*). Field dependency may be manifested during feeding activities. Individuals may start grabbing food items before having positioned themselves properly at the table. Individuals may also grab items as they are seen, although the items are inappropriate for the activity at hand.

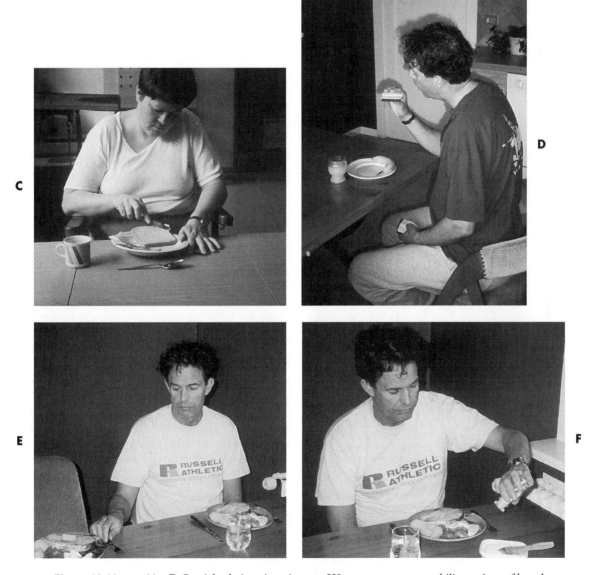

Figure 13-12, cont'd C, Spatial relations impairment. Woman attempts to stabilize a piece of bread but misjudges distances and grabs the side of the plate instead. **D,** Unilateral body neglect. Man does not attend to a piece of bread in left hand; hand slides unnoticed off table, and man grabs another slice with right hand. **E,** Unilateral spatial neglect. Man does not notice fork in his left visual field but solves problem by borrowing a fork from the next plate in the right visual field. **F,** Ideational apraxia. Man does not know what salt is used for and shakes it over butter container.

Functional Communication Performance Area

Functional communication is how the individual expresses needs and understands others' in the social environmental context. It includes, among other things, the ability to talk, comprehend, read, and write. If a dysfunction of sensorimotor components exists in the functional communication performance area, this may result in Broca's or expressive aphasia, in which the individual is not capable of verbal expression or has nonfluent speech. Dysarthria is a problem with articulation of speech musculature. It can be either due to primary motor or sensory involvement, resulting in slurred speech. Premotor perseverations of speech occur when an individual repeats the same words or syllables over and over, unable to shift to other words or syllables. A prefrontal perseveration may be at work when an individual repeats a concept from a previous question: for example, when the individual is asked about numbers, such as the length of the hospital stay, followed by a question regarding which month it is, the answer may be "the thirteenth," indicating a perseveration of the concept of numbers. An individual with auditory processing dysfunction resulting in sensory aphasia or Wernicke's aphasia, also termed receptive aphasia, may have difficulty comprehending spoken language: for example, the individual may not understand one- or two-step instructions, may not perform according to verbal instruction, or may have difficulty obtaining meaning from complex language. When this impairment is accompanied by jargon aphasia, the individual has fluent but unintelligible speech because the individual does not receive auditory feedback about personal performance.

Dysfunction of cognitive integration and cognitive components may present as the memory impairment anomia, in which the individual has fluent speech but has difficulty remembering names. An affected individual may present with paraphasia, in which words are misused or misplaced; this can be a problem with classification of concepts. An individual with paraphasia may use a word from the same group of concepts as the intended term but not the correct word. The individual may call apples oranges or claim to be going to school instead of the clinic. Mutism may occur if intention is affected. This will manifest as lack of an attempt to speak or communicate.

Pervasive Impairments

Some impairments are not necessarily tied to a particular performance area but can occur in relation to any performance area (see Table 13-2). Emotional and affective disturbance, such as apathy, depression, frustration, irritability, aggression, and lack of motivation, may affect task performance in different performance areas. Disorientation, memory disturbance, and the more severe cognitive impairment of confusion may come through during communication. Lack of insight is correlated with lack of judgment. However, it is addressed by specific questions about how the individual perceives his or her impairments

and how these impairments affect performance of daily activities. Memory impairments may involve both working memory, or short-term memory, and long-term memory. Memory disturbances are sometimes accompanied by confabulations (information, which may or may not be based on reality, used to fill in memory gaps). Anything that comes to mind may be expressed because of the individual's lack of inhibitions and lack of judgment regarding the content. The individual who confabulates will believe in what has been said, even though it is not true.

As stated earlier, different impairments have different effects on task performance. The behavioral examples described in this chapter are intended as guidelines to assist therapists in detecting impairments during activity analysis for assessment purposes. This information, used with the appropriate theoretical background and clinical reasoning, is important in determining intervention strategies. Occasionally it may be difficult, particularly for less experienced therapists, to differentiate between impairments with similar behavioral manifestations. Knowledge of neurologic function and of how impairments are grouped in different diagnostic categories may be valuable in such instances.

PATTERNS OF IMPAIRMENTS RESULTING FROM CEREBROVASCULAR ACCIDENTS

In the preceding section, many neurobehavioral impairments were defined and related to different cortical areas. Involvement of dysfunction affecting performance components depends on various pathologic conditions resulting in CVA and the different anatomic areas involved. The cerebral blood supply depends mainly on three arteries in each hemisphere: the middle and anterior cerebral arteries, which are branches of the internal carotid artery; and the posterior cerebral artery, which is a branch of the basilar artery, formed by the union of the vertebral arteries.[3,13,19] Two major types of cerebrovascular dysfunction cause neurologic lesions. These are (1) ischemia, or insufficient blood supply to the brain, which is responsible for 75% to 80% of all strokes; and (2) hemorrhage, or bleeding, due to a ruptured blood vessel, which accounts for the remaining 15% to 20% of strokes.[3,13,52] Hemorrhage results in swelling and compression of brain tissue. There are different subtypes of CVA. Ischemia is subdivided into thrombosis, or blood flow obstruction caused by a local process in one or more blood vessels; embolism, in which blood flow obstruction is caused by materials from distant parts of the vascular system; and decreased systemic perfusion, or hypoperfusion, in which low systemic perfusion pressure results in reduced blood flow.

Hemorrhage is subdivided into subarachnoid hemorrhage, which occurs at the surface of the brain and intracerebral; and intraparenchymal hemorrhage, or bleeding in the cerebral tissue.[3,13] Each type of CVA results in different patterns of impairment. The type of impairment and severity depend mainly on the anatomic location of the lesion.[13] These further depend on the rate of arterial occlusion, adequacy of the collateral circulation, resistance of brain structures to ischemia,[13] duration and severity of ischemia, hematoma size, and underlying mechanism of hypoperfusion,[55] as well as edema.

If the middle cerebral artery is occluded, affecting blood supply to the lateral aspect of the hemisphere, the impairments will vary depending on which of the artery's branches and which hemisphere is affected. If the insult affects the upper trunk of the middle cerebral artery, which supplies the lateral aspects of the frontal and parietal lobes, hemiplegia is to be expected on the contralateral body side, especially of the face and arm; and hemisensory loss, including both tactile and proprioceptive information. This type of insult may also cause impairment of a visual field to the opposite site of the lesion. If the right hemisphere is impaired, unilateral neglect of space and body may result, as well as attention deficits, including unilateral body inattention and unilateral spatial inattention, anosognosia, spatial relation dysfunction, unilateral motor apraxia of the left side (if not paralyzed), lack of judgment, lack of insight, field dependency, and organization of behavior and activity steps. Emotional disturbances such as apathy, lability, and depression may also be present. If the left hemisphere is involved, speech and language functions may be impaired, and bilateral motor apraxia may be present. Ideational apraxia and perseverations may also be present. Emotional disturbances such as depression and frustration may be present. If the lower trunk of the middle cerebral artery is affected, visual field defect of the contralateral visual field, Wernicke's aphasia due to involvement of the left hemisphere, and emotional disturbances may be present.[3,13]

If the anterior cerebral artery, which supplies the medial and superior aspects of the frontal and parietal lobes, is occluded, the paralysis and sensory loss will be greatest in the foot. Unilateral apraxia may result from dysfunction of the anterior part of the corpus callosum. Speech disturbance, or inertia of speech in a form of mutism, can be related to dysfunction of the supplementary motor area. Bilateral involvement of the anterior cerebral artery—or ruptured aneurysm of the anterior cerebral arteries or the anterior communicating artery, resulting in hemorrhage—may lead to behavioral disturbances related to dysfunction of limbic structures and the medial aspects of the frontal lobe.[3,13]

Occlusion of the posterior cerebral artery, which supplies the medial and inferior aspects of the temporal and occipital lobes, may result in homonymous hemianopsia or loss of a visual field. This loss results because of dysfunction of the visual cortex in the occipital lobe. Visual agnosia may be present (e.g., prosopagnosia, color agnosia, visual object agnosia). Left-sided lesions may cause alexia and associative visual agnosia or naming difficulties. Bilateral lesions cause cortical blindness. There may also be problems with spatial relations, as well as right-left discrimination, alexia, agraphia, acalculia, and memory.[3,10,13]

Dysfunctions affecting other arterial branches that supply structures adjacent to the cortex can cause lesions in the cerebellum, basal ganglias, caudate nuclei, thalamus, and the internal capsule. These lesions can result in various combinations of impairments.

Systemic hypoperfusion results in a diffuse cerebral dysfunction affecting the watershed regions or the border zones in the periphery of the major cerebral arteries. The hippocampus and the adjacent temporal structures on the medial side of cortex may also be involved. The cerebellum and brain stem nuclei are sometimes involved as well. The resulting impairments include agitation; simultanognosia, in which an object is seen as fragmented; brain stem reflexes; coma; confusion; memory disturbances with accompanying confabulations; restlessness; and occasional gait ataxia.[13] See Tables 13-3 and 13-4 for patterns of impairments as they are related to dysfunction of different cerebral arteries and different CNS areas as a result of various vascular pathologic conditions (see Chapter 1).

The case studies illustrated in Figures 13-13 and 13-14 describe two clients who sustained CVAs that resulted in different patterns of impairments based on involvement of different cerebral arteries. The A-ONE assessment was used to evaluate ADL performance, as well as the type of severity of neurobehavioral impairments that interfered with task performance. The studies demonstrate how neurobehavioral impairment interferes with ADL performance and how the two types of dysfunction—dysfunction of performance components and their impact on performance tasks—may be evaluated simultaneously as recommended by several authors.[3,23,37,51] The case studies show two individuals who both need physical assistance with all items in the dressing domain of the Functional Independence Scale of the A-ONE. The lack of functional independence is caused by different neurobehavioral impairments in each of the cases, resulting from different diagnoses. In Figure 13-13, *A*, Ms. Wilson has sustained a right CVA; unilateral body neglect, spatial relations impairment, unilateral spatial neglect, organization and sequencing problems, and left hemiplegia interfere with the dressing performance (as indicated by scores on the Neurobehavioral Specific Impairment Subscale of the A-ONE). In Figure 13-14, *A*, Mr. Johnson has, on the other hand, sustained left CVA; the impairments of ideational apraxia, motor apraxia, perseveration, organization and sequencing, and right hemiplegia interfere with dressing performance. The dressing domain is one of five domains on the Functional Independence Scale of the A-ONE. Summary sheets from the A-ONE indicating scores in the other functional domains and different neurobehavioral impairments are also shown for both of the individuals (Figure 13-13, *B* and *C* and Figure 13-14, *B* and *C*).

Table 13-3

Cerebral Artery Dysfunction: Cortical Involvement and Patterns of Impairment

ARTERY	LOCATION	POSSIBLE IMPAIRMENTS
Middle cerebral artery: upper trunk	Lateral aspect of frontal and parietal lobe	**Dysfunction of either hemisphere** Contralateral hemiplegia, especially of the face and the upper extremity Contralateral hemisensory loss Visual field impairment Poor contralateral conjugate gaze Ideational apraxia Lack of judgment Perseveration Field dependency Impaired organization of behavior Depression Lability Apathy **Right hemisphere dysfunction** Left unilateral body neglect Left unilateral visual neglect Anosognosia Visuospatial impairment Left unilateral motor apraxia **Left hemisphere dysfunction** Bilateral motor apraxia Broca's aphasia Frustration
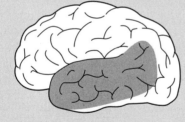		
Middle cerebral artery: lower trunk	Lateral aspect of right temporal and occipital lobes	**Dysfunction of either hemisphere** Contralateral visual field defect Behavioral abnormalities **Right hemisphere dysfunction** Visuospatial dysfunction **Left hemisphere dysfunction** Wernicke's aphasia
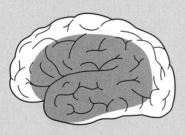		
Middle cerebral artery: both upper and lower trunks	Lateral aspect of the involved hemisphere	Impairments related to both upper and lower trunk dysfunction as listed in previous two sections

Table 13-3

Cerebral Artery Dysfunction: Cortical Involvement and Patterns of Impairment—cont'd

ARTERY	LOCATION	POSSIBLE IMPAIRMENTS
Anterior cerebral artery	Medial and superior aspects of frontal and parietal lobes	Contralateral hemiparesis, greatest in foot Contralateral hemisensory loss, greatest in foot Left unilateral apraxia Inertia of speech or mutism Behavioral disturbances

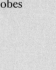

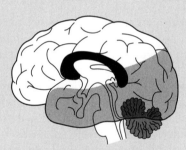

ARTERY	LOCATION	POSSIBLE IMPAIRMENTS
Internal carotid artery	Combination of middle cerebral artery distribution and anterior cerebral artery	Impairments related to dysfunction of middle and anterior cerebral arteries as listed above
Anterior choroidal artery, a branch of the internal carotid artery	Globus pallidus, lateral geniculate body, posterior limb of the internal capsule, medial temporal lobe	Hemiparesis of face, arm, and leg Hemisensory loss Hemianopsia[13]
Posterior cerebral artery	Medial and inferior aspects of right temporal and occipital lobes, posterior corpus callosum and penetrating arteries to midbrain and thalamus	**Dysfunction of either side** Homonymous hemianopsia Visual agnosia (visual object agnosia, prosopagnosia, color agnosia) Memory impairment Occasional contralateral numbness **Right side dysfunction** Cortical blindness Visuospatial impairment Impaired left-right discrimination **Left side dysfunction** Finger agnosia Anomia Agraphia Acalculia Alexia
Basilar artery proximal	Pons	Quadriparesis Bilateral asymmetric weakness Bulbar or pseudobulbar paralysis (bilateral paralysis of face, palate, pharynx, neck, or tongue) Paralysis of eye abductors Nystagmus Ptosis Cranial nerve abnormalities Diplopia Dizziness Occipital headache Coma[13]
Basilar artery distal	Midbrain, thalamus, and caudate nucleus	Papillary abnormalities Abnormal eye movements Altered level of alertness Coma Memory loss Agitation Hallucinations[13]

Continued

Table 13-3

Cerebral Artery Dysfunction: Cortical Involvement and Patterns of Impairment—cont'd

ARTERY	LOCATION	POSSIBLE IMPAIRMENTS
Vertebral artery	Lateral medulla and cerebellum	Dizziness
		Vomiting
		Nystagmus
		Pain in ipsilateral eye and face
		Numbness in face
		Clumsiness of ipsilateral limbs
		Hypotonia of ipsilateral limbs
		Tachycardia
		Gait ataxia[13]
Systemic hypoperfusion	Watershed region on lateral side of hemisphere, hippocampus and surrounding structures in medial temporal lobe	Coma
		Dizziness
		Confusion
		Decreased concentration
		Agitation
		Memory impairment
		Visual abnormalities due to disconnection from frontal eye fields
		Simultanognosia
		Impaired eye movements
		Weakness of shoulder and arm
		Gait ataxia[13]

USEFULNESS OF STANDARDIZED ASSESSMENT METHODS

The previous sections have described how neurobehavioral impairments can be detected during observation of task performance by the use of activity analysis based on the A-ONE theoretical framework. Functional assessments may include nonstandardized and standardized observations. According to Burke,[12] nonstandardized assessments "do not require specific instructions for administration. They are appropriate for a wide range of settings, situations, materials, and individuals. Their usefulness for generalizing results from one individual to another is limited, however, because the materials, time allotments, and assistance may all vary. Nevertheless, they are useful for measuring progress in one individual, provided that the therapist is able to replicate the same situation over time." Standardized assessments, on the other hand, have "...prescribed methods, materials, and instructions for collecting and analyzing performance. Assessment directions must be followed precisely to ensure that interpretation is consistent with that presented by the test authors. The materials and settings are carefully prescribed, and therapists often attend specific training programs."[12]

The information in this chapter has provided guidelines for the observation of CVA clients during task performance with the purpose of detecting impairments that interfere with independent performance. The conceptual and operational definitions provided here, based on the

A-ONE theory, are important to ensure consistency of the method. However, this information has limitations; as presented here, it is not standardized. In contrast, the A-ONE evaluation is standardized—that is, it includes detailed administration and scoring instructions and provides normative data and criterion references. Several studies of validity and reliability have been conducted to ensure the evaluation does what its developer claims it does and that it measures the traits consistently. The instrument requires a training seminar for therapists to ensure reliability. Thus the evaluation itself permits comparison across clients in addition to monitoring of progress, regardless of which trained therapist administers and interprets the evaluation. The results provide useful information for choice of treatment based on strengths and weaknesses of the client, from the perspective of performance components as well as task performance. Occupational therapists must gather valid, reliable information that can be used to build treatment guidelines. Therefore consistent terminology must be developed and as suggested by Holm and Rogers,[30] data collection must be made by use of valid, reliable instruments to ensure usefulness and integrity of the information.

In short the A-ONE instrument allows the therapist to detect impairments that interfere with task performance to understand factors underlying functional dependence. Such information aids therapists in understanding the reasons for the functional impairments. Subsequently, therapists can speculate about the best treatment for impair-

Text continued on p. 332.

Table 13-4

Cerebrovascular Dysfunction in Noncortical Areas: Patterns of Impairment

LOCATION	POSSIBLE IMPAIRMENTS
Anterolateral thalamus, either side	• Minor contralateral motor abnormalities • Long latency period • Slowness **Right side** • Visual neglect **Left side** • Aphasia[13]
Lateral thalamus	• Contralateral hemisensory symptoms • Contralateral limb ataxia[13]
Bilateral thalamus	• Memory impairment • Behavioral abnormalities • Hypersomnolence[13]
Internal capsule or basis pontis	• Pure motor stroke[13]
Posterior thalamus	• Numbness or decreased sensibility of face and arm • Choreic movements • Impaired eye movements • Hypersomnolence • Decreased consciousness • Decreased alertness **Right side** • Visual neglect • Anosognosia • Visuospatial abnormalities **Left side** • Aphasia • Jargon aphasia • Good comprehension of speech • Paraphasia • Anomia[13]
Caudate	• Dysarthria • Apathy • Restlessness • Agitation • Confusion • Delirium • Lack of initiative • Poor memory • Contralateral hemiparesis • Ipsilateral conjugate deviation of the eyes[13]
Putamen	• Contralateral hemiparesis • Contralateral hemisensory loss • Decreased consciousness • Ipsilateral conjugate gaze • Motor impersistence **Right side** • Visuospatial impairment **Left side** • Aphasia[13]
Pons	• Quadriplegia • Coma • Impaired eye movement[13]
Cerebellum	• Ipsilateral limb ataxia • Gait ataxia • Vomiting • Impaired eye movements[13]

Functional Independence Scale and
Neurobehavioral Specific Impairment Subscale

Name   Ms. Wilson   **Date**   6/13/96

Independence Score (IP):

4 = Independent and able to transfer activity to other
    environmental situations.
3 = Independent with supervision.
2 = Needs verbal assistance.
1 = Needs demonstration or physical assistance.
0 = Unable to perform. Totally dependent on assistance.

Neurobehavioral Score (NB):

0 = No neurobehavioral impairments observed.
1 = Able to perform without additional
    information, but some neurobehavioral impairment
    is observed.
2 = Able to perform with additional verbal assistance, but
    neurobehavioral impairment can be
    observed during performance.
3 = Able to perform with demonstration or
    minimal to considerable physical assistance.
4 = Unable to perform due to neurobehavioral impairment.
    Needs maximum physical assistance.

List helping aids used:

- Wheelchair
- Nonslip for soap and plate
- Adapted toothbrush
- Velcro fastening on shoes

PRIMARY ADL ACTIVITY   SCORING   COMMENTS AND REASONING

DRESSING	IP SCORE					COMMENTS
Shirt (or Dress)	4	3	2	(1)	0	Include one armhole, fix shoulder
Pants	4	3	2	(1)	0	Find correct leghole
Socks	4	3	2	(1)	0	One-handed technique, balance
Shoes	4	3	2	(1)	0	Balance
Fastenings	4	3	2	(1)	0	Match buttonholes, Velcro through loop
Other						

NB IMPAIRMENT	NB SCORE					COMMENTS
Motor Apraxia	(0)	1	2	3	4	
Ideational Apraxia	(0)	1	2	3	4	
Unilateral Body Neglect	0	1	2	(3)	4	Leaves out left body side
Somatoagnosia	(0)	1	2	3	4	
Spatial Relations	0	1	2	(3)	4	Finding correct holes, front/back
Unilateral Spatial Neglect	0	1	(2)	3	4	Leaves out items in l-vis. field
Abnormal Tone: Right	(0)	1	2	3	4	
Abnormal Tone: Left	0	1	2	(3)	4	Sitting balance/bilateral manipulation
Perseveration	(0)	1	2	3	4	
Organization/Sequencing	0	1	(2)	3	4	For activity steps
Other						

Note: All definitions and scoring criteria for each deficit are in the Evaluation Manual.

Figure 13-13   A, Árnadóttir Neurobehavioral Evaluation (A-ONE): sample from the dressing
domain of the functional independence (FI) scale and the neurobehavioral specific impairment (NB)
subscale for Ms. Wilson. (Courtesy G. Árnadóttir, Reykjavík, Iceland.)

Árnadóttir OT-ADL
Neurobehavioral Evaluation
(A-ONE)

Name ___Ms. Wilson___   **Date** ___6-13-96___

Birthdate ___4-15-1943___   **Age** ___53___

Gender ___Female___   **Ethnicity** ___Caucasian___

Dominance ___Right___   **Profession** ___Dressmaker___

Medical Diagnosis:
Right CVA 6/20/96. Ischemia.

Medication:

Social Situation:
Lives alone in an apartment building on third floor
Has two adult daughters

Summary of Independence:
Needs physical assistance with dressing, grooming, hygiene, transfer, and mobility tasks because of left-sided paralysis and perceptual and cognitive impairments. Is more or less able to feed herself if meals have been prepared. No problems with personal communication, although perceptual impairments will affect reading and writing skills. Also has lack of judgment and memory impairment, which affect task performance. Is not able to live alone at this stage. If personal home support becomes available, will need a home evaluation because of physical limitations and wheelchair use. Needs recommendations regarding removal of architectural barriers or suggestions for alternative housing. Unable to return to previous job as a dressmaker.

FUNCTIONAL INDEPENDENCE SCORE (optional)

FUNCTION	TOTAL SCORE	% SCORE
Dressing	1,1,1,1,1 = 5/20	
Grooming and Hygiene	1,2,1,1,3,0 = 8/24	
Transfer and Mobility	1,1,1,1,1 = 5/20	
Feeding	4,4,4,3 = 15/16	
Communication	4,4 = 8/8	

Figure 13-13, cont'd **B,** A-ONE summary sheet for the case of Ms. Wilson. (Courtesy G. Árnadóttir, Reykjavik, Iceland.)

LIST OF NEUROBEHAVIORAL IMPAIRMENTS OBSERVED:

SPECIFIC IMPAIRMENT	D	G	T	F	C
Motor Apraxia					
Ideational Apraxia					
Unilateral Body Neglect	3	3	3	1	
Somatoagnosia					
Spatial Relations	3	3	3	1	
Unilateral Spatial Neglect	2	2	3	1	
Abnormal Tone: Right					
Abnormal Tone: Left	3	3	3	1	
Perseveration					
Organization	2	2	2	1	
Topographic Disorientation			3		
Other					
Sensory Aphasia					
Jargon Aphasia					
Anomia					
Paraphasia					
Expressive Aphasia					

PERVASIVE IMPAIRMENT	ADL
Asterognosis	✓
Visual Object Agnosia	
Visual Spatial Agnosia	✓
Associative Visual Agnosia	
Anosognosia	
R/L Discrimination	✓
Short-Term Memory	✓
Long-Term Memory	
Disorientation	✓
Confabulation	
Lability	✓
Euphoria	
Apathy	
Depression	✓
Aggressiveness	
Irritability	
Frustration	

PERVASIVE IMPAIRMENT	ADL
Restlessness	
Concrete Thinking	✓
Decreased Insight	✓
Impaired Judgment	✓
Confusion	
Impaired Alertness	
Impaired Attention	✓
Distractibility	✓
Impaired Initiative	
Impaired Motivation	
Performance Latency	
Absent Mindedness	
Other	
Field Dependency	✓

Use (✓) for presence of specific impairments in different ADL domains (D = dressing, G = grooming, T = transfers, F = feeding, C = communication) and for presence of pervasive impairments detected during the ADL evaluation.

Summary of Neurobehavioral Impairments:

Needs physical assistance for most dressing, grooming, hygiene, transfer, and mobility tasks because of left-sided paralysis, spatial relations impairments (e.g., problems differentiating back from front of clothes and finding armholes and legholes), and unilateral body neglect (i.e., does not wash or dress affected side). Does not attend to objects in the left visual field and needs verbal cues for performance. Also needs verbal cues for organizing activity steps. Does not know her way around the hospital. Does not have insight into how the CVA affects her ADL and is thus unrealistic in day-to-day planning. Has impaired judgment resulting in unsafe transfer attempts. Leaves the water running after hygiene and grooming activities if not reminded to turn it off. Is emotionally labile and appears depressed at times. Is not oriented regarding time and date. Presents with impaired attention, distraction, and defective short-term memory requiring repeated verbal instructions.

Treatment Considerations:

Occupational Therapist:

A-ONE Certification Number:

Figure 13-13, cont'd C, A-ONE summary sheet for the case of Ms. Wilson. (Courtesy G. Árnadóttir, Reykjavík, Iceland.)

Functional Independence Scale and
Neurobehavioral Specific Impairment Subscale

Name Mr. A. Johnson   **Date** 7/5/96

Independence Score (IP):

4 = Independent and able to transfer activity to other environmental situations.
3 = Independent with supervision.
2 = Needs verbal assistance.
1 = Needs demonstration or physical assistance.
0 = Unable to perform. Totally dependent on assistance.

Neurobehavioral Score (NB):

0 = No neurobehavioral impairments observed.
1 = Able to perform without additional information, but some neurobehavioral impairment is observed.
2 = Able to perform with additional verbal assistance, but neurobehavioral impairment can be observed during performance.
3 = Able to perform with demonstration or minimal to considerable physical assistance.
4 = Unable to perform due to neurobehavioral impairment. Needs maximum physical assistance.

List Helping Aids Used:

• Wheelchair

PRIMARY ADL ACTIVITY   SCORING   COMMENTS AND REASONING

DRESSING	IP SCORE					COMMENTS
Shirt (or Dress)	4	3	2	(1)	0	Assistance with right arm
Pants	4	3	2	(1)	0	Stuck because of friction from shoe
Socks	4	3	2	(1)	0	One handed technique, balance
Shoes	4	3	2	(1)	0	Attempts without opening sock
Fastenings	4	3	2	(1)	0	Does not know how to handle buckle
Other						

NB IMPAIRMENT	NB SCORE					COMMENTS
Motor Apraxia	0	(1)	2	3	4	Left hand
Ideational Apraxia	0	1	2	(3)	4	Problems with belt, shoes before trousers
Unilateral Body Neglect	(0)	1	2	3	4	Stuck because of friction
Somatoagnosia	(0)	1	2	3	4	
Spatial Relations	(0)	1	2	3	4	
Unilateral Spatial Neglect	(0)	1	2	3	4	
Abnormal Tone: Right	0	1	2	(3)	4	Sitting balance/bilateral manip.
Abnormal Tone: Left	(0)	1	2	3	4	
Perseveration	0	1	2	(3)	4	Repeats pulling sleeve, sock
Organization/Sequencing	0	1	2	(3)	4	Assistance with activity steps
Other						Shoes before trousers

Note: All definitions and scoring criteria for each deficit are in the Evaluation Manual.

Figure 13-14 A, Árnadóttir Neurobehavior Evaluation (A-ONE): sample from the dressing domain of the functional independence (FI) scale and the neurobehavioral impairment (NB) subscale for Mr. Johnson. (Courtesy G. Árnadóttir, Reykjavík, Iceland.)

Árnadóttir OT-ADL
Neurobehavioral Evaluation
(A-ONE)

Name ___Mr. A. Johnson___ **Date** ___7-5-96___

Birthdate ___4-17-62___ **Age** ___34___

Gender ___Male___ **Ethnicity** ___Caucasian___

Dominance ___Right___ **Profession** ___Carpenter___

Medical Diagnosis:
Left CVA due to ruptured aneurysm and cerebral hemorrhage

Medications:

Social Situation:
Married with two sons, 3 and 5 years old. Lives in own house in a village, a 1-hour drive from the hospital. Worked as a carpenter. Wife works full time in office. Children in day care. Wife is supportive but under a lot of strain because of the present situation.

Summary of Independence:
Needs physical assistance with all dressing, grooming, and hygiene tasks because of right-sided paralysis, ideational apraxia, organization and sequencing impairment, motor apraxia, and perseverations. Slow performance. Has receptive aphasia so verbal instructions not sufficient. Uses pantomime to indicate needs because of inability to use verbal expression. Is able to maneuver in a wheelchair but needs physical assistance with all transfers. Is able to drink and feed himself if food has been prepared, cut, and buttered. Unable to use knife (to peel etc.) by using one-handed techniques, partially because of ideational apraxia, clumsy movements of left hand, and paralysis of right hand. Needs considerable assistance in most ADL tasks. Will need examination re architectural barriers at home and personal assistance before discharge. Unable to assume previous job and role of family provider.

FUNCTIONAL INDEPENDENCE SCORE (optional)

FUNCTION	TOTAL SCORE	% SCORE
Dressing	1,1,1,1,1 = 5/20	
Grooming and Hygiene	1,2,1,1,1,0 = 6/24	
Transfer and Mobility	1,1,3,1,1 = 7/20	
Feeding	4,4,4,1 = 13/16	
Communication	1,1 = 2/8	

Figure 13-14, cont'd **B,** A-ONE summary sheet for Mr. Johnson. (Courtesy G. Árnadóttir, Reykjavík, Iceland.)

LIST OF NEUROBEHAVIORAL IMPAIRMENTS OBSERVED:

SPECIFIC IMPAIRMENT	D	G	T	F	C
Motor Apraxia	1	3		3	
Ideational Apraxia	3	3	3	3	
Unilateral Body Neglect					
Somatoagnosia					
Spatial Relations					
Unilateral Spatial Neglect					
Abnormal Tone: Right	3	3	3	3	
Abnormal Tone: Left					
Perseveration	3	3		1	
Organization	3	3	3	1	
Topographic Disorientation				?	
Other					
Sensory Aphasia					✓
Jargon Aphasia					
Anomia					
Paraphasia					
Expressive Aphasia					✓

PERVASIVE IMPAIRMENT	ADL
Astereognosis	NT
Visual Object Agnosia	
Visual Spatial Agnosia	
Associative Visual Agnosia	
Anosognosia	
R/L Discrimination	
Short-Term Memory	NT
Long-Term Memory	NT
Disorientation	NT
Confabulation	
Lability	
Euphoria	
Apathy	
Depression	✓
Aggressiveness	
Irritability	
Frustration	✓

PERVASIVE IMPAIRMENT	ADL
Restlessness	
Concrete Thinking	✓
Decreased Insight	NT
Impaired Judgment	✓
Confusion	
Impaired Alertness	
Impaired Attention	✓
Distractibility	
Impaired Initiative	
Impaired Motivation	
Performance Latency	✓
Absent Mindedness	
Other	

Use (✓) for presence of specific impairments in different ADL domains (D = dressing, G = grooming, T = transfers, F = feeding, C = communication) and for presence of pervasive impairments detected during the ADL evaluation.

Summary of Neurobehavioral Impairments:

Has considerable ideational apraxia, sensory and expressive aphasia, and paralysis of right side, so requires extensive physical assistance in many ADL tasks. Limited use of left upper extremity for fine object manipulation due to motor apraxia. Takes long time to learn new skills because of ideational problems and comprehension. Incomplete testing of memory items because of communication problems. Appears depressed and frustrated at times, especially when unable to express self. Impaired judgment relating to inadequate organization and sequencing, as well as ideational apraxia. Brings electric razor toward running water. Attempts transfers without wheelchair brakes on.

Treatment Considerations:

Occupational Therapist:

A-ONE Certification Number:

Figure 13-14, cont'd   **C,** A-ONE summary sheet for Mr. Johnson. (Courtesy G. Árnadóttir, Reykjavík, Iceland.)

ments and for dysfunction for task performance (see Chapter 14). This decision can be based on information from the evaluation, as well as the therapist's knowledge of different treatment methods, be they focused on the level of performance tasks or the CNS level of the performance components. Different sensory stimuli can be provided with the aim of affecting neuronal processing (e.g., at the cortical level) on the basis of different theories. In other words the instrument aids the therapist in analyzing the nature or cause of a functional problem requiring occupational therapy intervention. However, it must be kept in mind that at present no functional assessment prescribes treatment and therefore clinical reasoning is necessary to combine evaluation results with available treatment choices. Furthermore, research studies are needed to test the efficacy of treatment and theories. For such testing, valid and reliable instruments are mandatory.

REVIEW QUESTIONS

1. Which kind of lesions may produce unilateral motor apraxia of the left side of the body?
2. What is the difference between the impairments of disorientation and confusion?
3. Which impairment(s) might cause an individual to place both legs in the same leghole of a pair of pants?
4. If an individual does not wash both sides of the body spontaneously, impairments such as unilateral body neglect, organization and sequencing problems, or ideational apraxia might be suspected. What information is needed to differentiate between the different possible impairments. How is this information gathered?
5. What is the difference between expected impairments in the presence of a right middle cerebral artery dysfunction compared with expected impairments of a left middle cerebral artery dysfunction?

■ COTA Considerations ■

- It is necessary to understand which performance components are necessary for performance of particular tasks and how dysfunction is manifested during task observation.
- It is important to understand the limitations of traditional pen and paper ("tabletop") evaluations on predicting functional independence.
- Utilize functional tasks to identify blocks to functional independence.
- Multiple neurobehavioral deficits can be evaluated simultaneously by using a single self-care task.
- Standardized evaluations, such as the A-ONE, stemming from occupational therapy literature are necessary to measure initial dysfunction and individual progress and to develop safe discharge plans.

REFERENCES

1. American Occupational Therapy Association: Uniform terminology for occupational therapy: third edition, *Am J Occup Ther* 48:1047, 1994.
2. American Occupational Therapy Association: Uniform terminology: third edition: Application to practice, *Am J Occup Ther* 48:1055, 1994.
3. Árnadóttir G: *The brain and behavior: assessing cortical dysfunction through activities of daily living*, St Louis, 1990, Mosby.
4. Ayres AJ: *Developmental dyspraxia and adult onset apraxia*, Torrance, Calif, 1985, Sensory Integration International.
5. Baddeley A et al: Closed head injury and memory. In Levin HS et al, editors: *Neurobehavioral recovery from head injury*, New York, 1987, Oxford University Press.
6. Barr ML, Kiernan JA: *The human nervous system: an anatomical viewpoint*, Philadelphia, 1993, Lippincott.
7. Bauer RM: Agnosia. In Heilman KM, Valenstein E, editors: *Clinical neuropsychology*, ed 3, New York, 1993, Oxford University Press.
8. Benson FD: Aphasia. In Heilman KM, Valenstein E, editors: *Clinical neuropsychology*, ed 3, New York, 1993, Oxford University Press.
9. Bogen JE: The callosal syndromes. In Heilman KM, Valenstein E, editors: *Clinical neuropsychology*, ed 3, New York, 1993, Oxford University Press.
10. Brust JCM: Stroke: diagnostic, anatomical and physiological conditions. In Kandel ER, Schwartz JH, editors: *Principles of neural science*, ed 2, New York, 1985, Elsevier.
11. Bryden MP, Lee RG: Right-hemispheric involvement in the perception and expression of emotion in normal humans. In Heilman KM, Satz P, editors: *Neuropsychology of human emotion*, New York, 1983, The Guilfold Press.
12. Burke JP: Selecting evaluation tools I. In Royeen CB, editor: *AOTA self study series: assessing function*, Rockville, Md, 1989, The American Occupational Therapy Association.
13. Caplan LR: *Stroke: a clinical approach*, ed 2, Boston, 1993, Butterworth-Heinemann.
14. Christiansen C: 1993 Continuing challenges of functional assessment in rehabilitation: recommended changes, *Am J Occup Ther* 47:258, 1993.
15. Christiansen C: Occupational therapy intervention for life performance. In Christiansen C, Baum C, editors: *Occupational therapy: overcoming human performance deficits*, Thorofare, NJ, 1991, SLACK.
16. Clark AF, et al: Occupational science: academic innovation in the service of occupational therapy's future, *Am J Occup Ther* 45:300, 1991.
17. Damasio AR, Anderson SW: The frontal lobes. In Heilman KM, Valenstein E, editors: *Clinical neuropsychology*, ed 3, New York, 1993, Oxford University Press.
18. Damasio AR: The frontal lobes. In Heilman KM, Valenstein E, editors: *Clinical neuropsychology*, ed 2, New York, 1985, Oxford University Press.
19. Daube JR, Sandok BA: *Medical neurosciences: an approach to anatomy, pathology and physiology by systems and levels*, Boston, 1978, Little, Brown.
20. Dickoff J et al: Theory in a practice discipline. I. Practice oriented theory, *Nurs Res* 17:415, 1968.
21. Dunn W et al: The ecology of human performance: a framework for considering the effect of context, *Am J Occup Ther* 48:595, 1994.
22. Dunn W et al: The ecology of human performance: a contextual perspective on human occupation. In Royeen CB, editor: *AOTA self study series: the practice of the future: putting occupation back into therapy*, Rockville, Md, 1994, American Occupational Therapy Association.
23. Fisher AG, Short-DeGraff M: Improving functional assessment in occupational therapy: Recommendations and philosophy for change, *Am J Occup Ther* 47:199, 1993.

24. Friedman RF, et al: Alexia. In Heilman KM, Valenstein E, editors: *Clinical neuropsychology*, ed 3, New York, 1993, Oxford University Press.

25. Geschwind N: Specialization of the human brain, *Sci Am* 241:80, 1979.

26. Goldberg E, Costa LD: Hemisphere differences in the acquisition and use of descriptive system, *Brain Language* 14:144, 1981.

27. Heilman KM, Gonzalez Rothi LJ: Apraxia. In Heilman KM, Valenstein E, editors: *Clinical neuropsychology*, ed 3, New York, 1993, Oxford University Press.

28. Heilman KM et al: Neglect and related disorders. In Heilman KM, Valenstein E, editors: *Clinical neuropsychology*, ed 3, New York, 1993, Oxford University Press.

29. Heilman KM, Watson RT: Intentional motor disorders. In Levin HS, Eisenberg HM, editors: Frontal lobe function and injury, New York, 1991, Oxford University Press.

30. Holm MB, Rogers JC: The therapists thinking behind functional assessment II. In Royeen CB, editor: *AOTA self study series: assessing function*, Rockville, Md, 1989, American Occupational Therapy Association.

31. Kaupfermann I: Hemispheric asymmetries and the cortical localization of higher cortical and affective functions. In Kandel ER, Schwartz JH, editors: *Principles of neural science*, ed 2, New York, 1985, Elsevier.

32. Levin HS et al: Acalculia. In Heilman KM, Valenstein E, editors: *Clinical neuropsychology*, ed 3, New York, 1993, Oxford University Press.

33. Llorens LA: Activity analysis: Agreement among factors in a sensory processing model, *Am J Occup Ther* 40:103, 1986.

34. Luria AR: *Higher cortical functions in man*, ed 2, New York, 1980, Basic Books.

35. Luria AR: *The working brain: an introduction to neuropsychology*, New York, 1973, Basic Books.

36. Martini R et al: ICIDH-PR: a potential model for occupational therapy, *Occup Ther Inter* 2:1, 1995.

37. Mathiowetz V: Role of physical performance component evaluations in occupational therapy functional assessment, *Am J Occup Ther* 47:225, 1993.

38. Nelson DL: Occupational form, occupational performance, and therapeutic occupation. In Royeen CB, editor: *AOTA self study series: the practice of the future: putting occupation back into therapy*, Rockville, Md, 1994, American Occupational Therapy Association.

39. Nelson CE et al: Adult physical dysfunction content in professional curricula, *Am J Occup Ther* 44:1079, 1990.

40. Pedretti LW: Occupational performance: a model for practice in physical dysfunction. In Pedretti LW, editor: *Occupational therapy practice skills for physical dysfunction*, ed 4, St Louis, 1996, Mosby.

41. Reynolds PD, *A primer in theory construction*, Indianapolis, 1971, Bobbs-Merrill Educational Publishing.

42. Rogers JC, Holm MB: The therapists thinking behind functional assessment I. In Royeen CB, editor: *AOTA self study series: assessing function*, Rockville, Md, 1989, American Occupational Therapy Association.

43. Siev E et al: *Perceptual and cognitive dysfunction in the adult stroke patient: a manual for evaluation and treatment*, Thorofare, NJ, 1986, SLACK.

44. Starkstein SE, Robinson RG: Neuropsychiatric aspects of stroke. In Coffey CE, Cummings JL, editors: *Textbook of geriatric neuropsychiatry*, Washington, DC, 1994, American Psychiatric Press.

45. Strub RL, Black FW: *The mental status examination in neurology*, ed 2, Philadelphia, 1985, FA Davis.

46. Townsend E et al: Using the World Health Organization's International Classification of Impairments, Disabilities, and Handicaps in occupational therapy, *Can J Occup Ther*, 57:16, 1990.

47. Trombly CA: Theoretical foundations for practice. In Trombly CA, editor: *Occupational therapy for physical dysfunction*, ed 4, Baltimore, 1995, Williams & Wilkins.

48. Trombly CA: Planning, guiding, and documenting therapy. Trombly CA, editor: *Occupational therapy for physical dysfunction*, ed 4, Baltimore, 1995, Williams & Wilkins.

49. Trombly CA: Clinical practice guidelines for post-stroke rehabilitation and occupational therapy practice, *Am J Occup Ther* 49:711, 1995.

50. Trombly CA: Occupation: purposefulness and meaningfulness as therapeutic mechanisms: 1995 Eleanor Clarke Slagle Lecture, *Am J Occup Ther* 49:960, 1995.

51. Trombly CA: Anticipating the future: Assessment of occupational function. *Am J Occup Ther* 47:253, 1993.

52. US Department of Health and Human Services: *Clinical practice guideline number 16: Post-stroke rehabilitation*. Rockville, Md, 1995, U.S. Department of Health and Human Services.

53. Walsh K: *Neuropsychology: a clinical approach*, Edinburgh, Scotland, 1987, Churchill Livingstone.

54. World Health Organization: *International classification of impairments, disabilities, and handicaps: a manual of classification relating to the consequences of disease*, Geneva, 1980, The Organization.

55. Yatsu FM et al: *Stroke: 100 maxims*, St Louis, 1995, Mosby.

56. Yerxa EJ: In search of good ideas for occupational therapy, *Scand J Occup Ther* 1:7, 1994.

SUGGESTED READING

Árnadóttir, G. *The brain and behavior: assessing cortical dysfunction through activities of daily living*, St Louis, 1990, Mosby.

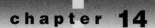

chapter **14**

Treatment of Neurobehavioral Deficits: A Function-Based Approach

key terms

cognition	apraxia	memory
perception	perseveration	attention
neurobehavior	unilateral neglect	concrete thinking
integrated functional approach	aphasia	insight
multicontextual approach	organization/sequencing	problem-solving
Affolter approach	spatial relations	

chapter objectives

After completing this chapter, the reader will be able to accomplish the following:

1. Understand the different approaches to treatment of cognitive and perceptual impairments and be aware of research conducted on each approach.
2. Recognize the importance of the environment, psychosocial issues, and meaningful activity in the context of treatment planning for this population.
3. Apply the multicontextual and Affolter approaches to treatment of cognitive and perceptual impairments.
4. Discuss different treatment approaches to individual neurobehavioral impairments.
5. Realize the relevance and importance of functional activities in the treatment of cognitive and perceptual impairments.

Few things are more interesting or frustrating to a therapist than observing a stroke patient with severe neglect or apraxia attempting unsuccessfully to perform a self-care task. It is difficult to imagine what is being felt by that person. The most important issue for occupational therapists is determining what can be done to improve the functional performance of stroke patients with cognitive or perceptual impairments.

In this chapter, studies and other literature on treatment approaches are reviewed and suggestions for treating cognitive and perceptual impairments that are frequently found in persons who have sustained a cerebrovascular accident (CVA) are discussed.

NEUROBEHAVIOR

Neurobehavior has been defined as any behavioral response resulting from CNS processing. It is considered the basis of task performance in activities of daily living (ADL).[5] In this chapter the term *neurobehavior* refers to cognitive and perceptual components of behavior, including praxis, attention, memory, spatial relations, sequencing, and problem-solving.

TREATMENT APPROACHES

Approaches to stroke rehabilitation can be directed at the level of impairment, disability, or handicap. Impairment refers to organ dysfunction, disability to task performance dysfunction, and handicap to social disadvantage. Approaches aimed at the level of handicap have the greatest impact on the stroke survivor's quality of life.[35] Unfortunately, in current practice, handicap is deemphasized, whereas impairment or disability is emphasized. Therapists must strive to provide service in all three areas of need while promoting issues relevant to the patient's quality of life.

Cognitive and perceptual impairments are commonly described in the literature, but the focus is often placed on assessment of these impairments. Controlled studies relating to treatment effectiveness in the stroke population are few,[52] and studies supporting specific treatment approaches for cognitive and perceptual impairments are even more rare. In a recent survey on cognitive and perceptual rehabilitation, most occupational therapists said they perceived a need for treatment guidelines and more treatment techniques and materials for this population.[56]

Treatment approaches to perceptual or cognitive impairments are generally classified in one of two categories: (1) the functional or adaptive approach, or (2) remediation or restoration. The functional or adaptive approach emphasizes techniques to assist the patient in adapting to deficits, changing the environmental parameters of a task to facilitate function, and using a person's strengths to compensate for loss of function. Remediation, or restoration, emphasizes the use of techniques to facilitate recovery of the actual cognitive or perceptual skills affected by the stroke. Each approach has strengths and limitations, and clinicians often use both approaches during stroke rehabilitation (Table 14-1).

Functional Approach

The functional approach uses repetitive practice in particular activities, usually daily living tasks, to help the patient become more independent. This approach is designed to treat symptoms rather than the cause of the dysfunction.[20]

Some occupational therapists believe their role in cognitive and perceptual rehabilitation lies solely in the realm of a functional approach, involving training in compensatory techniques and only with tasks directly related to functional performance.[44] This approach appears most compatible with research indicating that family members and financial providers rank independence in ADL as the highest priority for rehabilitation.[14,42]

Therapists use the functional approach to train patients to function by compensating. An example of compensation is the use of an alarm watch to remind someone with poor memory to take medication. Compensation circumvents the problem. Some clinicians believe its use should be limited to patients who have accepted the permanence of the perceptual or cognitive deficit.[46] Only persons who can benefit from compensation should be taught these strategies. That is, the persons must have a basic understanding of their skills and the permanence of their limitations because the use of compensation for disability requires that the individual recognize the need to compensate. The patient must be a self-starter, must be goal directed, and must want to learn new strategies. Successful compensation requires practice, repetition, and overlearning of the strategies.[58]

Environmental adaptation is more appropriate for those who cannot use compensatory strategies as a result of poor insight of disability.[58] Adaptation involves changing the characteristics of the task or environment. This technique is used in patients with poor learning potential. An example of adaptation is the use of contrasting colors for a plate and placemat for someone with figure-ground difficulties. Establishing a routine and constant environment with repeated participation in familiar activities is often the most successful strategy for these individuals. The adaptive approach relies on caregivers to implement treatment strategies.[58]

A significant limitation of the functional approach is the task specificity of the strategies and lack of generalizability to other tasks.[12] For example, the use of an alarm timer to take medications on time does not help the patient remember a repertoire of other activities, such as, to take a shower, start meal preparation, or get to a doctor's appointment unless the patient has specifically been trained to do so.

Remedial Approach

Remediation (or restoration or transfer of training) emphasizes restoration of the function or skill lost as a result of the stroke. Remedial treatment relies on several assumptions—the cerebral cortex is malleable and can adapt, and the brain can repair and reorganize itself after injury. Practice and repetition are assumed to result in learning. In turn, learning results in a more organized, functional system. Another assumption is that tabletop activities such as pegboard tasks or computer activities directly affect the underlying cognitive or perceptual skills required for the patient to perform those activities. The most important as-

Table 14-1

Comparison of Functional and Remedial Approaches

FUNCTIONAL/ADAPTIVE	REMEDIAL/RESTORATIVE
Emphasizes occupational skills	Emphasizes component skills
Targets symptoms of dysfunction	Targets cause of dysfunction
Uses compensatory techniques, environmental adaptation	Uses tabletop activities (pegboard/computer) to improve underlying cognitive and perceptual skills
Uses repetitive practice of daily living activities to improve performance	Assumes improved performance in pegboard or tabletop activity will translate into improved performance in everyday activities
Usually uses task-specific strategies that are not generalizable	Shows little generalizability to improved performance in functional tasks

sumption is that improved task performance of tabletop activities will be carried over to improved performance in functional activities.[12,20,36]

Although this approach has been successful when used in the initial stages of treatment,[20] most studies show only short-term results, generalization only to similar tasks,[52] or little effectiveness from remedial training for neurobehavioral impairments.[20,25] For this approach to be successful, treatment sessions must be frequent and lengthy. The U.S. Department of Health and Human Services Agency for Health Care Policy and Research will confront the issue of scientific evidence for effectiveness of remedial cognitive and perceptual training when *Practice Guidelines for Post-Stroke Rehabilitation*[52] is revised.

Neistadt[37] believes only those patients who show transfer of learning to tasks that are different in multiple characteristics are appropriate candidates for the remedial approach to cognitive and perceptual impairments. It is widely agreed that practice of a subcomponent skill, such as problem-solving or attention to task, must occur in multiple contexts for successful transfer of learning.[58] According to Neistadt,[38] therapists should always train for transfer of cognitive or perceptual retraining because the patient's home environment is always different from the clinic setting. Those who can transfer learning only to similar tasks should be restricted to a functional/adaptive approach to maximize their training potential.[37]

Recommended Approach

Determination of the appropriate treatment approach for the stroke patient with cognitive or perceptual impairments relies on the results of the assessment. Important questions include the following: Does the patient have the potential to learn? Is the patient aware of errors during task performance; and if so, does the patient have the potential to seek solutions to those errors? If the patient has poor learning potential and is unlikely to benefit from the use of cues or task modification, a strictly functional approach involving domain-specific training would be recommended.[50] Domain-specific training requires little or

no transfer of learning (generalizability) and involves repetitive performance of a specific functional task using a system of vanishing cues. (*Vanishing cues* are cues that are provided at every step of task performance but then gradually removed. The goal is to establish a program in which the patient can successfully perform the task with a minimum number of cues.) This type of training is hyperspecific, and the learning associated with it will persist only if the task and environmental characteristics remain unchanged.

Both the remedial and functional approaches involve teaching the patient new behaviors. The difference is in whether emphasis is placed on component skills or occupational skills. Research indicates that the use of one approach exclusively always has some disadvantages; therefore it is important to consider the patient's learning potential and ability to generalize information, the severity of the injury, and the overall health, age, and support systems.[37] Use of the functional training approach[39,47] or a combination of a functional approach with a cognitive or perceptual remedial approach[19,34,50] has been supported by research.

Traditionally the clinician has used either a restorative or functional approach; however, Abreu and colleagues[2] have proposed an integrated functional approach to treatment in which principles from both approaches are used simultaneously. In this approach, daily occupations and occupational environments are used to challenge cognitive and perceptual skill components. Because individuals engage in occupations as integrated wholes and not as separate attention machines, categorizers—or memory coders—treatments that are not aimed at real-life contexts are highly irrelevant to real life.[2] With this integrated functional approach, treatment may be focused on a subcomponent skill such as sustained attention, but daily occupations are used as the modality. For example, a self-feeding task can be used to improve sustained attention to task. Mealtime is often distracting. Eating can be a difficult task if attention deficits are present. A system of vanishing cues and a gradual increase in the amount of environmental dis-

Box 14-1

Tooth-Brushing Task: Treatment of Neurobehavioral Impairments

SPATIAL RELATIONS/SPATIAL POSITIONING

Positioning of toothbrush and toothpaste while applying paste to brush
Placement of toothbrush in mouth
Positioning of bristles in mouth
Placement of brush under faucet

SPATIAL NEGLECT

Visual search for and use of brush, paste, and cup in affected hemisphere
Visual search and use of faucet handle in affected hemisphere

BODY NEGLECT

Brushing of affected side of mouth

MOTOR APRAXIA

Manipulation of toothbrush during task performance
Manipulation of cap from toothpaste
Squeezing of toothpaste onto brush

IDEATIONAL APRAXIA

Appropriate use of objects (brush, paste, cup) during task

ORGANIZATION/SEQUENCING

Sequencing of task (removal of cap, application of paste to brush, turning on water, and putting brush in mouth)
Continuation of task to completion

ATTENTION

Attention to task (for greater difficulty, distractions such as conversation, flushing toilet, or running water may be added)
Refocus on task after distraction

FIGURE-GROUND

Distinguishing white toothbrush and toothpaste from sink

INITIATION/PERSEVERANCE

Initiation of task on command
Cleaning parts of mouth for appropriate period of time, then moving bristles to another part of mouth
Discontinuation of task when complete

VISUAL AGNOSIA

Use of touch to identify objects

PROBLEM-SOLVING

Search for alternatives if toothpaste or toothbrush is missing

---

traction can be used to address inattention to task and functional performance.

The use of a functional approach is supported by today's health care industry, which seeks documentation of patient's functional competence in ADL. Only cost-effective interventions that directly affect functional status will be embraced in today's health care environment.

Any functional task can be used to address myriad neurobehavioral impairments. It is imperative that occupational therapists use their skills in activity analysis to evaluate an activity for its effectiveness in addressing particular cognitive or perceptual deficits. Box 14-1 contains an example of using everyday function to address neurobehavioral skills.

TREATMENT CONSIDERATIONS

Many factors must be considered in the preparation of a treatment plan. A stroke patient may not have the same needs as a person with a closed-head injury, encephalitis, or a gunshot wound to the head. All have brain injury, but they have different patterns of behavior and recovery. Likewise, it must be remembered that no two stroke patients are alike. Each person with a CVA is a unique individual with special needs, goals, and problems.

Population

The patient's age should be considered; studies have found a functional decline with familiar and practiced tasks as adults age.[17] Expectations for functional level vary for different age ranges. A young stroke victim will surely have different goals and aspirations than one who is older than 65 years. The person's previous level of function must also be considered when goals are established. A person who was not independent before a stroke probably will not achieve independence after the stroke. Cultural differences often emerge during evaluation and should be supported during treatment planning. The importance placed on occupations varies among cultures, so care should be taken to ensure that goals and activities are culturally relevant to each patient.

Environment

The importance of the environment or setting where treatment takes place cannot be underestimated. Patients plan and perform ADL differently and with greater independence[43] at home than in the clinic setting.[40] Exposure to different environments requires patients to adapt strategies and solve problems,[29] leading to greater independence in a variety of situations.

The adaptation of purposeful activities to ensure success is of primary importance in occupational therapy. Success depends on the therapist's ability to analyze the activities and the patients' strengths, weaknesses, and needs to present the most relevant and challenging activity.

Psychosocial and Emotional Issues

Many factors influence quality of life after a stroke. OTs frequently measure quality by examining physical recovery and performance of self-care as the primary indicators.[45] However, research indicates that even with good physical and functional recovery, people show decreased socialization and leisure activity after a stroke.[4] Many patients sustain not only significant loss in functional ability after a stroke but difficulty adjusting emotionally to the new lifestyle. OTs must address all factors relating to quality of life. Enhanced quality of life should be the ultimate priority in the planning of treatment (see Chapter 3).

Group treatment has been suggested as a way to facilitate socialization and communication by patients.[18] Groups provide reinforcement for socially acceptable behaviors. In addition, a stroke survivor may be more inclined to share feelings and concerns with a group of other stroke survivors because they are more likely to understand those feelings. Many occupational therapists have established support groups for stroke victims and their families.[21,22]

Meaningful Activity

Although the underlying theory of occupational therapy revolves around the use of meaningful activity in treatment, it is still important to address the use of meaningful activity in the treatment of cognitive and perceptual impairments. Activities used in treatment should not only address the dysfunction but should also be meaningful and relevant to each patient.

In the early 1990s, greater emphasis was placed on the participation of patient and family in goal-setting. The health professions are recognizing that quality health care requires the patient and family to help establish a plan of care. The Joint Commission on Accreditation of Healthcare Organizations (JCAHO) and the Commission on Accreditation of Rehabilitation Facilities (CARF) require documentation of patient and family involvement in treatment planning, discharge planning, and education. Who knows better what activities and goals are meaningful and relevant than the patient and family?

NEUROBEHAVIORAL IMPAIRMENTS IN THE STROKE POPULATION

Perceptual and cognitive impairments in the stroke population are part of an interactive process involving the patient, the task at hand, and the environment in which the task is being performed.[50] Cognition and perception are constantly changing and reacting to both internal and external stimuli. Neurobehavioral impairments must be addressed in the context of the situation, according to the person's needs and goals. This is why a generic, general approach does not work for the patients included in this population.

Neurobehavioral impairments are often noted in CVA survivors. Localized lesions occurring in stroke may cause localized loss of function such as language comprehension. More often, strokes cause a variety of neurobehavioral impairments associated with the severity of the infarct. General treatment strategies for persons with cognitive and perceptual impairments after stroke are addressed. Commonly noted neurobehavioral impairments will be discussed individually later in the chapter.

INTERVENTION STRATEGIES

Treatment strategies for cognitive and perceptual impairments are common in the literature; however, very little research is available regarding the content and context validity or reliability of these approaches. The need for research studies to support the many approaches being used in this population is great. Until much of this research is conducted, we must rely on techniques and approaches that seem successful (but are not yet proven).

Activity Processing

Activity processing is especially helpful in cognitive rehabilitation because the purpose and results of the task are discussed with the patient. Awareness by the patient can be discerned from feedback provided during and after task performance. Activity processing enhances the patient's metacognition (knowledge of own cognitive ability and ability to monitor own performance) and general knowledge. Activity processing emphasizes the purpose of the activity in the rehabilitation process.[11] For example, when practicing spatial positioning during a dressing task, the patient should be instructed on the spatial requirements for each step of the task and the purpose of using the dressing task to improve on spatial skills. As the patient performs the task, the patient and the therapist should discuss performance and strategies to perform the activity.

Behavior Modification

Use of behavior-modification techniques such as prompting, shaping (reinforcing responses that increasingly resemble the sought-after behavior), and contingent reinforcement (reward contingent on an appropriate response) are common in the stroke and/or brain-injury population. Behavior-modification techniques with intermittent praise and reinforcement to improve independence in daily activity have been successful.[24,32]

Use of prompts and cues is key to successful cognitive and perceptual rehabilitation. Cues can be faded by reducing the number, frequency, or specificity of the prompts.[58] For example, a therapist may initially provide detailed cues at every step of task performance, such as "Look to the left to find the soap." Cues should be tapered and should become

less detailed as the patient progresses (e.g., "Have you remembered all the steps?"). Prompts and cues should be provided in a calculated and graded fashion. The use of cues and prompts is part of cognitive and perceptual rehabilitation and is an essential way of facilitating patient insight, error detection, and strategy development (Table 14-2).

Group Treatment

Group treatment in the stroke population is often effective. Group treatment can yield situations more like real life, because they are less structured and can generate unpredictable events and provide distractions. In a group, patients can get feedback from their peers (which is often more meaningful), share similar experiences, and exchange problem-solving and coping strategies. Group treatment allows patients to learn from others' mistakes, practice monitoring their own behavior, and see that their problems are not unique.

Two approaches to treatment of neurobehavioral impairments that are particularly relevant to occupational therapy are the multicontextual and Affolter approaches. Although many approaches specific to cognitive and perceptual intervention are described in the literature, these two approaches have broad potential for stroke patients with neurobehavioral impairments.

Multicontext Approach

The multicontext approach was developed by Joan P. Toglia, an occupational therapist, and is based on the dynamic interaction model of cognition.[50] This model views cognition as a product of constant interaction among the individual, the task, and the environment. In the multicontext approach the patient's processing abilities and self-monitoring techniques are used to facilitate learning for different tasks or environments (Box 14-2).

The ability to transfer information from one situation to another is an essential component of the multicontext approach. Toglia[51] believes transfer of skills must be taught throughout the learning process and during treatment sessions, not at the time of discharge. The ability to transfer learning across tasks can be facilitated by varying treatment environments or altering the nature of a task. Varying degrees of similarity between activities and having the patient practice a targeted strategy in different environments and with varying activities can also aid skills transfer. A near-transfer task is one that differs from the original task by only one or two surface characteristics (Box 14-3). If the original task is donning *shorts* in bed, a near-transfer task is donning a pair of *pants* in bed. Intermediate-transfer tasks change three to six surface characteristics and are not as readily identified with the original task. An example is donning underwear from a sitting position (type of clothing, type of material, positioning, and sequence of task have changed). Far-transfer tasks share just one, if any, surface characteristics but are still conceptually similar to the original task. The use of one-handed principles taught for lower-body dressing applied to upper-body dressing is an example of a far transfer. Very far transfer is the generalization or application of previously learned information in novel or spontaneous situations.[51]

Initially, the number of stimuli and complexity of tasks remain unchanged throughout the process of exposure to tasks with changing surface characteristics. As the patient shows consistent ability to use targeted strategies in a vari-

Table 14-2

Prompting Procedures

PROMPTS	RATIONALE
"How do you know this is the right answer/procedure?" or "Tell me why you chose this answer/procedure."	Refocuses patient's attention to task performance and error detection Can patient self-correct with a general cue?
"That is not correct. Can you see why?"	Provides general feedback about error but is not specific Can patient find error and initiate correction?
"It is not correct because . . ."	Provides specific feedback about error Can patient correct error when it is pointed out?
"Try this [strategy]" (e.g., going slower, saying each step out loud, verbalizing a plan before starting, using a checklist)	Provides patient with a specific, alternate approach Can patient use strategy given?
Task is altered. "Try it another way."	Modifies task by one parameter. Can patient perform task? Begin again with grading of prompting described previously.

Modified from Toglia JP: Attention and memory. In Royen CB, editor: *AOTA self-study series: cognitive rehabilitation*, Rockville, Md, 1993, American Occupational Therapy Association; Toglia JP: Generalization of treatment: a multicontext approach to cognitive perceptual impairment in adults with brain injury, *Am J Occup Ther* 45:505, 1991.

Box 14-2

Principles of the Multicontext Approach

- Transfer of skills must be taught, not just presumed to occur.
- Strategies taught to patients must be practiced in a variety of environments with many different tasks.
- Metacognitive skills are critical components of learning and the ability to generalize.
- Training of metacognitive skills and self-awareness is incorporated throughout treatment.
- Transfer of learning occurs through a graded series of tasks that decrease in similarity.
- Awareness questioning used to help the patient detect errors, estimate task difficulty and performance, and predict outcomes.

Modified from Toglia JP: Generalization of treatment: a multicontext approach to cognitive perceptual impairment in adults with brain injury, *Am J Occup Ther* 49:711, 1995.

Box 14-3

Examples of Task Surface Characteristics

- Color
- Shape
- Size
- Positioning
- Number of steps required
- Physical surroundings
- Spatial arrangement
- Familiarity of objects/task
- Sequence of steps

Modified from Toglia JP: Generalization of treatment: a multicontext approach to cognitive perceptual impairment in adults with brain injury, *Am J Occup Ther* 45:505, 1991.

ety of situations, the number of stimuli and the complexity of tasks are increased.

The multicontext approach emphasizes the use of functional activities, as well as a variety of gross motor, computer, and tabletop tasks. Treatment activities should be varied. Explicit teaching of the transfer from remedial to functional activities is essential.[36] Therefore, a patient must understand that scanning for coins on a tabletop promotes the use of visual scanning in everyday activities.

Awareness during task performance is a focal point of this approach. Emphasis is placed on teaching the patient to be more aware of cognitive or perceptual strengths and weaknesses and ways to compensate.[36] The use of awareness questions, estimation of performance, and strategy investigation should be used before and after task performance. The patient is questioned about the task's difficulty, the accuracy of task performance, and the amount of assistance needed. The patient should be given immediate feedback on the accuracy of responses to awareness questioning. Initially, the patient is asked these questions dur-

ing or after task performance. As improvement in accuracy of responses is noted, the patient is asked to predict task performance before engaging in the activity. The patient is also taught to ask questions such as "How am I doing?" "Am I implementing that strategy?" and "Am I forgetting anything?" The patient should also be given questions about the strategy used to complete the task, such as "How did you keep track of what to do next?"[48] The use of these techniques helps the patient detect errors, estimate task difficulty and performance, increase self-awareness, and use self-monitoring skills. Teaching processing strategies such as prioritizing, clustering related information, planning ahead, and time management, as well as awareness questioning, yield deeper and more organized processing of information.[51]

Transfer of training is more likely to occur in patients with localized lesions such as a stroke than in those with diffuse injury such as anoxia or closed-head injury. People with diffuse injury tend to have poorer information-processing skills. Someone with a localized pattern of injury is expected to retain better learning capacity than is one with diffuse injury.[36] Neistadt[36] believes that transfer of learning between tasks that are different in more than three to six characteristics is difficult for brain-injured subjects and that the likelihood of generalization of learning to different tasks is greater when greater emphasis is placed on explicit teaching for transfer.

The multicontext approach may be used when the patient shows potential for improvement through the use of environmental modification, assistance, or cues. This approach facilitates training techniques in a variety of task situations and environments to place increasingly difficult demands on the patient. The goal of this approach is to train the patient to use self-monitoring and compensation strategies to handle task performance in a variety of situations.[50]

Affolter Approach

The Affolter approach is a treatment approach based on tactile-kinesthetic (T-K) input provided to patients with cognitive and perceptual impairments. This approach was developed by Felicie Affolter, who has degrees in child psychology, audiology, and language pathology. Affolter has noted that the T-K sensory system is essential for interaction with the environment and that interaction with the environment results in increasingly complex skills.[9] Through T-K input, connections between movement and its effect on objects lead to information on cause-and-effect relationships. Cause-and-effect assists in the development of cognitive connections in daily activities.[16] Emphasis is placed on providing appropriate input to facilitate a problem-solving process rather than a focus on the end product or specific skills.[9,16] According to Affolter, therapists must be sure to teach problem-solving and not merely splinter skills, which are rarely carried over.[16]

Guiding is the main principle of the Affolter approach[9] (Box 14-4). The therapist places a hand over the patient's

Box 14-4

Guiding Principles

While guiding the patient, therapists should do the following:

- Place their hands over the patient's whole hand, down to the fingertips.
- Keep talking to a minimum.
- Guide both sides of the body when possible.
- Move along a supported surface to give the patient maximum tactile feedback.
- Involve the whole body in the task to challenge posture.
- Provide changes in resistance during the activity.
- Allow the patient to make mistakes to give opportunities to solve problems.

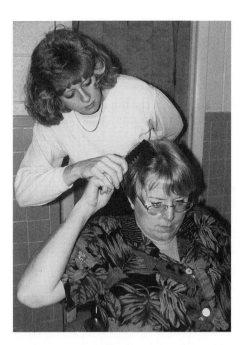

Figure 14-1   Patient is guided through a hair-brushing task.

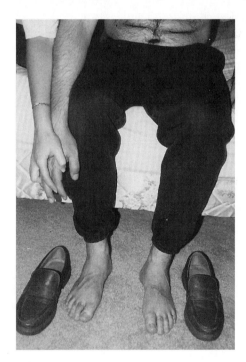

Figure 14-2   Guiding the patient's hand along a supported surface (leg) as he reaches for a shoe.

hand and guides the manipulation of objects as the patient performs the task.[16] The patient may respond with initial increased skeletal muscle activity, which often relaxes as the activity continues. Guiding often results in increased attention and sustained focus on the task at hand. Patients who were previously unable to brush their hair may begin to take over the purposeful movement and start to brush their hair while being guided by the therapist (Figure 14-1).[9] The amount of guiding fluctuates with the patients' change in muscle activity and active participation in the task. Guiding should initially be performed on a supported surface rather than through air. The surface provides tactile feedback, allow the patients to explore the environment, and provides feedback on distance and spatial relationships. For example, when assisting patients to reach for their shoes, the occupational therapist should guide the patients' hand along the surface of their leg to their foot (Figure 14-2). During a hygiene task, the occupational therapist can guide the patients' hand along the edge of the sink to reach for the faucet.[9]

When assisting the patient in solving problems, the therapist or caretaker must offer the patient possibilities, not solutions.[9] The therapist must create an environment that facilitates cognitive-perceptual learning by providing problems to be solved.[16] The patient must be allowed to make mistakes during treatment to use problem-solving skills. Therapists often correct mistakes too quickly. The patient may not even realize a mistake has been made or take the opportunity to address the problem (such as spilled milk on a tray or a washcloth dropped on the floor). Guiding the patient through the process of cleaning up the milk or picking up the washcloth may be the most meaningful part of the treatment session.

A good activity is one that does not rely on outside feedback but provides its own through its success or completion.[16] The change of resistance of the knife against the cutting board and the aroma of a freshly cut orange are cues that tell the patient the task is complete. Use of func-

tional and purposeful activities is essential to keep patients motivated. The environment should also be appropriate to the task: dressing in a bedroom, hygiene activity in a bathroom. Wiping a countertop that is not dirty or stacking cones is not purposeful because there is no problem to be solved.[9]

The Affolter approach deemphasizes talking because most or all of the feedback should come from the activity.[16] Communication is nonverbal, provided through the T-K sense. Instructions are not necessary to initiate guiding. It may be helpful for the therapist to say, "I'm going to guide your body/hands with my hands. My hands will tell you what I want you to do." Instead of telling the patient to grab the toothbrush, the therapist physically guides the patient through the process of reaching for the toothbrush and toothpaste.[9] As the patient begins to understand the purpose of the task through the T-K input, participation in the task increases. Refraining from speaking allows the patient to process information without excess stimulation.

Patients perceive the environment by being physically guided through task performance. Because the therapist is in direct contact with the patient, the therapist gains direct feedback about the patient's attention to task, sequencing, problem-solving, and muscle tone.[9]

Cognitive-perceptual training occurs regularly throughout the patient's day. Collaboration with other members of the health care team and education of families and caregivers on Affolter principles (Box 14-5) is vital because if the treatment plan is not supported and continued at home as well as in the clinical setting, the patient may experience conflict and confusion. Families often feel overwhelmed and helpless; training them to provide T-K input during task performance allows them to participate in the recovery of their loved one.[9]

TREATMENT APPROACHES FOR SPECIFIC NEUROBEHAVIORAL IMPAIRMENTS

Clinicians rarely observe perceptual or cognitive deficits in isolation. Usually these deficits overlap and are difficult to interpret because of their complexity. Little research has been conducted or published on outcomes of specific treatment approaches for isolated perceptual and cognitive deficits, with the possible exceptions of memory impairments and unilateral neglect. However, therapists continue to assess these impairments individually, and it does sometimes help to use a combination of general and specific treatment approaches to neurobehavioral impairments. It is with this thought in mind that information on distinct treatment approaches related to specific impairments follows (see Chapter 13).

Box 14-5

Affolter Principles

- Physically guiding the patient's hands/body in functional activities
- Emphasis on input rather than on output
- Less focus on skills; more focus on facilitation of problem-solving
- Purposeful, meaningful tasks; must be a problem to be solved

Apraxia

According to Ayres,[6] praxis is one of the most important connections between brain and behavior; it is what allows us to interact with our physical world. Apraxia is a dysfunction of purposeful movement that does not result primarily from motor, sensory, or comprehension impairments.[5] Although many different types of apraxia have been named and defined, the labels used to classify them are not universally accepted.[7] For relevance in this chapter, however, they fit into two general categories: motor and ideational apraxia.

Patients with apraxia are often unaware of their deficits, creating a dilemma when therapeutic interventions are planned. General treatment guidelines for patients with apraxia are listed in Box 14-6.

Motor Apraxia

Motor apraxia is a defect in symbolic or expressive gestures. It is the inability to produce the individual elements in a sequence of tasks even as the patient retains the concept or idea of the task. Árnadóttir[5] has described movements in patients with motor apraxia as clumsy and inflexible. Someone with motor apraxia has difficulty imitating a motor command and difficulty sequencing and orienting elements of a task together. It may be helpful for the therapist to give only general information about the activity goal and leave out the specific instructions.[7] For example, when working on morning ADL with the patient, a general statement of, "Let's get ready," should be used instead of step-by-step instructions for each task. It may be helpful to have the patient visualize task movements and sequences before carrying out the task. This visualization gives the patient a visual model to refer to in performing the task.

Ideational Apraxia

Ideational apraxia involves a disruption in the concept formation of action planning. The ability to select and organize movements to execute an action is impaired. This

Box 14-6

General Treatment Approaches for Persons With Apraxia

- Provide tactile, kinesthetic and proprioceptive input before and during the activity to help guide movements.
- Keep commands simple, with minimal wordiness.
- Make frequent use of spontaneous situations, keeping activity on a subcortical level.
- Perform activities in their usual environments.
- Work in a relaxed environment with few distractions.
- Use goal-directed activities to decrease confusion.
- Provide contextual and environmental cues.

impairment is often seen in a person's attempt to use objects: faulty or inappropriate tool use is the hallmark of ideational apraxia. Often the patient with ideational apraxia seems confused, stubborn, or uncooperative. Treatment considerations for this dysfunction include step-by-step commands for each task[7] because patients with this disorder cannot grasp the general concept or idea of the activity but may be able to perform individual components of the task on command.

Use of Affolter's guiding techniques for patients with motor apraxia can promote task continuation through the T-K sensation of smooth, rhythmical movement. Physical guiding provides the patient who has ideational apraxia with possibilities (not solutions). For example, as a patient is guided during a tooth-brushing task, the patient's hand should be guided toward objects at the sink but not directly at the appropriate object. The patient should be given the opportunity to plan and execute the appropriate movements.

Perseveration

Perseveration is demonstrated by the inability to shift from one concept to another or to change or cease a behavior pattern once it has been started. It also refers to the inability to translate knowledge into action (initiation of a task). The person is either "stuck in set"—unable to discard the previous set of behaviors—or unable to "activate" for a new situation. The person stuck in set is attempting to solve a problem with information relevant to a previous problem.

Bringing perseveration to a conscious level and training the patient to inhibit the perseverative behavior has been successful.[27] Other strategies include redirecting attention, assisting the patient in initiating a new movement or task, and engaging the patient in tasks that involve repetitive action (e.g., washing the face or body, stirring food, or sanding wood) to promote successful task participation.

Unilateral Neglect

Of all the neurobehavioral impairments discussed in this chapter, unilateral neglect has received the most attention in the health care literature (see Chapter 12 for information on visual field loss versus neglect). Not only does neglect occur in the horizontal plane, it is manifested in vertical and radial planes ("vertical" implying neglect of stimuli upward or downward and "radial" implying close to or far from the body). The existence of these phenomena requires clinicians to check for the presence of this disorder and implement a treatment program to include all neglected spaces.[31] The most widely supported theories explaining unilateral neglect involve the attention and arousal mechanisms of the brain. The attentional theories speculate that neglect results from impaired attention abilities. It is theorized that the right hemisphere is usually dominant for attentional skills and therefore that left-side neglect resulting from a right CVA is seen more frequently than right-side neglect from a left CVA, depending on hemispheric lateralization. Arousal theories state that left-side neglect occurs as a result of decreased stimulation to the injured hemisphere and overarousal in the noninjured hemisphere. According to this theory, the hyperaroused hemisphere pays greater attention to the contralateral space and body, and the unaroused hemisphere pays little attention to space and body contralateral to it. Research has not supported the arousal theory[13]; many clinicians support, at least in part, the attentional theories.

General treatment principles that have been recommended in the literature (but not supported by research) include use of visual markers, visual scanning training, cueing for visual anchoring, increased stimulation to the affected side, movement or activation of the affected extremity in the affected hemispace, and training awareness of neglect to facilitate compensation.[15,34,48]

Anosognosia, the impaired awareness of neglect or other deficits, is a fundamental problem in the rehabilitation of neglect. The ability to improve this lack of awareness by fostering understanding of the disability and its impact on function is a key component of treatment.[26]

Spatial Neglect

Neglect of the environment and space contralateral to the lesion site is referred to as *spatial neglect*. Visual scanning activities are the most common and successful treatment approaches for spatial neglect and visual field cuts. The focus of this approach is to train the patient to continually scan the environment for relevant stimuli and to attend to stimuli in the affected hemisphere. Principles guiding this approach include grading activities from simple to complex, providing consistent feedback, repetition of activities, and use of visual scanning in the context of functional activities.[28] Cognitive or perceptual training is generalized well to similar tasks; therefore continuous training with similar tasks in treatment will likely yield the greatest benefit with generalization. This principle was demonstrated in a group of studies involving a scanning machine and multiple wheelchair movement conditions to demonstrate improvement in wheelchair mobility and decreased contact with obstacles.[33,54,55] The ability to scan the environment decreases as the attention demands of the task increase[12]; therefore task performance must be kept simple when accurate scanning of the environment is necessary. Anchoring techniques are used to cue the patient and organize the scanning pattern. Warren[53] recommends combining scanning with manipulation of whatever is being scanned to increase success. Studies have found that an individual has a stronger mental representation of a visual image if the image or object has been explored by touch.[53]

Scanning training in combination with a scanning machine for treatment of spatial neglect has had some success. The scanning machine has a moving light that the patient visually tracks from one point to another.[12] A flashing stimulus light combined with verbal cues has also been successful in assisting patients to anchor the beginning and end of scanning movements.[12]

Greater improvement in neglect behaviors in patients with the most severe neglect has been demonstrated.[12,23] Persons who have severe impairments benefit from the use of external cues such as verbal reminders and colored anchors to improve function. Mildly impaired patients who show faulty scanning may be helped only if they can be trained to use internal cues to improve their scanning ability.[12] The ability to internalize strategies is the skill most pivotal and most difficult to achieve for the brain-injured population.

Activation or use by the impaired (usually left) hand, paired with perceptual anchoring, has been found to reduce the signs of neglect. This activation includes active and passive movement of the affected extremity. Whether the positive effect is a result of the actual movement of the arm or by a spaciomotor cueing process is a matter of controversy.[26]

Some examples of functional treatment activities focusing on visual scanning include scattering items for mealtime across both visual fields, using diminishing cues to help the patient find needed items during the meal, and strategically arranging items for grooming and hygiene so the patient must scan the neglected space for successful task performance. Again, the occupational therapist should provide diminishing verbal cues to teach the patient to visually scan independently.[28]

Although popular, the use of computers in the treatment of neglect has shown little promise.[47] Certainly the use of computers in the brain-injured population (as with any other neurobehavioral impairment) may be relevant if the patient uses computers for work or leisure activities. The use of computer games for the treatment of spatial neglect, however, has not been validated (especially the use of widely available software made specifically for "cognitive retraining"). These computer activities do not provide realistic or meaningful challenge for most patients, and they have been reported to have no generalizing effect.[39] Overall, the remedial or transfer of training approach for unilateral neglect has frequently been unsuccessful.[23]

Body Neglect

Inattention or neglect of body parts contralateral to the lesion site is termed *body neglect*. Activities requiring bilateral integration or use of both sides of the body have been used to treat the disorder. Affolter guiding techniques may also be useful. Guiding may allow a patient to perform a bilateral task with an otherwise nonfunctional extremity. Guiding the hemiparetic extremities can provide useful T-K input because the patient's body is taken through familiar movement patterns. Guiding may help increase at-

tention to the neglected side by "activating" the affected extremities. Tasks that provide increased sensory stimulation to the affected extremities (e.g., applying lotion or bathing with a washcloth) may also decrease neglect.

Compensatory strategies for body neglect include using a tactile stimulator (e.g., vibrating beeper) to draw attention to the unattended body side, a buzzer that sounds randomly to redirect attention to affected side, and auditory (verbal or nonverbal) stimulation through earphones to increase arousal to affected side. Attention to affected extremities during functional activities such as dressing or wheelchair transfers had not been shown to improve neglect (unless specifically set up for stimulation during those activities).

Aphasia

Language-processing defects are referred to as *aphasia*. Although treatment of aphasia is typically addressed by the speech pathologist, it is critical to understand how to facilitate communication with aphasic patients. Box 14-7 outlines helpful hints for use with aphasic patients and their caregivers.

Many of the techniques of awareness questioning described in the discussion of the multicontextual approach are not useful with aphasic patients. Approaches, especially cueing strategies, must be adjusted for the aphasic brain-injured population. Cues normally provided verbally may be more effective when provided by tactile or visual means for those with receptive aphasia. For example, instead of telling a patient to pay attention to the left arm, tapping the left arm or using gestures to indicate visual scanning to the left arm may be more successful. It may be helpful for therapists of patients with expressive aphasia to work closely with the speech therapist to establish a communication system that facilitates awareness questioning (e.g., use of writing, drawing, or gestures by patients, to give the

Box 14-7

Aphasia: Tips for Family Members

- It is easier for people with aphasia to understand speech when only one person talks to them at a time. Extra noise only creates confusion.
- Give the patient enough time to respond.
- Carefully phrase questions to make it easier for the patient to respond; for example, use yes/no and either/or questions.
- Use visual cues or gestures with speech to help the patient better understand.
- Never force the patient to respond.
- Use concise sentences.
- Do not rush communication. Rushed communication with a person who has aphasia can increase frustration and decrease the effectiveness of communication.

therapist information about their ability to estimate task difficulty, detect errors, or predict outcomes).

Sequencing and Organization Deficits

The ability to organize thoughts requires the integration of multiple skills including praxis, sequencing, and problem-solving. *Sequencing* refers to the ability to plan and carry out events in proper order, progression, and time.[5] Sequencing and organization deficits represent the breakdown of a complex integration of skills, including use of sensory feedback and organization. Patients with sequencing and organization deficits can be trained to use a daily planner, or tape recordings, or cue cards (depending on whether they perform better with auditory or visual cues) to help sequence the steps of daily tasks. Gradually increasing the number of steps in a task can increase a patient's tolerance and ability to perform more complex tasks (Box 14-8).

Spatial Relations Syndrome

Spatial relations syndrome is the label given to disorders with impairment in the perception of spatial relationship of objects. These disorders include impairments with figure-ground, position in space, spatial relations, and form and space constancy skills. Topographic disorientation is also sometimes classified as part of spatial relations syndrome. Recommendations for spatial impairments include training patients to move slowly through their environments, encouraging patients to touch objects in the environment frequently, teaching patients to handle objects by the base, and using verbal cues or feedback instead of gestures.[41] Perceptual impairments are often difficult for families to understand. Educating the caregivers about these disorders and instructing them on how they can help their loved ones (Box 14-9) is especially important.

Spatial Relation Dysfunction

Spatial relation dysfunction is an impairment in relating objects to one another or to the self. Some examples of functional activities for patients with spatial deficits include identification and orientation of clothing during a dressing activity. This includes matching buttons and buttonholes together on a shirt or working on the ability to orient shoelaces during a one-handed tie. Wheelchair transfers require the ability to position the body in relation to a bed or other object and spatial orientation to maneuver wheelchair brakes and armrests in the correct direction. Simple meal preparation is another activity that requires spatial orientation and positioning because of tasks as locating and selecting needed items, stirring food, and setting the table.[28]

The popular use of the computer for visuospatial retraining has little or no effect on visuospatial skills and no carryover to functional activities.[25] Thus the use of computer programs aimed solely at addressing visuospatial skill retraining appears to be an ineffective remediation technique. A computer screen provides information as a two-dimensional image. Spatial relation impairment is a three-dimensional problem. For persons who use the computer for work or leisure, however, the use of the keyboard or mouse while working on the computer can be an effective, challenging, and meaningful modality.

Spatial Positioning Impairment

The concept of spatial positioning involves accurate placement or positioning of objects, including body parts. That impairment, however, may be associated with impaired proprioception. This disorder is linked with language comprehension. Concepts such as "above," "in," and "under" are interpreted according to position in space and language skills.

Treatment for spatial positioning impairment should include increasing the patient's awareness of the impairment and teaching compensatory strategies. Matching colored markers for correct placement of objects can be helpful. Treatment ideas include having the patient practice placing a glass on top, in front, to the right, and to the left of a plate on command, placing certain objects (cups or utensils) in a row and having the patient identify which object is in a position different from those of the others. If language skills are impaired, the patient can be asked to create a place setting from a model. Repetition of specific spatial concepts, with emphasis on attention to detail and

---

Box 14-8

Sequencing Deficits: Tips for Family Members

- Frustration and error can be lessened by step-by-step directions written in a simple format (e.g., a checklist).
- Maps and diagrams may be useful.
- Visual aids often prove helpful, especially when combined with verbal instructions or physical guiding.
- Frequent, routine practice should help reinforce the sequencing of daily activities.

Box 14-9

Perceptual Problems: Tips for Family Members

- Overstimulation from visual information may increase the problem.
- Getting rid of unnecessary objects and equipment will lessen the demands on the patient and simplify the task. For example, the tabletop should be cleared of objects that look alike so that the patient does not confuse them.
- Slowing down while reaching for an object or walking into a new area is usually helpful.

compensatory strategies (e.g., Velcro shoe strap goes toward the colored marker), may be helpful.

Treatment techniques for right-left discrimination problems include providing activities that stress right and left differences, such as dressing and grooming. In addition, color or other markers may be used to distinguish the right from the left side of items such as clothing and shoes.

Figure-Ground Impairment

Figure-ground deficits involve the inability to distinguish the foreground from the background. Treatment strategies for figure-ground deficits should include teaching the patient to be cognitively aware of the deficit and to slow down enough during task performance to identify all the relevant objects or stimuli before handling or manipulating them. The environment can be adapted to make it simple and uncluttered (e.g., organizing drawers or shelves). The use of stark contrast between objects (e.g., the plate and table during mealtime) is extremely helpful for patients with this disorder. Sorting objects such as utensils from a kitchen drawer or nuts and bolts from a toolkit can be a good therapeutic activity; the sorting can be made more difficult with the addition of smaller and larger objects, thereby adding the element of size discrimination. The sorting should have a purpose, such as using the utensils for a cooking task.

Topographic Disorientation

Topographic disorientation is difficulty finding direction in space.[5] The use of compensatory techniques and environmental adaptation, progressively reduced as the patient demonstrates learning, is often successful in the treatment of this disorder. Markers such as colored dots can be used to identify a route the patient must travel every day. The cues are gradually removed as the patient memorizes the route. One successful treatment program described by Borst and Peterson[10] used the patient's intact skills of right-left discrimination and language to assist with functional mobility. In this treatment program the patient practiced following directional instructions (e.g., "Go left at the next door.") The patient was then asked to draw the path from room to room on a map of the clinic area. Such an exercise would be especially helpful in the home setting. At first the clinician may need to assist the patient with correctly orientating the map with each turn. Verbal cues should be slowly withdrawn. Next, the patient should attempt to go from room to room with only brief glances at the map. The last step is to withdraw the use of the map altogether. Generalization of this type of treatment is unlikely; therefore treatment should take place only in the most meaningful environment.

Agnosia

Agnosia is typically defined as the inability to recognize sensory stimuli. Agnosia presents as a defect of one particular sensory channel, such as visual, auditory, or tactile. Examples include finger agnosia, visual agnosia, somatoagnosia, simultanagnosia, and tactile agnosia. These disorders are rarely seen in isolation, and little data have been published regarding treatment techniques for agnosia. However, because the defining principle of agnosia is impairment of one specific sensory modality, treatment is usually focused on teaching the patient to use the intact sensory modalities. For example, in tactile agnosia—the inability to recognize objects by handling them—the patient is taught to use visual, olfactory, and auditory senses to recognize objects.

Somatoagnosia

Somatoagnosia is the decreased awareness of body structure and inability to recognize or relate body parts to each other. Treatment includes having the patient imitate body movements, identify and appropriately use body parts during task performance, and practice simple tasks that require two body parts working together (e.g., opening a jar).

Visual Agnosia

Visual agnosia can be broken down into visual object agnosia and visuospatial agnosia. Visual object agnosia is the inability to recognize objects through the visual senses, whereas visuospatial agnosia includes deficits of spatial relations, topographic orientation, and depth perception. Educating patients to use other intact sensory systems and avoiding reliance on visual information is the most successful treatment plan for patients with visual agnosia. One socially isolating agnosia is prosopagnosia—the inability to recognize familiar faces. Patients and their families must be educated to seek and provide other sensory information (e.g., voice recognition or familiar scents) to help the patient identify others.

Simultanagnosia

Simultanagnosia is the inability to grasp the association between multiple stimuli presented simultaneously, including interpretation or integration of elements into a meaningful theme. Persons with simultanagnosia may recognize individual items—such as shoes, socks, pants, and shirts—but have no understanding about how they are related. Therapy emphasizes the intact ability to recognize specific stimuli. Attempts to make persons with simultanagnosia understand the relationship between their shoe and their foot will probably be unsuccessful. For a successful outcome, patients can be taught to recognize both the shoe and the foot and instructed what to do. Step-by-step instructions for primary ADL are often necessary for such patients. Perhaps the use of tape-recorded instructions for morning routines would be successful (visual cues are not helpful because the patient cannot visually integrate or understand the cues).

Memory Impairments

Although memory impairments are not as common in persons who have sustained strokes as they are in those with closed-head injuries, dementia, or encephalitis, difficulty retaining information is nonetheless very common in the stroke population.

Fractionated memory loss, which is usually either material specific or modality specific, is the most common memory impairment in stroke survivors. These types of memory impairments are found in patients with focal lesions such as localized strokes and (less commonly) with diffuse brain diseases (such as dementia) or closed-head injury. Material-specific memory loss involves the loss of verbal or nonverbal memory as a result of unilateral damage to the medial temporal lobe. A stroke in the left medial temporal lobe leads to verbal memory loss, whereas a right medial temporal lobe infarct would result in nonverbal memory loss. Examples of verbal memory loss are the inability to recall a previous conversation or instructions given by a therapist. Examples of nonverbal memory loss are the inability to remember the route from home to the grocery store (or from the bedroom to the therapy gym) or the tune of a favorite song. When patients have material-specific memory loss, the therapeutic approach must take advantage of their intact systems. If verbal information is not being retained, the use of more gestures and body language may be effective. If spatial relationships are difficult to recall, it may be helpful to rely on the intact language system and use step-by-step verbal directions.

Modality-specific memory loss is associated with focal lesions of the fibers that connect the sensory processing areas (e.g., visual, tactile, sensory, auditory) to the medial temporal lobes. Therefore memory loss would correspond only to the affected sensory processing area. Treatment for modality-specific memory loss should also focus on using intact sensory systems to compensate for memory loss. For example, if during evaluation a patient was unable to recall any information that was given orally by the clinician, the treatment plan would be focused on training techniques involving frequent tactile and visual cues such as hand-over-hand techniques and drawings and written programs.

Short-term memory is closely tied to attention. Most people can hold about seven units of information in short-term memory. Short-term memory capacity can be increased by grouping information into more meaningful units ("chunking"). Long-term memory is believed to be coded and organized semantically or by meaning; therefore attaching specific meaning to information may aid retention of memories.

One strategy-based approach to improving memory involves the use of temporal tags. It is believed that when a memory is formed, it is associated not only with a certain context but also with a temporal tag (information about when memory occurred). If emphasis is placed on recalling *when* an event occurred, it may help the person recall the actual event that occurred. However, one of the hallmarks of most people with stroke-associated memory loss is their inability to form strategies to recall information; relying too heavily on rote memory is frequently the result.

Rehearsal (repeating information several times) refreshes or regenerates information. Use of visual imagery, first-letter mnemonics, and rehearsal have helped some patients remember things such as items on a shopping list and people's names. However, these techniques could not be generalized into everyday activities.[26] Patients should be trained to create their own personal prompts or reminders and taught the way to use them in everyday life. Spaced retrieval, a technique in which information is retrieved at progressively longer intervals, has been a successful memory technique; unfortunately it is limited by the small amount of material that can be retained.[26]

Although little evidence has been found showing that cognitive training can improve memory function, the functional use of memory aids has been repeatedly demonstrated.[26,30] Aids include calendars; log books; notes; tape recorders; time buzzers or alarms; and written, step-by-step instructions.

A patient with functional metamemory is able to process memories and monitor their content. More generally, the patient can appreciate, recognize, and assess the status of memory abilities. Metamemory (which is related to insight) therefore involves being aware of deficits and is clearly important in predicting the way a patient will approach a task. Treatment for a patient with metamemory deficits involves increasing the patient's awareness of the deficit; a patient who is unaware of a memory impairment will be unable to implement compensation techniques.

People remember better through recognition (e.g., remembering whether eggs or orange juice were on a grocery list) than cued recall (e.g., remembering whether breakfast foods were on a grocery list); they remember better through cued recall than free recall (e.g., remembering what was on a grocery list). It is therefore important to provide the particular environment and cues that facilitate successful recall for each individual.

Attention Deficits

Attention is an essential element in successful task performance. Poor ability to attend to a task is often misinterpreted as a lack of motivation or neglect. It is important to accurately assess an attention impairment to implement appropriate treatment techniques. One method that may be helpful in managing attention problems is changing the way occupational therapists speak to patients. The goal is to couple the patient's attention with the intended action; instructions should be in the logical sequence of the action. Instead of instructing a patient to "Scoot forward," the therapist would say, "Your bottom *(pause)*. Move it forward to the edge of the chair." The wording should correspond with the order in which the steps are to be executed and allow the patient to attend to each step. The pause is important to allow the patient enough time to shift focus and process the information.[12]

Use of systematic training incorporating a series of tasks with progressively increasing attentional demands has resulted in improvements in both memory and attention to task,[8] although other studies have failed to demonstrate support for remedial training in attention.[49]

Family members are often frustrated when their loved ones are easily distracted or unable to focus on a task. Family members must be informed that stroke survivors do not behave erratically on purpose. Teaching the family the way to create a supportive environment is important (Box 14-10).

Selective Attention Impairment

The ability to focus on relevant stimuli while screening out irrelevant stimuli is referred to as *selective attention*. Selective attention may be improved by training patients to react to certain environmental cues and ignore distractions. For example, a patient can be asked to follow audiorecorded instructions for a hygiene task (or meal preparation if a more complex task is desired). After the patient is able to successfully complete the task, elements of distraction such as a radio or television, can be added one by one.

Sustained Attention Impairment

Sustained attention is the ability to maintain attention over a period of time. Focusing and sustaining attention is improved by gradually increasing the attentional demands of activities, through choosing activities with longer duration and additional distractions. For example, a task such as combing hair in a quiet bathroom without a mirror may initially require less than 30 seconds of focused attention to complete (and have few inherent distractions). As the patient successfully completes these types of tasks, activities that require focused attention to detail and have more distractions should be chosen (e.g., straight razor shaving task with the radio playing in the background).

Alternating Attention Impairment

Alternating attention is shifting focus from one stimulus to another. For the brain-injured population, graded activities from simple to complex that initially require the patient to shift attention from one stimulus to another should be planned. For example, a simple activity may consist of participating in a ceramics painting project (in which the patient alternates attention from the paint to ceramic vase); a more complex task would be to have the patient perform a dressing task while watching the news on television and having the patient repeat important daily events after completing the task. Initially, tasks should only require attention shifts between two focal points. As the patient successfully completes these tasks, activities incorporating more focal points should be used (e.g., a meal-preparation task in which focus must alternate among planning, following directions, searching for supplies, monitoring other foods, timing, place-setting, etc.).

Concrete Thinking

Persons who use concrete thinking are characterized by inflexible thought processes. They have difficulty generalizing information from one situation to another and rely heavily on available sensory information.

Persons with impaired abstraction skills usually have poor ability to recognize and learn the cognitive and perceptual skills needed for a specific task. Therefore they may benefit only from learning splinter (nongeneralizable) skills in treatment and may demonstrate training only in those tasks that are very similar to those learned.[36] Box 14-11 reviews suggestions for family members to facilitate communication and task performance with this population.

Insight Problems

A patient's lack of awareness may lead others to think there is a lack of motivation. Insight is related to knowledge of self, abilities, and skills. Judgment and insight are frequently associated. Lack of insight can result in impulsiveness or an inability to plan for the future.[11] Treatment for decreased insight should focus on family education, use of feedback about skills, and self-awareness training.[11]

Lack of insight can be a significant limitation in the rehabilitation process. If someone cannot recognize the need for cognitive rehabilitation, it is likely there will be no motivation to learn. Pressure from family members or loved ones and use of positive reinforcement may help in these situations. Family and caregivers must understand the safety implications for those with impairments of insight, judgment, or abstraction skills. Frequently these patients need heavy supervision at home because of their lack of safety awareness. Providing a safe environment is the first priority, and instructing families on home adaptations is

Box 14-10

Distractibility: Tips for Family Members

- Help unclutter the environment. Turn off the television and close doors to decrease excessive noise.
- Allow only one or two visitors at a time.
- Establish eye contact.
- Make statements and questions as simple and uncomplicated as possible.

Box 14-11

Cognitive Inflexibility: Tips for Family Members

- Explain the reasons for certain procedures. The person may have difficulty understanding the long-term effects of therapy or medical procedures. Explain these with smaller goals that are easier to accomplish.
- If possible, structure tasks so they consist of a series of related tasks, rather than many unrelated tasks.

essential (Boxes 14-12 and 14-13). Feedback for this population should be immediate, concrete, and objective. Use of multiple media (visual, verbal, tactile) for feedback is most beneficial for retention of information.[11]

Impaired-Problem Solving Skills

Problem-solving is not a single function but an integration of multiple skills. New or unique circumstances require problem-solving skills; novel or different tasks in multiple contexts require a patient to call on these skills. Games and puzzles are often used to enhance problem-solving skills and are enjoyable and challenging for the patient. The use of games to practice newly learned problem-solving strategies is often less threatening than practice of ADL. The purpose of using a game to improve problem-solving skills should be understood by the patient. Strategies to practice include chaining (breaking down the sequence of component parts), performing one step at a time, and writing down each step of sequences.[58]

A case study by Yuen[57] involved a patient's decreased compliance in taking medication because of problem-solving and other difficulties. Compliance improved by structuring the environment, using assistive devices (e.g., pillbox timer), and cognitive cueing. Box 14-4 describes ways the family can assist patients with this impairment.

GOALS

The ability to appropriately document occupational therapy evaluation and treatment data is more important than ever. The insurance industry reimburses for occupational therapy services according to information provided to them through documentation; the goals that are set for a patient are critical to the support of the plan of care by the insurance company. Functional outcomes have gained increasing support and in many cases are required by insurance companies for reimbursement. Therefore goals should be meaningful and sustainable—it must be valued and carried out by the patient outside the clinical environment.[3] Allen et al[3] describes examples of goals and documentation criteria for use in the brain-injured population (Box 14-15).

Cognitive and perceptual rehabilitation has become a specialized area of practice for many occupational therapy practitioners. Specialization may result in decreased adherence to the roots of the profession and a focus on just one segment or function of the individual. It must be remembered that all cognitive and perceptual skills work together to produce an integrated and complex system of behaviors. The focus of occupational therapists should be on the way neurobehavioral impairments affect patients' lives. The overall intent should not be to increase patients' attention span but to improve their ability to perform meaningful, relevant activities.

There will never be a general approach that can be used for every stroke patient with cognitive or perceptual impairments. The approach taken to treat each person who has had a stroke must be an integration of the person's previous function, support system, severity of injury, and personal needs and goals. Cognitive and perceptual rehabilitation is a challenging and rewarding part of the rehabilitation process.

Box 14-12

Denial and Lack of Insight: Tips for Family Members

- Provide frequent reality orientation (e.g., explain why patient is in the hospital and what activities patient is having problems with).
- Be honest (but not critical) about the patient's condition or disabilities.
- If it is not dangerous, allow or even encourage the patient to try a desired activity. When the patient is unable to complete the task, calmly draw attention to it. Do not badger or gloat.
- Be patient. Remember that denial is a result of neurologic damage; it is not an effort to be stubborn on the part of the patient.
- Once you believe the patient can handle confrontation, it may be necessary to challenge the patient. Show that you can easily accomplish a task that the patient says no one can do.

Box 14-13

Impulsivity: Tips for Family Members

- Reward the patient for brief periods of self-control.
- Redirect the patient's attention to appropriate behavior.
- Place the wheelchair (or other equipment) out of sight to prevent the patient from being tempted to sit in it when alone.
- Ignore verbal outbursts whenever possible, and try not to take them personally.
- When the patient has some capability for control, be direct about your feelings but not critical. You may want to say things like, "My feelings are hurt when you talk to me this way" or "It embarrasses me when you tell other people things I have said to you about them."
- Keep dangerous objects such as knives and scissors in a safe place.

Box 14-14

Problem-Solving Impairments: Tips for Family Members

- Remove time restraints from tasks if possible.
- Provide written or verbal step-by-step instructions for tasks.
- Keep directions and tasks as simple as possible.

Box 14-15

Sample Goals for Patients With Neurobehavioral Impairments

- Patient will properly sequence dressing tasks involving the legs with fewer than two verbal cues in three out of three trials.
- Patient will use grab bars or other objects for stability and safety during dressing task in three out of three trials.
- Patient will demonstrate appropriate use of pillbox for medication schedule in three out of three trials.
- Patient will prepare a shopping list from a recipe with all needed ingredients in two out of three trials.
- Patient will use 75% of objects and eat 75% of food placed on left side of midline, without verbal cues, in three out of three trials.
- Patient will prepare a simple, familiar meal with 80% recognition of errors in three out of five trials.
- Patient will use objects with total appropriateness in hygiene tasks without assistance in two out of three trials.
- Patient will attend to and perform all steps of audio-cued grooming task in three out of three trials.
- Patient will plan and participate in community activities once a week in three out of five trials.

CASE STUDY

GW, a 49-year-old man, was working as a security guard at a prison when he sustained a massive right middle cerebral artery CVA. He was hospitalized for 7 days and subsequently underwent occupational therapy on an outpatient basis. GW's neurobehavioral deficits initially included severe left-side spatial and body neglect, anosognosia, and difficulty with spatial relationships, as well as severe spastic hemiparesis resulting in total dependence in mobility and all ADL except eating (for which he needed moderate assistance).

Initial treatment plans were focused on setting up functional activities such as eating, grooming, hygiene, and dressing. GW was required to visually scan the left side of space to find needed objects or use both arms to practice use of the left side of the body. (This was achieved through use of guiding techniques because no independent movement of left arm was present.) Diminishing verbal cues were used for GW to learn to attend to the left side of his body and left side of space during functional task performance. GW's greatest initial impediment was his steadfast denial that his left arm and leg belonged to him (known as anosognosia). Fortunately, this denial diminished and was no longer present 4 weeks after the stroke.

Compensatory techniques such as matching color markers were minimally successful in treating spatial deficits. However, adaptive devices, such as elastic shoelaces (to prevent the need to spatially execute one-handed shoelace-tying), and compensatory strategies, such as slowing down movements and keeping hands on supported surfaces while reaching, were highly successful in increasing GW's independence in daily task performance.

As GW's awareness of his disability improved, use of awareness questioning was emphasized. GW was initially questioned after (and then before) each task; he later learned to ask himself questions such as, "What do I do before I start?" "Do I see everything I need?" "Is there anything I forgot?" and "Did I pay attention to my left side?" Awareness questioning was the most successful technique for improving GW's ability to achieve independent performance of basic self-care and eventually perform instrumental ADL without assistance. GW received occupational therapy services for 13 months. Initially he lived with his mother and brother after the stroke, but he returned to independent living in his apartment and at the time of discharge was working with vocational rehabilitation services to find employment options.

CASE STUDY

MA, an 82-year-old man, sustained a left CVA at the age of 80 years and subsequently underwent right above-the-knee amputation as a result of peripheral vascular disease. MA was placed in a skilled nursing facility at that time and lived there during the occupational therapy evaluation. Neurobehavioral impairments noted at the time of evaluation included global aphasia, motor and ideational apraxia, and severe attention deficits. MA was dependent on others for all mobility and ADL skills, including eating. MA's family was supportive and visited him daily at lunch and dinner time. Much of the occupational therapy was focused on patient, family, and staff education. The family was taught to use Affolter guiding techniques, which they implemented at mealtime and for grooming and hygiene tasks. The family and staff were taught ways to facilitate communication through tactile and visual cues and guiding techniques, and ways to decrease environmental stimulation and distractions, and ways to approach MA to help him attend to tasks. MA responded well to guiding techniques, requiring only occasional tactile cues after initiating the task (through guiding) to eat, comb his hair, and wash his face in a low-stimulus environment. Occupational therapy continued for 7 weeks (because MA was also seen for contracture management), and MA was discharged to his family from the skilled nursing facility.

REVIEW QUESTIONS

1. How is the integrated functional approach different from traditional functional approaches, and why is it the recommended approach for cognitive and perceptual impairments?
2. What are the basic principles of the multicontextual and Affolter approaches, and why are they relevant to occupational therapy for cognitive and perceptual impairments?
3. What neurobehavioral components are required to perform a hair grooming task? How can this task be used in the treatment of motor apraxia?
4. How can caregivers adapt environments to assist loved ones with cognitive or perceptual impairments?
5. What do most research-based studies reveal about the use of computers for cognitive and perceptual impairments? When is the use of computers most relevant?

■ COTA Considerations ■

- Practicing functional tasks in multiple environments is the best means of treating persons recovering from stroke who have the ability to learn and generalize the information for use in daily activities through conventional means.
- When cognitive and perceptual deficits are so severe the patient cannot learn through conventional means, using previous habits to retrain the patient to function with the assistance of a caregiver is the best approach.
- Using a combination of remedial and functional learning is often the best treatment approach for most patients who will have persistent sequelae from a stroke.
- The positioning, tools, and approaches used to teach each patient to perform ADL depend on the combination of the patient's functional disability problems observed (see Box 14-1).

REFERENCES

1. Abreu B: Perceptual motor skills: assessment and intervention strategies. In Royeen CB, editor: *AOTA self-study series: cognitive rehabilitation*, Rockville, Md, 1994, American Occupational Therapy Association.
2. Abreu B et al: Occupational performance and the functional approach. In Royeen CB, editor: *AOTA self-study series: cognitive rehabilitation*, Rockville, Md, 1994, American Occupational Therapy Association.
3. Allen CK: Reporting occupational therapy services. In Allen CK, Earhart CA, Blue T, editors: *Occupational therapy treatment goals for the physically ill and cognitively disabled*, Rockville, Md, 1992, Occupational Therapy Association.
4. Ángeleri F et al: The influence of depression, social activity, and family stress on functional outcome after stroke, *Stroke* 24:1478, 1993.
5. Árnadóttir G: *The brain and behavior: assessing cortical dysfunction through activities of daily living*, St Louis, 1990, Mosby.
6. Ayres AJ: *Development dyspraxia and adult onset apraxia*, Torrance, Calif, 1985, Sensory Integration International.
7. Baggerly J: Sensory perceptual problems following stroke, *Nurs Clin North Am* 26:997, 1991.
8. Ben-Yishay Y, Piasetsky EB, Rattok J, editors: *A systematic method for ameliorating disorders in basic attention*, New York, 1987, Guilford Press.
9. Bonfils KB: The Affolter approach to treatment: a perceptual-cognitive perspective of function. In Pedretti LW, editor: *Occupational therapy: practice skills for physical dysfunction*, St Louis, 1996, Mosby.
10. Borst MJ, Peterson CQ: Overcoming topographical orientation deficits in an elderly women with a right cerebrovascular accident, *Am J Occup Ther* 47:551, 1993.
11. Bruce MA: Cognitive rehabilitation: intelligence, insight, and knowledge. In Royeen CB, editor: *AOTA self-study series: cognitive rehabilitation*, Rockville, Md, 1994, American Occupational Therapy Association.
12. Calvanio R, Levine D, Petrone P: Elements of cognitive rehabilitation after right hemisphere stroke, *Behav Neurol* 11:25, 1993.
13. Cermak SA et al: Effects of lateralized tasks on unilateral neglect after right cerebral vascular accident, *Occup Ther J Res* 11:271, 1991.
14. Condeluci A, Ferris LL, Bogdan A: Outcome and value: the survivor perspective, *J Head Trauma Rehabil* 7:37, 1992.
15. Cooke D: Remediation of unilateral neglect: what do we know? *Aust Occup Ther J* 39:19, 1992.
16. Davis JZ: The Affolter method: a model for treating perceptual disturbances in the hemiplegic and brain-injured patient, *Occup Ther Pract* 3:30, 1992.
17. Dickerson AE, Fisher AG: Age differences in functional performance, *Am J Occup Ther* 47:686, 1993.
18. Duncombe LW, Howe MC: Group treatment: goals, tasks, and economic implications, *Am J Occup Ther* 49:199, 1995.
19. Edmans JA, Lincoln NB: Treatment of visual perceptual deficits after stroke: single case studies on four patients with right hemiplegia, *Br J Occup Ther* 54:139, 1991.
20. Edmans JA, Lincoln NB: Treatment of visual perceptual deficits after stroke, *Int Disabil Studies* 11:25, 1989.
21. Evans R: Family stroke education, *Occup Ther Health Care* 2:63, 1985.
22. Friedland J: Social support for stroke survivors: development and evaluation of an intervention program, *Phys Occup Ther Ger* 7:55, 1989.
23. Fanthome Y et al: The treatment of visual neglect using the transfer of training approach, *Br J Occup Ther* 58:14, 1995.
24. Guiles GM, Clark-Wilson J: The use of behavioral techniques in functional skills training after severe brain injury, *Am J Occup Ther* 42:658, 1988.
25. Hajek VE: The effect of visuo-spatial training in patients with right hemisphere stroke, *Can J Rehabil* 6:175, 1993.
26. Halligan PW, Cockburn JM: Cognitive sequelae of stroke: visuo-spatial and memory disorders, *Crit Rev Phys Rehabil Med* 5:57, 1993.
27. Helm-Estabrooks N, Emory P, Albert ML: Treatment of aphasic perseveration, *Arch Neurol* 44:1253, 1987.
28. Jabri J: Providing visuoperceptual remediation treatment for stroke patients in the home setting, *J Home Health Care Pract* 4:36, 1992.
29. Jarus T: Motor learning and occupational therapy: the organization of practice, *Am J Occup Ther* 48:810, 1994.
30. Jennett SM, Lincoln NB: An evaluation of the effectiveness of group therapy for memory problems, *Int Disabil Studies* 13:83, 1991.
31. Kageyama S et al: Neglect in three dimensions, *Am J Occup Ther* 48:206, 1994.
32. Katzmann S, Mix C: Improving functional independence in a patient with encephalitis through behavior modification shaping techniques, *Am J Occup Ther* 48:259, 1994.
33. King T: Treatment of visual inattention using computerized overhead projection, *J Cognitive Rehabil* 11:32, 1993.

34. Lin K, Cermak SA: Cognitive perceptual intervention in poststroke patients with unilateral neglect: an annotated bibliography, *Phys Occup Ther Ger* 10:63, 1991.

35. Lincoln NB: Stroke rehabilitation, *Curr Opin Neurol Neurosurg* 5:677, 1992.

36. Neistadt ME: Perceptual retraining for adults with diffuse brain injury, *Am J Occup Ther* 48:225, 1994.

37. Neistadt ME: The neurobiology of learning: implications for treatment of adults with brain injury, *Am J Occup Ther* 48:421, 1994.

38. Neistadt ME: A meal preparation treatment protocol for adults with brain injury, *Am J Occup Ther* 48:431, 1994.

39. Neistadt ME: Occupational therapy treatments for constructional deficits, *Am J Occup Ther* 46:141, 1992.

40. Nygard L et al: Comparing motor and process ability of persons with suspected dementia in home and clinic settings, *Am J Occup Ther* 48:689, 1994.

41. Olson E: Perceptual deficits affecting the stroke patient, *Rehabil Nurs* 16:212, 1991.

42. Papstrat LA: Outcome and value following brain injury: A financial provider's perspective, *J Head Trauma Rehabil* 7:11, 1992.

43. Park S, Fisher AG, Velonzo C: Using the assessment of motor and process skills to compare occupational performance between home and clinic settings, *Am J Occup Ther* 48:697, 1994.

44. Radomski MV: Cognitive rehabilitation: advancing the stature of occupational therapy, *Am J Occup Ther* 48:271, 1994.

45. Radomski MV: There is more to life than putting on your pants, *Am J Occup Ther* 49:487, 1995.

46. Radomski MV et al: Case studies in cognitive rehabilitation. In Royeen CB, editor: *AOTA self-study series: cognitive rehabilitation*, Rockville, Md, 1994, American Occupational Therapy Association.

47. Robertson I et al: Microcomputer-based rehabilitation for unilateral left visual neglect: a randomized controlled trial, *Arch Phys Med Rehabil* 71:663, 1990.

48. Robertson IH, North NT, Geggie C: Spatiomotor cuing in unilateral left neglect: three case studies of its therapeutic effects, *J Neurol Neurosurg Psychiatry* 55:799, 1992.

49. Toglia JP: Attention and memory. In Royeen CB, editor: *AOTA self-studies series: cognitive rehabilitation*, Rockville, Md, 1993, American Occupational Therapy Association.

50. Toglia JP: A dynamic interactional approach to cognitive rehabilitation. In Katz N, editor: *Cognitive rehabilitation: models for intervention in occupational therapy*, Boston, 1992, Andover Medical Publishers.

51. Toglia JP: Generalization of treatment: a multicontext approach to cognitive perceptual impairment in adults with brain injury, *Am J Occup Ther* 45:505, 1991.

52. Trombly C: Clinical practice guidelines for post-stroke rehabilitation and occupational therapy practice, *Am J Occup Ther* 49:711, 1995.

53. Warren M: Visuospatial skills: assessment and intervention strategies. In Royeen CB, editor: *AOTA self-study series: cognitive rehabilitation*, Rockville, Md, 1994, American Occupational Therapy Association.

54. Webster J et al: Wheelchair obstacle course performance in right CVA victims, *J Clin Exp Neuropsychol* 11:295, 1989.

55. Webster J et al: Visual scanning training with stroke patients, *Behav Ther* 15:129, 1984.

56. Wheatley CJ: Cognitive rehabilitation service provision: results of a survey of practitioners, *Am J Occup Ther* 48:163, 1994.

57. Yuen HK: Increasing medication compliance in a women with anoxic brain damage and partial epilepsy, *Am J Occup Ther* 47:30, 1993.

58. Zemke R: Task skills, problem solving, and social interaction. In Royeen CB, editor: *AOTA self-study series: cognitive rehabilitation*, Rockville, Md, 1994, American Occupational Therapy Association.

SUGGESTED READING

Allen CK, Earhart CA, Blue T, editors: *Occupational therapy treatment goals for the physically and cognitively disabled*, Rockville, Md, 1992, American Occupational Therapy Association.

Árnadóttir G: *The brain and behavior: assessing cortical dysfunction through activities of daily living*, St Louis, 1990, Mosby.

Davies PM: *Starting again: early rehabilitation after traumatic brain injury or other severe brain lesion*, Berlin, 1994, Springer-Verlag.

Katz N, editor: Cognitive rehabilitation: models for intervention in occupational therapy, Boston, 1992, Andover Medical Publishers.

Royeen CB, editor: *AOTA self-study series: cognitive rehabilitation*, Rockville, Md, 1994, American Occupational Therapy Association.

Enhancing Performance of Instrumental Activities of Daily Living

key terms

occupation
performance
disability

instrumental activities of daily
living (IADL)
Canadian Occupational
Performance Measure (COPM)

Assessment of Motor and
Process Skills (AMPS)

chapter objectives

After completing this chapter, the reader will be able to accomplish the following:

1. Understand the concept of instrumental activities of daily living.
2. Recognize the impact of a stroke on a person's engagement in instrumental activities of daily living.
3. Understand the relationship between the degree of impairment and performance of instrumental activities of daily living and implications for evaluation and intervention.
4. Discuss the occupational therapy evaluation process for performance of instrumental activities of daily living.
5. Discuss the Canadian Occupational Performance Measure and the Assessment of Motor and Process Skills.
6. Understand the basics of goal writing for performance of instrumental activities of daily living.
7. Understand the adaptive approach to occupational therapy intervention for instrumental activities of daily living intervention.

Rehabilitation is a restorative and learning process that hastens and maximizes a patient's functional recovery after a cerebrovascular accident (CVA) by treating the resulting impairments, disabilities, and handicaps.[15] For all rehabilitation professionals the main objective is to restore functioning so that a patient can return or continue to live in the community. All rehabilitation disciplines also focus on a patient's functional status as well as the functional status of the patient's family.* For occupational therapy practitioners, however, function must be defined from an oc-

Box 15-1

Instrumental Activities of Daily Living

HOME ENVIRONMENT

Meal preparation tasks

Planning snacks and meals
Gathering food and materials
Opening food containers
Preparing food
Using tools and appliances
Re-storing food and materials
Setting the table

General household chores

Handling garbage and recycling
Performing minor repairs
Watering lawn and plants
Shoveling snow
Raking leaves

Communication activities

Using the telephone
Handling mail
Writing letters
Using a computer

Miscellaneous tasks

Operating light switches
Opening doors and using keys
Operating television and stereo
Caring for animals
Watering houseplants

House-cleaning routines

Vacuuming rugs
Dusting furniture
Washing windows
Mopping floors
Washing dishes
Sweeping floors

Laundry tasks

Washing, drying, and folding clothes
Making the bed
Changing bed linens
Ironing clothes

Financial responsibilities

Paying bills
Balancing checkbook

Emergency procedures

Responding to a fire
Communicating an emergency

COMMUNITY ENVIRONMENT

Mobility

Riding a bus or subway
Taking a taxi
Driving a car

Shopping

Buying groceries
Buying clothes
Handling monetary transactions

cupational therapy perspective to differentiate their services from those of other rehabilitation professionals.[29] From an occupational therapy practitioner's perspective, *function* is defined as a person's occupation—the engagement in daily activities that are meaningful and purposeful, including self-care, vocational, educational, and play and leisure activities, as well as instrumental activities of daily living (IADL).[2,6,11,28] Thus the main role of occupational therapy practitioners working with patients who have had a stroke is to facilitate the restoration of the ability to engage in daily occupation successfully so that the patient can return or continue to live in the community.[29] A patient's dysfunction in daily occupation—also termed *disability* (i.e., a restriction in or inability to perform daily life tasks)[44]—is the main focus of occupational therapy practitioners.

CVA AND INSTRUMENTAL ACTIVITIES OF DAILY LIVING

For patients who have had a stroke, a return to independent living in the community requires the ability to perform not only basic self-care tasks but also IADL tasks.[15]

Leslie Duran is gratefully acknowledged for her feedback and assistance throughout the preparation of this chapter. Appreciation for their assistance also is extended to Sally Huffman; Kathryn Kafalias; Stan Neiderhouse; Rehabilitation Institute of Oregon, Portland; and Eugene Good Samaritan Health Center, Eugene, Ore.
*The term *family* refers to all members of a patient's close-knit social group, which may include a spouse, a partner, relatives, and friends.

IADL are the more complex daily tasks that must be performed for the patient to continue living in the community. IADL do not include basic self-care tasks[15,20,33] (Box 15-1). IADL tasks are typically differentiated from play and leisure activities because the engagement in play and leisure, although important to a person's well-being, is not necessarily required for independent living in the community. Many patients who have had a stroke continue to engage in IADL despite the residual effects of the stroke. Studies performed in the United Kingdom indicate that many patients who have had a stroke achieve independence with the performance of various IADL tasks such as shopping, using public transportation, coping with money, ironing, hanging out the wash, making the bed, cleaning the house, and preparing a snack, hot drink, or meal.[9] However, more patients who have had a stroke attained independence with basic self-care tasks than with IADL tasks. The frequency of engagement in IADL tasks was significantly less than that before the stroke.[16] This trend is similar to one found in a study in the United States in which 1 year after a stroke, patients were generally sedentary, not involved in the routine care of the home, and isolated from friends and previous leisure activities.[39] Despite these discouraging findings, many patients who have had a stroke continue to engage in some IADL tasks as part of their daily occupations.

IADL require greater interaction with the physical and social environment and a greater degree of skill (e.g., problem-solving and social skills) than basic self-care tasks.[13,33,40] Therefore, any underlying impairments in a person's sensorimotor, cognitive-perceptual, or psychosocial capacity that may result from a CVA tend to affect the performance of IADL tasks to a greater degree than they affect basic self-care (Box 15-2). The presence of an impairment, however, is not predictive of a patient's level of performance of daily life tasks.[12,38] A Canadian study of patients with right- and left-side CVA[17] found that the ability to prepare a sandwich and cup of tea could not be accurately predicted from the extent of upper or lower extremity weakness, cognitive function, visuospatial abilities, somatosensory functioning, or motor planning dysfunction. A pilot study[35] investigated the meal-preparation skills (e.g., tuna salad or an omelette) of 10 ambulatory women with aphasia. No relationship was found between severity of aphasia and degree of cognitive-perceptual impairment, and all the women had retained some degree of meal-preparation skill. Indeed, 60% attained the highest rating for the meal-preparation task, indicating near-normal or independent performance.

Despite a tendency for persons with right-side CVA to have left inattention and visuospatial difficulties and for persons with left-side CVA to have apraxia and aphasia, the overall ability to perform daily living tasks may be similar for both types of patients.[3] IADL performance in patients with right- and left-side CVA revealed that the two groups did not differ significantly in their overall performance of IADL tasks despite the hemisphere-specific differences of their impairments. In other words, both groups were equally disabled with respect to performing IADL tasks.

OCCUPATIONAL THERAPY SERVICES FOR IADL PERFORMANCE

The critical issue with regard to the presence of underlying impairments resulting from a CVA and the performance of IADL tasks is whether occupational therapy intervention for a disability in IADL performance should be focused directly on improvement of a patient's underlying impairments. If a patient's IADL performance cannot be predicted from the degree of the impairment, changing a person's degree of impairment may not automatically improve IADL performance. Furthermore, other rehabilitation professionals focus their expertise on underlying impairments to reduce the degree of impairment and enhance functional status.[29] For example, a neuropsychologist addresses cognitive-perceptual function to formally evaluate the degree of a patient's left visual inattention. The presence of an underlying impairment is of concern to an occupational therapy practitioner when considering intervention for IADL performance, but the effect of an underlying impairment on a patient's ability to perform IADL tasks directs evaluation and intervention strategies.

Self-care and functional mobility are the most common variables used as outcome measures in studies of persons

with CVA.[17] These variables also reflect the intervention strategies commonly used by occupational therapy practitioners. In a survey of occupational therapy directors in adult physical rehabilitation facilities across the United States, the 10 most frequently used intervention activities, ranked in order of frequency, were the following[27]:

1. Self-care
2. Upper extremity exercise
3. Functional mobility
4. Neuromuscular function
5. Homemaking
6. Cognitive and perceptual training
7. Community living skills
8. Physical agent modalities
9. Sensory reeducation
10. Assistive technology

Because upper extremity exercise was ranked the second most common intervention strategy used by occupational therapy practitioners and homemaking and community living skills were ranked fifth and seventh, respectively, occupational therapy practitioners may not be doing enough to prepare their adult patients for successful reintegration to the community and should reorder their intervention priorities accordingly.[27] Meal preparation has been recommended for inclusion in rehabilitation intervention for stroke patients, particularly those with meal-preparation responsibility, because engagement in meal-preparation

Box 15-2

Potential Effect of Impairments on IADL Tasks Compared with Self-Care Tasks

- Paralysis of the arm may create more difficulty in opening a can of soup than in buttoning a shirt.
- Weakness in the leg may severely limit bending down to secure tools on a lower shelf in the garage but may be adequate to don a pair of slacks.
- Postural insecurity may result in a greater risk for injury when sweeping the floor than when standing to perform grooming tasks.
- Aphasia may make shopping for groceries at the local store more difficult than eating a meal at home.
- Visual inattention to the environment may make locating needed items in a kitchen more difficult than locating meal items on a table.
- Poor tactile sensation in the hand may lead to safety concerns about using knives to prepare vegetables for a meal but not about using a knife to butter toast for breakfast.
- Depression resulting from the stroke experience may decrease the patient's motivation and desire to engage in more complex IADL tasks that may seem overwhelming in their performance demands and energy requirements.

tasks may help foster a sense of usefulness and purpose, an important component of the rehabilitation process.[17,35]

In the inpatient rehabilitation setting, occupational therapy practitioners typically evaluate IADL tasks such as meal preparation at the end of a patient's rehabilitation stay (if at all)[17] and often after much emphasis and intervention has been directed at the performance of self-care tasks. Although the importance of enhancing a patient's level of performance in self-care tasks is not disputed, the amount of therapy time devoted to tasks that may involve only 1 or 2 hours of a patient's day is questionable, particularly because the patient has the rest of the day in which to occupy time meaningfully. Furthermore, some patients with physical impairments find that basic self-care tasks such as dressing and bathing are more difficult than some simpler IADL tasks such as getting a drink from the refrigerator or preparing a light snack.[10] Some patients who have had a stroke and their families may find more benefit in attaining independence in ADL tasks that are easy and more satisfying rather than concentrating on dressing or bathing independently.

Another issue arises when a patient has concluded inpatient rehabilitation and proceeds to outpatient or home health services, for which only a limited number of occupational therapy appointments may be reimbursed by a third-party payer. Given the growing presence of managed care, the length of stay is shorter for inpatient rehabilitation services and follow-up appointments for home health or outpatient services are frequently limited. The time frame under which the third-party payer will provide payment for services often affects the patient's desire and ability to reengage in desired daily life tasks. Patients who have had a stroke have commented that the stress of inpatient rehabilitation prevented them from benefiting completely from rehabilitation and that a period of time at home provided them with an opportunity to directly experience the ways the CVA had affected their lives.[39] These patients experienced renewed interest in improving skills and achieving independence in daily life tasks after time at home. Thus when stroke patients are motivated to enhance their skills, they may not be eligible to receive additional occupational therapy services.

Although engagement in daily activities may be dramatically different after a CVA, patients who have had a stroke clearly want and continue to engage in a variety of ADL despite the impact of the CVA. The role of the occupational therapy practitioner is to facilitate the patient's continued participation in meaningful and purposeful daily activities and adaptation to the changed status.[7-9] Ultimately, however, the quality of the patient's life is of the utmost importance. Occupational therapy practitioners who work in rehabilitation settings should not limit evaluation and intervention strategies to a patient's proficiency with basic self-care tasks or upper extremity function. They must expand the possibilities and assist each patient in engaging in an array of activities that will bring personal satisfaction.[32]

REHABILITATION EVALUATION PROCESS FOR IADL

Depending on the area of expertise, each rehabilitation professional fulfills a unique role during the evaluation process. For IADL tasks, however, patients are evaluated from a discipline perspective. Physical therapists may focus on a patient's ability to safely walk during IADL tasks such as riding the bus and watering the lawn. Social workers may focus on securing services to carry out IADL tasks if a patient is limited in the ability to perform these tasks and family members cannot take over the responsibility for them.

Despite the need for all rehabilitation professionals to focus on IADL tasks, appropriate standardized assessment tools with which to evaluate IADL performance are lacking.[10] Often the available assessment tools reflect the focus of a specific discipline and are therefore inappropriate for use by other rehabilitation professionals. Few self-care or IADL assessment tools were designed specifically for occupational therapy practitioners and based on an occupational therapy frame of reference.[18] Most IADL assessment tools have involved a self-report format—that is, the patient or a family member is asked a series of questions about a variety of IADL tasks that a patient is likely to be required to engage in at home. The Frenchay Activities Index,[16] developed in the United Kingdom, is a self-report assessment tool originally developed to gather information on the premorbid lifestyle of patients who have had a stroke and to record changes in the frequency of engagement in IADL tasks after a CVA. The assessment comprises 15 questions to which a person responds, using a 4-point scale to rate the frequency of engagement for each activity. The assessment, however, does not exclusively examine IADL tasks; leisure and vocational activities are also included (Figure 15-1). The accuracy of self-report assessment tools has been questioned, however.[4,34] Although self-report assessment tools may be useful in determining the need for support services and tracking a change in the level of IADL engagement, a self-report IADL assessment tool does not address reasons a person is unable or unwilling to engage in an IADL or the quality with which a person performs an IADL.

The IADL Scale[22,23] also examines a person's engagement in IADL tasks (Box 15-3). However, this scale has been adapted to be used as a self-report questionnaire and an observation of performance. The assessment comprises eight items that address a person's ability to use the telephone, shop, prepare food, perform housekeeping, do laundry, use public transportation, manage medications, and handle finances. Each task is rated on a 4-point scale of the level of assistance required and the quality of the performance. Again, the assessment does not identify the reasons a person may be experiencing difficulty with the performance of a particular IADL and is limited by the number of IADL tasks addressed. Little information is available regarding the use of the IADL Scale in the CVA population.[15]

Although these and similar IADL assessment tools can be valuable during the rehabilitation process to assess general outcomes and determine a need for support services, their utility is limited for occupational therapy practitioners. The main reason CVA patients are receiving occupational therapy services for IADL performance is that they have become disabled (i.e., a restriction in or ability to perform daily life tasks[44]) and they demonstrate the potential to become more able to perform IADL tasks.[29] For occupational therapy practitioners the evaluation process should focus on the abilities of the patient, as well as the disabilities. They should rely on their expertise and skills in observing IADL performance during the evaluation process and, when appropriate, use IADL assessment tools

---

During previous 3 months

Activity	Code
___ Preparing main meals	1 = Never
___ Washing up	2 = Under once weekly
	3 = 1-2 times a week
	4 = Most days
___ Washing clothes	1 = Never
___ Performing light housework	2 = 1-2 times in 3 months
___ Performing heavy housework	3 = 3-12 times in 3 months
___ Local shopping	4 = At least weekly
___ Going on social outings	
___ Walking outdoors for 15 minutes	
___ Pursuing active interest in hobby	
___ Driving a car or travelling on bus	

During previous 6 months

Activity	Code
___ Going on outings or car rides	1 = Never
	2 = 1-2 times in 6 months
	3 = 3-12 times in 6 months
	4 = At least weekly
___ Gardening	1 = Never
___ Maintaining household or car	2 = Light
	3 = Moderate
	4 = All necessary
___ Reading books	1 = None
	2 = 1 in 6 months
	3 = Less than 1 a fortnight (every 2 weeks)
	4 = More than 1 a fortnight (every 2 weeks)
___ Performing gainful work	1 = None
	2 = Up to 10 h/week
	3 = 10-30 h/week
	4 = More than 30 h/week

Total _____ : Factor 1 _____ , Factor 2 _____ , Factor 3 _____

Figure 15-1 Activities Index. (Modified from Holbrook M, Skilbeck CE: *Age Ageing* 12:170, 1983.)

Box 15-3

Instrumental Activities of Daily Living (IADL) Scale

A. Ability to use telephone
   1. Operates telephone on own initiative—looks up and dials numbers, etc.
   2. Dials a few well-known numbers.
   3. Answers telephone but does not dial.
   4. Does not use telephone at all.
B. Shopping
   1. Takes care of all shopping needs independently.
   2. Shops independently for small purchases.
   3. Needs to be accompanied on any shopping trip.
   4. Completely unable to shop.
C. Food preparation
   1. Plans, prepares, and serves adequate meals independently.
   2. Prepares adequate meals if supplied with ingredients.
   3. Heats and serves prepared meals, or prepares meals but does not maintain adequate diet.
   4. Needs to have meals prepared and served.
D. Housekeeping
   1. Maintains house alone or with occasional assistance (e.g., "heavy work—domestic help").
   2. Performs light daily tasks such as dishwashing, bed-making.
   3. Performs light daily tasks but cannot maintain acceptable level of cleanliness.
   4. Needs help with all home maintenance tasks.
   5. Does not participate in any housekeeping tasks.

E. Laundry
   1. Does personal laundry completely.
   2. Launders small items—rinses socks, stockings, etc.
   3. All laundry needs must be done by others.
F. Mode of transportation
   1. Travels independently on public transportation or drives own car.
   2. Arranges own travel via taxi, but does not otherwise use public transportation.
   3. Travels on public transportation when assisted or accompanied by another.
   4. Travel limited to taxi or automobile with assistance of another.
   5. Does not travel at all.
G. Responsibility for own medications
   1. Is responsible for taking medication in correct dosages at correct time.
   2. Takes responsibility if medication is prepared in advance in separate dosages.
   3. Is not capable of dispensing own medication.
H. Ability to handle finances
   1. Manages financial matters independently (budgets, writes checks, pays rent, bills, goes to bank), collects and keeps track of income.
   2. Manages day-to-day purchases, but needs help with banking, major purchases, etc.
   3. Is incapable of handling money.

From Lawton MP, Brody EM: Assessment of older people: self-maintaining and instrumental activities of daily living, *Gerontologist* 9:181, 1969.

developed for use by occupational therapy practitioners.[29] In the evaluation of a patient's IADL performance, occupational therapy practitioners must also consider any underlying impairments the patient is experiencing (e.g., hemiparesis, apraxia, visual inattention) because the rehabilitation evaluation process is affected by the interactive relationship among the deficits, impairments, and disabilities of the patient.[15]

OT Evaluation Process for IADL Performance

As occupational therapy practitioners bring their expertise in occupation to the rehabilitation team, they should focus the evaluation process on a patient's ability to resume the performance of daily life tasks in the environments in which the patient lives, works, and plays.[29] Therefore the evaluation process should begin with a focus on the daily life tasks of concern to the patient and family.[11] In addition, if occupational therapy practitioners use evaluation strategies reflective of their unique perspective on function—occupation—patients, families, and other health care professionals more readily identify their expertise in the health care field.[10]

Occupational therapy practitioners are also committed to client-centered practice—that is, the patient's knowledge and experience of daily life after a CVA is of central concern in rehabilitation services. Occupational therapy practitioners are guided by an ethical commitment to listen and respond to a person's priorities with regard to meaningful and purposeful occupation in daily life.[2,5,29] A client-centered approach to occupational therapy intervention requires an occupational therapy practitioner to actively seek information of concern to the patient and family.[5] The rehabilitation evaluation process is best begun with an interview of the patient, family, or both to identify those specific concerns.

Interview Process for IADL Performance

Occupational therapy practitioners should initiate the interview process by soliciting information regarding the daily life tasks of concern, including any IADL tasks a patient would like to be able to perform. Many interview formats can be used to gather this information. An informal conversation is the most casual and is often effective. For a more in-depth analysis of a patient's perspective on ADL, an interview based on the model of human occupation can yield specific insight into the patient's values, interests, and sense of personal causation—as well as habits and roles—with respect to IADL tasks[19] (Box 15-4).

Box 15-4

IADL Interview Questions Based on the Model of Human Occupation

These questions are intended to guide an occupational therapy practitioner's clinical reasoning with regard to the type of information desired and are not intended to be asked of a patient.

VOLITION

Personal causation

- Which IADL tasks can the patient perform?
- Which IADL tasks or aspects can the patient perform well?
- Which IADL tasks or aspects is the patient unable to perform?
- Does the patient feel capable of performing IADL tasks or certain aspects?
- What IADL tasks would the patient like to be able to perform?
- What prevents the patient from performing the desired IADL tasks?

Values

- What are the patient's values with respect to the ways IADL tasks should be performed?
- Is there a congruency between the patient's beliefs regarding the ways IADL tasks should be performed and their actual performance?
- Do family members support the patient's values regarding IADL performance?

Interests

- Are there IADL tasks in which the patient experiences pleasure, satisfaction, or investment?
- Are there IADL tasks from which the patient has a special source of motivation or joy?

HABITUATION

Habits

- What is the patient's daily routine, and are any IADL tasks an established part of this routine?
- What is the routine for the completion of IADL tasks within the home?

Roles

- What are the patient's current roles, and do any of these roles include a responsibility for IADL tasks?
- How important to the patient are the roles that entail a responsibility for IADL tasks?
- Which family members or other persons have assumed the roles that entail responsibility for IADL tasks in the household?

Mind-Brain-Body Performance

- What physical, emotional, or cognitive experiences are troubling for the patient with regard to IADL tasks?

Modified from Kielhofner G, Mallinson T, de la Heras CG: Methods of data gathering. In Kielhofner G, editor: *A model of human occupation: theory and application*, Baltimore, 1995, Williams & Wilkins.

During the interview process an occupational therapy practitioner should also gather information regarding the environment in which a patient will be performing IADL tasks.[29] Such an interview entails soliciting information about the physical layout of the home, particularly the kitchen. *A Consumer's Guide to Home Adaptation*[1] contains a framework with which to guide an interview focused on the patient's home environment. The information in this booklet details the types of daily life tasks that persons with disabilities are likely to engage in in their home and provides questions about tasks that are likely to be difficult. The booklet also provides information on home modifications and adaptations (see Chapter 20).

Canadian Occupational Performance Measure

One standardized interview format that is very useful in the evaluation process is the Canadian Occupational Performance Measure (COPM).[21] The COPM was developed from a client-centered perspective and can be used with anyone experiencing difficulty with the performance of daily activities, regardless of diagnosis or impairment. The COPM guides the occupational therapy practitioner through a semistructured conversation to identify the activities that the patient wants, needs, or is expected to do in

daily life and to identify problems or difficulties with those activities. The COPM also focuses on the patient's perception of the importance of performance of, and satisfaction with the identified activities of concern.

The format of the COPM guides the occupational therapy practitioner to ask questions about the person's engagement in daily activities, soliciting information about the person's morning-to-afternoon-to-evening routine. The COPM comprises six topic areas: (1) personal care, (2) functional mobility, (3) community management, (4) paid/unpaid work, (5) active recreation, and (6) socialization. The COPM also focuses intervention on the person's goals.

■

CASE STUDY*

KL, a 54-year-old woman, experienced visual blurring and partial left-side paralysis. She was taken to the hospital by her husband, where she was admitted and subsequently given the diagnosis of right-side CVA and moderate left-side hemipare-

*Modified from Park S, Duran L: AMPS intervention in rehabilitation settings. In Fisher A, editor: *AMPS intervention manual*, Fort Collins, Col, Three Star Press (in press).

sis. She stayed in the hospital for 6 nights. During her stay, KL rapidly made progress, spontaneously regaining much physical and cognitive-perceptual function, although the residual effects from the CVA were still apparent at discharge on day 7. Starting on the fourth day of her acute care hospitalization, she received physical therapy to evaluate her safety when walking. The physical therapist determined that although KL's gait pattern had some minor irregularity, she did not require a cane or walker. However, the physical therapist was concerned with the continued paresis of her left arm, mild left visual inattention, and short-term memory deficits. He recommended that she walk with supervision when outdoors and that she undergo outpatient physical therapy to address her irregular gait and improve overall physical function. Although the initial impact of the CVA had resolved substantially and KL was essentially independent in performing basic self-care tasks (the nursing staff having recommended supervision and adaptive equipment for bathing), her neurologist questioned her ability to safely engage in household tasks and community activities. Therefore he recommended to KL and her husband that she be supervised throughout the day and that she avoid more complex activities such as cooking and community outings. To further address the residual effects of the CVA, particularly the visual and cognitive issues of KL's ability to live safely in the community, the neurologist recommended that she receive outpatient occupational therapy.

KL went to her first outpatient occupational therapy appointment 16 days after the CVA. Her occupational therapist began the initial interview with a casual conversation, during which she gathered some general information about KL's role in the family and community and the impact of the stroke on KL's life, particularly the recommendation that she be supervised throughout the day. During this initial 20-minute conversation, the therapist realized the importance of KL's desire to resume her previous activities, particularly those associated with her role as a wife, mother, grandmother, homemaker, and hobbyist. The therapist also realized that KL was very unhappy with the prospect of continued supervision during the daytime. To further explore these areas of concern and gather more specific information about KL's perception of her ability to engage in self-care, work, and leisure activities, the occupational therapist chose to use the COPM to identify the specific activities of primary concern.

The occupational therapist explained the purpose of the COPM and then began by asking KL questions about the activities of her morning routine since her discharge from the hospital. She then continued with questions about other activities that KL wanted to or did engage in during the afternoon and into the evening. Throughout the interview, the therapist asked KL which activities she found difficult or was unable to do. By the end of the interview, KL had identified the six activities most important to her: (1) changing the bed, (2) preparing meals, (3) setting and combing her hair, (4) assisting her younger children with their homework, (5) sewing, and (6) playing with her grandchildren (Figure 15-2).

After hearing KL elaborate on the activities she identified during the interview, the occupational therapist realized that two of the activities of concern—changing the bed and meal preparation—were activities that she was not engaging in on the recommendation of the neurologist. KL had said that she did not feel physically capable of playing with her grandchildren and feared she might drop them. As for helping her children with their homework, KL believed she wasn't "smart enough now" because she occasionally became confused during conversations with her children. Finally, KL said she was frustrated with combing and setting her hair because "it just doesn't turn out the way it did before the stroke." This information from the COPM set the stage for the occupational therapist to begin identifying performance skills that would support KL's performance in daily life tasks and which performance skills might be limiting or preventing her participation in desired activities.

■

Observation of IADL Performance

Whether a formal or an informal interview procedure is used, the occupational therapy practitioner should continue the evaluation process with an observation of a patient performing some IADL tasks of concern.[29] Observation of such performance (as well as performance of other ADL) is an important component of every evaluation process, particularly because one valuable contribution the occupational therapy practitioners provide for the rehabilitation team is an evaluation of the ability to safely perform daily life tasks desired by or required of the patient to return and live safely in the community.[29]

The occupational therapy practitioner should not proceed with a direct evaluation of the degree of a patient's impairments such as muscle strength, mental status, and depression.[30] Patients with CVA may initially experience a multitude of underlying impairments such as hemiparesis, left visual inattention, aphasia, and hemianopsia. Direct measurement of the severity of these underlying impairments, however, does not provide the occupational therapy practitioner with the information necessary to determine the way the patient will perform IADL tasks. The interplay of a patient's impairments in the context of IADL performance and the environment in which those tasks are performed is the main focus of the occupational therapy practitioner.[29] Therefore impairments resulting from a CVA are best observed and evaluated in the context of a patient's task performance.[30,33] Occupational therapy practitioners should use evaluation procedures that capture the full spectrum of a patient's IADL performance ability and should limit evaluation procedures that address a patient's cognitive, sensorimotor, and psychosocial function.[29] This evaluation strategy reflects a "top-down" approach in which an occupational therapy practitioner begins with an evaluation of a patient's ability to perform daily life tasks

STEP 1A: Self-Care		IMPORTANCE
Personal Care (e.g., dressing, bathing, feeding, hygiene)	STYLING & COMBING HAIR	8
	TIME TO GET DRESSED	6
Functional Mobility (e.g., transfers, indoor, outdoor)	GETTING UP SAFELY FROM BATHTUB	8
Community Management (e.g., transportation, shopping, finances)	DRIVING	10

STEP 1B: Productivity		
Paid/Unpaid Work (e.g., finding/keeping a job, volunteering)	ASSISTING KIDS WITH HOMEWORK	10
Household Management (e.g., cleaning, doing laundry, cooking)	CHANGING SHEETS	9
	PREPARING MEALS FOR FAMILY	10
	FOLDING TOWELS	2
Play/School (e.g., play skills, homework)		

STEP 1C: Leisure		
Quiet Recreation (e.g., hobbies, crafts, reading)	SEWING	8
	NEEDLEPOINT	5
	MAKING X-MAS WREATHS	5
Active Recreation (e.g., sports, outings, travel)	PLAYING WITH GRANDKIDS ON THE FLOOR	9
	BOWLING	4
Socialization (e.g., visiting, phone calls, parties, correspondence)		

Figure 15-2 Results from KL's interview using Step 1 of the COPM. (Modified from Law M et al: *Canadian Occupational Performance Measure*, Toronto, 1994, CAOT Publications ACE.)

(the top) rather than beginning with an evaluation of a patient's underlying impairments (the bottom).[41]

Assessment tools with which to evaluate a patient's performance should evaluate a wide range of activities in the environment, and their use should permit systematic monitoring of progress throughout a patient's rehabilitation.[15] Many self-care and IADL assessment tools, however, have limitations: many (1) are not sensitive to a change in patients with high levels of functional disability, (2) fail to detect improvements in specific activities, and (3) fail to identify the effects of specific underlying impairments or diseases on the patient's performance. The Assessment of Motor and Process Skills (AMPS)[10] is one assessment tool for occupational therapy practitioners that reflects the recommendations for the use of assessment tools in rehabilitation.

Assessment of Motor and Process Skills

The AMPS is a client-centered, task-oriented performance assessment of a person's disability in IADL performance and not the person's underlying impairments.[3,10] It was developed specifically for use in OT and has been standardized internationally and cross-culturally on more than 7000 people. The AMPS tests the ability of a person to perform IADL tasks and the quality of efficiency with which the person performs the tasks. Although the AMPS does not directly measure a person's underlying impairment, its use does help clarify whether underlying impairments are influencing the ability to effectively perform IADL tasks and at what point in the performance the impact from the impairment may be occurring.[3] The AMPS can be used with any person who (1) desires to perform, even if at a marginal level, simple daily living tasks; (2) has at least assisted mobility; and (3) is familiar with at least two of the AMPS tasks.[10] Moreover, the AMPS is not restricted to any specific diagnosis and has been used extensively with persons with CVA.

The AMPS requires no specialized equipment and can be conducted in any IADL-relevant setting within 60 minutes. The occupational therapy practitioner who uses the AMPS must attend a 5-day AMPS training course to become certified in its use.* For the assessment the person chooses two or three IADL tasks that are culturally appropriate, familiar, and relevant to daily life. The choices range from simple to complex meal-preparation tasks such as getting a drink from the refrigerator and preparing juice and cereal to preparing a tossed salad or an omelet, toast, and a beverage, and from simple to complex household tasks such as folding laundry and washing dishes to vacuuming a rug or changing sheets on a bed (Box 15-5). The IADL choices also reflect various cultural backgrounds and include tasks reflecting American, British, Hispanic, and

Scandinavian cultures. The AMPS-trained occupational therapy practitioner ensures that the tasks chosen by the person are sufficiently challenging so that the practitioner can observe the ability to perform IADL tasks and note any difficulties. The task is performed in the person's usual manner to discern the natural ability to perform such tasks.[10]

Because the AMPS is a standardized measurement tool, to evaluate a person's performance accurately, an AMPS-trained occupational therapy practitioner must compare the performance against the criteria for the specified task.[10] For example, one task choice is to prepare scrambled eggs, toast, and a beverage. According to the criteria for this AMPS task, the person should use one or two eggs to make the eggs, use two slices of bread with one spread to prepare the toast, and pour a glass of juice or milk or a cup of coffee. The person prepares the eggs in a skillet or frying pan on a stove and uses a standard toaster or toaster oven. Finally, the person serves the eggs, toast, and beverage in appropriate dishes at a counter or table and restores the workspace to its original condition.[10] No restrictions are placed on the way the task should be performed. The person is free to choose any method that accomplishes the objective of the specific AMPS task.

Box 15-5

Task Choices in the Assessment of Motor and Process Skills

MEAL-PREPARATION TASKS

Drink from the refrigerator
Toast and boiled or brewed coffee or tea
Peanut butter and jelly sandwich
Luncheon meat or cheese sandwich
Fried ripe bananas (*plátanos*)
Grilled cheese sandwich and beverage
Juice and cold cereal
Beans and toast
Tossed salad and dressing
Eggs, toast, and Cuban coffee
Tea or coffee with cookies
French toast and beverage

HOUSEHOLD CHORES

Sweeping the floor
Making a bed
Ironing a shirt
Repotting a plant
Changing sheets on a bed with a duvet
Hand-washing dishes
Folding laundry
Vacuuming
Setting a table

From Fisher AG: *Assessment of motor and process skills*, Fort Collins, Col, 1995, Three Star Press.

*Both occupational therapists and occupational therapy assistants are eligible to become certified in the use of the AMPS.

After observation of a person's IADL performance, the occupational therapy practitioner rates the performance on 16 motor and 20 process skill items (Box 15-6). Motor skills are observable actions a person uses to move the body or objects during all task performance. Process skills are observable actions a person uses to sensibly organize and adapt the actions of task performance as the process unfolds over time. Process skills include actions that determine (1) what tools and materials are used by the person, (2) how the tools and materials are used during task performance, and (3) when, where, and how those actions occur to effect logical and competent task performance. Process skills also include actions that determine a person's effectiveness in overcoming any problems encountered during task performance or compensating for any underlying sensorimotor or cognitive-perceptual impairments possibly affecting the efficiency of IADL performance.[10]

Process skills should not be equated with a person's cognitive capacity, such as attentional, memory, motor planning, and problem-solving skills. Cognitive skills reflect the person's underlying capacity for performance (i.e., the mind-brain-body system in the model of human occupation) and support the way a person organizes and adapts actions during task performance.[10] For example, the ability to gather tools and materials to a workspace requires many underlying cognitive skills such as attentional, memory, and problem-solving skills. These cognitive skills, however, are not directly observed during IADL performance. What is observed while a person gathers tools and materials is the behavioral output (occupational performance) of the person's underlying capacity (cognitive skills). Similarly, motor skills (as defined in the AMPS) also reflect the behavioral output of a person's underlying motor capacity and should not be equated with traditional motor skills such as muscle strength, range of motion, postural control, and motor planning.[10]

Because motor and process skills are observable actions expressed in the context of occupational behavior, each skill item is evaluated in terms of the way it contributes to the logical progression and outcome of task performance.[10] Thus each motor and process skill item is rated on a 4-point scale, in which 4 is competent, 3 is questionable, 2 is ineffective, and 1 is deficit. The person is rated on the competency of performance in each skill item. For example, an inpatient rehabilitation patient is shown to have moderate hemiparesis of the right upper extremity and a mild motor planning deficit as on a standardized assessment of impairment. An AMPS-trained occupational therapy assistant observed the patient preparing a grilled cheese sandwich for an AMPS assessment and scored this performance according to the criteria and examples in the AMPS manual. During the task, the patient was readily and consistently able to locate the needed tools and materials in the familiar occupational therapy clinic kitchen and thus received a score of 4 (competent performance) on the skill item *search/locates*. The patient received a score of 3 (questionable performance) on the process skill item *chooses* because the occupational therapy assistant questioned the appropriateness of using a steak knife to effectively spread butter on a piece of bread. The patient received a score of 2 (ineffective performance) on the motor skill item *manipulates* because of difficulty manipulating the twist-tie for the bag of bread, which was dropped on the counter two times. Finally, the patient received a score of 1 (deficit performance) on the motor skill item *grips* because the package of cheese being grasped in the patient's right hand fell to the floor. "Well" persons are also expected to occasionally receive a score of 2 or even 1 on a few skill items. The AMPS does not have a ceiling for motor or process skill abilities. Thus the AMPS detects a change in ability even in persons with higher functional abilities who still experience some difficulty with IADL performance.[10]

Once the items are scored for each task, the results are entered in the AMPS computer scoring program.[14]* The computer analysis of the motor and process skill scores results in motor ability and process ability measurements. The ability measurement represents the placement of the person on a continuum of motor or process ability.[10] Per-

Box 15-6

Motor and Process Skills

MOTOR SKILLS	PROCESS SKILLS
Stabilizes	Paces*
Walks	Uses
Coordinates	Inquires
Moves	Sequences
Calibrates	Gathers
Paces*	Navigates
Aligns	Adjusts
Reaches	Attends
Manipulates	Handles
Transports	Initiates
Grips	Terminates
Positions	Organizes
Bends	Notices/responds
Flows	Benefits
Lifts	Chooses
Endures	Heeds
	Continues
	Searches/locates
	Restores
	Accommodates

From Fisher AG: *Assessment of motor and process skills*, Fort Collins, Col, 1995, Three Star Press.
*Paces is considered both a motor and a process skill.

*The AMPS computer scoring program is available only to occupational therapy practitioners who have completed the 5-day AMPS training course.

sons with higher motor ability measures are more skilled in their ability to move themselves and objects during task performance, and persons with higher process ability measures are more skilled in their ability to sensibly organize and adapt the actions of task performance to achieve an effective outcome. Because the AMPS is a sensitive measurement tool, any change in the ability of a person to perform IADL tasks results in a change in the person's process or motor ability measure, or both. Therefore the AMPS is ideally suited to evaluate a change in IADL performance resulting from occupational therapy intervention.[10]

The measurement model used to develop the AMPS and analyze a person's motor and process skill scores also accounts for (1) the relative challenge of each task the person performed and (2) the severity of the AMPS-trained rater who observed and scored the person's task performance.[10] Thus no matter which tasks a person chooses to perform for the assessment, the resulting motor and process ability measures are adjusted accordingly. Further, no matter which occupational therapy practitioner scores the person's task performances, the motor and process ability measurements are adjusted accordingly. Impartiality is particularly useful if rehabilitation patients are receiving services on a continuum of care; a patient's progress with IADL performance can be objectively measured throughout service delivery if AMPS-trained occupational therapy practitioners work within the various programs.

The administration of the AMPS, however, does not conclude with the computer generation of the motor and process skill ability measures. The occupational therapist or occupational therapy assistant (in collaboration with an occupational therapist) must still interpret the ability measures and the specific motor or process skill item scores in light of other information the practitioner has gathered about the person to use the results of the AMPS to plan occupational therapy intervention.*

■

CASE STUDY—CONT'D†

At the conclusion of the COPM interview with KL during her first outpatient appointment, her occupational therapist learned that the activities of primary concern to her were (1) changing the bed, (2) preparing meals, (3) setting and combing her hair, (4) assisting her children with their homework, (5) sewing, and (6) playing with her grandchildren. She learned that KL was concerned with the recommendation that she not engage in complex household or community activities and with being supervised during the day. (Her sister-in-law was staying with KL

---

*Basic self-care tasks are now included in the AMPS.
†Adapted from Park S, Duran L: AMPS intervention in rehabilitation settings. In Fisher A, editor: *AMPS intervention manual*, Fort Collins, Col, Three Star Press (in press).

while KL's husband worked.) However, the occupational therapist needed more objective information to begin intervention planning. Rather than informally observe KL using the stove in the occupational therapy clinic, her occupational therapist wanted to use the AMPS to evaluate KL's IADL performance ability and solicit objective evidence to determine whether KL was indeed safe in staying home alone and engaging in more complex IADL tasks. She also wanted to determine how KL's underlying impairments (partial paralysis of the left arm, mild left visual inattention, and mild short-term memory deficits) might be affecting KL's performance. The occupational therapist asked KL whether she would be willing to perform some IADL tasks during the second outpatient appointment so that she could observe KL's performance, and KL agreed.

To conclude KL's first outpatient appointment, her occupational therapist conducted a 10-minute AMPS interview following the interview guidelines as detailed in the AMPS manual. After this interview, KL chose to perform two tasks for the AMPS: (1) changing standard sheets on a freestanding bed and (2) preparing scrambled eggs, toast, and a beverage. During the interview, the occupational therapist ensured that these tasks were familiar to KL; that they would be of sufficient challenge to her, given the mild residual effects of her right-side CVA; and that they were appropriate for the occupational therapy clinic. The occupational therapist stressed that because this was a formal assessment, she and KL needed to agree to specific criteria for each task as specified in the AMPS manual. To prepare eggs, toast, and a beverage, KL understood and agreed that she would use two eggs, adding some milk, salt, and pepper; two slices of whole wheat bread with margarine for the toast; and a glass of orange juice. She also understood she was to serve the eggs, toast, and orange juice at the table and clean her workspaces but that she did not have to wash dishes or utensils. In changing the sheets, KL understood and agreed that she was to remove the blanket, bedspread, sheets, and pillowcases; replace the sheets and pillowcases with clean sheets from the closet; place the blanket and bedspread on the bed; and dispose of the soiled sheets and pillowcases in the laundry hamper.[10] Although KL's occupational therapist stressed that these conditions had to be met, she also stressed that KL could perform the tasks in her usual manner, using the tools, materials, and methods she preferred. During the AMPS interview process, the occupational therapist also determined which tools and materials KL would like to use during the assessment—particularly in preparing the eggs, toast, and beverage in the kitchen—to ensure that all needed tools and materials would be available during the second appointment when KL would be performing both IADL tasks.

When KL returned 2 days later for her second outpatient appointment, the occupational therapist explained the assessment procedures again and oriented KL to the kitchen and bedroom. Although these tasks were familiar to KL, she had not performed them in the outpatient clinic and the occupational therapist wanted to ensure KL knew where all the needed tools and materials were in the kitchen and how the stove and toaster worked. She even asked KL to place needed tools and materials in locations in the kitchen approximating their locations in KL's home. To further approximate KL's home environment, her occupational therapist ensured that extra tools and materials, such as various cookware items, dishes, utensils, and food items, were stocked in the kitchen. After ensuring that KL was fully oriented to the kitchen, her occupational therapist began the assessment by stating, "You agreed to prepare scrambled eggs, using two eggs, milk, salt and pepper; two pieces of toast, using whole wheat bread and margarine; and a glass of orange juice and to serve it at the counter. Please leave your workspace as you found it; however, you do not need to wash the dishes. If you have any questions, please feel free to ask. When you are finished, just let me know."[10]

KL then proceeded to prepare the eggs, toast, and beverage while her occupational therapist observed her performance and took notes to refer to in scoring the performance (Figure 15-3). KL finished the task in approximately 12 minutes, after which she took a 5-minute coffee break while her occupational therapist scored her task performance on the 16 motor and 20 process skill items. Then the occupational therapist gave her the instructions for the second task—changing the sheets—which KL performed while her occupational therapist again observed her performance. KL took approximately 8 minutes to complete this task. Afterward, her occupational therapist again scored KL's performance. After the completion of both tasks, KL and her occupational therapist discussed KL's perception of her performance, particularly with reference to awareness of safety issues. KL reported that she felt she was safe in using the stove and that her performance was fairly good because the eggs and toast were edible. KL did note her frustration at feeling slow and awkward while changing the sheets. The occupational therapist said she also believed KL's use of the stove was safe but that she would have more information after the results of the AMPS were entered in the computer scoring program. She also promised KL that she would share those results with her during the next appointment.

Because the occupational therapist did not have a formal assessment tool with which to observe the other activities of concern to KL (sewing, setting and combing her hair, assisting with her children's homework, playing with her grandchildren), she asked KL if she could observe her engaging in sewing and setting and combing her hair during the third appointment. On the basis of the information she gained by observing KL perform the two AMPS tasks, however, the occupational therapist believed she had some good information regarding KL's motor and process skill abilities and that she could not only conduct an informal evaluation of these activities but begin intervention to address KL's concerns.

Later that afternoon, the occupational therapist entered the scores from both task performances into the computer scoring program. The AMPS Graphical Report showed KL's motor ability measure was 0.9 and her process ability measure was 1.2 (Figure 15-4). KL's motor ability measure reflected that she experienced some mild difficulty in (1) positioning her body appropriate to the task, (2) coordinating her arms to stabilize task objects, (3) manipulating task objects with her left hand, (4) executing smooth and fluid left arm and hand movements, (5) lifting heavy objects, (6) calibrating the force and extent of her left arm movements, and (7) gripping objects with her left hand. KL's motor ability score of 0.9 indicated she would probably need some physical assistance to live in the community; 83% of all persons with a motor ability measure of 2.0 or lower require some kind of assistance.[10] Despite KL's diminished motor ability to move herself and objects, her actions did not place her at risk for injury or a fall, and she was successful in achieving the desired outcome—preparing a meal with the use of a stove and changing the sheets on a bed. The occupational therapist reasoned that given KL's current motor abilities, KL possessed the skills to engage in a variety of activities despite the impact of the CVA. In fact, the therapist reasoned that continual engagement in various activities throughout KL's day would help improve her overall motor ability.

When the occupational therapist interpreted KL's process ability measure, she was encouraged by the results. This measure of 1.2 indicated that she probably required only minimal assistance to live in the community; only 7% of all persons who receive a process ability measure of 1.0 or higher require some level of assistance to live in the community.[10] During both AMPS tasks, KL demonstrated good awareness about avoiding injury or damage, and her occupational therapist reasoned that given KL's current ability to organize and adapt her actions over time, KL would not be at great risk for an accident during household chores and meal-preparation tasks. This did not mean KL's task performance was flawless. She did experience some mild difficulty in (1) choosing the tools and materials need for the tasks (e.g., she did not choose orange juice for eggs, toast, and beverage and she chose extra pillows from the closet when changing the sheets), (2) heeding the goal of the task (e.g., she did not serve orange juice with the eggs and toast), (3) logically sequencing the steps of the task (e.g., she prepared the eggs and then had to wait for the bread to be toasted), and (4) restoring tools and materials (e.g., the margarine was not returned to the refrigerator). These problems also suggested KL was experiencing some mild difficulty accommodating her actions to overcome problems, although minor ones, as they arose during her IADL performance. Her occupational therapist reasoned, however, that these issues were not related to an underlying impairment of KL's judgment but more to her mild memory deficit. The occupational therapist also reasoned that although KL had demonstrated mild left visual inattention during a neurologic examination performed by her neurologist, this residual impairment did not appear to affect her performance during the assessment.

Given the objective results of the AMPS and the information she gathered during the initial interview, from a review of KL's medical chart, and from a discussion with KL's physical therapist, the occupational therapist was confident that KL could begin to initiate and independently perform some IADL tasks

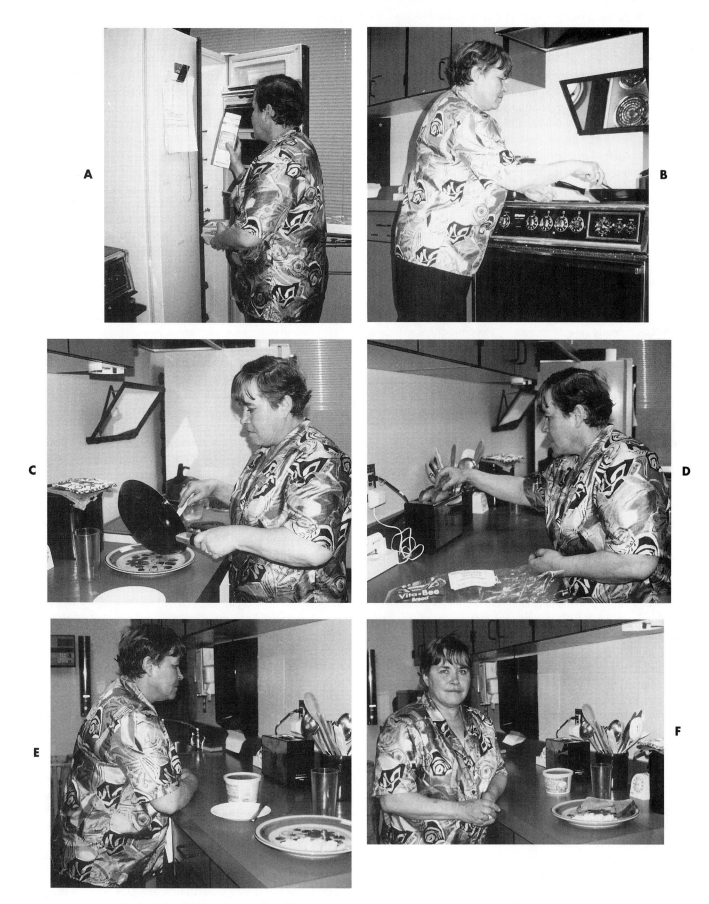

Figure 15-3 Performing the task of preparing eggs, toast, and a beverage for the AMPS. **A,** *Choosing* needed items for the task. **B,** Ineffective *positioning* of self; standing too far away to stir eggs. **C,** *Coordinating* two body parts in the same action. **D,** *Initiating* a step of the task. **E,** Ineffective *sequencing* of steps for task results in a delay. **F,** Ineffective *heeding* of the task goal; no orange juice was served.

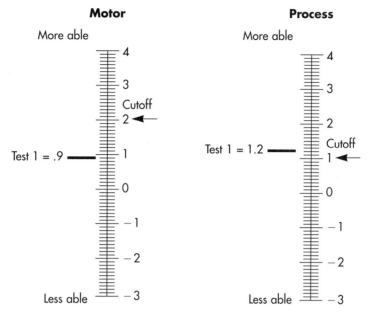

Figure 15-4 Computer-generated graphic report of KL's AMPS results. AMPS motor and process ability measures are plotted in reference to AMPS scale cutoff values that indicate problems affecting performance.

at home on a trial basis. The occupational therapist called KL's neurologist, shared the results of her evaluation, and indicated that she would work with KL and her husband to set up a trial program at home, gradually expanding KL's repertoire of independent activities. When KL returned for her third outpatient appointment, her occupational therapist shared the results of the AMPS and her professional opinion of KL's ability to begin engaging independently in home and community activities. Although the issue of community activities remained to be explored, KL and her occupational therapist developed a plan for reengagement in favorite home activities and set goals to mark KL's progress toward a return to safe, independent living in the community.

■

GOAL-SETTING FOR REHABILITATION INTERVENTION

Thorough, consistent, well-documented evaluation procedures at each stage of a patient's rehabilitation are critical in guiding a professional's clinical reasoning to establish realistic rehabilitation goals, plan interventions, and monitor a patient's progress.[15] After a rehabilitation professional has conducted a thorough evaluation that reflects the professional's area of expertise and focuses on the areas of concern to the patient and family, the patient, family, and rehabilitation team members should collaborate to establish goals for the current phase of the patient's rehabilitation. The goals should be agreed on by the patient, the family, and the rehabilitation professionals and should be

clearly understood by the patient and family.[15] If a patient and family members do not understand the rehabilitation goal, the goal is probably not appropriate or should be defined in functional terms that the patient and family members understand and find meaningful.

One current concern in the rehabilitation setting is that professionals may not be considering the patient's personal goals when planning intervention.[25,28,38] Evidence suggests more effort could and should be made to promote more collaboration between patients and rehabilitation professionals in the development of goals. If rehabilitation professionals agree to realistic goals that are important and meaningful to the patient and they make a concerted effort to initiate intervention directly related to those goals, the professionals provide a purposeful experience that is immediately relevant to their patients' lives.[24] Rehabilitation goals should be realistic in terms of the patient's current level of ability (or disability) and potential for recovery from the CVA.[15] Rehabilitation professionals should collaborate with the patient to develop goals for which the professionals can use their expertise to facilitate the accomplishment of those goals. Each rehabilitation professional possesses skills unique to the discipline, and depending on the goals of the patient, a particular professional may be more suited to facilitate the accomplishment of a patient's goal. For example, if a patient with severe right leg hemiplegia decided the most important goal was to walk independently, a physical therapist would be the most qualified rehabilitation professional to collaborate with the patient and determine whether this goal was realistic. Finally, goals should be documented in explicit, measurable terms so that they serve as yardsticks by which to measure whether a patient is benefiting from rehabilitation services.[15]

Goal-Setting for Occupational Therapy Intervention

For occupational therapy practitioners, the process of establishing goals begins with the initial interview, which focuses on daily life tasks of concern to the patient and family. No matter the stage of rehabilitation (inpatient, outpatient, or home health), the initial interview should always address the daily life tasks of concern to the patient, including IADL tasks when appropriate. The opportunity for any patient with a CVA to pursue enhanced quality of performance or independence with IADL tasks should always be available.

To ensure that IADL goals are both measurable and essential, occupational therapy practitioners should include a description of the patient's baseline performance and the reasons the patient is experiencing difficulty[30] (Table 15-1). This is typically a description of a patient's impairments and the effect of those impairments on the patient's performance. "Patient will safely and independently prepare a simple lunch using the stovetop" is an appropriate IADL goal. Before the inclusion of this goal in the documentation, the occupational therapy practitioner should state the patient's baseline performance for that goal: for example, "Patient is unsafe and requires moderate verbal supervision when preparing a simple meal in the kitchen as she demonstrates postural insecurity when ambulating, placing her at mild risk for a fall. She also is at a mild risk for injury as a right visual field cut is impacting her effec-

tiveness and safety when searching for and locating objects in the kitchen." The goal is compared with the patient's baseline IADL performance at admission to determine whether the patient is benefiting from rehabilitation intervention. For example, if the occupational therapy practitioner failed to document that the patient required moderate supervision during meal-preparation tasks and was at risk for a fall or an injury, there would be no baseline by which to "measure" whether the patient had reduced the risk of a fall or injury or required less supervision when preparing a simple lunch using the stovetop. Even though the patient's risk for a fall or an injury might have been reduced substantially by discharge and the patient was now able to perform simple meal-preparation tasks safely and without supervision, the patient's actual progress would be unsubstantiated.

To establish that the goals are realistic, occupational therapy practitioners should also include information regarding a patient's current capacities and abilities. For example, to justify the goal, "Patient will safely and independently prepare a simple lunch using the stovetop," the occupational therapy practitioner should document that the patient demonstrates a capacity to learn new skills and an awareness of postural insecurity and is cognitively capable of recognizing and responding to obvious safety hazards in the kitchen in the intact visual field. The inclusion of such information establishes that the patient is capable of benefiting from rehabilitation services and shows that goals are realistic and obtainable.

Typically, IADL goals are written to reflect the level of physical or verbal assistance a patient will receive while

Table 15-1

IADL Baseline Performance and Goals

BASELINE PERFORMANCE	GOAL
• Patient requires *moderate physical assistance* to prepare a breakfast and is at *mild risk* for injury because of ineffectiveness in retrieving, transporting, and organizing needed items.	• Patient will *independently and safely* prepare a light breakfast.
• Patient requires *moderate verbal cueing* to set the table because of left inattention to the environment.	• Patient will *independently* and correctly set table for dinner, requiring *no verbal cueing*.
• Patient experiences *moderate difficulty* when vacuuming because of *ineffective* capacity to move vacuum and furniture resulting from poor motor planning capacity.	• Patient will experience only *minimal difficulty* with vacuuming, demonstrating ability to *effectively* move vacuum and furniture.
• Patient is *unsafe* when washing windows because of poor judgment, which places the patient at risk for a fall.	• Patient will *safely* and *independently* wash indoor windows.
• Patient displays *poor ability* to use a computer keyboard because of incoordination resulting from a severe right arm tremor.	• Patient will be *able to effectively* use a computer keyboard to write a one-page letter.
• Patient is *unable* to operate light switches on wall because of inability to reach and grasp switches when sitting in a wheelchair.	• Patient will be *able to independently* operate light switches on the wall.
• Patient requires *moderate verbal assistance* to ride the bus because of poor ability to plan route and communicate needs during trip.	• Patient will ride the bus to the local post office, requiring only *minimal verbal assistance*.

Italicized words reflect baseline performance and the next level of ability the patient is expected to achieve.

performing a task. However, a patient may be able to perform an IADL task independently, requiring no physical or verbal assistance but still have unacceptable quality of performance.[30] For example, although a patient may be physically independent when washing dishes, observation of the performance indicates a concern with (1) safety (e.g., a plate was dropped on the floor but did not break), (2) efficiency (e.g., 20 minutes was required to wash 10 items, and obvious signs of fatigue were present), and (3) the degree of difficulty encountered (e.g., significant incoordination resulted in substantial motor effort to reach, grasp, move, manipulate, and place objects during the task). The goal that focused on washing dishes would need to reflect an improvement with the level of safety or efficiency or a reduction in difficulty. For example, a goal such as, "Patient will safely wash dishes, experiencing only minimal difficulty," would be appropriate only if the patient's baseline performance clearly established a lack of safety for the patient when washing dishes and moderate difficulty with the task; reasons for the difficulty should also be included. The occupational therapy practitioner must describe the patient's current performance difficulties in terms of safety, efficiency, and degree of difficulty to establish that the goal reflects an improvement in the quality of the patient's performance and not just a reduction in the level of assistance.

Goals specific to occupational therapy should also reflect the unique perspective of occupational therapy—that is, a patient's occupational performance, which is not the perspective of other professionals.[30] For example, a goal such as "Patient will achieve 120 degrees of shoulder flexion to place objects in upper kitchen cabinets" is not an appropriate IADL goal. The statement "Patient will achieve 120 degrees of shoulder flexion" reflects a framework based on physical movement.

IADL goals should not describe the type of intervention the occupational therapy practitioner intends to use to achieve the goal.[30] From the previous example, the statement "Patient will achieve 120 degrees of shoulder flexion to place objects on upper kitchen cabinets" reflects the occupational therapy practitioner's intervention strategy; that is, the plan to focus on improving the patient's underlying muscle strength to enhance the patient's active range of motion. If the goal is to place items on upper kitchen cabinets (a reflection of the patient's actual IADL performance), a variety of interventions are available with which to achieve this goal, not just to enhance the patient's active range of motion. An appropriate IADL goal in this example would be "Patient will safely and easily place objects in upper kitchen cabinets." Such goals reflect the daily life tasks that patients perform, the expected outcome of occupational therapy intervention.

Concern exists that including goals reflecting IADL performance will not be honored by third-party payers. Under Medicare, Part A, guidelines, if a home health occupational therapy practitioner documents that a patient is experiencing problems with IADL tasks and fails to document that the patient also is experiencing problems with basic self-care tasks, the occupational therapy services may not be eligible for reimbursement because the documentation suggests the patient is not "disabled enough" to be considered homebound.[37] A similar situation also may occur in the inpatient rehabilitation setting. Thus if the goals solely reflect a patient's performance with IADL tasks to the exclusion of basic self-care tasks or other activities of daily living, some difficulty with reimbursement for occupational therapy services may occur. This typically, though, is not an issue for outpatient settings.

REHABILITATION INTERVENTION FOR IADL

The patient and family members must be actively involved in all stages of recovery.[15] The intervention plan and goals should incorporate the role of the patient in the family constellation. If a patient's prior role responsibilities included home and community IADL, the rehabilitation team should encourage the family to involve the patient in the process of deciding to whom these responsibilities should be delegated. Many times a patient derives great satisfaction from engaging in an IADL with the assistance of family members or other individuals even though independent performance is not possible. For example, although a patient may not be able to independently prepare a batch of her grandson's favorite cookies because of mild impairment in motor planning, she may be able to assist her son with parts of the task.

The rehabilitation team should also ensure that family members continue to maintain their roles in the family despite any new caregiving responsibilities that may be required. Assuming the role of a caregiver and taking over household chores and responsibilities can be stressful, and the rehabilitation team should not assume that all family members are capable of performing the IADL tasks that the patient previously performed. Rehabilitation professionals must be aware of the shifting roles and responsibilities in the family and actively work with the family to manage their new roles and responsibilities (see Chapter 25).

Occupational Therapy Approaches for IADL Intervention

Intervention strategies used by occupational therapy practitioners for patients with CVA tend to fall in two categories: (1) a remedial approach, in which a practitioner focuses intervention on the patient's underlying capacity (e.g., active range of motion, memory skills, motor planning, visual attention) necessary to perform functional activities, and (2) an adaptive approach, in which a practitioner focuses intervention on the patient's ability to perform a specific activity.[26,27] The use of a remedial approach assumes that targeting a specific underlying impairment (e.g., visual inattention to the left environment) and focusing intervention on enhancing the patient's underlying capacity (e.g., attending and responding to visual stimuli in the left environment during visual training exercises) will be transferred to other activities in which the patient engages during the day and will result in overall improved performance of daily activities (see Chapter 14).

In contrast, the use of an adaptive approach assumes that patients have difficulty transferring learning across activities. For example, an adaptive approach for a patient with visual inattention of the left environment assumes that improving the patient's ability to visually locate a moving target on a computer screen will not transfer well and will not improve the ability to visually locate a family member walking in a grocery store. Consequently, occupational therapy practitioners who follow an adaptive approach believe intervention should be focused on the skilled practice of the specific daily life tasks of concern to the patient and that this will promote independent living.[26] Because the skills and knowledge being taught during rehabilitation should be meaningful to the patient,[15] an adaptive approach directly relates the patient's goals to the intervention strategy and is particularly relevant as patients understand their disabilities in terms of the precipitating event and their ability to function.[27]

When implementing an adaptive approach, an occupational therapy practitioner may consider three aspects to promote a patient's IADL performance: (1) modifying the task, (2) modifying the method of accomplishing the task, and (3) modifying the environment[40] (Table 15-2). Modifying the task entails changing the performance requirements such that the overall objective of the task remains the same but the performance demands are better matched

to the patient's abilities. For example, a home health patient with substantial right hemiparesis and low endurance wanted to shop for clothes but knew a trip to the local department store was not feasible. The occupational therapy assistant suggested that the patient consider sending away for some catalogs from which to shop. The occupational therapy assistant has modified the task of shopping such that the performance demands of shopping for clothes (in this case, by catalog rather than at the store) match the patient's current abilities. When modifying a task, an occupational therapy practitioner assists a patient in identifying those tasks that can be performed.

In contrast, modifying the method of accomplishing the task requires that a patient learn new ways of performing the same task. In other words, the characteristics of the task remain the same, but the way the patient performs the task is adapted. For example, a 58-year-old patient receiving outpatient services was experiencing a memory impairment that affected his role as a father. He wanted to be able to call and talk with his three sons and two daughters, all of whom lived out of state, but he was embarrassed because he occasionally forgot to whom he was talking and often could not remember the significant events that he wanted to share with his children. The occupational therapist worked with him to develop a new routine in which he would write each of his children's names on a piece of paper and below each name those significant events he wanted to share. When he made a phone call, the name at the top of the page reminded him to whom he was talking and the notes below helped him remember what he wanted to say. In essence, the task of calling and carrying on a con-

Table 15-2

Adaptive Approaches to Intervention for IADL Performance

MODIFYING THE TASK	MODIFYING THE METHOD	MODIFYING THE ENVIRONMENT
Problem: Difficulty Manipulating Objects When Preparing Breakfast (Because of Diminished Physical Capacity)		
Use filters that are prepackaged with coffee rather than coffee grounds that must be scooped from a can.	Slide utensils to edge of the counter so that the handle may be grasped rather than attempt to use fingers to pick up utensils from a flat surface.	Purchase large clips to seal bread bags rather than use small store fasteners.
Problem: Difficulty Sequencing Actions When Preparing Breakfast (Because of Diminished Cognitive Capacity)		
Prepare only simple breakfasts such as cold cereal or frozen breakfast entrees rather than breakfasts that require extensive cooking.	Learn a routine to gather items first and organize them on the counter before initiating food preparation rather than approaching task without a plan.	Post written instructions on the wall above the stove that describe steps to prepare scrambled eggs rather than attempt to remember the sequence of steps.

Modified from Trombly CA: Retraining basic and instrumental activities of daily living. In Trombly C, editor: *Occupational therapy for physical dysfunction*, Baltimore, 1995, Williams & Wilkins.

versation remained the same, but the strategy required him to learn and implement a new method when making a telephone call. When considering modifying the method of the way a task is accomplished, an occupational therapist also considers a patient's capacity to learn and adapt actions to new performance demands.

Modifying the environment entails making some change in the physical or social environment to facilitate the patient's performance of the task. Suggesting modifications to the home for improved accessibility is an example of modifying the physical environment to enhance a patient's performance. The use of adaptive equipment, such as one-handed can openers and over-the-stove mirrors, is an aspect of modifying the environment—specifically, the tools and materials with which to perform the task. Modifying the social environment entails bringing another person into the environment whose presence can facilitate the person's performance. For example, a patient with moderate hemiparesis was receiving outpatient occupational therapy services in which she was focusing on preparing meals for her family. She reported to her occupational therapist that the one aspect of meal preparation she could not do at home was using the built-in microwave above the stove. The occupational therapist and patient discussed and tried various ideas, all of which were rejected by the patient as too costly (e.g., remodeling the kitchen) or too difficult (e.g., lifting the food items with a reacher adapted to hold microwave containers of food). In the end, the occupational therapist suggested that perhaps the patient needed to get assistance from one of her family members when she needed to use the microwave. Although the patient was initially reluctant, she also realized that, of the suggestions, this was the most reasonable. Through further discussion with the occupational therapist, she recognized that she did not have to perform all tasks independently to retain her sense of competency and worth within the family.

Modifying the task, modifying the method of accomplishing the task, and modifying the environment are not mutually exclusive approaches. Using a long-handled duster (i.e., modifying the environment) when cleaning furniture also may entail a patient learning a new one-handed technique (i.e., modifying the method). Preparing cereal and juice for breakfast rather than eggs, toast, and coffee (i.e., modifying the task) also may require that needed items be placed on shelves within easy reach (i.e., modifying the environment). Taking a taxi rather than a bus to the local grocery store (i.e., modifying the task) also may entail a patient learning a new routine to pay the cabdriver, such as calling ahead, asking for the fare, and then placing the money in a shirt pocket for easy access (i.e., modifying the method). No matter which aspect of adaptation an occupational therapy practitioner considers, however, the capability of the patient is always the focus.

When suggesting adaptive approaches for IADL performance, occupational therapy practitioners should be aware that suggestions are most effectively made in a way that promotes discussion between the patient and the practitioner and that promotes the creation of a variety of options from which to choose.[42] Of particular concern is the issue that learning new methods of performing tasks may compete with previous habits and preferences of performance.[42] For example, an occupational therapist working in home health suggested to a patient with significant right arm hemiparesis that she use a wheeled cart to transport dishes from the kitchen to the dining room table. This suggestion was met with considerable resistance by the patient because she insisted that the cart would be too complicated to use and that it would take up too much room in the kitchen. Considering the patient's preference for the way she believed the task should be performed, the patient and occupational therapist devised an alternative method whereby the patient was able to transport the dishes to the counter, then to a side table, and then to the dining room table.

Another issue to consider is that any new method of performing tasks must be reinforced in the patient's home environment,[42] particularly if the tasks are learned in an inpatient rehabilitation setting. Without the assistance of family members to reinforce and assist with the new methods, the emotional and cognitive demands of changing performance, transferring new methods of performance from the clinic to the home, and developing new patterns of performance in the home may be more difficult.[42] Finally, when occupational therapy practitioners make suggestions about adaptations to the home environment, these suggestions must incorporate not only the physical layout of the home but the patient's current ability, personal feelings about the home adaptations, and the possible impact of adapting the home on family members.[42]

Occupational therapy practitioners should be cautious when extrapolating a patient's IADL performance in the rehabilitation setting to the home.[15] Intervention strategies that rely on adapted methods of performance only work if the patient is also taught the way to adapt performance in a variety of environments. If a patient is only taught the way to make meals using a microwave oven in the rehabilitation clinic and will be using a stovetop and oven at home to prepare meals, the patient may not be able to generalize the information unless the occupational therapy practitioner has focused on the patient's skill in adapting performance to different environments. Conversely, a patient may have difficulty mastering simple meal preparation in the outpatient occupational therapy clinic because of its unfamiliarity, but adaptive skills in performing the same meal-preparation activities at home may be more apparent in the familiar environment.[43] Some objective evidence exists that older adults perform better at home with regard to adaptive strategies when performing IADL tasks, although this has not been confirmed for persons with CVA.[31] The specific setting of the intervention should also be conducted in as realistic a context as possible. For example, although practicing the component tasks of meal preparation such as cutting vegetables and opening cans of food is feasible in a dining room with just a table and the appropriate utensils, the same room would not be a realistic context in which to prepare a sandwich and a can of soup for lunch. IADL intervention, particularly when focusing on the patient's efficiency and safety during performance, should be conducted in as realistic a context as possible to recreate the rich complexity of options available when the patient is performing IADL tasks in a naturalistic environment.

A potential conflict may exist for occupational therapy practitioners who use an adaptive approach, particularly when providing services in inpatient settings for patients newly diagnosed with CVA. Some rehabilitation professionals recommend that adaptive devices be used only if other methods of performing the task are not available or cannot be learned.[15] They also assert that a patient mastering a method of performing the task without the use of adaptive devices will experience greater flexibility, satisfaction, and independence. From an occupational therapy perspective, the belief that adaptive devices should be a last resort is uncertain. Waiting to engage in certain activities until a patient's underlying impairments have improved or resolved can be discouraging for patients who want to begin engaging in specific activities. When adapting an activity to include the use of an adaptive device, an occupational therapy practitioner can facilitate a patient's ability to carry out an activity successfully, which may promote the patient's intrinsic recovery of underlying impairments.[7,8] For example, the use of a can opener designed for one-handed operation does not exclude the use of bilateral arm and hand movements. If movement is possible in the affected arm, a patient can and should use that movement when using the one-handed can opener. Thus the use of an adaptive device can help meet the goal of being able to open a can of food and promote a patient's intrinsic physical function at the same time. As such, occupational therapy practitioners should work closely with other rehabilitation professionals to explain their rationale for using an adaptive approach and should coordinate their intervention approach with other rehabilitation approaches.

On the basis of a recent review of rehabilitation outcome studies, evidence suggests that adaptive intervention approaches do improve a patient's performance of daily living tasks and level of independence and are more effective than remedial intervention approaches.[27] Occupational therapy practitioners focus on purposeful activities that have value and meaning as their "modality" of intervention and actively seek the engagement of the patient rather than a passive response.[7,8] A patient's engagement in meaningful occupation requires more than just the ability to regain and control movement after a CVA. It also requires interest, motivation, cognitive and perceptual function, and support of the patient's family and community. The

value of interventions for a patient's IADL performance that focus specifically on a patient's underlying motor impairments is questionable.[3] To limit the focus of intervention to a patient's motor performance limits the patient's chances of successfully engaging in desired IADL tasks on returning to the community. An adaptive approach that considers the sensorimotor, cognitive-perceptual, and psychosocial aspects of task performance, and the physical and social environments in which the task performance occurs is more consistent with the holistic philosophy of occupational therapy and more effective in assisting a patient in achieving desired goals in IADL performance.[27]

Use of the AMPS to Guide IADL Intervention

Assessment tools are valuable in assisting an occupational therapy practitioner in identifying the status of a patient's disability and can assist the practitioner in making decisions about intervention strategies. One distinct advantage of the AMPS is the generation of an objective measure of a person's motor and process skill ability (see Figure 15-4). This information allows the occupational therapy practitioner to determine whether a person appears to be experiencing greater difficulty with motor or process skills and to plan intervention accordingly. For example, if a person has a low motor ability measure but a high process ability measure, an occupational therapy practitioner should consider whether the person could use these process skills to work around limitations of motor skills.[30] Conversely, if a patient has a low process ability measure and the occupational therapy practitioner believes little improvement is possible with a patient's underlying impairments and the person's potential for learning new skills is limited, the practitioner can consider focusing intervention on training a person's family to assist with and support the patient's IADL performance.[30]

An assessment tool, however, should provide more information that just a number. "To guide an intervention program, a tool should identify not only a patient's functional status, but also the specific factors that led to such a determination."[36] The AMPS reflects this principle because it assists an occupational therapy practitioner in focusing on the specific actions of task performance (i.e., the specific motor or process skills) with which a person is experiencing difficulty and also the relative competencies a person possesses with regard to performance.[30] To readily identify the motor and process skills that support or limit a person's IADL performance, the occupational therapy practitioner can examine the AMPS computer-generated report (Figure 15-5). Those motor or process skills that are effective for a person are identified as *adequate*, those skills that are relatively ineffective are identified as *difficulty*, and those skills that are particularly problematic are identified as *markedly deficient*.

No "recipe" exists that an occupational therapy practitioner can follow to determine which intervention

Client:	MR. STUART	**Therapist:**	
ID:	3597-34	**Gender:**	Male
Age:	80	**Evaluation Date:**	05/23/95

The Assessment of Motor and Process Skills (AMPS) was used to determine how MR. STUART'S MOTOR and ORGANIZATIONAL/ ADAPTIVE (process) capabilities affect MR. STUART'S ability to perform functional DAILY LIVING TASKS necessary for COMMUNITY LIVING. The tasks were chosen from a list of standard functional activities rated according to their level of complexity. MR. STUART chose to perform the following tasks that MR. STUART considered to be meaningful and necessary for functional independence in the community:

Task 1: F-2 Luncheon meat or cheese sandwich
Task 2: L-1 Folding a basket of laundry

The level of complexity of the tasks chosen was easier than average or average. Overall performance in each skill area is summarized below using the following scale: ADEQUATE SKILL: no apparent disruption was observed, DIFFICULTY: ineffective skill was observed, MARKEDLY DEFICIENT SKILL: observed problems were severe enough to be unsafe or require therapist intervention.

The following strengths and problems were observed during the administration of the AMPS:

Adequate = A   Difficulty = D   Markedly Deficient = MD

MOTOR SKILLS:

Skills needed to move self and objects

	A	D	MD
Posture:			
STABILIZING the body for balance		X	
ALIGNING the body in a vertical position	X		
POSITIONING the body or arms appropriate to the task		X	
Mobility:			
WALKING: moving about the task environment (level surface)		X	
REACHING for task objects		X	
BENDING or rotating the body appropriate to the task		X	
Coordination:			
COORDINATING two body parts to securely stabilize task objects			X
MANIPULATING task objects		X	
FLOWS: executing smooth and fluid arm and hand movements		X	
Strength and Effort:			
MOVES: pushing and pulling task objects on level surfaces or opening and closing doors or drawers		X	
TRANSPORTING task objects from one place to another		X	
LIFTING objects used during the task		X	
CALIBRATES: regulating the force and extent of movements		X	
GRIPS: maintaining a secure grasp on task objects		X	
Energy:			
ENDURING for the duration of the task performance		X	
Maintaining an even and appropriate PACE during task performance		X	

Figure 15-5 Computer-generated AMPS report. *Continued*

strategies will work best given the configuration of a person's motor and process skills.[30] The occupational therapy practitioner's clinical reasoning guides the practitioner to decide which intervention strategies will be used to assist a patient in achieving the stated IADL goals. The use of an adaptive approach, however, is highly recommended for use with the AMPS because the AMPS readily identifies those motor and process abilities that are relatively intact and applicable to daily life tasks.[30] For example, from a computer-generated report, an occupational therapy assistant learns that a person is relatively able to initiate the steps of a task without hesitation (the process skill termed *initiates*). Using the AMPS as a framework by which to guide intervention, the occupational therapy assistant can develop intervention strategies that present a comfortable challenge to the person and that requires competency in initiating the steps of a particular task. The recommendation is that the tasks to

PROCESS SKILLS:
Skills needed to organize and adapt actions to complete a task

	A	D	MD
Energy:			
Maintaining an even and appropriate PACE during task performance		X	
Maintaining focused ATTENTION throughout the task performance	X		
Using Knowledge:			
CHOOSING appropriate tools and materials needed for task performance		X	
USING task objects according to their intended purposes	X		
Knowing when and how to stabilize and support or HANDLE task objects		X	
HEEDING the goal of the specified task		X	
INQUIRES: asking for needed information	X		
Temporal Organization:			
INITIATING actions or steps of task without hesitation		X	
CONTINUING actions through to completion		X	
Logically SEQUENCING the steps of the task	X		
TERMINATING actions or steps at the appropriate time		X	
Space and Objects:			
SEARCHING for and LOCATING tools and materials		X	
GATHERING tools and materials into the task workspace		X	
ORGANIZING tools and materials in an orderly, logical, and spatially appropriate fashion			X
RESTORES: putting away tools and materials or straightening the workspace			X
NAVIGATES: maneuvering the hand and body around obstacles	X		
Adaptation:			
NOTICING AND RESPONDING appropriately to nonverbal task-related environmental cues			X
ACCOMMODATES: modifying actions to overcome problems			X
ADJUSTS: changing the workspace to overcome problems		X	
BENEFITS: preventing problems from reoccuring or persisting			X

Figure 15-5, cont'd   Computer-generated AMPS report.

be mastered by the persons are tailored to their abilities to avoid stress.[15] The use of the AMPS supports this principle because it helps the occupational therapy practitioner identify performance skills that a person possesses and skills that are more problematic.

Because the AMPS readily identifies the motor and process abilities that are difficult or markedly deficient for the person, the occupational therapy practitioner can develop intervention strategies to assist the person in (1) enhancing ability with a specific motor or process skill and (2) adapting to the diminished skill ability by using other motor or process skills.[30] For example, a person with poor postural control has difficulty stabilizing her body while sitting in a wheelchair during IADL task performance (the skill item termed *stabilizes*). The occupational therapist may consider intervention strategies that enhance the person's ability to stabilize her body or adapt to the loss of stability by using other motor or process skills. To enhance the person's ability to stabilize her body while seated in the wheelchair, an occupational therapist may consider adapting the wheelchair (i.e., modifying the environment) with a seating system that promotes greater stability after discussion with a physical therapy practitioner (see Chapter

19). To use the person's process skills to adapt to her diminished ability to stabilize her body, an occupational therapist might consider the implementation of a new strategy for the person to overcome her problem with instability (i.e., modifying the method of performance)—that is, she may need to learn to place the affected arm on the wheelchair armrest to adequately stabilize the trunk when reaching for objects with the unaffected arm. In either scenario, the occupational therapy practitioner is using an adaptive approach for intervention.

The use of the AMPS during intervention can also assist an occupational therapy practitioner in modifying a task, particularly when examining the relative demand of IADL tasks and attempting to find tasks suited to the person's current abilities. The 56 IADL tasks included to date in the AMPS manual have been analyzed and placed on a hierarchical scale from easier to harder for both motor and process abilities.[10] An AMPS-trained occupational therapy practitioner can readily identify which IADL tasks are easier (or harder) with respect to motor or process skills and begin IADL intervention with the tasks that present an appropriate challenge to the person's motor or process skill ability. For example, folding a basket of laundry is an easier than average task with respect to process skill ability than the task of preparing a fruit salad, which is a harder than average task.[10] For a person with diminished process skills, a more appropriate challenge is to begin IADL intervention with easier-than-average tasks, such as folding laundry, and the other IADL tasks that are found at this end of the AMPS task hierarchy. As a person improves IADL task performance, more challenging tasks may be identified from the AMPS task hierarchy. Because rehabilitation intervention may be guided by the level of task difficulty with less complex or demanding tasks addressed first so that a patient experiences success,[15] the AMPS is ideally suited to use during rehabilitation intervention. This assumes, of course, that a patient is interested in pursuing a variety of IADL tasks for intervention and sees the relevancy of the intervention tasks to stated goals.

Repetition and practice between training sessions when the patient is on the unit or at home is also recommended for patients with CVA.[15] Because the AMPS motor and process skills are universal skills that are used in all IADL task performances,[10] the skill items may be emphasized in a variety of tasks and contexts. For example, the motor skill termed *positions* is the action of positioning the body or arms appropriate to the task, including the wheelchair relative to the task demands. The occupational therapy practitioner and other rehabilitation team members or family members may focus on this skill during a variety of tasks, facilitating a patient's ability to position the wheelchair while retrieving a carton of milk from the refrigerator, wiping the dinner table, or making the bed. The motor skill *positions* is also used during the performance of self-care tasks and the occupational therapy practitioner may emphasize the repetition and practice of this skill during the morning self-care routine.

Finally, the AMPS may be given at any time during rehabilitation intervention and as often as warranted to determine whether a patient is making progress in IADL task performance. If a positive change occurs in a patient's motor or process ability measure, objective evidence is obtained that the patient is improving. The determination of a patient's progress, however, should not be based solely on the improvement in a patient's specific ability measure. The true benchmark by which progress should be judged is whether a patient is achieving the desired goals with regard to daily life tasks.[30]

■

CASE STUDY*

One morning, Stuart, an 80-year-old retired railroad mechanic and watch repairman, awoke to discover that he could not move his left arm and leg to get out of bed. His wife called for an ambulance, and on his arrival at the local hospital, Stuart

*Modified from Park S, Duran L: AMPS intervention in rehabilitation settings. In Fisher A, editor: *AMPS intervention manual*, Fort Collins, Col, Three Star Press (in press).

was found to have sustained a right CVA resulting in left hemiplegia. Initially, the impact of the right CVA was severe; Stuart experienced extensive hemiplegia on his left side, including facial paralysis, visual inattention to the left environment, and tactile inattention to the left side of his body. Over the next 5 days, Stuart's condition improved somewhat. He started to regain some movement in his left hip and knee, although his left arm remained flaccid, and his attention to the left side of his body improved. Stuart's medical team believed a course of rehabilitation would be beneficial; however, given their knowledge of Stuart's health before the CVA (diabetes mellitus, hypertension, mild chronic obstructive pulmonary disease [COPD], and glaucoma) and his premorbid activity level (fairly sedentary), they decided a course of rehabilitation at a local skilled nursing facility (SNF) was a better choice than transferring Stuart to the regional inpatient rehabilitation unit, located 80 miles away. Although Stuart expressed a strong desire to return home to live with his wife, the medical team was concerned that the couple had a limited community support system—a close friend who lived 6 blocks away and the manager of the assisted living complex where they lived. (Stuart and his wife had no children.) Although their friend and the manager volunteered to help out when Stuart returned home, the medical team was apprehensive about the success of this plan. They believed, however, that Stuart should remain in the community where he lived, and so plans were made for Stuart to undergo an anticipated 5-week stay on the skilled rehabilitation unit of a local nursing facility.

On Stuart's admission at the SNF, the occupational therapist and occupational therapy assistant working on the skilled unit received a referral accompanied by Stuart's medical history. After deciding to initiate the evaluation process with an interview, they scheduled a half-hour that afternoon for the occupational therapy assistant to interview Stuart. She planned to focus on Stuart's roles, routines, values, and interests with regard to his daily occupation, the environments in which he typically occupied his time, and his concerns with regard to the impact of the CVA on his daily life.

During the interview, the occupational therapy assistant discovered that Stuart lived in a small, rural town with his wife of 56 years. After his retirement from the railroad company in 1975, Stuart began a second career as a watch repairman. He and his wife managed a small repair shop for many years in the downtown shopping area of the town where they lived until his wife, because of frail health, could no longer assist with the business. Stuart reported that because his own health had been declining with the onset of diabetes mellitus, hypertension, mild COPD, and glaucoma, they subsequently sold the business and moved to an assisted-living complex where they would no longer be responsible for the upkeep of a home. Their mornings consisted of rising around 7 AM, dressing, eating a breakfast that Stuart generally prepared, and watching a favorite television program at 10 AM. Two or three times a week, Stuart also took a shower in the morning. After their favorite program, Stuart and his wife enjoyed playing cards or taking short walks on the grounds of the complex. Together,

Stuart and his wife prepared a light lunch, generally followed by a short rest. During the afternoon, Stuart and his wife completed light household chores such as general cleaning and laundry or pursued more sedentary leisure activities such as listening to the radio or reading large-print books from the local library. For the more demanding household chores, such as cleaning the bathroom and vacuuming, they used the services of a cleaning agency. Because dinner was provided in the complex's dining room, the evening was available for relaxation. Stuart and his wife often played cards again or watched television before retiring around 9 PM. Once a week, in the afternoon, the couple took a taxi to the local grocery store, although Stuart reported that this was becoming more difficult because his wife relied increasingly on the use of a wheelchair for community excursions. Finally, Stuart revealed that it was important for he and his wife to be together; although a neighbor and their close friend were looking in on his wife, Stuart believed her health would decline further if he was not at home with her.

The morning after the initial interview the occupational therapist continued the evaluation process with a performance assessment of Stuart's self-care skills. She discovered Stuart required maximal assistance in donning his underwear, pants, shoes, and socks because his left hemiplegia interfered greatly with his ability to transfer, stand, and move his body. With his T-shirt and button-down shirt, however, Stuart only required moderate assistance. When dressed and seated in a wheelchair, Stuart required minimal assistance with his grooming in front of a wheelchair-accessible sink, in addition to a few verbal cues to thoroughly shave the left side of his face and to comb the hair on the left side of his head. After Stuart's morning routine, his occupational therapist accompanied him to the dining hall, where she provided some physical assistance with Stuart's food preparation and a few verbal cues to draw Stuart's attention to food items located on the left side of his placemat.

Throughout the evaluation of Stuart's self-care skills the occupational therapist noted that Stuart was able to sit independently in the wheelchair, although his dynamic balance in reaching for items was poor. He required moderate assistance to stand, but he was capable of following her instructions to enhance his stability. She noted that Stuart displayed no movement in his left arm, although she did not observe any gross neglect of his arm or other parts of his body that might result in an injury. Throughout his morning routine, she observed that Stuart initiated many of the required steps, indicating he knew what needed to occur next, although he required overall minimal verbal assistance to improve the quality of his performance because his techniques to perform tasks one-handed were awkward. He also needed minor assistance to more quickly locate needed objects in his left visual field.

When the occupational therapist and occupational therapy assistant shared information from their sessions during their scheduled consultation time, they discovered that Stuart had voiced several concerns about going home. He believed it was important that he be able to help out around the house and

not just sit all day long. Although he knew he and his wife would need assistance when he was discharged, he did not want to move from his current apartment to have someone live with them. Therefore Stuart and his wife needed to be able to manage on their own at night and at least during part of the day. (The social worker had already discussed with Stuart the possibility of someone assisting with Stuart's morning self-care routine if necessary and to perform other necessary tasks.) Both occupational therapy practitioners realized that Stuart was frustrated with his dependence on others for his morning routine and his lack of engagement in activities with his wife. As Stuart had repeated to both of them, "It's just me and my wife," and he obviously missed spending time with her since his CVA, particularly because his wife was not able to make daily trips to the SNF as a result of her poor health. Stuart had also mentioned to the occupational therapy assistant that he was frustrated in not being able to call his wife on his own. When questioned further, Stuart said he often couldn't reach the telephone in his room, particularly from his bed, and he kept getting a wrong number or was disconnected.

After their discussion, the occupational therapist met briefly with Stuart in the afternoon to discuss potential goals. Stuart expressed an interest in being able to get ready in the morning with less assistance, to telephone his wife daily, to eat without anyone watching over him, and to play cards with his wife when she was able to make a trip to the SNF. To pursue more information on Stuart's performance skills, the occupational therapist asked Stuart whether she could observe him while he telephoned his wife in his room. Stuart agreed, and he proceeded to dial his home telephone number. The occupational therapist realized that Stuart was unable to locate and press the correct buttons. She wondered whether this was due to a problem with Stuart's vision or visual attention and made a mental note to pursue more information in his medical chart. She also observed Stuart did not have much difficulty using only his right arm and hand, although she did note the placement of the telephone in the room was not accessible when Stuart was in bed. When someone answered the telephone and Stuart realized it was not his wife, he abruptly hung up the phone. Before additional frustration set in, Stuart's occupational therapist dialed the number for him and left the room for a few minutes to allow Stuart to talk privately with his wife.

After Stuart finished his telephone call, his occupational therapist returned and asked Stuart to play cards to observe whether he experienced any difficulties. She explained that she was curious as to whether Stuart was experiencing difficulty with his vision and the best way for her to explore this further was to again observe Stuart while he engaged in an activity. She further explained that she had an adapted card holder that would allow Stuart to hold his cards without the use of his hands. Because Stuart's favorite game was double solitaire, he said a card holder would not be necessary, although he said he might be interested in the device for other games. During the 5-minute game of solitaire, the occupational therapist observed that Stuart did not readily notice cards to be played on the left as frequently as he noticed cards on the right. She made a mental note to seek a referral to an optometrist to obtain more information.

With the information from Stuart's medical chart and initial interview and observations of Stuart's morning self-care routine, use of the telephone, and playing of a game of cards, both occupational therapy practitioners had gathered enough information with which to write the initial occupational therapy evaluation. From that evaluation, the following goals were set for the next week: (1) patient will locate food items when eating a meal without verbal cueing, (2) patient will don underwear and pants with moderate assistance, (3) patient will don shirt with minimal assistance, and (4) patient will independently and successfully use the telephone in his room to call his wife daily. Both occupational therapy practitioners discussed the intervention plan for Stuart for the next week, which focused on the daily practice of the tasks Stuart valued—including a daily morning routine of dressing, grooming, and eating and practicing using the telephone in his room. They worked with Stuart twice a day and, as the week progressed, noted improvement with Stuart's self-care ability and his ability to use the telephone. This was due in part to the modifications made to Stuart's physical environment; they obtained a telephone with enlarged buttons and rearranged the placement of the telephone in his room for easier access. Stuart was becoming more competent in using the phone, and by the end of the week he was successfully calling his wife with no assistance.

After 10 days his occupational therapy practitioners began to address the other concerns Stuart had expressed—his desire to perform some IADL tasks so that he would not just sit around when he returned home. Stuart's physical capacity was improving; he now required only moderate to minimal assistance for dressing, and his visual attention to the left environment appeared to be improving. They decided that the occupational therapy assistant would administer the AMPS to not only gain some objective information regarding Stuart's ability to live independently in the community but further clarify Stuart's competencies and limitations with regard to the performance of IADL tasks.

After Stuart had spent 12 days in the SNF, his occupational therapy assistant conducted an AMPS interview in the morning. She knew the biggest challenge Stuart would face was his fairly limited physical capacity to perform IADL tasks. Although Stuart was fairly successful moving his wheelchair around the SNF, his endurance was poor, only limited movement was available in his left leg, and no movement had been observed in his left arm. She wanted to limit the AMPS task choices to those that would be easier than average with respect to motor abilities. The AMPS interview focused on the IADL tasks that Stuart had performed before his CVA and that currently were of concern to him with regard to living at home. On the basis of types of IADL tasks that Stuart had performed in the past and was willing to perform for the assessment, she offered five choices to Stuart: (1) folding a basket of laundry,

(2) getting a drink from the refrigerator, (3) preparing a meat sandwich, (4) polishing shoes, and (5) watering a plant. All the tasks, with the exception of preparing a meat sandwich, were easier than average with respect to motor skills.[10] Because Stuart was concerned about meals at home, he chose to prepare a meat sandwich; because his wife hated to fold the laundry and "someone had to do it," folding a basket of laundry was his second choice.

That afternoon, Stuart's occupational therapy assistant initiated the first AMPS observation. The SNF did not have a laundry room similar to the one in Stuart's complex, but Stuart said he and his wife occasionally folded the laundry at the dining room table in their apartment when the laundry room was crowded. The occupational therapy assistant determined that the best place for the assessment was in a dining hall free from distractions. Before having Stuart start the task, she again explained the task criteria and observed Stuart as he folded approximately 20 items of laundry. Stuart took almost 20 minutes to fold the basket of laundry and was visibly fatigued on completing the task. The occupational therapy assistant decided it would be better if Stuart waited until the next day to perform the second AMPS task. After Stuart returned to his room, she scored his performance.

The administration of the AMPS continued the next morning in a small kitchen on the rehabilitation unit, where Stuart prepared a bologna sandwich with mayonnaise and white bread. Before beginning the task, Stuart said he would use his wheelchair lap tray. Although the occupational therapy assistant was skeptical that Stuart would be able to maneuver his wheelchair and reach for objects in the kitchen, she allowed him to decide the way he would perform the task. She again observed Stuart; he took 17 minutes to prepare the sandwich. Although at times she was concerned about the risk for injury (e.g., Stuart used a paring knife to spread the mayonnaise), she did not intervene because she saw no obvious signs of imminent risk for injury and she wanted to evaluate Stuart's abilities with regard to the way he would perform the task, not how she believed it should be performed. Again, Stuart was fatigued at the end of the task and returned to his room for a rest. She scored his performance and entered his scores from both tasks into the AMPS computer scoring program.[14]

The results of the computer analysis were not surprising to Stuart's occupational therapy assistant. Stuart's motor ability measure of −1.0 was substantially below 2.0; 84% of all individuals scoring 2.0 or below require some kind of assistance to live in the community. Stuart's limited physical capacity as a result of the CVA was reflected in his low motor ability measure. Stuart's process ability measure of −0.4 was also below 1.0; 93% of individuals scoring 1.0 or below require some level of assistance to live in the community.[10] Stuart's cognitive capacity had been affected by the CVA but not to the same degree as his physical capacity. Although Stuart scored low on the process ability scale (relative to a process ability measure of 1.0 that reflected a greater ability to live independently in the community), his occupational therapy assistant believed

Stuart's significant motor skill difficulties were also affecting his ability to effectively organize and adapt his actions during IADL performance. She also believed Stuart demonstrated potential to learn the way to adapt to his current motor skill difficulties and, in doing so, would be enhancing his process skills.

Later that afternoon, before putting the computer-generated AMPS report in the medical chart (see Figure 15-5), the occupational therapy assistant shared the results with the occupational therapist, and they spent a few minutes discussing the implications for Stuart's intervention plan. On the basis of their discussion, the occupational therapy assistant modified the intervention plan to include the practice of IADL tasks during her afternoon session with Stuart. They also included the following goals, in addition to Stuart's ongoing self-care goals, in the weekly progress note: (1) patient will safely and efficiently transport needed items when setting a table, and (2) patient will efficiently organize his workspace when folding laundry. Both goals were chosen because Stuart had indicated that he wanted to perform some household chores and meal-preparation tasks when he returned home. Both goals reflected the performance of IADLs tasks that were easier than average with respect to motor skills and within Stuart's current physical capacity, although both tasks would still present a challenge. On the basis of her observations of his performance, the occupational therapy assistant noted that Stuart's difficulty with transporting items appeared to limit his options as to where and how a task was performed and that his organizational skills as to where objects were placed in the workspace made tasks more difficult. In the weekly note accompanying the goals, the occupational therapy assistant included this information and her assessment that Stuart was demonstrating poor efficiency with both skills as a result of his limited physical capacity and his lack of experience performing tasks with one hand and from a wheelchair.

In modifying the intervention plan to include a focus on IADL performance, both occupational therapy practitioners realized Stuart would not make great gains with his motor skills or become independent with the performance of IADL tasks. Yet they reasoned that if Stuart could perform some IADL tasks at home, he would rely less on outside services. Stuart would be pleased to remain at home, assisting with household chores and meal-preparation tasks as much as he was able. (Stuart particularly enjoyed activities involving food.) Because they were able to examine the AMPS hierarchy to determine which tasks were easier, they could also use an adaptive approach of modifying the tasks to present a comfortable challenge to Stuart in learning new skills. Finally, the motor and process skills that would be emphasized in the context of practicing IADL tasks could also be emphasized during Stuart's self-care activities.

To begin IADL intervention with Stuart, the occupational therapy assistant thoroughly examined the AMPS report. She began with Stuart's motor skills because these presented the greatest challenge to Stuart. She knew, however, that for Stu-

art to enhance his motor skills, he would have to rely on his process skills to change the way he performed IADL tasks.

Of the first three motor skills, *positions* presented the most difficulty for Stuart. To enhance Stuart's ability to position himself more effectively and reduce the need to stabilize his trunk while bending and reaching for objects, his occupational therapy assistant engaged Stuart in a variety of IADL tasks during their afternoon session and practiced positioning his wheelchair and his body relative to the demands of the task. In some cases a head-on approach with his wheelchair worked best; in others, a 45-degree angle was better. She provided feedback to Stuart regarding his performance and frequently solicited Stuart's opinion as to how he felt about the practice. She also asked Stuart to practice this skill when he attended his favorite weekly activities such as the gourmet tasting and popcorn party offered by the SNF activity program.

Although Stuart experienced some difficulty stabilizing his body, the motor skill termed *stabilizes,* the occupational therapist knew Stuart's physical therapy practitioners were focusing on Stuart's postural control, and she reported to them the difficulties Stuart was experiencing during the performance of IADL tasks. They also discussed some modifications to the seating of the wheelchair to help promote better stabilization of his trunk. His occupational therapy assistant also reasoned that if Stuart learned to better position himself relative to the demands of the task, the need for trunk stability would be less. Finally, because Stuart's ability to maintain an upright posture in the wheelchair—the motor skill termed *aligns*—was adequate, she did not need to address this area.

When looking at the next three motor skills, *walks, reaches,* and *bends* (Figure 15-6), Stuart's occupational therapy assistant reasoned that these skills, although difficult for Stuart, were not of great hindrance to his performance. Stuart had received

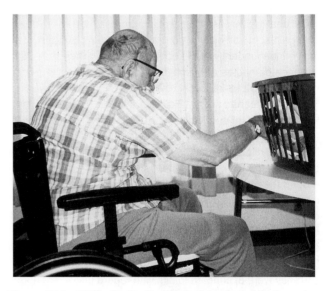

Figure 15-6   Difficulty *bending* the body and *reaching* for task objects.

a score of 2 on *walks* for both tasks because he required a wheelchair for mobility, per the scoring criteria outlined in the AMPS manual.[10] His occupational therapy assistant reasoned that minor modifications could be made to Stuart's home environment, such as rearranging the kitchen cupboards and hall closets to reduce the demand for reaching and bending. She discussed these modifications with Stuart, and they made plans to meet with the complex's manager because she had agreed to help out when Stuart returned home. Finally, with regard to Stuart's ability to reach and bend, his physical therapy practitioners were focusing on enhancing his underlying physical capacity, which would help support his ability to reach and bend, although Stuart would most likely not regain full physical function during his 5-week rehabilitation stay.

Of all the motor skills, *coordinates* was the only one identified as markedly deficient on the report. This reflected the lack of functional use of the left arm, which made holding and stabilizing objects that typically required the use of two hands difficult. With this in mind, the occupational therapy assistant considered two adaptive approaches. First, she focused on modifying the method by which Stuart attempted to hold and stabilize objects. This entailed focusing on the use, whenever possible, of Stuart's left arm to serve as a "weight" or "block" to secure objects. During both IADL tasks for the assessment, Stuart made no attempt to use his left arm. This was due in part to Stuart's perception that his left arm was of no use. He had not yet learned that in some cases, his arm could be used as a weight to hold objects on his lap or a flat surface and as a block against which an object could be wedged. Because Stuart's left arm showed no signs of spasticity, this new method was feasible for him.

The second adaptive approach for the motor skill *coordinates* involved modifying the environment with the use of adaptive devices. Particularly for meal-preparation tasks, Stuart and his occupational therapy assistant explored options for adaptive devices that would allow him to perform certain components of an IADL without struggling to stabilize objects during task performance. The use of a modified cutting board and devices to stabilize dishes on the counter and pans on the stove were explored, and those of interest to Stuart were used when he practiced preparing simple snacks and light meals during the afternoon. The occupational therapy assistant again recognized that the use of adaptive devices also entailed Stuart learning how to use them, reflecting a need to modify the method by which he accomplished a task. This relied on his process skill abilities to adapt and organize his actions despite the fact that the focus was on a motor skill.

With regard to the motor skill *manipulates* (Figure 15-7), Stuart's occupational therapy assistant chose an adaptive approach that again focused on modifying the environment. For example, Stuart had some difficulty manipulating objects with his right hand, such as when he was putting the fastener back on the bag of bread. This task typically requires the use of two hands, and Stuart's score of 2 was reflective of his difficulty in

performing such a task with only one hand. For IADL tasks that relied more on his fine-motor capacity, Stuart and his occupational therapy assistant explored adaptive devices within his abilities, such as a clothespin to seal the bag of bread rather than the tiny fastener or twist-tie that typically comes with a bag of bread. The motor skill *flows,* the ability to execute smooth and fluid arm movements, also presented some difficulty for Stuart. Because his CVA was fairly recent, more spontaneous recovery was likely, and this motor skill was not interfering greatly with Stuart's performance, the occupational therapy practitioners decided not to emphasize this motor skill during intervention.

Of the next five motor skills—*moves, transports, lifts, calibrates,* and *grips*—only *transports* was chosen for particular emphasis during intervention. This reflected the occupational therapy practitioners' assumptions that Stuart's low scores on these motor skills reflected his underlying capacity (i.e., his diminished muscle strength) and that in the short time remaining for his inpatient rehabilitation, Stuart's overall strength would probably not increase significantly. Stuart's physical therapy practitioners developed an exercise program for Stuart, and he was actively engaging in many other activities at the SNF. These other opportunities to develop underlying physical capacity would support Stuart's ability to move, lift, and grip objects.

One significant issue, however, was Stuart's ability to transport objects from one place to another while moving the wheelchair. Although his wheelchair lap tray presented a stable platform on which to secure an object when moving it from one area of a room to another, it also presented some obstacles to the efficiency of Stuart's performance. Stuart's occupational therapy assistant recommended that he not use the lap tray while performing IADL tasks. Instead, she explored with Stuart different styles of wheelchair bags to hold the objects he needed to transport. Stuart also learned some new methods by which to transport objects, including sliding heavier objects along the countertop rather than transporting them in his wheelchair. The biggest issue, however, arose when

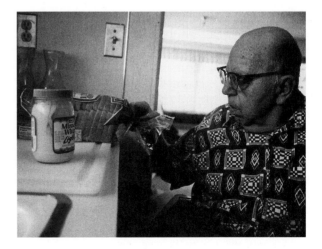

Figure 15-7 Difficulty *manipulating* task objects.

Stuart attempted to transport food items once he had retrieved them from the refrigerator. Again, Stuart relied on practice to learn to retrieve food items, place them in a wheelchair bag or secure them in his lap, and safely transport them to a counter or table.

With the last of the motor skill items, *endures* and *paces,* Stuart's occupational therapy assistant recognized this would be an ongoing issue for Stuart. He became fatigued quite easily after 10 minutes of performing easier-than-average IADL tasks. Again, she reasoned that his underlying capacity (i.e., his cardiopulmonary endurance) was fairly compromised, particularly because of his history of mild COPD, and that Stuart would need to adapt his daily routine to his limited capacity. Therefore she and Stuart explored the need to pace his activities throughout the day and not attempt to do too much at one time. This limitation presented a challenge to Stuart because he preferred to try as hard as he could during his therapy to get better faster and get home sooner. His occupational therapy assistant explained the need to temper his activity level so that he wouldn't run out of energy by the end of the day, when his wife would need his assistance the most. Stuart reluctantly agreed, but from the occupational therapy assistant's perspective, he continued to push himself too hard while at the SNF.

The occupational therapy assistant next turned to the scores on Stuart's process skills and examined them with regard to potential intervention strategies. One reason she surmised Stuart would be able to benefit from therapy was his ability to maintain focused attention throughout the task, the process skill *attends.* Although persons with right CVA have a greater tendency to distractibility, this was not the case with Stuart. In fact, during her discussion with the occupational therapist, Stuart's occupational therapy assistant learned that Stuart's tendency to delay his response to what was occurring in his left visual field (e.g., playing cards within his left visual field when playing solitaire) was probably reflective not of his ability to maintain his focused attention but his ability to appropriately notice and respond to nonverbal, environmental cues in his environment, the process skill *notices/responds.* As the optometrist had confirmed, his visual capacity was also diminished, which complicated his ability to notice environmental information to which he needed to respond.

Of the next five process skills, *chooses, heeds,* and *handles* presented some difficulty for Stuart. His occupational therapy assistant, however, was not concerned with the process skills *chooses* and *heeds* relative to the demands of the types of IADL tasks Stuart would engage in at home. On the AMPS report, *chooses* and *heeds* were identified as difficult (equivalent to a score of 2 [ineffective performance]) because he chose wheat bread to make the sandwich instead of white bread and did not sort the socks into pairs while folding the laundry, as specified in the task criteria to which he agreed before beginning each task. Yet these actions were not of major concern to the occupational therapy assistant because the consequences of his actions were relatively minor. If Stuart

ended up making a sandwich at home with mustard rather than the mayonnaise he originally considered, the consequences would not be of major concern. Stuart's occupational therapy assistant also believed that if Stuart were presented with more challenging situations in which he needed to remember information and act on it, the consequences might be of more concern.

With regard to Stuart's ability to know the way to stabilize and support task objects, the process skill *handles,* his occupational therapy assistant surmised that this was the result of Stuart's inexperience with performing tasks one handed. As he practiced various methods of stabilizing and support task objects to adapt to his significantly diminished motor skill *coordinates,* Stuart learned more ways to effectively stabilize and hold objects. Because Stuart demonstrated an ability to use task objects according to their intended purpose—the process skill *uses* (Figure 15-8)—and an ability to effectively ask for needed information—the process skill *inquires*—the occupational therapy assistant did not need to address these skills.

Similar to the previous items, the process skills *initiates, continues, sequences,* and *terminates,* although presenting some difficulty for Stuart, were not of major concern. Stuart demonstrated the ability to logically sequence the steps of a task—the process skill *sequences*—and although he displayed some hesitation when initiating some actions (the process skill *initiates*), his occupational therapy assistant surmised that this was Stuart trying to "figure out" the way he was going to perform a specific component of the task with his motor skill limitations. For example, the occupational therapy assistant had observed that Stuart hesitated for about 6 seconds before opening the refrigerator door. When she questioned Stuart after the assessment, he responded that he was trying to figure out how to get the door open with only one hand and also move his wheelchair. Similarly, Stuart would stop in the

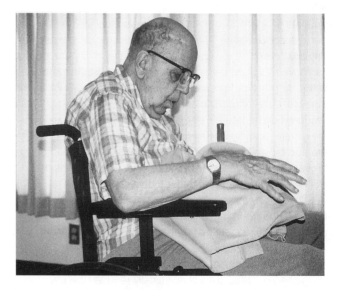

Figure 15-8 *Using* task objects according to their intended purpose.

middle of an action, such as spreading the mayonnaise on a slice of bread, close the bag of bread, and then return to spreading the mayonnaise, a behavior reflecting the process skill *continues.* Stuart also spent a significant amount of time spreading the mayonnaise on the bread, reflecting ineffective performance in stopping actions at an appropriate time, the motor skill *terminates.* Although these skills were interfering with Stuart's overall efficiency in performing a task, they did not interfere greatly with the overall quality or outcome of the task. Consequently, these four process skills were not emphasized during Stuart's therapy.

The process skill *search/locates,* in contrast, was a skill that Stuart's occupational therapy practitioners believed should be emphasized during therapy. Both occupational therapy practitioners surmised that Stuart's diminished visual capacity (i.e., acuity, saccades, pursuits) was affecting his ability to search for and locate needed items. They also believed Stuart's ability to visually attend to the environment, as observed on his admission to the SNF, may still be affecting his performance. For example, if Stuart initially didn't "see" an item on a shelf, he quickly began looking on the next shelf down. To help Stuart develop a more effective search pattern, the occupational therapy assistant worked with Stuart to slow down when looking for items and to examine each area in his visual field carefully before moving on to the next area. She also made some recommendations—both to Stuart for his home and to the SNF administrator for the facility—to modify the environment to ensure that adequate lighting was available.

The process skill *gathers* was also emphasized during intervention, in part as a way of adapting to Stuart's diminished motor skills (Figure 15-9). If Stuart were able to employ more efficient strategies with which to gather items, less reliance on his motor skills to transport items would be required. The same reasoning was applied to the process skill *organizes* (Figure 15-10). If Stuart were able to learn more efficient strategies with which to organize the tools and materials in his workspace, the demand on his motor skills would be reduced. For example, when he folded the laundry for the assessment, Stuart had requested that the basket of laundry be placed on the table, where he proceeded to move it closer to him. This left a small space on which to fold clothing. As Stuart folded more items, the space became crowded with the folded clothes, leaving him less space in which to fold clothes. By the end of the task, Stuart was folding the clothes on his lap because the table had no more space. Although this reflected Stuart knowing that a lap could be used as a surface from which to fold clothes (see Figure 15-8), it created additional difficulty when performing the task. Focusing on this process skill, as reflected in his second IADL goal, required great patience on Stuart's part. He was not used to organizing his workspace, and he reported to his occupational therapy assistant that he typically worked within the "mess" he created and didn't pay much attention to having a "neat" workspace. His occupational therapist explained the reasoning for trying to organize his workspace a bit better, referring to the example with the bas-

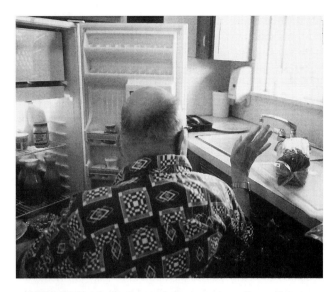

Figure 15-9 *Gathering* needed materials in the workspace.

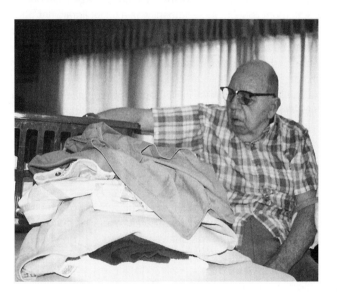

Figure 15-10 Ineffectively *organizing* materials in the workspace results in limited work surface on which to fold clothes.

ket of laundry. She mentioned that had Stuart moved the basket of laundry to a different location, more space would have been available in which to fold the clothes. This challenging goal took considerable attention during their therapy sessions together because it was a hard habit for Stuart to break.

As with the process skill *organizes,* the process skill *restores* had been identified as markedly deficient on the report. After discussion, Stuart's occupational therapy assistant realized that this too was probably related to Stuart's previous habits. He reported that he generally did not restore items right away and his wife frequently badgered him to clean up. Because this was a natural behavior of his, Stuart's occupational therapy assistant made little attempt to emphasize this process skill, except to point out to Stuart occasionally that he might save some time and energy if he restored items throughout the task.

To the surprise of both occupational therapy practitioners, Stuart's score on the process skill *navigates,* his ability to maneuver his hand and body around obstacles, had been identified as adequate on the report. They both believed the presence of visual inattention to the left environment might create some difficulty for Stuart during IADL tasks. They were correct, however, in their assumption that Stuart's underlying impairment with visual attention to the left environment did affect his ability to notice nonverbal environmental cues and respond appropriately; the process skill *notice/responds* was identified as markedly deficient on the report. To address this issue, the occupational therapy assistant again suggested modifying the environment to ensure adequate lighting. When she eventually spoke with Stuart and the manager of the assisted-living complex, she emphasized the need to simplify the visual environment to make it easier for Stuart to notice environmental cues. For example, Stuart mentioned that the tablecloth on the dining room table in his apartment was a bright floral print. Stuart's occupational therapy assistant explained that this might make it more difficult for Stuart to visually note items on the table and that a plain white tablecloth would be a better choice.

The last three process skills—*accommodates, adjusts,* and *benefits*—were the most important of the process skills because they reflected Stuart's ability to effectively deal with problems as they arose during task performance. Two of three process skills were identified as markedly deficient. Yet both occupational therapy practitioners needed to interpret this in light of Stuart's overall abilities. His low process scores on these items were in part reflective of his inability to effectively overcome and adapt to the many difficulties with motor skills. In other words, Stuart had only recently begun to practice new skills with his changed body since his CVA. Because this was the first time Stuart had attempted to perform IADL tasks, his difficulties were expected. For example, when preparing the sandwich, Stuart chose to keep the lap tray on his wheelchair while he worked in the kitchen. This presented additional problems because Stuart was not able to bend as far forward to reach objects, and the presence of the lap tray required additional maneuvering of the wheelchair to avoid hitting the countertop with the edge of the tray.

Stuart's underlying impairments were affecting his ability to adapt to problems as they arose. His occupational therapy practitioners surmised that Stuart's delay in turning over the knife he was using to cut the meat sandwich in half (i.e., not readily recognizing that he was using the knife incorrectly) may have resulted from his diminished visual capacity to see the knife blade (Figure 15-11). As such, this may have been affecting the process skill *accommodates.* Although Stuart's scores on *accommodates, adjusts,* and *benefits* were low, both occupational therapy practitioners believed Stuart still possessed the underlying cognitive capacity with which to learn to adapt and organize his actions more efficiently. They

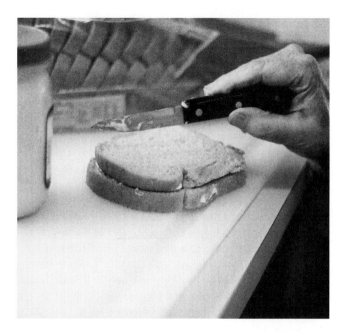

Figure 15-11 Ineffectively modifying actions *(accommodates)* results in a delay turning over the knife.

surmised that if Stuart concentrated on developing strategies with which to enhance his ability with specific motor or process skills or to adapt to his diminished motor skills by using his process skills, a greater repertoire of strategies with which to deal with problems should be available to Stuart.

Over the final 3 weeks of inpatient rehabilitation, Stuart's goals for occupational therapy intervention focused on achieving greater independence with self-care skills and improved quality of performance with IADL tasks. He continued to practice performing IADL tasks, preparing simple snacks and light meals in the kitchen, watering houseplants, folding laundry, dusting, and cleaning countertops and tables. Throughout, Stuart's occupational therapy assistant focused on the way Stuart performed the task, working with him to develop strategies to more efficiently accomplish the task. Although this required Stuart to learn new methods, regaining movement was not the primary focus of the intervention. The focus was on Stuart's need to be able to engage in simple IADL tasks so that he and his wife could continue living in their home.

By the end of the Stuart's 5 weeks in the SNF rehabilitation unit, Stuart had made significant although not outstanding progress. As a result of a consistent morning self-care routine monitored by the occupational therapist, Stuart only required minimal assistance to get ready in the morning. (He did, however, require moderate assistance with showering.) Once Stuart was ready for the day, he was able to engage in simple IADL tasks such as washing a few dishes, getting a drink from the refrigerator, and setting the table without great difficulty. The rehabilitation team believed Stuart and his wife would be able to manage at home, with less assistance than they originally thought.

Just before Stuart's discharge, his occupational therapist used the AMPS to reevaluate him. This time, however, Stuart chose to set the table and iron a shirt as his two task choices. Neither the occupational therapist performing the AMPS (the occupational therapy assistant having performed the first assessment) nor Stuart's choosing different IADL tasks invalidated the results of the AMPS because the computer program accounted for both factors in the analysis. The results showed that his motor ability measure had improved from -1.0 to -0.7, a slight improvement. His process ability measure, however, improved from -0.4 to 0.3, indicating that he was better able to organize and adapt his actions during task performance than he had been on admission. Stuart demonstrated an enhanced ability to more effectively search for and locate items in his environment, handle and support objects, pace his performance, coordinate his body parts to hold and stabilize objects, transport and manipulate objects, and overcome problems as they arose during task performance. All these abilities supported Stuart's goal to return home and live in the community. Because his goal had been achieved, his rehabilitation was considered successful.

■

REVIEW QUESTIONS

1. Describe the perspective on function of occupational therapy practitioners compared with other rehabilitation professionals.
2. What do research studies reveal regarding the impact of a CVA on a person's engagement in IADL tasks?
3. What is the relationship between a person's degree of impairment resulting from a CVA and ability to perform IADL tasks?
4. Compare occupational therapy IADL assessments with those from other rehabilitation disciplines. What are the differences?
5. What are the advantages of using the COPM with respect to a focus on IADL tasks?
6. Why is the use of IADL performance assessments recommended for use by occupational therapy practitioners?
7. What are the key elements that must be included in the documentation when writing goals for IADL performance?
8. Compare the adaptive and remedial approaches to occupational therapy intervention for IADL performance.
9. Describe the different aspects of adaptation that an occupational therapy practitioner considers when using an adaptive approach to IADL intervention.
10. What are the advantages of using the AMPS to guide intervention for IADL performance?

■ COTA Considerations ■

- To return to the community, people must be able to perform instrumental ADL (IADL) tasks such as shopping, using public transportation, handling money, ironing, doing laundry, making the bed, cleaning the house, and preparing a snack. After a stroke, IADL are often more difficult to perform than BADL (basic ADL).
- Occupation means the engagement in daily life activities that are meaningful and purposeful to the individual.
- The ability to perform a task cannot be accurately predicted by the extent of upper or lower extremity weakness, cognitive function, visuospatial abilities, somatosensory function, or motor planning disturbance. Ability to perform a task is determined by observation of the individual during the performance of that task.
- The COPM is a standardized, patient-centered assessment that assesses personal care, functional mobility, community management, paid or unpaid work, active recreation, and socialization. It can be used to develop patient-driven treatment programs, to document patient satisfaction with task performance, and as an outcome measure.
- A "top-down" approach to ADL assessment begins with a person's abilities to perform daily life tasks rather than focusing initially on impairments.
- The AMPS is a standardized assessment that focuses on the performance of IADL. It helps clarify whether underlying impairments influence performance ability. Individuals perform two or three familiar activities in a culturally appropriate context, and they are asked to perform the activities in their usual manner. The assessment is scored according to criteria defined in the AMPS manual and is scored by computer.

REFERENCES

1. Adaptive Environments Center: *A consumer's guide to home adaptation,* Boston, 1993, The Center.
2. American Occupational Therapy Association: Uniform terminology for occupational therapy—third edition, *Am J Occup Ther* 48:1047, 1994.
3. Bernspang B, Fisher AG: Differences between persons with right or left CVA on the Assessment of Motor and Process Skills, *Arch Phys Med Rehab* 76:1144, 1995.
4. Branch LG, Meyers AR: Assessing physical function in the elderly, *Clin Geriatr Med* 3:29, 1987.
5. Canadian Association of Occupational Therapists: *Occupational therapy guidelines for patient-centered practice,* Toronto, 1991, The Association.
6. Christensen C, Baum C: *Occupational therapy: overcoming human performance deficits,* Thorofare, NJ, 1991, SLACK.
7. Eakin P: Occupational therapy in stroke rehabilitation: implications of research into therapy outcomes, *Br J Occup Ther* 54:326, 1991.
8. Eakin P: The outcome of therapy in stroke rehabilitation: do we know what we are doing? *Br J Occup Ther* 54:305, 1991.
9. Edmans JA, Towle D: Comparison of stroke unit and non-stroke unit inpatients on independence in ADL, *Br J Occup Ther* 53:415, 1990.
10. Fisher AG: Assessment of motor and process skills, Fort Collins, Col, 1995, Three Star Press.

11. Fisher AG: Functional measures. 1. What is function. what should we measure, and how should we measure it? *Am J Occup Ther* 46:183, 1992.

12. Fisher AG: Functional measures. 2. Selecting the right test, minimizing the limitation, *Am J Occup Ther* 46:278, 1992.

13. Foti D, Pedretti LW: Activities of daily living: section 1: self-care/home management. In Pedretti LW, editor: *Occupational therapy: practice skills for physical dysfunction*, St Louis, 1996, Mosby.

14. Gershon R: *AMPS computer scoring program (version 1.1)* (software) Chicago, 1995, Computer Adaptive Technologies.

15. Gresham GE et al: *Post-stroke rehabilitation: clinical practice guideline, no 16*, Rockville, Md, 1995, U.S. Department of Health and Human Services, Public Health Service, Agency for Health Care Policy and Research, AHCPR publication no 95-0662.

16. Holbrook M, Skilbeck CE: An activities index for use with stroke patients, *Age Aging* 12:166, 1983.

17. Jongbloed L, Brighton C, Stacey S: Factors associated with independent meal preparation, self-care and mobility in CVA patients, *Can J Occup Ther* 55:259, 1988.

18. Kelly FA, Kawamoto TT, Rubenstein LZ: Assessment of the geriatric patient. In Kiernat JM, editor: *Occupational therapy and the older adult: a clinician manual*, Gaithersburg, Md, 1991, Aspen.

19. Kielhofner G, Mallinson T, de las Heras CG: Methods of data gathering. In Kielhofner G, editor: *A model of human occupation: theory and application*, Baltimore, 1995, Williams & Wilkins.

20. Law M: Evaluation of occupational performance. In Trombly C, editor: *Occupational therapy for physical dysfunction*, Baltimore, 1995, Williams & Wilkins.

21. Law M et al: *Canadian occupational performance measure*, ed 2, Toronto, 1995, Canadian Association of Occupational Therapists.

22. Lawton, MP: Scales to measure competence in everyday activities, *Psychopharmacol Bull* 24:609, 1988.

23. Lawton MP, Brody EM: Assessment of older people: self-maintaining and instrumental activities of daily living, *Gerontologist* 9:179, 1969.

24. Levine RE, Gitlin LN: A model to promote activity competence in elders, *Am J Occup Ther* 47:147, 1993.

25. Neistadt ME: Methods of assessing patients' priorities: a survey of adult physical dysfunction settings, *Am J Occup Ther* 49:428, 1995.

26. Neistadt ME: Occupational therapy treatment for constructional deficits, *Am J Occup Ther* 46:141, 1992.

27. Neistadt ME, Seymour SG: Treatment activity preferences of occupational therapists in adult physical dysfunction settings, *Am J Occup Ther* 49:437, 1995.

28. Northern JG et al: Involvement of adult rehabilitation patients in setting occupational therapy goals, *Am J Occup Ther* 49:214, 1995.

29. Park S: Restoring occupational performance: rehabilitation services for older adults. In Larson KO, Pedretti LW, Stevens-Ratchford RG, editors: *ROTE: the role of occupational therapy with the elderly*, Bethesda, Md, 1996, AOTA.

30. Park S: Treatment planning. In Fisher AG, editor: *Assessment of motor and process skills*, Fort Collins, Col, 1995, Three Star Press.

31. Park S, Fisher AG, Velozo CA: Using the Assessment of Motor and Process Skills to compare occupational performance between clinic and home settings, *Am J Occup Ther* 48:697, 1994.

32. Radomski MV: There is more to life than putting on your pants, *Am J Occup Ther* 49:487, 1995.

33. Rogers JC, Holm MB: Assessment of self-care. In Bonder BR, Waner MB, editors: *Functional performance in older adults*, Philadelphia, 1994, FA Davis.

34. Rubenstein LZ et al: Systematic biases in functional status assessment of elderly adults: effects of different data sources, *J Gerontol* 39:686, 1984.

35. Sarno MT, Buonaguro A: Factors associated with independent meal preparation in aphasic females: a pilot study, *Occup Ther J Res* 3:23, 1984.

36. Settle C, Holm MB: Program planning: the clinical utility of three activities of daily living assessment tools, *Am J Occup Ther* 47:911, 1993.

37. Spector M: Assessing status and function. In May BJ, editor: *Home health and rehabilitation*, Philadelphia, 1993, FA Davis.

38. Steinberg FU: Medical evaluation, assessment of function and potential, and rehabilitation plan. In Felsenthal G, Garrison SJ, Steinberg FU, editors: *Rehabilitation of the aging and elderly patient*, Baltimore, 1994, Williams & Wilkins.

39. Tangeman PT, Banaitis DA, Williams AK: Rehabilitation of chronic stroke patients: changes in functional performance, *Arch Phys Med Rehab* 71:876, 1990.

40. Trombly CA: Retraining basic and instrumental activities of daily living. In Trombly C, editor: *Occupational therapy for physical dysfunction*, Baltimore, 1995, Williams & Wilkins.

41. Trombly C: The issue is—anticipating the future: assessment of occupational function, *Am J Occup Ther* 47:253, 1993.

42. Wilcock AA: *Occupational therapy approaches to stroke*, Melbourne, 1986, Churchill Livingstone.

43. Woodson AM: Stroke. In Trombly C, editor: *Occupational therapy for physical dysfunction*, Baltimore, 1995, Williams & Wilkins.

44. World Health Organization: International classification of impairments, disabilities, and handicaps (ICIDH), Geneva, 1980, The Organization.

susan l. pierce

chapter 16

Driving

chapter objectives

After completing this chapter, the reader will be able to accomplish the following:

1. Discuss the legal issues associated with interventions aimed at independent driving for the stroke survivor.
2. Identify performance deficits that interfere with driving after stroke.
3. Understand the comprehensive driver evaluation and treatment procedures currently used for the stroke survivor.

In the continuum of activities of daily living (ADL), mobility must be considered by the occupational therapist in the rehabilitation process of the patient recovering from cerebrovascular accident (CVA). Treatment planning centers on independent mobility for the patient in and around the house and community. Studies of housing patterns of the elderly in 1970 and 1980 showed a dramatic move from rural to urban living with the accessibility offered by cars and federal mortgage assistance programs after World War II. By 1980 the parents of today's baby boomers moved away from their parents' homes in the city and to the suburbs where they are now "graying in place." This movement pattern greatly changes the nature of the transportation needs of the elderly today and will continue to be a significant factor when the baby boomers move into the elderly category.[22]

A century ago, people could walk to work, shops, friends' homes, churches, and most other destinations. Today, with the primary mode of transportation being the personal vehicle and the separation between homes and businesses in the suburbs, few destinations are now within walking distance. Physical infirmity caused by a CVA or age can further shorten distances traversable on foot. Conference planners were surprised at the 1971 White House Conference on Aging when delegates ranked transportation third in importance, preceded only by income and health. Research confirms that in general older persons are not satisfied with their abilities to get around in the community.[5] Because people must go into the community for almost all their needs, the existence of facilities and services is meaningless without accessibility. Automobiles provide vital access to widely scattered services and facilities. Reduced mobility can be accompanied by lower self-esteem, feelings of uselessness, loneliness, unhappiness, and depression.

Skills necessary for safe driving begin to deteriorate around the age of 55 and dramatically decline after 75.[19] Approximately 72% of strokes occur in people older than 65. The brain damage from a cerebral infarct and its clinical manifestations also can affect the person's driving skills. The specific motor, sensory, and cognitive effects depend on the location and severity of the cerebrovascular damage. This damage can cause one or more temporary or permanent impairments. Of the approximately 80% of people who survive the initial period, 75% are left with residual perceptual-cognitive dysfunction.[15] Although these impairments may affect safe driving, each patient recovering from CVA must be evaluated individually because the location and nature of the stroke can produce different problems and deficits.

Independent transportation should be considered an instrumental ADL. Frances Carp, a California psychologist who has studied older drivers, explains "well-being, as contrasted with mere existence, depends on satisfaction of two categories of needs: those with satisfaction is requisite to independent living and those whose satisfaction is necessary to give life an acceptable and positive quality."[5] Carp's conceptual model in Figure 16-1 reflects life-maintenance needs, including nourishment, clothing, medical care, banking, and pharmaceuticals. Community resources for meeting these needs include grocery and drug stores, department stores, physician's offices, and banks. If a person has no access to these resources, independent living is impossible. Other needs, labeled *higher order,* include needs for social interaction, usefulness, recreation, and religious experience. Carp's research of investigative studies supports the idea that "if life is to have an acceptable quality higher-order needs such as those expressed in trips for relaxation and enjoyment and religious activities are also essential."[5]

The threat of losing a driver's license may have devastating effects on a stroke survivor's motivation to maintain

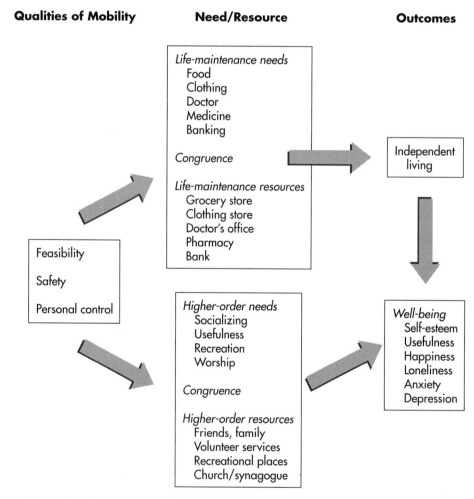

Figure 16-1 The determinants and dynamics of emotional and social well-being. (Modified from Transportation Research Board—National Research Council, Special Report 218, *Transportation in an aging society,* Washington, DC, 1988.)

independence in other areas of daily living. The primary fear of elderly people is not death but losing their independence and becoming burdens to their loved ones.[3] Carp states the following[5]:

Loss of license is a serious fear among drivers, a threat to their autonomy, usefulness, and self-esteem. . . . A century ago people could walk to work, shops, others' homes, religious services, and most destinations. Few destinations [today] lie within walking distance for any person. . . . Mobility is a key influence on the congruence term in the model. . . . Satisfaction of life-maintenance and higher order needs require going out into the community. . . . The loss of a license would mean inability to go where they needed to go and therefore meet their needs independently. . . . Just as receipt of the first driver's license is an important rite of passage to adulthood and independence, license loss formally identifies one as "over the hill."

Driving is inseparable with being one's own person and taking care of oneself. The issue is more than just one of losing mobility. Rendering an opinion as to whether the patient recovering from CVA is capable of driving is serious and demands careful attention by the rehabilitation team. Furthermore, the professional involved in the driving evaluation and decision phase should have the proper knowledge and skill to be able to provide reliable recommendations compassionately, mindful of the implication of the results for the patient's life.

THE OCCUPATIONAL THERAPIST AS A DRIVER REHABILITATION SPECIALIST

The occupational therapist is concerned with the performance level of ADL for the patient recovering from CVA. The focus for ADL retraining varies depending on whether the patient walks or uses a wheelchair. The daily living task of mobility may involve bed and wheelchair mobility, transfers, walking, and driving. These tasks allow an individual to function independently by moving from one place to another. Community mobility depends on the patient's ability to drive or use alternative transportation.

The occupational therapist must understand the significance of community mobility for the total well-being of the patient recovering from CVA. A holistic view presents driving as a vital link between the patient and the outside world. Because driving is an ADL, it should be considered by the rehabilitation team (Figure 16-2). Just as patients must practice and relearn safe techniques for dressing, walking, and other self-care, they also must learn and practice techniques relating to the proper use of an automobile. Driving requires skill in physical, visual, perceptual, and cognitive performance areas; the occupational therapist is the logical team member to assist in evaluating the patient's abilities in these areas. The occupational therapist's background and training in evaluation and treatment in these areas provides a unique understanding of diagnostic and age-related problem areas and

their implications for driving. A comprehensive driving evaluation involves a team process (Figure 16-3). The driver rehabilitation specialist (DRS) generally coordinates the team and all services required for evaluation and follow-up. Communication with team members is crucial. The therapist must consider the activity of driving whether the patient is seen in a rehabilitation setting, a temporary residential care facility, or through a home health agency. If an older person is not being seen for rehabilitation, the primary care physician is often the first professional to identify deficits in skills that may affect driving performance. The Department of Motor Vehicles may demand an evaluation if the older driver is involved

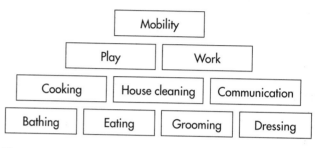

Figure 16-2 Pyramid model for rehabilitation of activities of daily living.

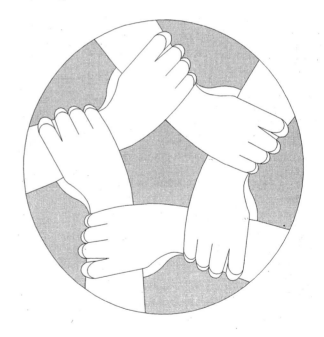

- Client
- Funding source contact
- Driver rehabilitation specialist
- Adaptive equipment installer
- Physician

Figure 16-3 A successful outcome—driving independently—relies on the interdependence and interactions of the mobility team.

in a collision, receives a ticket, or is reported for unsafe driving behavior. In either case the physician or Department of Motor Vehicles should know the community resources that offer driver rehabilitation services. The social and ethical dilemma faced by medical professionals and the Department of Motor Vehicles is to strike a balance between protecting the older adult's privilege to drive and the safety of other road users, including pedestrians, other drivers, and vehicle passengers.

The impact of persisting sensory, perceptual, motor, and cognitive deficits on driving risk levels must be addressed through a driving evaluation and special training and equipment. A thorough clinical examination of the skills needed for driving is necessary to determine whether the patient is ready for an on-the-road evaluation. A DRS must know and understand problems that can occur with the patient recovering from CVA, and the implications each deficit may have for the driving task. The clinical occupational therapist serving in this role requires additional training and knowledge in the field of driver education and driver rehabilitation services.

The Association of Driver Educators for the Disabled (ADED) can be a helpful resource in obtaining more information about this field. It has more than 450 members; a large number of them are from the occupational therapy profession. The ADED offers annual educational conferences with presentations for new and advanced driver rehabilitation specialists. It also offers a certification examination process leading to designation as a Certified Driver Rehabilitation Specialist (CDRS). Several institutions and businesses besides the ADED also offer annual educational programs and workshops for driver rehabilitation specialists. Driver education courses can be obtained from many local universities and community colleges or from a local Traffic Safety Council (Box 16-1).

DRIVING AS AN ACTIVITY OF DAILY LIVING SKILL

Community mobility is paramount to the patient recovering from CVA and attempting to maintain a productive lifestyle in the work or social arenas. Because of its complexity, driving should be one of the last ADL resumed during rehabilitation. Because driving is an ADL that is potentially dangerous to the patient, the therapist, and other road users, a full assessment should take place after the patient is discharged from inpatient rehabilitation and is receiving outpatient treatment. Few patients have strokes and are able to demonstrate normal functioning in all areas within a 1- or 2-week period. The medical team treating the patient should determine collectively when the patient is ready to drive again or be reevaluated.

Personal functioning should be optimized before the patient is scheduled for a driving evaluation. Patient and family education before discharge from inpatient treatment is important. The patient and family should be educated in the complete evaluation process and when and where it will take place; the occupational therapist should recommend that the patient abstain from driving until results are determined from the evaluation. Input from all team members should be sought, and the physician should provide medical clearance when the patient is ready for evaluation. Timeliness of referral is crucial to ensure the evaluation takes place before the patient resumes driving.

After a complete driving evaluation, final recommendations should be thoroughly explained to the patient and family members. The referring physician should receive written notification of the outcome of the evaluation. Documentation of the results, recommendations, and patient caregiver education should be noted in the patient's chart. The client should sign the written recommendations to demonstrate legal proof of explanation of the findings. If

---

Box 16-1

Resources for Educational Seminars and Materials

AAA
Traffic Safety
1000 AAA Drive
Box 78
Heathrow, FL 32746-5080

Association of Driver Educators for the Disabled (ADED)
109 West St.
Edgerton, WI 53534
Secretariat: Ric Cerna
608-884-8833

Adaptive Mobility Services, Inc.
116 East Gatlin Ave.
Orlando, FL 32806-6908
407-855-8050

Louisiana Tech University
P.O. Box 3185
Ruston, LA 71272
Biomedical Engineering Department
318-257-4562

National Safety Council
1121 Spring Lake Drive
Itisca, IL 60143-3201
708-285-1121

Veterans Administration
Glenn Ramsey
Department of Veterans Affairs
PM & RS/VA Headquarters
225 Humphreys Blvd.
Memphis, TN 38120

the results of the evaluation are negative, a team member may inform the proper driver licensing authority in the patient's state of residency. Some states allow any health care professional to report to the driver licensing authority, whereas other states only accept a physician's report. Moreover, some states provide immunity to the reporting person, and others do not. Research by the DRS into each state's reporting and licensing regulations is necessary.

LIABILITY CONSIDERATIONS FOR DRIVING ASSESSMENT PROGRAMS

In the past 20 years, court precedent has established that physicians have responsibility for protecting the public health even if it conflicts with the patient's right to privacy and confidentiality. This duty to warn society for the greater good has been upheld by the courts. Consequently, the physician's liability to inform third parties has been increased. The inherent responsibility may be mitigated by the nonspecific nature of the person to be warned. As America's passion for lawsuits continues to rise, the physician and other treating professionals of drivers recovering from CVA should be careful to consider recommending a safe driving assessment if any question exists about the patient's skill level. Failure to address these issues with the patient and concerned others may expose a health care provider to a charge of negligence.

In a March 1993 American Occupational Therapy Association (AOTA) physical disabilities special interest section newsletter, the legal considerations for driver rehabilitation programs were discussed in terms of the responsibility of the patient, physician, and DRS.[20] The driver has an ethical responsibility to avoid harming self or others. Each state's Department of Motor Vehicles grants a person the privilege of a driver license based on criteria and regulations that vary from state to state. The driver must realize that the driving privilege can lead to potential disaster through injury to people and destruction of property if residual functional deficits interfere with driving skills. Patients recovering from CVA who cannot master the operational, tactical, and strategic skills necessary to operate a motor vehicle safely present a clear risk of injury to themselves, their passengers, pedestrians, and other operators of motor vehicles.[2]

Many states do not require a driver to report a new medical episode resulting in disability between license renewals. Furthermore, testing procedures in driver examination offices do not fully evaluate all skills related to driving. Examiners may not have knowledge of an applicant's diagnoses unless the person informs them or a physician provides written notification. They do not have an understanding of possible implications for driving. For example, a person with a complete right homonymous hemianopsia, a common vision deficit seen after stroke, has at best 90° of total intact visual field. Most states require a minimum of 140°; however, states' typical methods of vision testing measure only visual acuity not visual fields. A person can have 20/40 visual acuity, which is acceptable; however, the driver examiner may never know the person also has homonymous hemianopsia unless the person says so.

To avoid any legal difficulties with the driver's insurance, the car insurance company should be notified about the stroke, the results of the driving evaluation, and the validation of the person's driving ability by the Department of Motor Vehicles. If the insurer requires an assurance of good health for policy application or renewal, a failure to notify the insurance company may result in a claim of fraud if the client has an accident. As a result the stroke survivor who is driving may be held completely or partially liable for costs rewarded in court judgments for property damage, bodily damage, pain, suffering, and loss of any parties involved in the accident because of contributory negligence.

Some states have mandatory reporting laws. A physician must report a new disability or diagnosis to the Department of Driver Licensing. In states that lack this law, some physicians overlook, ignore, or are hesitant to report a patient for fear of losing a patient. They may feel a loyalty toward patients they have treated for many years. Patients may influence their decisions by saying they are the only drivers in their families and driving is crucial to their independent living. Although all of these may seem like good reasons to overlook findings, the physician's first thought should be the safety and protection of the patient and the public. An intermediate level of reporting may occur with the family or concerned others who may be driven by this person or are in a position to assist with the person's mobility needs. If the physician is unsure the patient will comply with the recommendation, the patient should be reported to the Department of Driver Licensing. The Code of Ethics of the American Medical Association states the following:

A physician may not reveal the confidence entrusted to him in the course of medical attendance or the deficiencies he may observe in the character of clients, unless he is required to do so by law, or unless it becomes necessary to protect the welfare of the individual or the community.

The physician's decision to report a patient should be based on the amount of risk involved in allowing the patient to continue driving. The physician should protect patients from further harm or injury to themselves or others if necessary. The state of Florida, for example, protects a professional or layperson from being sued for slander or character defamation for reporting a patient to the Department of Driver Licensing. To further protect reporting persons, their names are not revealed to the licensee. The professional is protected by state statute in reporting confidential information about a patient.

A team or family member should never hesitate to report the patient to the Department of Driver Licensing if the patient does not comply and is deemed unsafe to self or the public while driving. If the physician is hesitant to address driving concerns to a long-term patient or thinks liability may be avoided by not addressing the issue, another team member should contact the Department of Driver Licensing. Each state differs in the requirements for reporting a person, so the DRS should investigate the procedure for the patient's resident state. Obtaining a copy of the state's statute is important, as is talking to the Department of Driver Licensing or Medical Review Board.

Clinicians must remember that protective privilege ends where public peril begins. The issue of driving should be considered by every physician and rehabilitation facility. If the facility does not have a driving program, a referral to a qualified program in the community should be made and documented in the chart. The ADED can be contacted for members or resources at national and international locations.

A review of past court opinions and judgments reveals rulings both for and against physicians. Jacobs,[13] in a 1978 article entitled "Reporting the Handicapped Driver" cited several lawsuits against physicians. In a 1920 invasion of privacy lawsuit, *Simonsen v. Swenson*, the physician was vindicated of any wrongdoing by proving that the public welfare was being protected. In *Freese v. Lemmon, 210 N.W.2d 576 (Iowa, 1973)*, a physician was found guilty of malpractice because he failed to warn and counsel a patient about the possible effects a medical condition might have on driving ability. In this case the patient had been diagnosed with epilepsy. The physician did not advise the person to stop driving. The patient had a seizure while driving and struck a pedestrian. In a 1986 lawsuit, *Tarasoff v. Regents of the University of California (551 p. 2d334, at 344 [1986])*, a psychologist working in the student health department on campus was held liable because of his failure to alert and advise campus authorities properly when a student reported to him an intention to murder his girlfriend. The court ruled the psychologist had a duty to break confidentiality and warn the potential victim. The court's opinion concluded that the "protective privilege ends where the public peril begins." The court also stated the following[3]:

> The doctor treating a mentally ill patient, just as a doctor treating a physical illness, bears a duty to use reasonable care to give threatened persons such warnings as are essential to avert foreseeable danger arising from his patient's condition or treatment.

Antrim and Engum,[2] in an article entitled "The Driving Dilemma and the Law: Patients Striving for Independence Versus Public Safety," describe other legal cases illustrating practitioner liability. In *Naidu v. Laird, 539 A.2d 1064 (Del. 1988)*, the court heard that Laird was killed in a car accident by a known psychotic person who had been involved in several similar accidents in which he drove his car deliberately into someone else's car. When taking his medication, the psychotic person was generally manageable, appropriate, and capable of living semi-independently. When not taking his medication, he had violent tendencies that presented a risk of harm to himself and others. Laird's widow sued the psychotic person and the treating physician, Dr. Naidu, for wrongful death. The court ruled in favor of the plaintiff. The court stated that "a psychiatrist owes an affirmative duty to persons other than the patient to exercise reasonable care in the treatment and discharge of their patients." Antrim defines *reasonable care* as the degree of care, skill, and diligence that a reasonably prudent psychiatrist engaged in a similar practice and in similar conditions would ordinarily have exercised in like circumstances.

Antrim and Engum further discuss the California case of *Myers v. Quesenberry, 144 Cal.App.3d 888 (1983)*, which involved a car accident of a patient of Dr. Quesenberry's who was being treated for diabetes and receiving prenatal care. The doctor knew that his patient had been seriously affected during two previous pregnancies that resulted in one stillbirth. During the third pregnancy the patient's diabetes could not be stabilized. During an office examination the physician discovered the fetus had died. Dr. Quesenberry advised the patient to have a dilation and curettage procedure. He instructed her to drive immediately to a hospital. Emotionally distraught, the patient suffered a diabetic attack enroute and lost control of her car, striking a pedestrian, Myers. The court noted that a fundamental principle of tort law held physicians liable for injuries caused by their failure to exercise reasonable care. A physician must warn a patient if the patient's condition or medications renders certain conduct such as operating a motor vehicle dangerous to others.[2]

A physician must appreciate the complexity and dangers of driving and understand that certain conditions or deficits may impair driving performance. Physicians should recognize their limitations in their abilities to fully evaluate the patient's driving skills in the office or hospital. Physicians should be informed about the expertise and role of the DRS so that they can refer their patients for full driving evaluations, including clinical and on-the-road assessments.

The DRS's responsibility can be as great and serious as is the physician's. An occupational therapist serving in this role has a much greater degree of vulnerability to liability lawsuits compared with an occupational therapist in clinical practice. First, the nature of the job, in which they take clients out in traffic has inherent risks. The therapist risks personal danger and the public's safety. Second, therapists must adequately credential themselves to enhance their clinical reasoning, case management, and the value of their professional opinion. The therapist must have a strong working knowledge of each step of a comprehensive driving evaluation and possess all necessary clinical and vehicle tools, tests, and skills to pass judgment fairly and accurately on a person's driving future. The therapist should evaluate a patient's driving ability fully, considering the safety of the patient and the public at large. The therapist should avoid zealousness as an advocate for the patient whose skills are in question. Rather, the studied and influential analysis of disabilities on driving ability should be respected.

Antrim is a practicing attorney and a member of the board of reviewers of the journal *Cognitive Rehabilitation*. He strongly suggests that current legal authority appears ready to impose liability on health care professionals for negligence in failing to address their patients' abilities to drive. Antrim recommends that health care professionals use a standard of care in making these recommendations and their evaluation process should include guidelines for making those decisions reasonably and responsibly.[2] No standardization is currently available for driving evaluation, so each DRS develops a technique and process for each individual program. The industry lacks consistency. The ADED offers recommended practices for driver rehabilitation services, but the practices are written in general terms and do not identify the specific procedures or tests that must be used in the clinic or evaluator vehicle (Box 16-2). The therapist must rely on a thorough literature search, available educational materials, other DRS's opinions and personal judgment regarding the driving skills to be tested and the means for testing them. For legal protection, therapists should have their own profes-

sional liability insurance in addition to coverage from the employer.

The therapist should have strong clinical experience and confidence in the ability to assess a patient's skill in each performance area of physical, visual, visuoperceptual, cognitive, and communication skills. The therapist must then know the way the patient's performance level in each area may affect driving performance. Activity analysis is a useful tool. Because driving requires certain abilities in each of the performance areas, the DRS also should know the way to assess performance levels in each area in the evaluation vehicle and dynamic traffic situations (Box 16-3).

The on-the-road portion of the driver evaluation is crucial to the final decision about a person's driving abilities. The DRS must not only have a driver education background but also have working knowledge of medical diagnosis and medications and their relationships to the driving task. Many hospitals and rehabilitation centers decide to use a commercial driving school instructor or a retired driver educator from a school to complete the on-the-road assessment. This can result in an inadequate outcome if the assessor does not understand diagnoses, disabilities, and the way to assess each skill level in the car. The person's educational background, personal references, work history, and knowledge of diagnoses should be carefully considered. In Florida a person can obtain a commercial driving instructor license by having a high school degree, a good driving record with no criminal record, and proof of good medical health. Except for a 2-day required driver education course, no other specialized

Box 16-2

The Association of Driver Educators for the Disabled's Recommended Practices for Driver Rehabilitation Services

A driver rehabilitation program must have a qualified driver rehabilitation specialist and the appropriate vehicles and equipment to provide comprehensive services in the following areas:
1. Clinical evaluation—Applicable testing in the areas of physical functioning and visual/perceptual/cognitive screening; wheelchair and seating assessment
2. Driving evaluation—An on-the-road performance assessment of the patient in an actual driving environment using equipment similar to that being prescribed
3. Vehicle modification and prescription—Prescriptions based on the patient's demonstrated performance in an actual driving experience with equipment similar to that being prescribed, including appropriate descriptions and dimensions of the patient's vehicle and wheelchair
4. Driver Education—Includes sufficient practice and training to enable the patient to operate a motor vehicle with the prescribed equipment at a level that meets the client's needs for a driver's license
5. Final Fitting—A final fitting and operational assessment in the patient's modified vehicle

(Courtesy ADED, Edgerton, Wis)

Box 16-3

Examples of Driving Behaviors to be Observed During the In-Traffic Assessment

Visually searching traffic environment (20-30 seconds ahead)
Demonstrating safe physical control of the vehicle at all times
Maintaining safe speeds
Smooth braking
Demonstrating good lane selection
Maintaining a safe following distance
Backing the vehicle
Making turns
Navigating curves
Changing lanes and merging
Judging gaps at intersections
Making passing maneuvers
Performing parallel and angle parking
Interacting with traffic in a low-risk manner
Entering and exiting expressways
Using turn signals appropriately
Demonstrating proper use of all mirrors
Checking blind spots

training is required. Many driving schools exist to teach new drivers the way to pass a road test so that they can obtain driver licenses. Little information is given to analyze driving behavior. This assessor is usually not a professional, has no understanding of disabilities, and tends to concentrate on teaching a person to pass a road test. The assessor's motivation is often to provide a revenue-generating service. A driver *educator* usually has a professional college degree with special study in driver education. This person is able to evaluate a person's driving capabilities objectively. The therapist can apprise the driver educator of the client's strengths and weaknesses and probable behaviors that may be observed or expected. The therapist also can assist the driver educator in handling particular problem areas and provide recommendations for appropriate remedial training to see whether the driver can compensate for these problems.

If driving instructors or driver educators have little or no experience working with persons with disabilities, the therapist is needed to complete the clinical portion of the evaluation. Therapists must remain closely involved with the in-vehicle evaluator to ensure that proper and continued understanding of the driver's deficits and progress or lack of progress is evidenced. The therapist may need to be in the evaluator vehicle only for the first or last session, but the therapist's observations and concurrence with the in-car instructor's recommendations and findings are crucial. The therapist, as the supervisor of the in-car instructor, is responsible for any decisions or actions made by this person. Although the employer has the "deep pocket" in terms of finances and assets, the therapist and in-car instructor also can be brought into a lawsuit. Their actions and decisions would then be scrutinized by the plaintiff's attorney, a judge, and possibly a jury to determine whether they followed a standard of care, showed reasonable judgment, and did not demonstrate any negligence or malpractice in their work or decisions. Any accidents or collisions in an evaluation car can produce a potential litigation case against all parties associated with the driver evaluation.

In a 1986 article, Steich[27] explained that the law holds professionals to a higher standard than it does the public because professionals consider themselves more highly skilled in their particular fields of expertise. For example, the DRS owes a greater duty of care to a patient and the public than does a parent teaching a child to drive. Steich goes on to explain that the occupational therapist must do something wrong or fail to do something that should have been done to be held liable.[27] If the program's policies and procedures define the steps that should be done to complete a comprehensive driver assessment but the therapist fails to use the tool or procedure defined, the therapist may be held liable for omitting that portion of the test. The wording of the driving program policies and procedures should be reviewed by legal counsel. The wording that "the following test may be used" leaves the therapist free to

decide to use whatever tests or procedures necessary for a particular patient.

The therapist is responsible for ensuring that all evaluative or testing equipment is working when needed. For example, several commercially available devices can be used to test visual acuity and night vision. If the machine that measures night vision is not working when the therapist evaluates a patient with a diagnosis in which night vision could be a suspected problem (such as glaucoma), the therapist may be found negligent for not having the machine fully functioning when the client was evaluated. The therapist may make a statement in the summary indicating that rendering an opinion on the issue was impossible; however, in making a final conclusion regarding the person's driving ability, night vision should be tested appropriately.

Documentation of a driving evaluation is crucial and necessary for several purposes. The evaluation and training report can be used to justify an adaptive equipment purchase for a third-party payor, inform the Department of Motor Vehicles and a physician of the patient's driving performance, and help defend the therapist in a court of law or during a deposition in which professional judgment or expertise is deposed. The therapist should keep in mind that if something is not documented on paper, in the eyes of the court it was not done. This documentation is more vulnerable than usual because it is scrutinized far more than is the documentation of in-house therapy for ADL training not related to driving. Because driving is an ADL that can kill, the risk is greater that documentation for a driving program will be subpoenaed by an attorney searching for liability justification in a suit brought by a former patient or by an individual not necessarily related to the patient who was injured by the patient or suffered property damage.

Occupational therapists should write their notes and summaries within 24 hours of assessment. Adherence to this recommendation ensures that memory of the information is fresh and subsequently documentation is more thorough and accurate. The notes should document in detail interactions with the patient, the way the patient performed in each step, and the clinical reasoning inherent in the decision-making regarding the patient's driving potential or performance. Statements such as "the patient has potential to be a safe driver" should be avoided. Rather, the therapist must have enough confidence in the patient and in professional judgment to document "the patient is a safe driver." Another method of documentation is to say "today the patient drove safely in the following situations." The documentation should account for the time and days spent with a patient. Positive and negative observations or scores should be noted. Brief, incomplete, and poorly written documentation is hard to defend in court if an expert witness is used to judge the DRS's work and decisions. As with the physician's cases noted previously, an expert witness with similar practice to the therapist may be called to testify regarding standard procedure in similar conditions. This witness may not be able to testify that the DRS acted with a reasonable care of duty if the documentation cannot support conclusions with evidence. Also, the background, training, and experience of the DRS is often compared against those of other DRSs in the country. Attendance at related workshops and ADED conferences and continual updating of the therapist's knowledge can validate the therapist's credentials.

The DRS must appreciate the importance of driving to a patient and work in the patient's best interest to keep the patient licensed if reasonably safe. To protect themselves legally, DRSs should consistently document and ensure that a complete and objective assessment was done. The therapist's final decision should be based on objective observations. The occupational therapist should be aware of the potential liability in this role and the way to maximize protection from harm, prevent claims, and defend oneself if necessary. ADED and AOTA membership, participation

in educational opportunities, reading books and literature available on the subject, taking a defensive driving course, and becoming involved in Transportation Research Board activities help keep the therapist up to date with the profession.

DRIVING ASSESSMENT

Multiple decisions must be made constantly, and information must be correctly and quickly interpreted for safe driving (Figure 16-4). Smith states the following[26]:

Driving a modern passenger vehicle on a clear day in light traffic does not overtax any dimension of performance (perceptual, cognitive, or physical). However, in heavy traffic at high speed, at night on poorly marked roads, at a complex intersection, or in a potential accident situation, the demands placed on drivers can exceed their abilities.

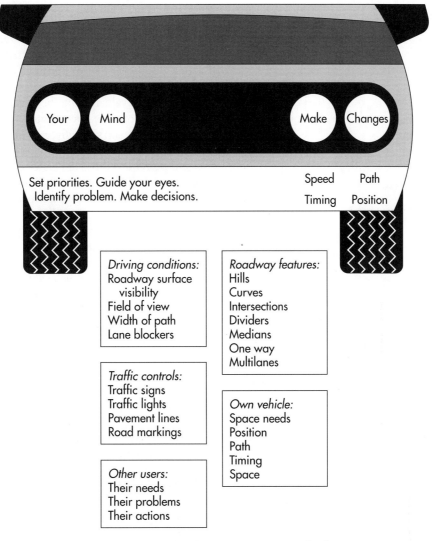

Figure 16-4 Visual and cognitive processing for driving.

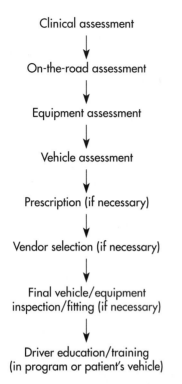

Figure 16-5 Driving assessment for a patient recovering from CVA.

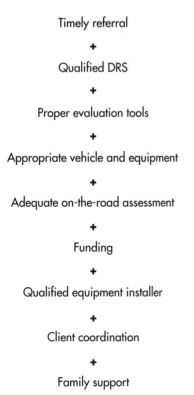

Figure 16-6 Factors that influence a successful driving evaluation.

He describes a step procedure necessary for safe driving[26]:

1. The driver must see or hear a situation developing (stimulus registered and sampled at the visual, auditory, or perceptual level).
2. The driver must recognize it (stimulus recognition at the cognitive level).
3. The driver must decide the way to respond (cognitive level).
4. The driver must execute the physical maneuver (motor level).

Age-related changes complicated by a stroke should raise concerns by the health care professional regarding the patient's ability to perform all the described steps thoroughly and quickly.

Driving is one of the most complex activities a person may perform. It requires integration of many performance areas. With abbreviated inpatient rehabilitation stays for stroke survivors becoming the norm, the driving evaluation should not take place until the patient has been discharged from the outpatient treatment program or has recovered to a maximal level of independence in the performance of other ADL. A timely referral by the physician or other team members may reduce the likelihood that the patient may begin driving with no supervision from a family member or friend. The physician should effectively communicate the driving restrictions that are in place until an evaluation has been completed. This recommendation should be documented and verbally communicated to the person's caregivers. For liability protection of the rehabilitation facility and team members, the patient should be required to sign a form demonstrating understanding of the recommendations given and indicating willingness to comply. Each team member that has verbally given the same recommendations to the patient should document in their progress or discharge summaries the instructions given to the patient.

The therapist should caution the client against practicing a week or so before the evaluation appointment. This strategy is unsafe and needless and puts the patient at risk to be sued by parties for driving while impaired, which can cause personal and property damage. In addition, insurance companies may be able to claim fraud and violation of their regulations, so that they are not monetarily responsible for any damages ordered by a court. The potential consequences are not worth the risk and associated liability.

A comprehensive driving assessment for a person who has had a stroke may include the steps illustrated in Figure 16-5. A successful driving evaluation depends on factors influenced by all members of the mobility team (Figure 16-6).

Clinical Assessment

When structuring the clinical assessment the therapist should be guided by common sense to determine the specific clinical tests and techniques to be used. A lengthy clinical assessment should not be performed before the driving assessment because no correlation or relevance to driving performance has been ascertained. Patients recovering from CVA, who are generally older than 55, may feel threatened by a person who has the power to take away their driver's licenses. Patients may be more cooperative with the clinical assessment if they appreciate its relevancy to the driving task. For example, the patient may feel frustrated and angry working on a puzzle or paper maze during a driving evaluation but may understand the importance of a test that provides specific data related to driving such as reaction time, steering control, and diverted attention. The physical and visual assessment is generally easy for the therapist to set up because the training and techniques used in these areas are similar to those used in other settings and with disabilities.

During the clinical assessment phase the DRS should perform an interview with the patient. Because a person's driver's license is a matter of public record, the DRS should check the license, make sure it is still valid, and note any restrictions already placed on the license. Most Departments of Motor Vehicles do not allow a person to drive if the license has been suspended or has expired. A complete medical history should be reviewed with the patient to assess any pertinent information that should be considered during the driving evaluation. Driving abilities may be impaired as a result of adverse drug effects or age-related factors such as physiologic changes and age-associated diseases and conditions, including arthritis, cataracts, memory loss, and hearing loss. Knowledge and perspective of problems with other coexisting medical conditions in areas that may not necessarily be related to the CVA diagnosis should be explored at this time for an understanding of the total person. For example, if the person also has a history of diabetes and has had the right leg amputated, the therapist would be prudent to explore the potential problems that may occur in the patient's left leg. This may affect equipment recommendations in terms of a left foot gas pedal or a set of hand controls. Finally, the DRS should explore the patient's driving experience and driving history, need to drive, amount of driving, type of traffic environments, and time of day in which driving occurs.

The next step in the clinical phase is to evaluate the patient's physical, visual, visuoperceptual, and cognitive performance with a functional perspective toward driving performance. Engum et al define basic operational and behavioral skills as "attention, concentration, rapid decision-making, stimulus discrimination/response differentiation, sequencing, visual-motor speed and coordination, visual scanning and acuity and attention shifting."[8] To assess these individual categories properly, the DRS should know the way specific areas in each category relate to specific driving tasks. In the *Post-Stroke Rehabilitation Practice Guide-line*, results of neurologic findings that most strongly influence rehabilitation decisions were charted. Using selected deficits seen most often in the patient recovering from CVA, the DRS addresses the way these deficits may affect driving performance. For example, the DRS addresses the way impulsive behavior and poor insight relate to driving a vehicle and the way upper or lower extremity sensory loss affects the ability to use the gas and brake pedals.

Physical Assessment

The physical assessment should involve a brief functional look at the patient's active range of motion, muscle strength, bilateral and unilateral gross and fine motor coordination, and any abnormalities such as spasticity, stereotypical patterns, associated reactions, and lack of any sensory modality. A slowing of physical functioning can affect reaction time in responding to stimuli in the environment. Slower reaction time among older drivers may be caused by strength and motor change or a slower decision-making process. The loss of strength and range of motion can prevent the person from safely operating the vehicle's primary or secondary controls. Decreases in physical function seen in the patient recovering from CVA can be accommodated with various kinds of adaptive equipment and driving aids (Figure 16-7). If this is not effective, patients may need to learn another method of driving, for example, using the left hand for inserting and turning the ignition key or operating the gear shift lever and using special panoramic mirrors to accommodate limited neck range of motion (Figures 16-8 and 16-9). If a flaccid arm or strong flexion pattern is noted in the movements of the arm that affect isolated control, the person may have only one hand to use on the steering wheel and may require a spinner knob. Some states require a spinner knob even if the person can palm the wheel and control it well with the remaining good arm. However compensatory techniques with special equipment for driving can only assist with the task of controlling a vehicle and do not resolve the older driver's other declining performance areas.

Visual Assessment

A vision assessment is crucial because driving is so dependent on visual skills. A vision assessment is more than mere checking of a client's visual acuity and depth perception. Scheiman, a rehabilitation optometrist who works with patients with various diagnoses, states that good vision is more than clear vision: "the individual must have the ability to use his eyes for extended periods of time without discomfort, be able to analyze and interpret the incoming information, and respond to what is being seen."[23] His experience indicates that nearly half of the patients admitted to a rehabilitation center with CVA or traumatic brain injury have visual system deficits, primarily in the area of binocular vision and accommodation. Other commonly re-

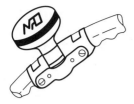

Spinner knob

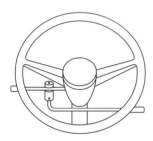

Left foot accelerator

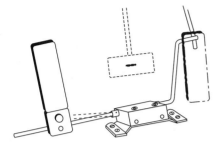

Turn signal crossover

Figure 16-7 Typical driving aids for a person recovering from CVA. (Courtesy Mobility Products and Design, Crow River Industries, Minneapolis, Minn.)

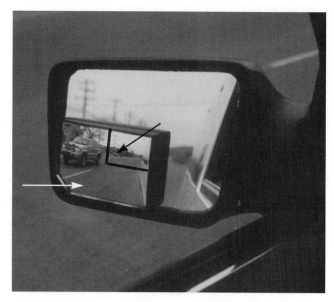

Figure 16-8 SmartView Mirror by Interactive Driving Systems. This mirror eliminates the confusion noted in the typical spot convex mirror and increases rear vision by dividing the mirror into two areas. The outside half of the SmartView mirror (*white arrow*) shows objects in the vehicle's blind spot, or Danger Zone. If a car is detected in the Danger Zone, the driver must not move in front of it. In this photograph the car shown is detected by the mirror to be in the driver's Danger Zone. The upper inside quadrant of the mirror (*black arrow*) is boxed and shows the Safe Zone. If a car is seen in the box—and stays in the box—the driver may move in front of it. (Courtesy Interactive Driving Systems, Cheshire, Conn.)

ported vision problems include reduced visual acuity, decreased contrast sensitivity, visual field deficits, visual neglect, strabismus, oculomotor dysfunction, and accommodative and stereopsis dysfunction.[23]

During the initial visual assessment, patients should be evaluated according to their respective states' vision requirements for licensing. This usually includes visual acuity of 20/40 in at least one eye and a total field of vision of at least 140°. Eye test charts can be used to ascertain visual acuity. A commercially available stereoscopic vision tester that is self-contained and often used by driver licensing agencies may be applicable to a clinical setting (Box 16-4). In addition to visual acuity, these machines also screen for depth perception, or stereopsis, contrast sensitivity, road sign recognition, phoria, fusion, and field of vision. These machines have limitations that must be taken into consideration by the therapist using them and interpreting the results. For example, stereoscopic vision testers often rely on binocular vision; if clients do not possess this skill, some of the findings will not be valid. These machines are a

starting point to assess these areas. If any suspicion of problem areas arises, the patient should be referred to an eye care specialist (Box 16-5). If basic state requirements are not met, the patient should be seen by an eye care specialist before having an on-the-road assessment. Some states allow a loss of vision in the lower quadrant as long as the lateral median in the superior quadrant is normal (Figure 16-10).

Lateralized visual field loss is common in patients recovering from CVA. The exact degree of visual field available in each eye should be assessed quantitatively. Gianutsos and Suchoff[10] have suggested that perimetric and functional visual fields also are important to assess. A patient with complete homonymous hemianopsia may have only 90° of total visual field. An occupational therapy clinic generally cannot afford expensive perimetric machines that can quantitatively measure exact degrees of visual fields in all quadrants.

Peripheral vision is an important visual function for safe driving. Whenever a DRS suspects that a patient has peripheral loss, an eye care specialist should evaluate the DRS's suspicion with an objective test using machines such as the Goldman or Humphrey perimeter tests. The speed of a vehicle also can affect visual acuity and side vision. For

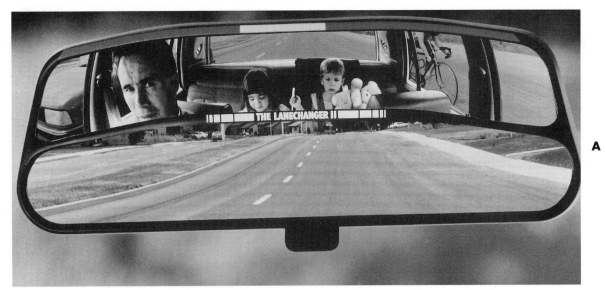

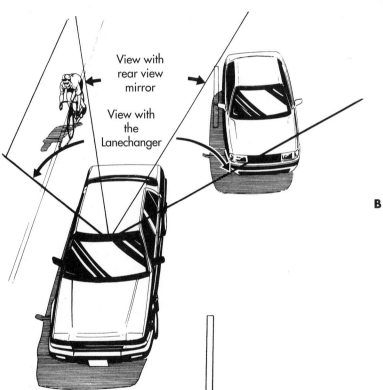

Figure 16-9   A, The Lanechanger mirror combines a standard rearview mirror with a convex mirror. **B,** This provides a wider angle of vision and increased safety. (Courtesy The Lanechanger, Quebec, Canada.)

example, if a person has 200° of visual field, at 20 miles per hour it is reduced to 104°, at 40 miles per hour it is 70°, and at 60 miles per hour it is 40°. Speed also decreases visual acuity; the faster the speed the less time available to react to visual stimuli in the environment.[25]

Aside from visual deficits that may occur because of the CVA, the DRS also must consider the normal change in vision skills occurring as a result of the person's age. As does any organ in the body, the eye loses some of its capability with age. The pupil of the eye becomes less elastic and restricts the amount of light let into the retina. Many elderly patients complain of difficulty driving at night or during weather conditions when the illumination is poor, such as in rain, fog, or snow. Cataracts and glaucoma are

Box 16-4

Vision Testing Equipment

Keystone View
Division of Mast Development
2212 East 12th St.
Davenport, IA 52803

Porto-Clinic
Driver Testing Equipment
1309 South Main Ave.
Scranton, PA 18504

Stereo Optical Company
3539 North Kento Ave.
Chicago, IL 60641

Titmus Optical Company
1015 Commerce St.
Petersburg, VA 23803-2934

Vistech Consultants, Inc.
1372 North Fairfield Rd.
Dayton, OH 45432

Box 16-5

Resources

College of Optometrists and Vision Development
(COVD)
P.O. Box 285
Chula Vista, CA 92012
619-592-6191

American Academy of Optometry
4330 East West Highway
Suite 1117
Bethesda, MD 20814
301-718-6500

Box 16-6

Common Driving Errors in Older Drivers

Difficulty backing up and making turns
Not seeing traffic signs or other cars quickly enough
Difficulty in locating and retrieving information from
    dashboard displays and traffic signs
Delayed glare recovery when driving at night
Not checking rearview mirrors and blind spots
Bumping into curbs and objects
Not yielding to oncoming traffic or right-of-way vehicles
Irregular or slow vehicle speeds

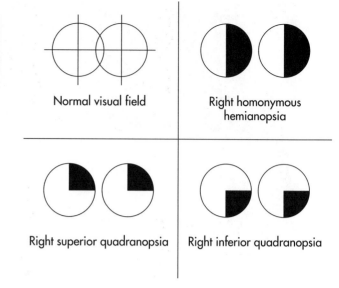

Figure 16-10 Representation of normal visual field in the eyes and typical visual field defects.

common among elderly persons. Cataracts, a clouding of the lenses, also can affect night driving and produce hazy vision during the day. Cataract surgery has a 90% success rate in a healthy older person who does not have comorbidities. Glaucoma, an increase in ocular pressure that results in damage to the optic nerve and retinal nerve fibers, begins to affect side vision first and then eventually compromises central vision. Glaucoma is a treatable condition, and a referral to the appropriate eye care specialist is important before performing a complete driving evaluation. Diabetic retinopathy should be considered for a person with a history of diabetes. Visual scanning, awareness, and attention should be assessed in the clinic by using some of the subtests in the visuoperceptual and cognitive tests discussed later in this chapter and in the vehicle and dynamic moving traffic environment (see Chapter 12).

Visuoperception and Cognitive Assessment

Common driving errors committed by elderly drivers may be related to vision, visuoperception, cognitive dysfunction, or an overall decline (Box 16-6). The driver must not only see objects in the path of travel but also understand their implications for safety to adjust driving accordingly. The most frequent citations for older drivers, noted by McKnight in his report "Driver and Pedestrian Training," involved failure to heed stop signs, traffic lights, no left turn signs, and other signs and signals.[17] Underwood notes that "safe driving requires complex cognitive skills, including vigilance, rapid visual scanning with attention to environmental detail, rapid processing of multiple stimuli in several sensory modalities, adequate judgment, and rapid decision-making."[30]

The purpose of the visuoperception and cognitive assessment is to attempt to identify problem areas and address these areas in relation to driving with minimal risk to the patient and therapist. The therapist should attempt to use clinical tools and tests that have the most significance to the driving task but not deny a patient the driving test based on these findings. A commonly accepted (but not researched) practice in driver rehabilitation in which occupational therapists are involved is to use a battery of familiar paper tests that assess specific visuoperceptual or cognitive areas although not in a manner analogous to driving. The DRS may spend 2 hours with the patient and still only be able to make an assumption regarding significant deficits and the way they may interfere with on-road performance. Because research shows little correlation between these tests and driving performance, the DRS must structure the clinical assessment with more driver-related tasks and tests that are currently available on the market (Box 16-7).

According to Toglia, the limitation to the deficit-specific approach to perception is that "it equates difficulty in performance of a specific task with a deficit … [and] does not consider the underlying reasons for failure or the conditions that influence performance."[29] For example, a patient may score low on a typical occupational therapy clinical test of visuoperceptual skills; nevertheless, the results may be a result of reduced visual acuity or accommodation and not necessarily a specific visuoperceptual deficit.

A stroke survivor who has serious visuoperceptual deficits will have difficulty throughout the rehabilitation process.[31] Documentation and observations of deficits should be performed by the clinical occupational therapist during routine evaluation and treatment procedures and functional tasks such as dressing, bathing, and cooking. The patient should probably not be referred for a driving evaluation until the deficit areas no longer interfere with basic ADL. If the therapist understands the definition of each visuoperceptual category and the way deficits in each area affect a person's basic self-care skills, a further analysis of driving tasks can show the way persistent problems in these areas can interfere with driving performance (see Chapter 13).

Driving requires a combination of perceptual skills in which cognitive performance plays a major role. Strong cognitive abilities are fundamental to attentiveness in the driving task, recognition of stimuli, and choice of the appropriate way to respond.[1] A decline in cognitive abilities can significantly influence a person's ability to plan, judge, and act adequately. A cognitively impaired person may have difficulty maneuvering a vehicle through rapidly changing traffic with many unexpected actions and reactions from other drivers, passengers, pedestrians, and bicyclists. Cognitive impairment has been linked to higher motor vehicle crash rates in elderly individuals.[1] Problem areas may involve attention, orientation, concentration, learning (short-term memory), and problem-solving. Diffuse cognitive deficits occur more frequently in patients with large frontal strokes, visuospatial deficits in right hemisphere strokes, and apraxia in left hemisphere strokes.[33] Unilateral neglect has been reported in half of the patients with right brain damage and in 20% to 25% with left brain damage.[28] Diller and Weinberg report that "patients with left hemiparesis often experience accidents that are related to difficulties in dealing with space, while accidents in patients with right hemiparesis are often related to slowness in processing information."[6]

Patients are generally more aware of motor problems than they are of cognitive problems.[12] Gresham et al note that "unawareness of the stroke (or its manifestations) is often found in patients with lesions in the nondominant hemisphere. It can lead to impulsive, unsafe behavior in a patient who may otherwise appear relatively normal with respect to physical functioning."[11] Patients' poor insight into their own problem areas can be dangerous because patients may not be aware of serious driver errors and the potentially fatal consequences of their actions. A neuropsychology evaluation performed by a psychologist or neuropsychologist can provide information regarding the cognitive performance of a patient; however, this is not often done with an elderly patient with a CVA. The occupational therapist may decide to use some common verbal and written tasks to assess orientation, concentration, reasoning, and problem-solving, but these tests are static and two dimensional and do not begin to simulate the dynamics of the driving task. The most effective way an occupational therapist who is a DRS can evaluate the effect of cognitive deficits on driving is via the driving task. Table 16-1 describes several performance areas and the way deficits in these areas can affect driving performance.

Table 16-1

Effects of Various Deficits on Driving Performance

TYPE OF DEFICIT	EFFECT ON DRIVING PERFORMANCE
Higher cognitive functions, memory, ability to learn	Cannot remember route to take to location or loses way if makes wrong turn; may not remember road names but can remember the route; severe deficits in higher functions may impede safe driving; unless the patient recovering from CVA is a new driver, the inability to learn new tasks may not impede safe driving; may require directions to be repeated
Motor	Usually does not impede safe driving because compensatory driving techniques or adaptive driving aids can be used
Disturbances in balance and coordination	May impede car transfers or loading of mobility device (e.g., wheelchair, walker); steering device, left-foot accelerator, or turn signal adaptation may compensate for inability to use the upper or lower extremity
Somatosensory	Does not generally interfere with driving because a person does not use an extremity with lack of sensation or with limiting pain while driving
Vision disorders	Severe visual loss or ocular motility disturbances may impede safe driving; the deficit may lead to the patient not meeting driver licensing requirements; persons with homonymous hemianopsia are not allowed to drive in most states; other age-related deficits such as glaucoma, cataracts, and diabetic retinopathy may impede safe driving
Unilateral neglect	A contraindication for safe driving
Speech and language	Expressive aphasia, dysarthria, or apraxias of speech are usually not problems in driving, although attempting to carry on a conversation while driving may cause distraction; receptive aphasia may impede the driver from understanding directions or conversation
Pain	The unaffected extremities may be used to drive; does not impede driving unless it is so severe it causes a distraction

In fairness to the patient the therapist's decision regarding the patient's visual, perceptual, and cognitive abilities for driving should not be based solely on a clinical test or solely on an on-the-road test. In a 1994 review of driver assessment methods at the Jewish Rehabilitation Center in Montreal, Canada, the chief of research and her associates found that 95% of their patients were given on-the-road tests because no clear cut-off score based on typical clinical tests was reliable in predicting whether a person was unsafe to drive.[15] Research by Gianutsos[9] and Engum et al[8] indicates a significant correlation in the elemental driving simulator (EDS) and cognitive behavioral driver's inventory (CBDI). These researchers believe that their results confirm the reliability and validity of their clinical driving assessment programs (Figure 16-11).

Gianutsos states that "road tests lack the basic psychometric requisites of tests—standardization, reliability and empirical validity."[9] She describes the EDS as a "computer-based quasi-simulator that is based on objective, norm-referenced measures of the cognitive abilities regarded as critical for driving."[9] These include mental processing efficiency, simultaneous information processing, perceptual-motor skills, and impulse control. The EDS also attempts to measure insight and judgment by comparing self-appraisal with performance.[9]

Egnum and associates note the following[8]:

Knowing the patient's diagnosis or pathology typically does not yield predictions about the patient's ability to drive. . . . Even loss of brain mass is not deemed to be an exact predictor of driving skills . . . neuropsychological tests which can detect gross organic impairment or provide useful catalogs of patients' impairments and abilities do not seem to assess driver potential.

Their 4-year research project with more than 230 brain-damaged patients led to the development of the CBDI. Their results demonstrated that more than 95% of the patients receiving passing scores on the CBDI were independently judged by an on-the-road driving test as safe to operate a motor vehicle. Conversely, all patients who failed the CBDI were judged as unsafe drivers in the independently administered road test.[8] A subsequent study by some of the same authors in 1988 completed a double-blind test of the validity of the CBDI. Again, a high correlation was found between the results of the CBDI and the independent road test.[7] However, although the CBDI is psychometrically strong, it has no face validity. So although the CBDI is useful, the EDS has face validity and may be better understood by patients as being relative to driving because it involves operating simulated primary car controls.

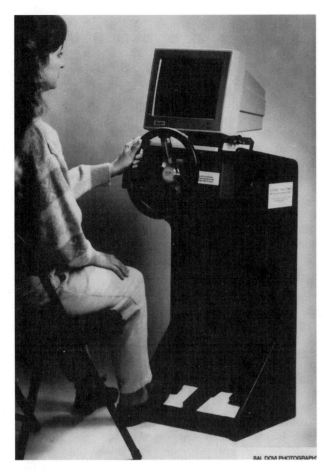

Figure 16-11 The elemental driving system. (Courtesy Life Science Associates, Bayport, NY.)

By using the EDS or CBDI the therapist not only obtains objective data but also recorded information relevant to the driving task. More importantly, data from these tests have demonstrated reliability and validity with published norms and standardized rules. This ensures that every patient is evaluated equally and the final judgment is not based solely on observation or a "gut feeling." The final judgment of the driving ability of a patient recovering from a CVA is difficult to defend in court if the decision is based on subjective means and not supported by objective data.

An appropriate end to the clinical assessment is a road rule and road sign test. Some DRSs also use the driver performance test (DPT), which is distributed by the Advanced Driving Skills Institute. This video of simulated "real world" driving scenes provides insight into the patient's perceptual capabilities, psychomotor responses, and decision-making strategies. Using a driver education defensive driving technique of identifying, predicting, deciding, and executing, the DPT requires the patient to search for hazardous situations or conditions, identify potential and immediate hazards, predict the effect of the hazard, decide the way to evade the hazard, and execute evasive

driving actions.[32] The drawback to this test is that it takes about 45 minutes to administer. Additional time is then necessary to review the answer video with the patient, an essential step for any learning or understanding to take place either by the patient or the therapist. Because the DPT has no statistical validity, the therapist should decide whether to use valuable time administering it or opting for a road test. The DPT also may be stress producing to the patient recovering from a CVA, because it requires quick problem solving and decision-making, quick marking on an answer sheet, and information retention. The test taker has only a few seconds to choose an answer and then must go on to the next traffic scene because no delay or pause is built into the video. If test takers get behind, they may become disorganized and not be able to respond to the next scene. Although quick thinking and reaction are important for driving, the DPT may be a better tool to use after the patient has passed all clinical tests and on-road tests. In other words, it may be a more effective tool to use when the therapist determines that the patient needs more practice, training, or review in the areas tested by the DPT.

On-the-Road Assessment

The value of the in-vehicle, in-traffic or on-the-road assessment cannot be underestimated. This portion of the driving evaluation is crucial and ideally should be conducted by a qualified professional who has an adequate medical background to understand the underlying diagnosis and disability. The evaluator also should have driver education knowledge and understand the purpose of taking a specific route, what to look for, the way to elicit underlying behaviors. The evaluator must have verbal, visual, and physical skills required to control the driver and the vehicle throughout the test. The road test has the following purposes:

1. To assess the driver's ability to enter and exit the vehicle safely and store any mobility aids efficiently
2. To assess the driver's understanding and operation of all vehicle primary and secondary controls
3. To assess in the moving vehicle the driver's need for adaptive devices or techniques for driving safely (e.g., using two feet to operate the gas and brake pedals may be safer than using the right leg on both pedals if the patient has a leg brace, hip flexion weakness, or slow reaction time)
4. To assess the driver's operational and strategic abilities in various traffic, speed, and road conditions
5. To assess the driver's memory for the roads and paths to various common locations
6. To support the findings of the clinical assessment and be able to accept and comply with specific recommendations based on driving performance in the real dynamic driving environment

Each individual should be given the opportunity for a behind-the-wheel evaluation, with the exception of persons not meeting state driver licensing guidelines. Even if the evaluation consists only of driving range maneuvers, the mistakes observed on the range may demonstrate to the patient the potential danger in actual traffic. According to Gianutsos,[9a] The New York State Vocational and Educational Services for Individuals with Disabilities (VESID) committee that addressed this issue concluded in its report on August 13, 1993, that no candidate should be advanced to driving without a behind-the-wheel test. Numerous studies have investigated driving after a stroke or head injury. These patients can be most difficult to assess for driving because they may not have physical disabilities that are readily seen, but may have more subtle visual, visuoperceptual, or cognitive problems not easily seen in typical clinical tests. More than half of all stroke survivors who drove cars before their strokes stop driving afterward.[16] Factors that are most commonly associated with driving cessation are older age at the time of stroke and the presence of cognitive deficits.[11] Wilson and Smith[34] investigated the driving performance of patients after stroke using two control groups on a planned driving course. The results indicated that the patients recovering from stroke performed more poorly than did the controls. Specific problems identified included difficulties entering and leaving an interstate, lack of awareness of other potential interacting vehicles, and difficulty in reacting to emergency situations. Analyses of the more likely performance components causing the driving errors were concluded to be difficulty in visual scanning, lane positioning, appropriate speed, coordination of separate visual scans, interaction with same directional traffic, and maintaining a safe distance from other vehicles.[34]

Earlier studies suggest that persons who pass tests for cognitive deficits do not require road tests.[18,24] Experienced certified DRSs and other more recent studies have found that clinical testing alone is insufficient and recommend a mandatory driving test.[4,14,35]

A simple 5- to 10-minute road test given by the driver licensing examiner is not adequate to assess fully all areas that must be considered in driving after a stroke. The examiner is primarily evaluating physical control of the vehicle during basic skills tests such as perpendicular or parallel parking, backing up, three-point turns, and right and left turns. Many times drivers are not even tested in traffic, or if they are, traffic exposure is light and short. The U.S. Department of Health and Human Resources' panel for post-stroke rehabilitation guidelines reflected in their report that "stroke survivors may be able to pass a driving test despite having visuospatial deficits or problems with easy distractibility, impulsive behaviors, or slowed decision making that may impair their ability to drive safely under unpredictable road conditions."[11] The driver examiner rarely has knowledge of all the adaptive equipment available for physical deficits. This lack of knowledge may be apparent. Proper evaluation and training in a dual-

controlled vehicle is necessary. Few states provide this type of evaluation and training through the driver licensing branch.

VEHICLE AND EQUIPMENT ASSESSMENT

Before taking a patient on the road, the DRS must complete the clinical portion of the vehicle and equipment assessment to decide what equipment should be set up for the driver's use in the evaluation vehicle. Determination of the vehicle and adaptive driving equipment appropriate for each patient depends largely on the physical and functional assessment results. Final determination of equipment needs takes place in the vehicle; however, the patient's own vehicle must be considered at some point. Fortunately, the elderly driver typically owns a vehicle with automatic transmission, which is required for the installation of most driving aids. Usually the driving equipment needed by a patient with left or right hemiplegia is minimal and not very costly (between $30 and $200). The patient requires special instructions and training on the devices in a dual-controlled vehicle. This training and practice should help prevent any accidents and allow the patient to become familiar with the devices. Proper use of the equipment also should be ascertained in a dynamic situation; however, the driver should be given sufficient learning time before being taken into complex traffic situations. A driving range or neighborhood with light traffic and speeds of 15 to 25 miles per hour is a safe, undemanding, and nonthreatening environment in which to start. Even if the patient has no equipment needs, this environment provides time to become familiar with the evaluator vehicle and the directions of the driver evaluator or instructor.

The driver recovering from a CVA generally requires a longer period of training because compensation or adaptation involves breaking habits (i.e., using hand controls instead of the feet for pedal operation). Driving is an overlearned skill for the experienced elderly driver, so the on-road test does not generally require teaching the patient to drive. Many operational components come back naturally to the patient unless a residual memory problem associated with dementia or agnosia or apraxia is evident. Patients' strategic skills may be impaired by any visual, visuoperceptual, or cognitive deficits that remain.

The goals, objectives, and structuring for the in-traffic assessment must be understood and planned. Every mile of road the patient is requested to drive should have a purpose. Ramsey,[21] a driver educator from West Virginia who has more than 30 years' experience working with people with diverse disabilities, states that if driver evaluators or educators go straight for more than a mile, they are "taking a joy ride" and not effectively assessing a person's ability to drive. Driving straight is easier than making vehicle and speed adjustments for left and right turns and merging.[21] The visual and mental demands on the driver are greatly increased in executing multiple-step procedures with divided attention demands. A planned route on which every patient is evaluated can be used. The route for a patient who has had a stroke should focus on problem areas seen with the patient's particular deficit areas. Driving tasks also may bring out the common errors seen in elderly drivers. Routes familiar and unfamiliar to the patient may have to be used to expose the patient to many complex driving situations. If possible, the evaluator should start or end the test at the patient's home environment, because the patient will likely perform better and be more relaxed on familiar roads. Also, the DRS can get an understanding of the traffic and roads that the patient normally encounters during driving.

The therapist must be flexible on the road, guiding the patient on and off the planned route to observe driver error. For example, if a patient with poor insight and visual awareness is running stop signs or doesn't show any reaction to a lane ending sign, this person should be taken off the route to practice this skill to see whether improvement is possible. This driver should not be taken into more complex driving situations in which a hazard may be posed to other road users until correction is seen. A patient with expressive and receptive aphasia may be distracted from the driving scene while attempting to process the therapist's verbal directions during driving. In this case, the patient may benefit from being taken around the familiar home environment and allowed to self-direct in driving from one destination to another such as the bank, drugstore, or doctor's office.

ADAPTIVE EQUIPMENT PRESCRIPTION

After the patient has been through the clinical assessment, vehicle and equipment assessment, and in-traffic assessment, the occupational therapist should write an evaluation summary supporting licensure or specifying equipment recommendations or a prescription. Webster's dictionary defines *prescription* as "a formula directing the preparation of anything." In the context of driving, a prescription may include directing the patient, the equipment installer, and possibly a funding source to the specific equipment needs of the client. The document should be easily read and understandable, written specifically for the patient and the patient's vehicle. Sometimes the therapist may need to be more descriptive than just recommending a left foot gas pedal. In other words, if the patient prefers a quick-release model so a spouse can drive the car without worrying about inadvertently stepping on the left gas pedal, a specific brand must be specified, because not all brands provide this convenient feature. The prescription should be inclusive, considering every aspect of a vehicle or control such as the way the driver operates the steering column controls, the way the driver loads or carries a manual wheelchair or quad cane, or the way the driver opens the door or trunk of the vehicle.

The prescription should not be guesswork or an estimation. It should be based on a thorough and objective assessment in stationary and dynamic modes after the patient was observed using each piece of equipment or device safely, efficiently, and easily. Finally, the prescription should not be written until the patient has had sufficient time in a moving assessment or training to demonstrate safe driving skills and safe use of the equipment. Many patients, particularly those who have had strokes, often may need several driving sessions until they are deemed safe drivers. If the therapist writes the prescription too soon, the patient may go to an installer and have the equipment put in the vehicle before the patient is ready to drive. The prescription should indicate to all significant parties that the patient has successfully completed a comprehensive driving assessment, the evaluator has made an objective determination that the patient can drive safely, and the equipment prescribed is the only necessity for the patient to return to driving.

Guiding the patient to a competent and qualified mobility equipment dealer and installer is important. The DRS should identify all the dealers in the communities in which the driving program operates so that an appropriate referral can be made. The dealer should be factory trained or certified by the equipment manufacturer to install the specific devices prescribed. The dealer should respect the therapist's expertise and role so as not to overstep boundaries and install equipment without a prescription or substitute, delete, change, or add items on the document.

The final task for the DRS is to provide any necessary follow-up steps. These may include but are not limited to the following:

1. *Additional driver training in the evaluation vehicle or the patient's own vehicle after the prescribed equipment has been installed*—If training is completed in the patient's vehicle, a rental training brake should be installed or the patient should be close to finishing the training and the therapist should not perceive a need for a brake.

2. *Equipment inspection and adjustments*—Inspection and adjustment of equipment should be done after the installation of the equipment and before the patient is released to drive the vehicle. The therapist should ensure that all prescription items have been installed and are working properly. The driver should be observed using the equipment so that any adjustments or fitting may be completed by the mobility equipment dealer. The dealer does not have the knowledge about the patient that the therapist has and may not know or understand the way to adjust equipment for a particular patient's needs. Equipment may be installed properly and still not work optimally for the client if it has not been ad-

justed for safe use. For example, the therapist may prescribe a spinner knob at the 5 o'clock position on the steering wheel. The dealer may ignore or forget the location specified and place the knob at 1 o'clock. The patient has a weak right shoulder and fatigues quickly if the arm is held suspended against gravity for a long period. The lower position on the wheel allows the patient to maintain the arm in a resting position while steering straight and keeps the knob easily available for curves and turns. The patient may wear a size 12 shoe, but if the vendor ignores this factor when determining the location of the left foot gas pedal in relation to the brake, the pedals may be so close that the patient inadvertently steps on both pedals simultaneously.

3. *Driver licensing or relicensing*—Informing the patient of the law's requirements and providing assistance if necessary by obtaining a valid driver's license with the appropriate restrictions are other therapist activities. The patient may need to be taken for a road test in the evaluation vehicle or may require the DRS's guidance and assistance to communicate with the medical review board to have the driver license reinstated after a suspension.

4. *Communicating with the physician, other team members, and the family so they know the outcome of the driving evaluation*—It is important for the physician, team members, and family to understand and support any follow-up services that may be necessary after the initial evaluation period. If the patient has a progressive condition such as the beginning of cataracts, multiple sclerosis, Parkinson's disease, senile dementia, or Alzheimer's disease, the doctor and medical review board should be notified of the need for periodic reevaluation of the patient's driving skills, the time frame of the reevaluation, and the need for education on events that may indicate a need for reevaluation at a given point.

When the patient can no longer drive safely, the appropriate party should gently inform the patient with compassion. The loss of a driver's license changes a person's life dramatically. The person may no longer be able to live alone or remain in the house that has been home for 30 or 40 years. The person may become dependent on others for transportation and may have to cut out many social activities. The patient may be forced to get to destinations important for purchasing services and goods for daily living by using a taxi, walking to a public bus stop, or calling on the cheaper but often unreliable local transportation services for the disabled that are available in many city communities. The patient should be informed that taxis are expensive means of transportation but still cheaper than owning a car and paying for maintenance, gas, and insurance.

The patient recovering from CVA should not be told

about the inability to continue driving without follow-up. Transportation needs and options should be discussed with the person and family members or other caregivers. The following recommendations are suggested means to ease the frustration:

1. The person should be given a frank and honest description of observable driving behaviors or problems areas that do not allow for safe driving. Discussion of the EDS personalized report is helpful at this point because time is needed for the information and consequences to be processed; the patient should be given an opportunity to discuss problems and ask questions.

2. A significant other should be present with the patient for psychological support, to help the patient decide the best way of securing transportation, and perhaps to discuss selling the vehicle.

3. Available counseling through the doctor, psychologist, or other senior health counselor should be sought to assist the patient psychologically. The patient will likely go through an expression of a variety of feelings and emotions such as denial, anger, resentment, and depression. Family members and friends should be available to check on the patient in case depression becomes deep enough to require frequent and formal counseling.

4. Transportation problems must be resolved for the patient. Family members or friends should be recruited for personal errands and appointments. Information about optional transportation for senior citizens and persons with disabilities should be given in detail and in writing to the patient. If necessary, the patient should be taken on a city bus route to one of the patient's appointments and instructed in the way to use the route and bus map guide. The therapist may discuss the option of keeping the personal car and hiring a neighbor or friend to drive it several days of the week for any necessary trips.

SUMMARY

Driving after a stroke is possible for some patients. A comprehensive driving evaluation with a qualified DRS is paramount to any decision regarding the patient's driving ability. Patients and their families must be educated early in rehabilitation by the physician and other team members of the necessity and importance of the evaluation. Liability and insurance issues arising from driving without a valid license, without the doctor's approval, without necessary equipment, or without a documented evaluation should be explained, with the emphasis on the detrimental effects on the patient's finances, assets, and security if an accident occurs. The occupational therapist is the logical team member to coordinate and be directly involved in driver evaluation procedures. Necessary specialized education and a period of practice and learning must take place to ensure the occupational therapist is confident and competent to make the important judgment regarding a patient's ability to drive. A patient who has had a CVA presents unique problems that must be looked at individually. The final decision regarding the patient's driving future must be made on as much reliable, objective information as can be obtained.

REVIEW QUESTIONS

1. Describe at least five activities that illustrate the importance of community mobility to a patient who has had a CVA.
2. What specific areas should be evaluated during a driving assessment for a patient with left hemiplegia from a CVA?
3. Describe the liability issues the physician, therapist, and facility face when performing a driving assessment?
4. Give four driving behaviors or errors that may be seen in a patient with left side neglect.
5. Give specific performance components (e.g., visual, perceptual, cognitive, physical) used in the following steps of each driving task:
   Lane change to the right
   Rearview mirror check
   Right outside mirror check
   Right turn signal
   Right head check
   Gradual and small turn of wheel to right
   Cancel turn signal
   Accelerate as appropriate
6. List at least six factors influencing a successful driving evaluation.
7. What is the purpose of the driving prescription? List all its uses.
8. What adaptive driving equipment may be used for the following deficits?
   Use of one hand only for steering
   Nonuse of right lower extremity
   Nonuse of left upper extremity
   Lack of neck motion (particularly rotation)
9. What challenges should the DRS present to the patient recovering from CVA during the in-traffic assessment?

REFERENCES

1. *Aging and performance: transportation in an aging society*, Committee for the Study on Improving Mobility and Safety for Older Persons—vol 1, Transportation Research Board, Washington, DC, 1988.
2. Antrim MJ, Engum ES: The driving dilemma and the law: patients striving for independence versus public safety, *Cognitive Rehab*, pp 16-19, March/April 1989.
3. Blum J: Keeping seniors on the move, *Columbus Monthly* 8:72, 1993.
4. Brooke MM et al: Driving evaluation after traumatic brain injury, *Am J Phys Med Rehabil* 71:177, 1992.
5. Carp FM: Significance of mobility for the well-being of the elderly, *Transportation in an Aging Society* 2:2, 1988.
6. Diller L, Weinberg J: Evidence for accident-prone behavior in hemiplegic patients, *Arch Phys Med Rehabil* 51:358, 1970.
7. Engum ES: Criterion-related validity of the cognitive behavioral driver's inventory: brain-injured patients versus normal control, *Cognitive Rehab* 8:20, 1990.
8. Engum ES et al: Cognitive behavioral driver's inventory, *Cognitive Rehab*, pp 34-50, Sept/Oct 1988.
9. Gianutsos R: Driving advisement with the elemental driving simulator (EDS): when less suffices, behavior research methods, *Instruments and Computers* 26:183, 1997.
9a. Gianutsos R: Personal communication, September 1996.
10. Gianutsos R, Suchoff IB: Visual fields after brain injury: management issues for the occupational therapist. In Scheiman M, editor: *Vision: screening and intervention techniques for occupational therapists*, Thorofare, NJ, 1996, SLACK.
11. Gresham GE et al: *Post-stroke rehabilitation. Clinical practice guideline*, No 16, Rockville, MD: US Department of Health and Human Services. Public Health Service, Agency for Health Care Policy and Research. AHCPR Publication No. 95-0662, May 1995.
12. Hibbard MR et al: Awareness of disability in patients following stroke, *Rehabil Psychol* 37:103, 1992.
13. Jacobs S: Reporting the handicapped driver, *Arch Phys Med Rehabil* 59:387, 1978.
14. Katz RT et al: Driving safety after brain damage: follow-up of 22 patients with matched controls, *Arch Phys Med Rehabil* 71:133, 1990.
15. Korner-Bitensky N: Assessing ability to drive following an acute neurological event: are we on the right road? *Can J Occup Ther* 61:141, 1994.
16. Legh-Smith J: Driving after a stroke, *JR Soc Med* 79:200, 1986.
17. McKnight JA: *Driver and pedestrian training*, Transportation Research Board.
18. Nouri FM: Cognitive ability and driving after stroke, *Int Dis Stud* 9:110, 1987.
19. Persson D: The elderly driver: deciding when to stop, *The Gerontologist* 33:88, 1993.
20. Pierce S: Legal considerations for a driver rehabilitation specialist, *AOTA Physical Disabilities Special Interest Section Newsletter* 16:1, 1993.
21. Ramsey B: *Take the wheel: a driver education course for the therapist*, Course notes, Orlando, Fla, 1996.
22. Rosenbloom S: The mobility needs of the elderly, *Transportation in an Aging Society* 2:26, 1988.
23. Scheiman M: *Understanding and managing visual deficits: theory screening procedures, intervention techniques*, Course notes, Atlanta, 1996.
24. Sivak M et al: Driving and perceptual/cognitive skills and behavioral consequences of brain damage, *Arch Phys Med Rehabil* 62:476, 1981.
25. Slavin S: *Association of driver educators for the disabled conference presentation*, Orlando, FL, 1987.
26. Smith EE: *Choice research time: an analysis of the major theoretical positions*, *Psych Bull* 69:77, 1968.
27. Steich T: Malpractice insurance important for occupational therapy personnel, *OT Week* 40, 1986.
28. Stone SP et al: The assessment of visuo-spatial neglect after acute stroke, *J Neurol Neurosurg Psych* 54:345, 1991.
29. Toglia JP: Visual perception of objects: an approach to assessment and intervention, *Am J Occup Ther* 43:587, 1993.

30. Underwood M: The older driver: clinical assessment and injury prevention, *Arch Intern Med* 152:737, 1992.

31. Warren M: A hierarchical model for evaluation and treatment of visual perceptual dysfunction in adult acquired brain injury, part 2, *Am J Occup Ther* 47:55, 1993.

32. Weaver J: *Driver performance test*, Palm Harbor, FL, 1989, Advanced Driving Skills Institute.

33. Wilson B: Development of a behavioral test of visuospatial neglect, *Arch Phys Med Rehabil* 68:98, 1987.

34. Wilson T, Smith T: Driving after stroke, *Int Rehabil Med* 5:170, 1983.

35. Van Zomeran AH: Acquired brain damage and driving: a review, *Arch Phys Med Rehabil* 68:697, 1987.

anne marie skvarla
roberta ann schroeder-lopez

chapter **17**

Dysphagia Management

key terms

dysphagia
bedside evaluation
modified barium swallow
fiberoptic endoscopic evaluation
of swallowing

aspiration
penetration
silent aspiration
bolus

alternate nutrition
feeding trials
auscultation

chapter objectives

After completing this chapter, the reader will be able to accomplish the following:

1. Describe the normal anatomy and physiology of the swallowing mechanism.
2. Demonstrate the effects of stroke on the swallowing mechanism.
3. Describe the psychosocial effects of dysphagia.
4. Describe various techniques used to treat dysphagia after a stroke.
5. Describe the symptoms of dysphagia that occur after a stroke.
6. Discuss the implications of various treatment approaches and their possible outcomes.

Dysphagia (dis-fá-je- ə) comes from the Greek prefix *dys*, meaning *difficult*, and the Greek term *phagein*, meaning *to eat*. The occurrence of dysphagia (swallowing difficulty) after stroke is common, with a reported incidence as high as 47%.[36] Problems associated with dysphagia following stroke include aspiration pneumonia, compromised nutritional status, dehydration, and death.

Aspiration refers to the penetration of food or liquid into the airway, below the level of the vocal folds, before, during, or after the swallow. Penetration refers to the entrance of food or liquid into the larynx, above the level of

the vocal folds.[39] Silent aspiration is defined as the penetration of saliva, food, or liquid below the level of the true vocal folds without a cough or any outward sign of difficulty.[19] Causes of aspiration include gastric reflux, food, liquid, and saliva.[17,33]

Veis and Logemann[68] estimate that approximately one third of all stroke patients with dysphagia aspirate. Aspiration is common in the acute phase following stroke, with a greater incidence in severe strokes and pharyngeal sensory loss.[15] Horner and associates[20] report that approximately 30% of all patients who have strokes experience dysphagia, and silent aspiration goes unnoticed. Approximately 40% of patients with dysphagia who aspirate do not exhibit symptoms of aspiration during the bedside evaluation.[19] Of patients selected for a videofluoroscopic study, 40% to 70% were shown to actually aspirate.[20] Veis and Logemann[68] found that 75% of their subjects had more than one swallowing disorder, with a delayed swallow reflex usually causing aspiration before the swallow and decreased laryngeal adduction generally causing aspiration during the swallow. They also found that 32% of the subjects aspirated from pharyngeal dysphagia, which cannot be detected during the bedside evaluation.[68] Thus videofluoroscopic studies appear to be essential in the identification of aspiration after stroke.

Aspiration can lead to pneumonia. Langmore[33] reports that aspiration of gastric reflux can quickly lead to pneumonia because of the burn-like damage resulting from the acidic contents of the stomach. Acute respiratory distress can occur within hours. Food entering the airway can lead to pneumonia within a week. Liquids are particularly damaging when they are acidic. Saliva can be very dangerous if infected with pathogens and can lead to pneumonia in several weeks.[26,27]

Dehydration is another possible consequence of dysphagia,[56] although Smithard et al.[63] report that changes in hydration are not statistically significant. Schmidt et al.[60] were unable to identify an increased risk of dehydration for patients with aspiration compared with those who did not aspirate. Schmidt et al.[60] also reported that as documented by modified barium swallow, aspiration after stroke is associated with a significant increase in the risk of pneumonia and death but not dehydration. They also reported that the odds ratio for death is 9.2 times greater for patients who aspirated thickened liquids or more solid consistencies compared with those who did not aspirate or aspirated thin liquids only.

Nutritional status may also be compromised by stroke.[3,44] Many variables may be involved, including dysphagia, loss of appetite, decreased mental status, depression and other psychosocial factors, and medication interactions.

SITE OF LESION

The correlation of stroke location with aspiration remains unclear.[1,17,45] Teasell and associates[66] report that aspiration occurred in at least 9.9% of all patients who had unilateral right hemispheric strokes, 12.1% of those who had unilateral left hemispheric strokes, 24% of those who had bilateral hemispheric strokes, and 39.5% of those who had brain stem strokes. Horner and associates report that aspiration occurred two times more often in bilateral cerebrovascular accidents (CVA) compared with unilateral CVAs. The most common reason for aspiration after bi-

lateral stroke was incomplete laryngeal elevation and closure, which encourages aspiration during the swallow and reduces pharyngeal peristalsis after the swallow, affecting aspiration of residue.[20] Alberts et al.[1] reported that patients with only small vessel infarcts had a decreased incidence of aspiration compared with those who had both large and small vessel infarcts. The highest frequency of aspiration occurred with large vessel pontine lesions, followed by infarcts in the middle cerebral artery and posterior cerebral artery. These findings suggest that patients who have experienced stroke should be evaluated on a case-by-case basis for dysphagia regardless of type, location, and size of the infarct.[4,6,7,18,55] Aspiration pneumonia is an important complication of stroke.[42,43,51] If left untreated, it often results in hospitalization or death. The optimal management of patients with dysphagia should focus on the prevention of aspiration by early intervention and treatment. Wallenburg's syndrome, or lateral medullary syndrome, is one of the most frequently recognized syndromes of brain stem stroke. Although dysphagia is usually diagnosed as mild, it is occasionally severe enough to warrant feeding by nasogastric tube. Ipsilateral palatal paralysis and hoarseness secondary to ipsilateral vocal fold paralysis are sometimes noted. Reduced sensation to pain and temperature on the opposite side of the body is noted as well. This is important to patients with dysphagia because of the oral-pharyngeal bolus sensation.[58] Lacunar infarcts are not always associated with specific dysphagic symptoms; however, lacunar infarcts may eventually lead to multi-infarct dementia, which may influence swallow functioning secondary to cognitive deficits.

NORMAL ANATOMY AND PHYSIOLOGY OF THE SWALLOWING MECHANISM

A prerequisite for successful management of patients with dysphagia is knowledge of the anatomy and physiology of the swallowing mechanism. Figure 17-1 represents a midsagittal view of the anatomic landmarks of the head and neck important in swallowing. Figure 17-2 represents anatomic landmarks of the oral cavity. The act of swallowing may be divided into three separate stages: oral, pharyngeal, and esophageal. Figure 17-3 illustrates the division of these three stages. The oral stage is preceded by an oral preparatory phase.

Oral Preparatory Stage

At the oral preparatory stage, patients should be able to demonstrate the following skills: tray set-up and preparation, orientation to bolus, transport of the bolus to the mouth, adequate mouth opening, bolus containment in the oral cavity, oral sensation for the bolus, and manipulation of the bolus using the muscles of mastication, jaw, and soft palate.

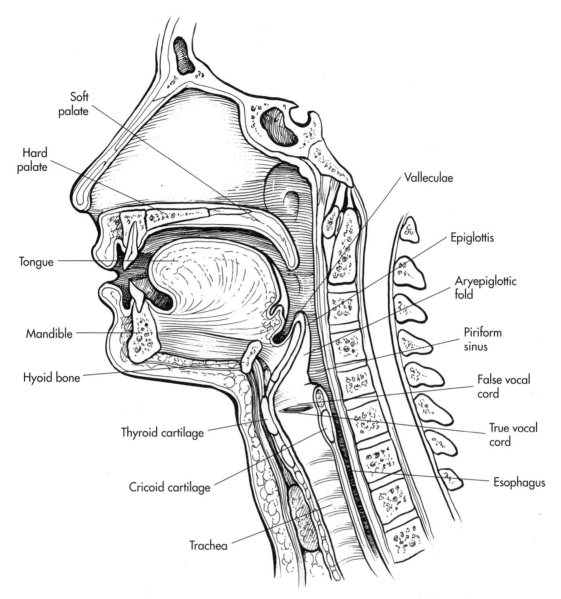

Figure 17-1 Midsagittal view of swallowing landmarks.

Oral Stage

During the oral stage of the swallow, the food or liquid enters the oral cavity. The muscles of mastication prepare the bolus for transport (Figure 17-4, *A*). The lips and buccal muscles contract and propel the bolus posteriorly as the tongue strips the bolus against the hard palate, propelling it into the oropharynx and beginning the pharyngeal stage of the swallow (Figure 17-4, *B*).

Pharyngeal Stage

During this stage of the swallow, the soft palate elevates, closing off the nasopharynx. The vocal folds close, protecting the airway from aspiration and penetration. The epiglottis folds over the laryngeal vestibule (Figure 17-4, *C*), again preventing airway penetration and directing the bolus toward the piriform sinus. The larynx rises and the pharyngeal peristalsis squeezes the bolus downward through the pharnyx toward the cricopharyngeal muscle (Figure 17-4, *D*). The cricopharyngeal muscle, which is at the superior aspect of the esophagus, relaxes and allows the bolus to pass into the esophagus, the third stage of the swallow[25] (Figure 17-4, *E*).

Cranial Nerves/Swallow Function

Six cranial nerves are involved in the swallow process[32,52] (Box 17-1).

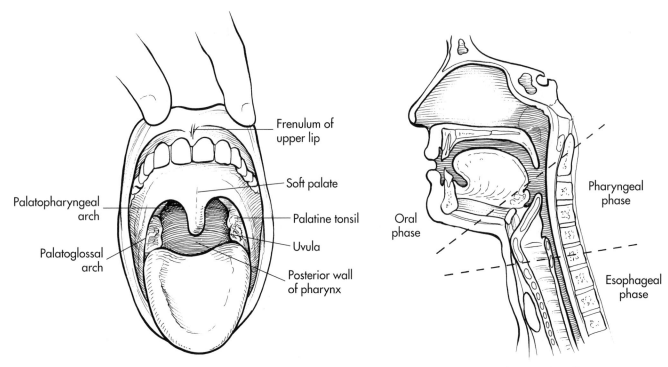

Figure 17-2 Landmarks of the oral cavity.

Figure 17-3 Stages of a normal swallow: sagittal view.

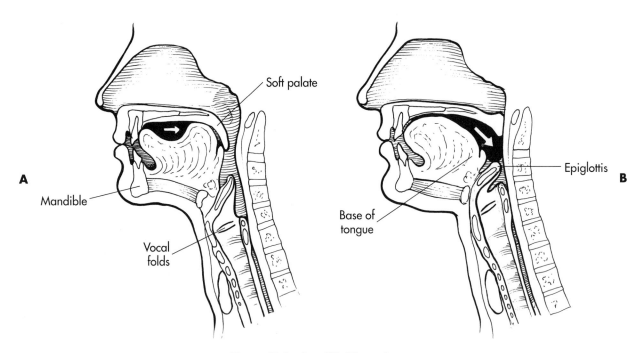

Figure 17-4 **A** and **B,** The oral stage.

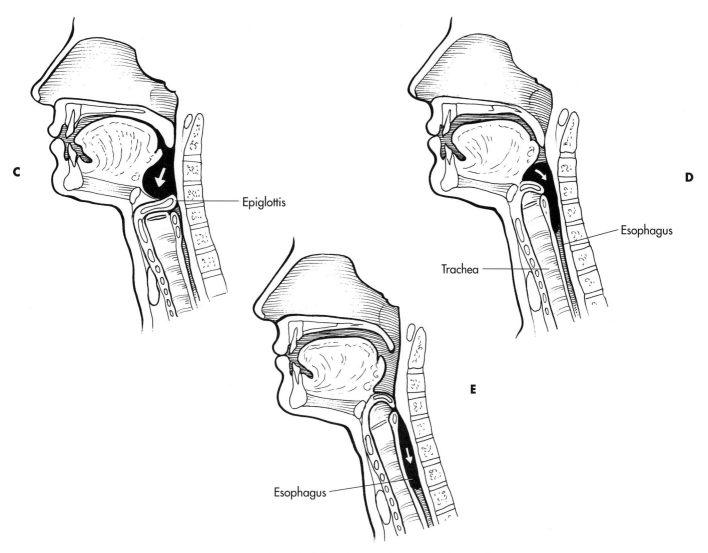

Figure 17-4, cont'd   **C** and **D**, The pharyngeal stage. **E**, The esophageal stage.

Box 17-1

Cranial Nerve Functions

ORAL STAGE

CN V Trigeminal—tactile and proprioceptive sensation and motor

CN VII Facial—taste and motor

PHARYNGEAL STAGE

CN IX Glossopharyngeal—taste, pharyngeal peristalsis, salivation, taste

CN X Vagus—taste and motor, intrinsic laryngeal muscles, pharyngeal peristalsis, swallow initiation

CN XI Accessory—pharyngeal peristalsis, head and neck stability

ORAL AND PHARYNGEAL STAGE

CN XII Hypoglossal—lingual movement, laryngeal and hyoid movement

ROLE OF THE SWALLOW TEAM

The optimal swallow evaluation and management of dysphagia are performed by a multidisciplinary team.[47] The team plays an important role in the identification, evaluation, diagnosis, treatment, and overall management of patients with dysphagia.

The multidisciplinary team[48,69] should include the speech-language pathologist, occupational therapist, nurse,[34] physician, respiratory therapist, and nutritionist.[44] The patient and caregivers should also play an active role in decision-making. For management of the dysphagic patient to be successful, *all* persons involved in the patient's care should understand the dysphagic impairment and the management techniques employed.[9,10,24] Ongoing education and follow-up is necessary.[2]

Evaluation of Swallowing

According to Sonies,[64] "swallowing is a complex, sequential behavior with a variety of interdependent patterns of motor activity that occur simultaneously and rapidly in a predetermined order." Dysphagia occurs when something interferes with this behavior.

Dysphagia can be evaluated by observation or the use of instruments. *Instrumental evaluation* refers to diagnostic testing such as videofluoroscopy and fiberoptic endoscopic evaluation of swallowing (FEES) exams.[5,31] Sonies[64] believes that "accurate assessment of the activity of the oral, pharyngeal, and esophageal areas during swallowing requires the use of instrumental diagnostic imaging techniques to view the intrinsic physiology." However, many of these evaluation procedures are invasive and uncomfortable and expose the patient to radiation. Some do not show the anatomy during swallowing or evaluate only part of the swallow process. Thus the risks and benefits must be considered before subjecting a patient to such procedures.

Videofluoroscopy is a dynamic evaluation of the complete swallow that produces a picture of the anatomy during swallowing. Ultrasound is a noninvasive, dynamic evaluation of swallowing that also shows the anatomy. Normal foods and liquids are used in this procedure, and it is safe for infants and patients who are comatose or uncooperative. This procedure evaluates only part of the swallow, however. Neither electroencephalogram (EEG) nor electromyogram (EMG) show anatomy. EEG is invasive and can detect laryngeal elevation. It is more often used for research. EMG, although noninvasive, is better used to evaluate for muscular paralysis. Scintigraphy is expensive and not readily available because it requires an MD trained in nuclear medicine. Scintigraphy is best used to assess aspiration with tracheostomy patients. FEES has historically been used by otolaryngologists to assess vocal cord function. It has been used increasingly in dysphagia to determine whether residual food is present on the vocal cords or pooled in the vallecula or sinuses after a swallow. The negative aspects of this evaluation are that the endoscopic tube inhibits a normal swallow and produces a static view of only part of a swallow. This procedure is contraindicated for patients with cardiac arrhythmias, respiratory distress, bleeding disorders, anatomic deviations (narrow nasal passage), agitated or hostile patients, or patients with movement disorders.[64]

Observational evaluations include bedside and clinical evaluations (see Chapter 17 Appendix). Perlman et al.[54] describe bedside evaluation as a screening tool and the clinical evaluation as a more thorough examination of the patient. This chapter focuses on clinical evaluation, which includes information from the medical chart, patient and caregiver interviews, and evaluation of mental status, respiratory system, and oral, motor, and swallow function. Although Splaingard et al[65] report that the bedside evaluation is a poor indicator of risk for aspiration, risk of

complication, or need for further investigation, other studies dispute this finding. The 3-oz water test screening, along with a clinical checklist of symptoms can determine the evidence of aspiration and whether more comprehensive testing is necessary.[12]

The Burke dysphagia screen test, which identified 11 of 12 patients who developed pneumonia, obstructed airway, or death, is a fast and cost-effective way to identify patients at risk for aspiration.[13]

Clinical Evaluation

When dysphagia is suspected, the physician or general nurse practitioner can order a bedside swallow evaluation. Nursing staff, allied health professionals, the patient's family or caregiver, the patient's roommate, or the patient may identify the need for this evaluation. The benefit of a bedside swallow evaluation is it assists the therapist in determining the patient's risk for aspiration and other factors that may contribute to a decrease in oral intake. The appropriate referrals can be made to further assess the dysphagia, and interventions for treatment may be implemented.

Chart Review

The therapist must first carefully review the patient's chart to ascertain pertinent facts from the medical and feeding history. The therapist must determine the reason that the physician has requested a swallowing evaluation and then ask the patient or caregivers specific questions regarding the patient's eating habits. The following questions may be relevant:

- Has a change occurred in the type or amount of food eaten? (If so, note when this occurred and any symptoms of dysphagia.)
- Has dysphagia or aspiration pneumonia been diagnosed previously?
- Has the patient experienced weight loss or other factors that may explain the patient's difficulty eating?

Often the information obtained during chart review reveals that the decrease in oral intake is caused not by a problem with the swallowing mechanism but by other reasons, including depression, pain, inability to eat independently, incorrect diet, or food dislikes.

Certain types of information are particularly important during chart review. The following list identifies key areas to emphasize:

- Age[41]
- Previous evaluations and tests indicating current function (positive infiltrate on chest x-ray examination; ear, nose, and throat evaluation)
- Primary diagnosis and date of onset
- Past medical history and secondary diagnosis
- Previous history of aspiration pneumonia

- Aspiration precautions
- Respiratory therapy involvement
- Current method of nutritional intake
- Current type of diet ordered (dysphagia diet)
- Calorie count
- Length of time on current diet
- Dietary restrictions (diabetic: no concentrated sugars; cardiac: low sodium)
- Food allergies
- Current respiratory status

When reviewing the chart, the therapist must consider the patient's ability to participate in the evaluation, which determines the appropriateness of oral feeding. Mental and respiratory status play an important role in a person's ability to eat. Logemann[38] states that medical and behavioral factors can affect oral intake regardless of the presence of dysphagia. She cites combative behavior, hypersensitivity at or around the mouth when being fed, impulsivity when eating independently, fatigue, and distractibility as examples. Factors to consider for mental status are as follows: primary language spoken, level of alertness, ability to follow directions, insight into swallowing difficulty, cognitive and perceptual status, and ability to communicate needs. Because eating requires a coordination of breathing and swallowing, respiratory problems may affect a person's ability to eat safely. The following factors should be considered when evaluating the patient's ability to eat orally: excessive oral secretions, tracheostomy type (including whether it is cuffed), ventilator dependence and ability to wean, chest physical therapy involvement, and frequency and route of suctioning.

Patient/Caregiver Interview

Initial contact begins at the nursing station and in the patient's room, where the practitioner may ask questions of the patient, nurse, aide, physician, caregivers, and visitors regarding the patient's past and present eating function. The patient may cough during or after meals or eat in suboptimal positions. Obtaining this type of information in advance can expedite and enhance the evaluation process.

Informal observation begins as soon as the practitioner enters the patient's room. The therapist should observe the room for any types of food that may indicate the patient's recent diet. Details to observe include the presence of an untouched meal tray; residual food on the patient's face, clothing, bed, or tray; and wet or hoarse breath sounds and abnormal vocal quality. The position of the patient's body, head, neck, and arms is also relevant. The therapist should note whether the patient seems alert and able to communicate.

Functional Status

Functional status refers to the patient's ability to move in space and make use of the environment. A key to the swallowing evaluation is positioning for eating. If patients are unable to self-adjust to achieve an upright sitting position, they may require assistance. The therapist should determine the amount of assistance required to position patients in the bed or chair and whether they are able to maintain the position independently. Ideally the patient is sitting upright in a chair with the pelvis in a neutral-anterior tilt, forearms weight bearing on the tabletop, and the head and neck slightly forward flexed. Hand function is also evaluated because it relates to the ability to control upper extremity movement and eat independently.

Adaptive equipment or environmental adaptations may enable patients to feed themselves if indicated. Adaptations to position include supporting feet that do not reach the floor with a telephone book or foot rest, increasing chair height with cushions, and elevating the table height by placing a telephone book under the food tray. Adaptive equipment may also include wheelchairs with removable or swing-away armrests that allow the patient to eat at the table. Other helpful items are dycem to prevent the plate from slipping, a rocker knife and plate guard for one-handed eating, a covered cup or straw for bringing beverages to the mouth without spilling, and built-up utensils for weakened and uncontrolled grasp.

Oral Motor Exam

An oral motor exam of the lips, cheeks, tongue, jaw, and palate must be administered before presenting food to the patient. The therapist should determine whether range of motion, strength, and sensation (both intra- and extraorally) are decreased, increased, or within normal limits.

Primitive Reflexes

If present, primitive reflexes can interfere with feeding. These reflexes must be identified and the feeding process adapted accordingly to ensure success and prevent caregiver frustration. Primitive reflexes include the bite reflex, rooting reflex, jaw jerk, and the asymmetric tonic neck reflex.

Clinical Evaluation of Swallow Function

Once the initial observation components of the evaluation are complete, the clinical assessment may proceed (see Chapter 17 Appendix). Occasionally a request is made to evaluate a patient who is NPO (not eating food by mouth). In this case, recommendations for prefeeding therapy may be based solely on observational and oral/motor/vegetative findings. Physician's orders would be necessary for PO (taking food/liquid by mouth) trials with this patient.

PO Trials

PO trials are appropriate for patients with fair motor control who are alert, able to follow commands, and medically stable. Factors that may contraindicate PO trials include absence of or significantly reduced laryngeal elevation during dry swallows, moderate to severe dysarthria, lethargy or severely impaired mental status, severe pulmonary compromise, and absence of a protective cough.[54] Again, the patient's physician should always be consulted before initiation of PO trials to rule out any contraindications.

Patients may be observed in a formal evaluation setting or informally at mealtime. Informal mealtime observation provides an efficient indication of the patient's eating ability. It allows the evaluator to assess the patient's ability to concentrate despite distractions and interruptions. It allows for observation of the rate of intake and the patient's reaction to the presentation of the meal.[54] If the evaluation takes place in a formal setting, trials should begin with foods that are unlikely to be aspirated, such as purée. The evaluation then progresses to include foods of more difficult consistencies, depending on the patient's tolerance and medical status. The usual progression of consistencies is shown in Box 17-2 (from easiest to most difficult).

The therapist may evaluate all the consistencies shown in Box 17-2 or begin at the consistency the patient is currently tolerating. For patients beginning PO trials, purée is the consistency of choice. During the PO trial the therapist should pay close attention to the following indicators of laryngeal function:

1. Cough: In normal swallowing, penetration occurs more frequently than aspiration. Material that is penetrated is cleared from the larynx during elevation and usually does not result in any audible laryngeal reaction (cough). However, laryngeal reaction to aspirated material below the true vocal folds is normally a cough, which should expel the aspirated material.[62] On evaluation a strong cough is necessary to protect the airway. Horner et al[18] report that a weak cough is more likely to occur in aspirating patients than in nonaspirating patients.
2. Laryngeal elevation: Perlman et al[54] concluded that reduced hyoid elevation impairs the pharyngeal stage of the swallow, thereby increasing the risk of vallecular residue and pharyngeal stasis. These factors may result in aspiration.[54] Figure 17-5 demonstrates the proper positioning of the examiner's hand and digits on the patient's neck for palpation of the larynx to assess laryngeal elevation.

Box 17-2

Consistency Progression
The usual progression of consistencies (easiest to most difficult)

SOLIDS	LIQUIDS
Purée	Spoon-thick
Souffle/semisolid	Honey-thick
Soft solid	Nectar-thick
Regular	Thin

3. Breath and vocal quality: These may be assessed via cervical auscultation with a stethoscope. Cervical auscultation is achieved by placing the flat head of the stethoscope against the lateral side of the neck, preferably the weaker side, in the laryngeal region. Placement may be adjusted until cervical breath sounds are heard. The normal pharyngeal stage includes swallow initiation promptly after oral transit, an apneic period during the swallow, and exhalation immediately after the swallow, with clear breath sounds and vocal quality.[70] Breath and vocal quality differ in patients with dysphagia and are often characterized by gurgling sounds, increased throat clearing, and a "wet" vocal quality (Figure 17-5).

Zenner and associates[70] concluded that cervical auscultation is an imprecise clinical method for the evaluation of aspiration. However, it deserves further study because it is an inexpensive and readily available evaluation option in the absence of more sophisticated assessment tools.

4. Vocal quality: As previously stated, a wet, gurgly vocal quality can indicate dysphagia. Linden-Castelli[32] reports a high correlation of aspiration and dysphonia after stroke. Dysphagia is used to describe a "wet-hoarse" quality thought to be caused by the accumulation of saliva in the laryngopharynx. Horner and associates[20] suggest that the presence of any types of

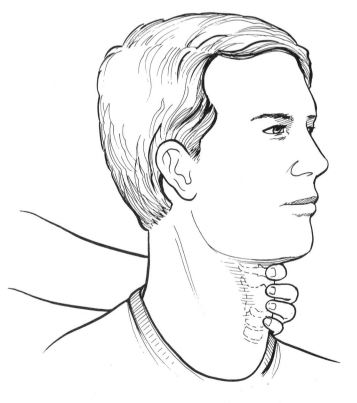

Figure 17-5 Palpation during the swallowing evaluation.

dysphonia may increase the possibility of aspiration in neurogenic dysphagia. The authors deduced that dysphonia may not only be present in laryngeal dysfunction but may in fact be a secondary result of upper-airway weakness, generalized weakness, and pharyngeal dryness in NPO patients. They suggest that the presence of a wet vocal quality may signal aspiration; although aspiration should not be ruled out in the absence of a wet vocal quality.[21]

5. Gag: Logemann[36] asserted that the presence or absence of a gag reflex in patients with neurologic impairments is not an accurate indicator of the patient's ability to swallow. Horner et al.[21] that a poor gag reflex proved to be a poor indicator of prognosis. The gag is not a protective mechanism for the swallow. Food does not trigger a gag because it is not a foreign substance or a noxious stimulus.[36]

The stages of swallow portion of the Continuation Sheet shown in Appendix D identifies the specific actions to be observed during the stages of swallowing. Observations relating to these actions should be made for each consistency presented. Final recommendations will be based on this information as well as the medical history.

Evaluation Impressions and Recommendations

After gathering information from the clinical assessment, the clinician must determine whether further instrumental evaluation of swallowing is warranted. Instrumental evaluation refers to diagnostic procedures such as the modified barium swallow and fiberoptic endoscopic evaluation of swallowing.[65]

Modified Barium Swallow

The modified barium swallow (MBS) videofluoroscopic evaluation of swallowing is the technique most widely used because it allows the clinician the opportunity to examine the oral preparatory, oral, pharyngeal, and esophageal aspects of the dynamic swallow (see Chapter 17 Appendix). The MBS also allows the clinician to observe aspiration before, during, and after the swallow.[37] The ability to recognize risk factors associated with aspiration is vital to the development of treatment plans.[53] The modified barium swallow is ideally performed by the radiologist and members of the dysphagia team, primarily the occupational therapist, the speech-language pathologist, or both. Food and liquid boluses are laced with barium contrast and presented to the patient. The swallows are recorded via videofluoroscopy and viewed by the team. The MBS not only allows the clinician to view swallow function and rule out aspiration but also provides useful information regarding compensatory strategies. Strategies include chin-tuck, head-turn, and supraglottic swallow and may reduce the risk of aspiration. When used creatively, the MBS includes alteration in bolus volume, texture, and delivery, as well as more specific quantification of the amount, frequency, quality, and clearance of the aspirant. These modifications provide valuable information regarding management of oropharyngeal dysphagia and aspiration.

Ultrasound

Ultrasound is the method of choice if only oral function is to be assessed. It is a noninvasive, dynamic evaluation of swallowing that shows the anatomy. This procedure uses normal foods and liquids and is safe to use with comatose, uncooperative, and infant patients.[64]

Fiberoptic Endoscopic Evaluation of Swallowing

Fiberoptic endoscopic evaluation of swallowing (FEES) allows the examiner to evaluate laryngeal function, assess the amount of hypopharyngeal residue, and observe aspiration before and after the swallow. However, FEES cannot always explain the reason that aspiration is occurring. FEES is particularly useful for patients who cannot undergo a modified barium swallow or require frequent reassessment.

Clinical benefits of FEES include assessment of airway protection when vocal fold involvement or impaired adduction is suspected, assessment of laryngeal/pharyngeal sensation, and evaluation of anatomy when it is believed to be a contributing factor in dysphagia. During a FEES evaluation the endoscope is passed transnasally through the nasopharynx and hypopharynx and positioned in the laryngopharynx above the false vocal folds, superior to the epiglottis. Liquid and solid boluses are dyed with green food coloring for easy visualization.

Aspiration occurs in 45% of normal adults during sleep. However, pneumonia does not develop when pulmonary defense mechanisms are intact. Tolerance appears to be individual-specific and depends on the frequency, volume, and character of the aspirate. Often, the degree of aspiration tolerance becomes the focus during discussions about patient care. Information regarding who may tolerate aspiration and in what parameters is scarce. Therefore counseling patients on the risks of continued oral intake is difficult because little data exists to support or negate its consequence.

Whether feeding should be oral (PO) or nonoral (NPO) is a decision to be made by the team,[14,35,57] which should always include the patient and caregiver or significant other. When making this decision the team should consider the following: medical history, physical status, and diagnostic test results. Langmore[33] lists the following factors relevant to the risk for aspiration:

• Activity level
• Level of consciousness
• Past aspiration with or without resultant pneumonia
• Prognosis of medical condition
• Prognosis for dysphagia to improve

She also states that tube feeding increases the risk of tooth decay, reflux, and irritation from the tube and generally leads to a decrease in oral hygiene.

The team should consider the impact of an NPO decision on the patient and family.[29],[30] The caregivers and patient provide information about the patient's quality of life and preferences regarding medical intervention. If PO feeding is initiated against medical advice, mealtime management guidelines are provided to improve safety and emphasize the consistency least likely to be aspirated. Purée is the consistency normally recommended.

ALTERNATIVE MEANS OF NUTRITION

Patients who are not candidates for oral feeding require alternative means of nutrition.[8] The medical team must determine the length of time the patient will be NPO and the optimal nutritional route. Two primary feeding routes are generally used: enteral, which uses the gastrointestinal route, and parenteral, which uses the intravenous route.

Enteral Feedings

1. Noninvasive tube feedings: Most appropriate for short periods of time. Nasogastric tube (NG tube): Tube is placed through the nose, pharynx, and esophagus into the stomach. Food passes through the tube into the stomach (Figure 17-6).
2. Invasive feeding methods: Best for prolonged, indefinite periods. Gastrostomy tube (G tube)[23]: An external opening is made into the abdomen, and a tube is placed directly into the stomach. The food passes through the tube into the stomach.

Parenteral Feedings

1. TPN: total parenteral nutrition is the administration of a complete metabolic diet through a central vein.

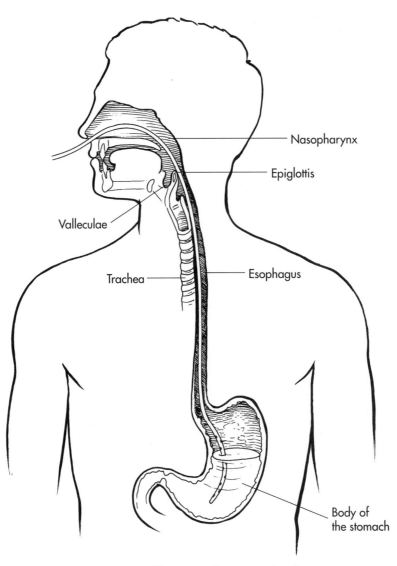

Figure 17-6   Placement of a nasogastric tube.

2. PPN: peripheral parenteral nutrition is administered through a peripheral vein.

The risks and benefits associated with oral, enteral, and parenteral nutrition are outlined in Table 17-1.

PRACTICAL MANAGEMENT

In the acute phase after a stroke, patients may require daily reevaluation because their status may change daily. Mirro and Patey[47] believe that in addition to the swallowing mechanism itself, the level of cognition, alertness, orientation, and ability to follow directions and learn new tasks must also be examined. All the previously listed skills are prerequisites for the treatment of dysphagia. Logemann[36,39] describes behavioral and cognitive methods used to prepare a patient for the task of eating. The patient must be in an alert state and not fatigued. Eating five smaller meals throughout the day rather than three large meals may help patients conserve energy. The patient should also be oriented to person, place, and time because confusion can lead to combative behavior. Impulsivity and poor judgment can cause patients to stuff their mouths with food or burn their mouths and may necessitate close supervision. Poor memory can lead to missed meals or overeating. Memory can also affect the ability to learn and use swallowing maneuvers and the need for supervision and cueing. The patient must be able to use visual perception to distinguish the food from the plate, identify the food as edible, and recognize the need to bring it to the mouth to eat. Mirro and Patey[47] support a team approach to the treatment of dysphagia because factors such as depression, emotion, and behavior (impulsivity) have an effect on eating.

Practical management of dysphagia[28,46,50] is contingent on the information provided to the patient and caregivers. The education process begins with initial contact with the patient and caregivers and continues with follow-up visits, informational pamphlets, and referrals to other health care professionals. Patients and caregivers must understand the concept of dysphagia, including the causes and consequences of aspiration, because they cannot follow recommended treatment without knowledge of the problem and its possible consequences. Anatomic pictures, handouts, and verbal explanations are useful educational tools. Precautionary signs placed by the bed may also be helpful in reinforcing the need to follow mealtime management guidelines.

Table 17-1

Risks and Benefits Associated with Oral, Enteral, and Parenteral Nutritional Support

TYPE OF NUTRITIONAL SUPPORT	RISKS AND DRAWBACKS	BENEFITS
Oral	Tracheal aspiration	Psychologically pleasurable
	Inability to ingest sufficient calories	Provides socialization experience
	Poor patient satisfaction (limited diet)	Promotes normal digestion
Nasogastric	Ulceration	Routine procedure
	Bleeding	Affordable
	Fistula	Begins immediately
	Gastroesophageal reflux	Easily reversible
	Oropharyngeal discomfort	
	Poor patient satisfaction and compliance	
Gastrostomy	General anesthesia	Common procedure
	Bleeding	Good for long-term care if gastrointestinal tract is inaccessible
	Gastroesophageal reflux	Easily replaceable
	Diarrhea	Removes tube from head/neck region
	Stomal irritation	Nonsurgical placement available
Jejunostomy	Peritonitis	Minimizes gastroesophageal reflux
	Diarrhea	Can be used when stomach cannot tolerate diet
	Difficult to replace	Nonsurgical placement available
Total parenteral nutrition (TPN)	Sepsis	Fewer complications in patients with dysphagia and malnutrition
	Infection at site	For use in nonfunctioning gastrointestinal tract
	Short-term alimentation	Minimizes risk of aspirating stomach contents
	Pneumothorax	
	Expensive	

Modified from Groher ME: Formulating feeding decisions for acute dysphagic patients, *Occup Ther Practice* 3:27,1992, Aspen.

Compensatory strategies and therapeutic feeding techniques are often helpful. Many compensatory techniques exist that can help patients achieve a more efficient and therefore safer swallow.* Logemann reports that "postural strategies can be effective in eliminating aspiration in 75% to 80% of patients . . ." and that swallowing therapy procedures, including swallowing maneuvers, sensory input, and exercise programs, may eliminate the aspiration immediately or with therapy.[39]

Compensatory strategies include the following:

1. Chin-down posture: Shanahan et al[62] finds the chin-down posture is beneficial in decreasing aspiration in persons who experience a delayed pharyngeal swallow and reduced airway closure if the source of aspiration is material pooled in the valleculae. The posture did not decrease risk of aspiration with pooling in the pyriform sinus. Because the posture causes shortening and narrowing of the pyriform sinus, material pooled there is likely to spill over into the airway.

2. Head rotation: maximal rotation of the head causes the bolus to move away from the direction of rotation. Rotation of the head to the far right causes the bolus to move laterally to the left. Rotation is an effective postural tool in treating dysphagia caused by unilateral dysfunction. An efficient swallow has "decreased resistance at the pharyngoesophageal junction."[40] Head rotation decreases the resistance by opening the cricopharyngeal spincter to a near-normal size.

Swallow maneuvers include supraglottic swallow, super-supraglottic swallow, effortful swallow, and the Mendelsohn maneuver.[39] Logemann states that sensory input can increase oral awareness and improve the quality of the swallow. Examples of sensory stimulation include use of a spoon to apply pressure to the tongue and presentation of a cold or textured bolus.[37] Facial exercises target oral structures such as lips, tongue, cheeks, and jaws, the movement and strength of which are required for eating. Examples of oral exercises include the following:

- Lips: Patient purses lips and holds tongue depressor between lips
- Tongue: Patient licks lips and pushes them against a tongue depressor anteriorly and laterally
- Cheeks: Patient blows bubbles through a straw, drinks thick liquids through the straw, and provides resistance to zygomaticus by smiling

Selley et al.[61] describe the use of the palatal training appliance (PTA) in the treatment of dysphagia. The device itself is a U-shaped wire attached to dentures or fabricated into an appliance that can be mounted onto existing teeth.

It extends back in the mouth to the soft palate, where it exerts no pressure on the structures. The appliance is tolerated only by patients with decreased sensation between the faucial arches. Theoretically, this appliance provides sensory feedback and helps prevent the "humping" tongue movements seen with decreased tongue control, which interferes with the swallow. The study found that the use of the appliance in conjunction with therapy and, if applicable, proper refitting of dentures improves the swallowing of 8 of 13 patients fitted with the device. The exact mechanism whereby the PTA improves the swallow is not yet known.[61]

The eating environment and food presentation are important considerations.[22] The patient may require set up, adaptive equipment, or thickener in preparation for eating. Weiss and associates[67] describe many factors that influence the eating environment. For personal comfort, patients should have their eyeglasses, hearing aid, and dentures; in addition, all appliances should fit and work properly. Compensatory techniques for visual and perceptual deficits should be employed during the meal. Environmental considerations include increasing the light in dim areas and reducing glare in bright areas. Distractions should be minimized as much as possible. The meal should also offer an opportunity for interpersonal interaction.

While feeding the patient, caregivers should be aware of signs and symptoms of aspiration and be proficient in the therapeutic feeding techniques mentioned previously. Weiss and associates[67] state that a supportive attitude is important to the therapeutic process and helps the patient gain independence. Caregivers may bring favorite foods to a patient, but they must first check with the team.

Follow-up is recommended to determine whether caregivers and patients understand and are complying with the recommendations. Patients should be monitored to ensure that they are receiving the correct food and liquid consistencies for dysphagia.[16] Caregivers and patients should be reassured that favorite foods and beverages, such as coffee, may require modification but can still be enjoyed. As indicated, a reevaluation may be administered.

A review of the literature reveals little research on the topic of the psychologic impact of dysphagia. Facial assymetries are prevalent among dysphagic patients. Many of the mastication muscles are also used to express emotion. Davies[11] explains that the face has great social importance, as shown by media advertisement. The effects of dysphagia on a patient's ability to participate in social and traditional activities are not documented. Teasell and associates[66] report that stroke recovery is influenced by the victim's reaction, and many survivors feel depressed, exhibit lability, and try to avoid thinking about the stroke by not participating in the rehabilitation effort. Furthermore, stroke can lead to isolation[59] because of factors such as decreased mobility and complications such as incontinence.[67] Morawski[49] reports no formal research has been done that

*Treatments for dysphagia include therapeutic techniques, postural changes, diet modification, adaptive equipment, and supervision.[11,22,32,34,37,39,46,50,62]

measures psychologic impact affecting a patient's overall performance. She compares the psychologic impact to that produced by other embarrassing incidents such as having food stuck in your teeth or a pimple on your face or even being unable to speak clearly with a numb tongue. The craving for foods eliminated from the diet are similar to those people feel when travelling, or preparing for medical procedures.[49] However, whereas the preceding examples are temporary, the diagnosis of dysphagia may mean a permanent change in a patient's diet. Therapists must be empathetic to the effect this change may have on a patient.[49] Food is more than a necessity for life. It is associated with family gatherings, celebrations, social events, and cultural traditions. The smell of food stimulates the olfactory, gustatory, and visual senses. Morawski[49] states that problems with facial expression produce feelings such as "embarrassment, self-consciousness, anger, wanting to isolate yourself,... [and] craving." These emotions, combined with the fact that dysphagia may alter an individual's ability to participate in activities surrounding food, frequently cause decreased self-esteem, self-concept, and self-image.

REVIEW QUESTIONS

1. Describe the clinical symptoms of aspiration.
2. Describe the concepts of aspiration in contrast to those of penetration.
3. Describe the four stages of swallowing. Indicate three symptoms of dysphagia at each stage.
4. Name the cranial nerves and identify their functions in swallowing.
5. Name 10 items important for chart review.
6. Describe two advantages of FEES.
7. Describe two advantages of MBS.

■ COTA Considerations ■

- Be familiar with and aware of the signs and symptoms of dysphagia during the initial feeding evaluation of your patients.
- Postural strategies are often effective in decreasing the symptoms of dysphagia.
- Facial paralysis has an adverse effect on not only swallowing function but also psychosocial factors such as body image, expression of emotions, and the embarrassment associated with spillage of food and secretions.
- Respect cultural differences when diet modifications are required.
- Patient and family education are a critical component of dysphagia management.
- A thorough chart review and patient/family interview form the basis of the dysphagia evaluation.

REFERENCES

1. Alberts MJ et al: Aspiration after stroke: lesion analysis by brain MRI, *Dysphagia* 7:170, 1992.
2. Arsenault JK, Atwood J: Development of a competency-based training model for dysphagia management in a medical center, *Semin Speech Language* 12:236, 1991.
3. Axelsson K et al: Eating problems and nutritional status during hospital stay of patients with severe stroke, *J Am Diet Assoc* 89:1092, 1989.
4. Barer DH: The natural history and functional consequences of dysphagia after hemispheric stroke, *J Neurol Neurosurg Psychiatry* 52:236, 1989.
5. Bastian R: The videoendoscopic swallowing study: an alternative and partner to the videofluoroscopic swallowing study, *Dysphagia* 8:359, 1993.
6. Buchholz DW: Clinically probable brain stem stroke presenting primarily as dysphagia and nonvisualized by MRI, *Dysphagia* 8:235, 1993.
7. Buchholz DW: Dysphagia associated with neurological disorders, *Acta Otorhinolaryngol Belg* 48:143, 1994.
8. Ciocon JO: Indications for tube feedings in elderly patients, *Dysphagia* 5:1, 1990.
9. Curran J, Groher ME: Development and dissemination of an aspiration risk reduction diet, *Dysphagia* 5:6, 1990.
10. Cox MS: The challenges of an interdisciplinary dysphagia clinic and educational program, *Physical Disabilities Special Interest Section Newsletter* 17:3, 1994.
11. Davies PM: *Steps to follow*, New York, 1985, Springer Verlag.
12. DePippo KL, Hosas MA, Reding MJ: Validation of the 3-oz water swallow test for aspiration following stroke, *Arch Neurol* 49:1259, 1992.
13. DePippo KL, Hosas MA, Reding MJ: The Burke dysphagia screening test: validation of its use in patients with stroke, *Arch Phys Med Rehabil* 75:1284, 1994.
14. Groher ME: Determination for the risks and benefits of oral feeding, *Dysphagia* 9:233, 1994.
15. Groher ME, Bukatman R: The prevalence of swallowing disorders in two teaching hospitals, *Dysphagia* 1:3, 1986.
16. Halper AS: Developing quality assurance monitors for dysphagia: continuous quality improvement, *Semin Speech Language* 12:288, 1991.
17. Holas MA, DePippo KL, Reding MJ: Aspiration and relative risk of medical complications following stroke, *Arch Neurol* 51:1051, 1994.
18. Horner J et al: Dysphagia following brain-stem stroke: clinical correlates and outcome, *Arch Neurol* 48:1170, 1991.
19. Horner J, Massey EW: Silent aspiration following stroke, *Neurology* 38:317, 1988.
20. Horner J, Massey EW, Brazer SR: Aspiration in bilateral stroke patients, *Neurology* 40:1686, 1990.
21. Horner J et al: Aspiration following stroke: clinical correlates and outcome, *Neurology* 38:1359, 1988.
22. Hotaling D: Adapting the mealtime environment: setting the stage for eating, *Dysphagia* 5:77, 1990.
23. Hull MA et al: Audit of outcome of long-term enteral nutrition by percutaneous endoscopic gastrostomy, *Lancet* 341:869, 1993.
24. Hutchins BF, Giancarlo JL: Developing a comprehensive dysphagia program, *Semin Speech Language* 12(3):209, 1991.
25. Johnson ER et al: Dysphagia following stroke: quantitative evaluation of pharyngeal transit times, *Arch Phys Med Rahabil* 73:419, 1992.
26. Johnson ER, McKenzie SW, Sievers A: Aspiration pneumonia in stroke, *Arch Phys Med Rehabil* 74:973, 1993.
27. Kalra L et al: Medical complications during stroke rehabilitation, *Stroke* 26:990, 1995.

28. Kasprisin AT, Clumeck H, Nino-Murcia M: The efficacy of rehabilitative management of dysphagia, *Dysphagia* 4:48, 1989.

29. Kidd D et al: Aspiration in acute stroke: a clinical study with videofluoroscopy, *Q J Med* 86:825, 1993.

30. Kidd D et al: The natural history and clinical consequences of aspiration in acute stroke, *Q J Med* 88:409, 1995.

31. Kidder TM, Langmore SE, Martin BJW: Indications and techniques of endoscopy in evaluation of cervical dysphagia: comparison with radiographic techniques, *Dysphagia* 9:256, 1994.

32. Linden-Castelli P: Treatment strategies for adult neurogenic dysphagia, *Semin Speech Language* 12:255, 1991.

33. Langmore SE: Managing the complications of aspiration in dysphagic adults, *Semin Speech Language* 12:199, 1991.

34. Layne KA: Feeding strategies for the dysphagic patient: a nursing perspective, *Dysphagia* 5:84, 1990.

35. Lo B, Dornbrand L: Understanding the benefits and burdens of tube feedings, *Dysphagia* 5:77, 1990.

36. Logeman JA: *Evaluation and treatment of swallowing disorders,* Boston, 1983, Little, Brown.

37. Logemann JA: Criteria for studies of the treatment for oralpharyngeal dysphagia, *Dysphagia* 1:193, 1987.

38. Logemann JA: Factors affecting ability to resume oral nutrition in the oropharyngeal dysphagic individual, *Dysphagia* 4:202, 1990.

39. Logemann JA: Noninvasive approaches to deglutitive aspiration, *Dysphagia* 8:331, 1993.

40. Logemann JA et al: The benefit of head rotation on pharyngeoesophageal dysphagia, *Arch Phys Med Rehabil* 70:767, 1989.

41. Logemann JA: Effects of aging on the swallowing mechanism, *Otolaryngol Clin North Am* 23:1045, 1990.

42. Lorish TR, et al: Stroke Rehabilitation evaluation and management, *Arch Phys Med Rehabil* 75:S47, 1994.

43. Martin BJW et al: The association of swallowing dysfunction and aspiration pneumonia, *Dysphagia* 9:1, 1994.

44. Martin KU, Martin JO: Meeting the oral health needs of the institutionalized elderly, *Dysphagia* 7:73, 1992.

45. Miller AJ: The search for the central swallowing pathway: the quest for clarity, *Dysphagia* 8:185, 1993.

46. Miller RM, Langmore SE: Treatment efficacy for adults with oropharyngeal dysphagia, *Arch Phys Med Rehabil* 75:1256, 1994.

47. Mirro JF, Patey C: Developing a dysphagia dietary program, *Semin Speech Language* 12(3):218, 1991.

48. Mody M, Nagai J: A multidisciplinary approach to the development of competency standards and appropriate allocation for patients with dysphagia, *Am J Occup Ther* 44:369, 1990.

49. Morawski D: Dysphagia: its psychological impact, *Physical Disabilities Special Interest Section Newsletter Am J Occup Ther* 17:1, 1994.

50. Neumann S: Swallowing therapy with neurologic patients: results of direct and indirect therapy methods in 66 patients suffering from neurologic disorders, *Dysphagia* 8:150, 1993.

51. Noll SF, Roth EJ: Stroke rehabilitation. I. Epidemiologic aspects and acute management, *Arch Phys Med Rehabil* 75:538, 1994.

52. Perlman AL: The neurology of swallowing, *Semin Speech Language* 12(3):171, 1991.

53. Perlman AL, Booth BM, Grayhack JP: Videofluoroscopic predictors of aspiration in patients with oropharyngeal dysphagia, *Dysphagia* 9:90, 1994.

54. Perlman et al: Comprehensive clinical examination of oropharyngeal swallowing function: Veteran's Administration procedure, *Semin Speech Language* 12(3):246, 1991.

55. Robbins J et al: Swallowing after unilateral stroke of the cerebral cortex, *Arch Phys Med Rehabil* 74:1295, 1993.

56. Robbins J, Levine RL: Swallowing after unilateral stroke of the cerebral cortex: preliminary experience, *Dysphagia* 3:11, 1988.

57. Rogers B, Msall M, Shucard D: Hypoxemia during oral feedings in adults with dysphagia and severe neurological disabilities, *Dysphagia* 8:43, 1993.

58. Sacco RL et al: Wallenberg's lateral medullary syndrome: clinicalmagnetic resonance imaging correlations, *Neurology* 50:609, 1993.

59. Sandin KJ, Cifu DX, Noll SF: Stroke rehabilitation. IV. Psychologic and social implications, *Arch Phys Med Rehabil* 75:552, 1994.

60. Schmidt J et al: Videofluoroscopic evidence of aspiration predicts pneumonia and death but not dehydration following stroke, *Dysphagia* 9:7, 1994.

61. Selley WG et al: Dysphagia following strokes: clinical observation of swallowing rehabilitation employing palatal training appliances, *Dysphagia* 10:32, 1995.

62. Shanahan TK et al: Chin-down posture effect on aspiration in dysphagic patients, *Arch Phys Med Rehabil* 74:736, 1993.

63. Smithard DG et al: Complications and outcome after acute stroke: does dysphagia matter? *Stroke* 27(7):1200, 1996.

64. Sonies BC: Instrumental procedures for dysphagia diagnosis, *Semin Speech Language* 12:186, 1991.

65. Splaingard ML et al: Aspiration in rehabilitation patients: videofluoroscopy vs. bedside clinical assessment, *Arch Phys Med Rehabil* 69:637, 1988.

66. Teasell RW, Bach DB, McRae M: Prevalence and recovery of aspiration poststroke: a retrospective analysis, *Dysphagia* 9:35, 1994.

67. Weiss DR, Conyers KH, Epstein CF: A systems approach to eating skills programming in long-term care, *Occup Ther Pract* 3(2):65, 1992.

68. Veis SL, Logemann JA: Swallowing disorders in persons with cerebrovascular accident, *Arch Phys Med Rehabil* 66:372, 1985.

69. Williams-Santa K: The dysphagia program of the national rehabilitation hospital, *Physical Disabilities Special Interest Section Newsletter* 17:5, 1994.

70. Zenner PM, Losinski DS, Mills RH: Using cervical auscultation in the clinical dysphagia examination in long-term care, *Dysphagia* 10:27, 1995.

Pathophysiology of Dysphagia After CVA

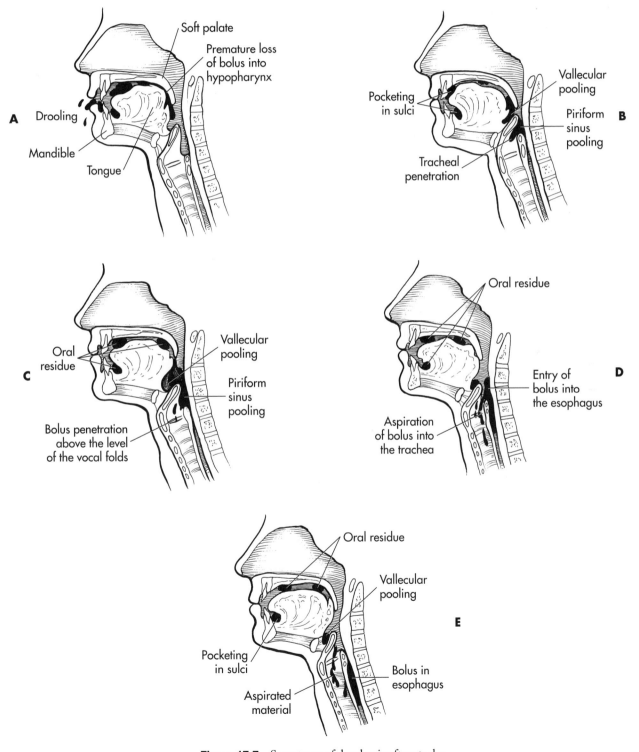

Figure 17-7 Symptoms of dysphagia after stroke.

Dysphagia Symptoms Associated With the Stages of Swallowing

STAGE	BEDSIDE EVALUATION SYMPTOMS	MODIFIED BARIUM SWALLOW SYMPTOMS	PHYSIOLOGIC SYMPTOMS
Oral prep	• Reduced orientation to bolus • Inability to separate edibles from nonedibles • Inability to recognize food • Poor sitting posture • Poor tray set-up • Inability to open packages • Inability to prepare/cut food on plate • Inability to get bolus to mouth • Reduced mouth opening • Reduced lip control • Drooling • Perioral residue (food/liquid on lips)	— • Suboptimal view • Loss of bolus onto lips • Decreased ability to form bolus —	• Reduced cognition • Perceptual deficits/field cut (sensation, sight, smell, etc.) • Visual agnosia • Poor trunk control • Poor muscle control • Poor hand function/coordination • Apraxia/ataxia • Reduced oral-motor strength/tone/range • Reduced perioral sensitivity
Oral	• Drooling • Pooling • Pocketing • Oral residue • Reduced tongue elevation • Reduced anterior to posterior tongue movement/bolus propulsion • Reduced mastication • Slow oral transit time • Tongue thrust • Disorganized tongue movements • Use of fingers to manipulate the bolus posteriorly • Deficient salivation • Lengthy mealtime • Fatigue • Holding of food in the mouth	• Oral residue on tongue and sulci/lips/palate • Incohesive bolus • Tongue pumping • Disorganized/uncoordinated tongue movements • Ineffective mastication • Ineffective anterior to posterior bolus transport	• Reduced/absent intraoral sensation • Reduced/absent muscle control • Apraxia/ataxia • Reduced cognition • Abnormal reflexes • Reduced muscle strength
Pharyngeal	• Coughing/choking • Wet/gurgly breath and vocal quality • Weak cough • Complains of food sticking in throat • Increased throat clearing • Multiple swallows • Nasal regurgitation • Absent swallow reflex • Difficulty initiating a swallow • Head/neck extension • Complains of pain on swallow • Avoidance of problematic foods • Lengthy mealtime • Increase in salivation • Awaking with a wet pillow	• Premature loss of bolus into hypopharynx • Delayed or absent swallow reflex • Valleculae/piriform sinus pooling • Penetration of bolus into trachea above level of vocal folds • Aspiration of bolus into trachea below level of vocal folds • Ineffective cough; cannot clear aspirated material • Ineffective multiple swallow to clear residue • Pharyngeal wall residue • Reduced epiglottal movement	• CN X/IX—reduced/absent swallow • CN IX/X—reduced/absent sensation • Reduced pharyngeal peristalsis • Reduced upper esophageal sphincter tone • Bilateral or unilateral vocal fold paralysis • Decrease in cranial nerves IX and X function • Reduced respiratory support/capacity • Muscle weakness • Abnormally increased muscle activity
Esophageal	• Reflux, regurgitation, sour taste, burning	• Rarely observed although may see reflux	• Esophageal/gastric reflux

jessica farman
judith dicker friedman

chapter **18**

Sexual Function and Intimacy

key terms

aging

disability

sexual dysfunction

sexual function

sexuality

sexuality counseling

sexuality rehabilitation

stroke

chapter objectives

After completing this chapter, the reader will be able to accomplish the following:

1. Identify and describe the normal human sexual response cycle and the changes that occur during the aging process.
2. Understand the effects of stroke on sexual function.
3. Identify the occupational therapist's role in sexuality intervention.
4. Understand and apply the levels of the PLISSIT model that are appropriate for occupational therapists.
5. Identify sexual impairments in functional terms.
6. Plan treatment interventions for impairments affecting sexual function.

A discussion of sexuality includes not only specific sexual practices but the attitudes, behaviors, thoughts, and feelings associated with sex and sexuality. This includes but is not limited to an individual's perception of self as a sexual being, body image, self-esteem, participation and roles in relationships (sexual and other), sexual orientation (that is, heterosexual, homosexual, or bisexual), and beliefs and attitudes toward a wide range of sexual behaviors, including masturbation, coitus, oral-genital sex, cuddling, and sensuality. Romano defines it expertly:

Sexuality is more than the art of sexual intercourse. It involves for most . . . the whole business of relating to another person; the tenderness, the desire to give as well as take, the compliments, casual caresses, reciprocal concerns, tolerance, the forms of communication that both include and go beyond words . . . sexuality includes a range of behavior from smiling through orgasm; it is not just what happens between two people in bed.[39]

Everyone can enjoy sex. Health care professionals must be aware of their own attitudes toward sexuality. Our patients may be different from ourselves—they may be older, may be of a sexual orientation different from our own, or they may have permanent or temporary disabilities. And just as differences among human beings are inherent, the variances in sexual behaviors, preferences, and beliefs among individuals must be considered and respected.

NORMAL HUMAN SEXUAL RESPONSE

An understanding of the normal human sexual response cycle must be achieved before an individual can explore the relationship between sexuality and disability. Masters and Johnson[27] divided the human sexual response cycle into four segments: (1) excitement, (2) plateau, (3) orgasm, and (4) resolution. In each phase definite physical changes occur in both sexes. During the excitement phase, physiologic reactions occur as a result of somatosensory or psychogenic stimulation. In females, the nipples become erect, the vagina swells and becomes lubricated, the clitoris and the labia minora and majora swell, and the uterus and cervix retract. In males, the penis grows erect and the testicles rise. In both sexes blood pressure and heart rate increase.

During the plateau phase respiration increases and blood pressure and heart rate increase further. In females the areola surrounding the nipple swells, the orgasmic platform forms (vasocongestion of the outer two thirds of the vagina), and the color of the labia minora deepens from pink to red. In males a full erection is achieved as the testes elevate further and Cowper's gland secretes preejaculatory fluid.

Orgasms differ between the sexes; some women can achieve multiple orgasms. In both sexes peak pulse rate, blood pressure, and respiration increase, as does muscle tone. Rhythmic contractions of the orgasmic platform and the uterus occur in women, and rhythmic contractions of the penis project semen forward in males.

Cardiac response was recorded by Masters and Johnson, who found peak heart rates of 110 to 180 beats per minute during orgasm.[27] However, the mean maximum heart rate during sexual activity was 117.4 beats per minute in a study of middle-aged men with postcoronary disease.[23] During sexual activity, systolic and diastolic pressure increase (from 30 to 80 and 20 to 40 mm Hg, respectively).[27] Respiration rates of up to 40 breaths per minute have been recorded, depending on the level of intensity and duration of sexual activity.[27]

The resolution phase is characterized by the return to preexcitement status, including reductions in blood pressure, heart rate, and respiration. The genitals and breasts return to preexcitement size.

Aging and the Human Sexual Response Cycle

In normal human development changes occur during the aging process. Such changes affect sexuality[36] in males and females and may already affect patients who have sustained cerebrovascular accidents (CVAs).

Women

Generally between the ages of 40 and 50 women experience menopause, the cessation of menstruation caused by a lack of production of estrogen that occurs over a period of several months to a few years.[25] The major effects of menopause are as follows:

1. Vasomotor syndrome ("hot flashes")[25]
2. Atrophic vaginitis (thinning of the vaginal walls)[25]
3. Osteoporosis[25]
4. A decrease in the rate, amount, and type of vaginal fluid, which can cause pain during intercourse and may lead to infection[45]
5. Loss of contractility of vaginal muscles, which can cause shorter orgasms[45]
6. Decreased size of the uterus and clitoris and atrophy of the clitoral hood[25]
7. Loss of elasticity in breast tissue, causing sagging

According to Laflin, regular muscle contractions help maintain the integrity of vaginal muscle tone, and "contact with the penis helps preserve the shape and size of the vaginal space."[25] Therefore an active sex life can have a positive effect on genital function.

Men

As men grow older the following changes occur:

1. Erections are often less full, take longer to achieve and may require direct stimulation.[45]
2. Ejaculatory control increases, ejaculation may only occur every third sexual episode and is less forceful, and loss of erection after orgasm may occur faster.[25,45]
3. It may take 12 to 24 hours before another erection can be achieved.[25]
4. Sperm volume decreases and the ejaculation may be less intense, which may affect the intensity of orgasm.[24,45]
5. The size and firmness of the testes diminish.
6. The testosterone level decreases.

Many elderly people continue to enjoy sexual activity; however, a decline in sexual activity among elderly people is not uncommon. Older people do not necessarily lose their desire for sex, but circumstances can make it difficult for them to engage in active sexual relationships. Leading causes of altered sexual activity in the older adult include difficulty finding partners, illness, medication effects, widowhood, divorce, biases about masturbation, societal attitudes about sex and the elderly and even their own biases and prejudices toward sexuality.[38] Elderly people may view sex as something that only young, attractive people do.

SEXUALITY AND NEUROLOGIC FUNCTION

Sexual function is controlled by the brain, spinal cord, and peripheral nerves, whereas control of libido and sexual pleasure are mediated by several areas in the cortex, midbrain, and brain stem.[34] Men experience reflexogenic and psychogenic erections. Reflexogenic erections are caused by direct stimulation to the penis and may occur without conscious awareness, even in the absence of penile sensation. Psychogenic erections originate from mental activity such as sexual fantasies and stimulating visual input and do not require direct penile stimulation. Reflexogenic erections are controlled by the nervous system through the sacral roots, and psychogenic erections involve the sympathetic nerves between T11 and L2.[48] Female sexual function is similar to that of males with regard to nerve innervation.[48] The parasympathetic nerves, S2 to S4, influence the clitoris and vaginal lubrication. "Contraction of the vaginal sphincter and pelvic floor occur with stimulation of the somatic aspect of the pudendal nerves (S2-S4)."[48] Neurologic disability can cause organic impotence by altering the blood flow needed for penile erection, as well as problems with emission and ejaculation in males and with lubrication, clitoral engorgement, and orgasm in females.[48] Some of the subcortical structures theorized to be involved in the neurology of sexuality are the reticular activating system and the hippocampus, amygadala, and hypothalamus.[48] According to Zasler,[48] the thalamus and basal ganglia are hypothesized to be involved with the mediation of sexual function. Some of the cortical areas involved are the frontal lobes and the nondominant temporal lobe. "Lesions in the dominant hemisphere may produce aphasia or apraxia both of which could impede sexual activity. Nondominant hemisphere injury may result in . . . visuoperceptual deficits, denial and impulsiveness, all of which could impede expression of sexuality."[48] Sexual stimulation is caused by stimulation of the brain or peripheral nerves, the former of which is a result of thoughts and psychological processes and the latter of which is a result of direct physical stimulation.[31,48]

Effects of Stroke on Sexual Function

The literature shows that common effects of stroke on sexual function are decreased libido, impaired erectile and ejaculatory function, decreased vaginal lubrication, impaired ego and self-esteem, and depression. However, the reasons for these dysfunctions are not clear.[6,11,15,16,19,40-42] Research has been focused mainly on relating sexual dysfunction to the location of the lesion. To date, no research has been reported on the causes of poststroke sexual dysfunction. Most of the scientific literature fails to provide treatment interventions, tends to focus solely on intercourse as a sexual behavior, and does not include the effects of stroke on oral-genital sex, kissing, mutual masturbation, or other forms of sexuality. As a result, clinicians are left with insufficient information to adequately treat sexual dysfunction.

Monga, Lawson, and Inglis[30] found that among men and women who had sustained strokes, libido was decreased, abilities to achieve erection and vaginal lubrication were impaired, and the frequency of intercourse was diminished. Isolated cases of hypersexuality and abnormal sexual behavior were found to occur in individuals with temporal lobe lesions and concurrent histories of poststroke seizure activity.[31]

In a study of 13 female stroke survivors it was found that the most common complaint was a decreased desire for sexual activity after the stroke; only 5% of the women reported actual impairment in the production of vaginal secretions after the stroke.[2] Most of the women reported no changes in the abilities to achieve orgasm or in their menstrual periods. In addition, although the stroke itself impaired sexual desire, physiological function remained unimpaired. It was concluded that nondominant hemispheric stroke is related to decreased desire; five of seven patients with decreased desire had right brain involvement.

The authors of several studies have attempted to determine cerebral hemisphere dominance on sexual function. Although some investigators found a greater decline in sexual function with left CVA, others found little or no difference between right and left cerebral hemisphere strokes.[6,11,16,40] Garden[17] concludes, "There seems to be an overall consensus that stroke patients maintain prestroke sexual desire but commonly experience sexual dysfunction including erectile and libido problems. Changes in coital frequency and libido are also common. As a result there can be great potential for depression and loss of self esteem."

The individual's prestroke sexual activity is usually a better indicator of poststroke activity.[7,16,19,22] If the individual was leading an active sex life before a stroke, the likelihood of returning to sexual activities is good. Age is also a predictor of resumption of sexual activity, although less so.[22] Individuals who were without a partner before a stroke have less opportunity to develop new partnerships and resume sexual activity after a stroke. This decreased opportunity has to do with the effects of stroke itself, as well as an individual's impaired social contact, possible placement in a nursing home or other long-term setting, depression, altered self-image, and the multitude of psychologic effects caused by stroke (see Chapter 3).

Impotence or difficulty maintaining a full erection may occur as a direct result of stroke.[22,40] It may also occur in men whose sexual partners have sustained strokes because of fear of causing another stroke or hurting the partner or averse feelings toward the disabled partner.[16,19,20] In women vaginal lubrication may be insufficient, causing painful intercourse.[2,16,17]

Initiation of sexual activity after discharge from the hospital may be difficult. A couple may delay sexual activity because each partner waits for the other to initiate sex.[19,20] In a study by Goddess, Wagner, and Silverman[19] one couple put off sexual activity for 15 months after the husband's stroke. The man was unsure whether his wife would find him attractive or a suitable partner, and the wife was concerned that sexual play for her husband may be unsafe.

Sensory impairment is common after stroke. Considering the significant role of touch in sexual expression, its dysfunction may also contribute to sexual dysfunction.[15] Again, the research is inconclusive, although a recent study of 15 male stroke patients showed that disturbed superficial and deep sensation were not correlated with decreased desire.[1]

Motor impairment can affect sexual function. Decreased range of motion, strength, endurance, balance, abnormal skeletal muscle activity, impaired coordination, and oral motor dysfunction may interfere with intercourse or other sexual activities. However, some research suggests that the degree of hemiplegic impairment is not a major factor in sexual dysfunction.[15,16]

Cognitive deficits may also affect the stroke survivor's social and sexual function. Fundamental cognitive abilities such as attention and concentration are prerequisites for social and sexual activities; distractability and overstimulation may cause anxiety and agitation, which prevent interaction. Decreased initiation, impulsivity, poor memory, decreased speed of processing, and impaired executive functions are all possible effects of neurologic dysfunction and can clearly affect sexual relations.[43]

McCormick, Riffer, and Thompson[29] note that sexual activity is itself a form of human communication. When verbal or nonverbal communication is impaired, sexual activity may be affected.[48] One study found that sexual adjustment was easiest for physically intact individuals with aphasia with spared comprehension and nonverbal communication.[47] However, in one study involving 110 subjects no correlation between aphasia and poststroke sexual activity was found.[42]

The effect of stroke on psychologic function is enormous. The loss of function, including hemiparesis, sensory and balance disorders, pain, and cognitive, perceptual, and impaired communication skills may have an enormous negative effect on an individual's self-image. As Strauss[43] notes, the formulation of relationships, sexual or other, requires some level of self-esteem. An impaired image of one's body and appearance can affect the ability to make new relationships or maintain existing ones. Loss of confidence and decreased self-esteem may result from the following:

- Changes in appearance, including facial asymmetries and diminished facial expression
- Changes in clothing style (inability to don pantyhose or walk in high heels as a result of required ankle-foot orthosis [AFO]
- Need for adaptive equipment or assistive devices such as a splint, wheelchair, or cane

- Dependence in activities of daily living (ADL), such as the need to have food cut and to have assistance with toileting

In addition to changes in self-perception, the stroke survivor may suddenly find a new role in relationships. For instance, a wife may discover that she is no longer able to carry out the functions related to her role as wife as a result of the effects of a stroke. The stroke survivor may be more dependent on other family members. Role changes could affect the quality of an existing relationship.[8,38] Such changes may be confusing and stressful for the patient and the partner, particularly if the stroke survivor requires assistance with self-care activities such as toileting or bathing. Dependence in ADL is a major predictor of sexual activity level after a stroke. In a study conducted by Sjogren and Fugl-Meyer, subjects who were dependent in ADL reported a decrease or cessation of sexual activity.[42]

Impaired bladder function may also affect sexual activity. Medications used to treat incontinence have side effects such as dry mouth, which can make kissing or other oral activities unpleasant. If the individual is taking additional medication for other reasons (for example, diuretic agents), urine output may be increased.[24] For the individual with mobility impairments, quick and frequent access to the bathroom may be difficult, resulting in episodes of incontinence. Incontinence may affect self-esteem and may be a source of embarrassment.[24] Bowel incontinence is less common after CVA because stroke patients are typically constipated as a result of immobility and inactivity, as well as poor food and fluid intake, which can cause bloating and discomfort.[46]

Individuals who have had strokes often have history of other medical problems, including heart disease, which alone can cause functional impairments related to sexual activities. Often, individuals with a history of myocardial infarction (MI) or bypass surgery fear the resumption of sexual activities.[23,26,32] Muller et al[32] studied 858 patients who were sexually active in the year preceding MI and found that although the risk of MI increases in the 2 hours following sexual activity, the risk is almost equivalent in patients with and without heart disease. The research indicated that the risk of MI caused by sexual activity is 2 in 1 million for a person with heart disease, and that individuals who experience periods of anger or heavy exertion have a greater increase in actual risk because these behaviors occur with more frequency than sexual activity. However, the overall risk of MI is lower for patients who engage in regular exercise, which has been shown to decrease the amount of cardiac work required during sexual activity.

From a cardiac rehabilitation perspective, a patient is "safe" to resume sexual activity when two flights of stairs can be climbed or the length of a city block or its equivalent can be walked at a brisk pace, with no discomfort.[23,26] This parameter may be difficult to assess in some stroke patients because of mobility deficits, and alternative activities may have to be explored (for example, propelling a wheelchair at a brisk pace with the use of unaffected arms and legs).

The effect of stroke on sexual function is difficult to assess without examining the types of medications patients are taking (see inside cover of book). Antihypertensive agents have been found to cause impotence, impede ejaculation, and decrease libido.[10,15,16] Some β-blockers are known to affect erectile function and cause depression.[10] One antihypertensive diuretic medication, spironolactone, is known to cause breast tenderness, galactorrhea (excessive secretion of the mammary glands), and gynecomastia (overdevelopment of the mammary glands), which is not always reversible in men.[10] In a study by Aloni,[2] six of the seven women who reported decreased sexual desire were taking anticoagulant drugs, suggesting that the medications may affect sexual function.[2] Medications other than those prescribed for stroke management or hypertension may have additional side effects such as rashes and feelings of fatigue that may affect a patient's desire to participate in sexual activities. Considering the potential side effects of various medications on sexual function and informing patients as necessary is the rehabilitation team's responsibility.

Societal Attitudes

Attitudes on the part of the public or the patient's family members may also emotionally or psychologically affect the patient. Although the Americans with Disabilities Act has resulted in some improvement in public attitude, the fact remains that many people still harshly judge individuals who appear "different" from the rest of society and regard disabled individuals with fear and shame. Stroke survivors and people with other disabilities perceive these attitudes and, as a result, avoid social or public situations. The media seldom depict people with disabilities as full partners in sexual relationships. The stroke patient and partner, family members, and others may share the view that people with disabilities are sexless, "different," and undeserving of social and sexual fulfillment. These attitudes can affect patients' existing relationships, as well as their willingness to pursue new relationships.

ROLE OF OCCUPATIONAL THERAPY

When people experience changes in sexual function, they may require professional intervention to cope with these changes in sexual function and sexuality. What is the role of occupational therapy in sexuality intervention for these patients, and what is required to fulfill this role?

Sexuality has long been considered an appropriate area for occupational therapy intervention. Andamo[4] states that "sexual function should be included in the occupational therapy evaluation as it relates to the identification of the patient's abilities and limitations in his daily living neces-

sary for the resumption of his various roles." Neistadt[34] notes that as "holistic caregivers, dedicated to facilitating quality lives, occupational therapists should be prepared to address sexuality issues with their adolescent and adult patients."[34] The American Occupational Therapy Association has confirmed the role of occupational therapy by including sexual expression, defined as "engaging in desired sexual and intimate activities"[3] in its ADL list in the *Uniform Terminology for Occupational Therapy—Third Edition.*

Occupational therapists are well prepared to address sexuality problems in stroke patients; the sensory, motor, cognitive, and psychosocial impairments that interfere with sexual function are the same ones that affect other performance areas addressed by occupational therapy, including other ADL and work and leisure activities. Occupational therapists' skills of activity analysis and adaptation, holistic orientation, and knowledge of biologic and behavioral sciences help them deal effectively with patients' sexual difficulties.[13] Research indicates that dependence in ADL is a major factor in decreased sexual activity after stroke,[42] further supporting the role of occupational therapists in sexual rehabilitation by restoring patients to the highest possible level of independence and role function.

Most occupational therapists receive some training in sexuality intervention. Even before sexual expression was made an official part of occupational therapy's domain by inclusion in the *Uniform Terminology*, the authors of a 1988 study reported that 88% of 50 occupational therapy programs included formal classroom training about sexual function, with an average of 3.5 hours of class time devoted to this subject.[37]

Team Approach

Although occupational therapists must be involved in sexual health care, effective sexual rehabilitation, like all rehabilitation, requires a team approach. The rehabilitation team must address all the individual's problems in a holistic way, and all team members should be knowledgeable about sexual issues and treatment options.[48] If each member of the treatment team is knowledgeable and skilled in this area, the patient can choose the team member with whom he or she is most comfortable to address sexual issues. In addition, each team member has different expertise from which the patient may benefit. Problems related to erectile dysfunction may be best addressed by a physician, relationship changes may require social work intervention, and communication difficulties may be best addressed by the speech and language pathologist.

In reality, sexuality issues are often ignored by the health care team, especially for the stroke population. A support group of 37 wives of stroke patients at a Veterans Administration center reported that no one had spoken to them about poststroke sexuality.[29] In a 1988 study of sexuality counseling in an inpatient rehabilitation program, only 20% of non–spinal cord injured patients (55% of whom had a diagnosis of stroke) had received written materials on sex. Sexuality information was voluntarily given to 32%.[12] Rehabilitation professionals cite various reasons for not addressing sexuality with their patients, with the most common responses being that another team member is responsible for this intervention and that their knowledge is inadequate.[33] The physician, social worker, and psychologist are most often cited as responsible for sexuality intervention.

Besides being neglected in the clinic, sexual rehabilitation has received little attention in research. However, a general positive correlation has been found between successful sexual rehabilitation and positive adjustment to disability. The literature shows that patients with disabilities are interested in the inclusion of sexuality in rehabilitation and give sexuality a high priority.[18]

In clinical rehabilitation, "a job title does not always define competencies," and "no job title . . . excludes discussion of sexuality."[9] The qualities necessary in a competent sexuality counselor for people with disabilities have been variously described. Chipouras et al[9] emphasize comfort with sexuality, including one's own; comfort with disability; empathy; nonprojection of one's own morals onto the patient; awareness of available resources; basic knowledge of human sexuality; and awareness of one's own competency and willingness to refer to others as necessary. The foundation of sexuality counseling consists of awareness and knowledge, which can be gained through reading, inservice education, coursework, and workshops. Skill in sexuality counseling must be developed through practice, like all clinical skills. Discomfort in dealing with sexuality need be no different than discomfort with other difficult disability issues. Occupational therapists address many personal and sometimes painful issues with their patients. Increased competency, skill, and comfort comes with practice. Practice of sexuality interventions through role play with other staff members may be helpful in achieving greater comfort in conducting sexuality interventions.

PLISSIT

Various frameworks and models may be used to address sexuality issues in health care. Among the earliest and most prevalent is the PLISSIT model, developed by psychologist Jack Annon.[5] *PLISSIT* is an acronym for four levels of intervention: Permission, Limited Information, Specific Suggestions, and Intensive Therapy (Figure 18-1). Using this model, the practitioner can determine the type and extent of sexuality intervention needed, whether he or she has the skills to perform the intervention, and whether to refer to a more qualified counselor.

Permission

Permission is the most basic and most frequently required intervention. It consists of reassuring patients that their ac-

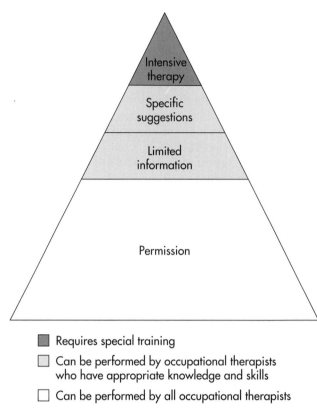

Figure 18-1 The PLISSIT model.

tions and feelings are normal and acceptable. All occupational therapists should strive to perform permission-level sexuality interventions. Recognizing that sexual behavior varies widely and not projecting one's own values or morals onto the patient is most important.

The practitioner must be proactive to provide patients with permission. Waiting for the patient to bring up sexual issues is not enough; the therapist must let the patient know that it is acceptable to express sexual concerns. The simplest way to do this is to ask: "People who have had strokes sometimes have concerns or questions about how they will be affected sexually. Do you have any concerns or questions in this area?" This line of questioning serves to normalize the concerns and gives patients the opportunity to say no if they are not comfortable discussing sexuality with that person at that time. It also lets patients know that sexual concerns are considered legitimate and gives them permission to bring up sexual issues again if their needs change. The therapist should ask questions in a language appropriate for the patient's understanding, including the use of slang terms if necessary.

The best time to bring up sexuality is usually at the initial evaluation, when other ADL issues are also being addressed. If this is not feasible because of time constraints or because the evaluating therapist will not be treating the patient, sexuality should be brought up as soon as is comfortable. Sexual concerns should be explored before home visits and in the formulation of discharge plans because the patient's needs and concerns change throughout rehabilitation.

Opportunities to give patients permission to express themselves as sexual beings often occur spontaneously. On one rehabilitation unit, a 38-year-old Hispanic man with a diagnosis of right CVA was playing a "getting-to-know-you" game with the other patients, all of whom were older women. As part of the activity, each member of the group was asked to name something they liked. The women named things such as chocolate, flowers, and pets. The man said, "I like women." After a few seconds of silence, the occupational therapist running the group said, "Of course you do; what could be more natural?" The group members all nodded, and the activity continued.

Limited Information

Sometimes simply reassuring patients about sexuality is not enough. If patients do have concerns or questions, they may require Limited Information, specific information related to their stated concerns. Most occupational therapists are qualified to provide patients with limited information. This level of intervention is often concerned with dispelling myths or misconceptions about sexuality. It may be related to facts about the effect of disability on sexuality and sexual function. Handouts and pamphlets as well as group education programs are good ways to provide limited information. The patients may read and absorb information on their own and ask the practitioner for clarification as needed. The important issue is to limit the information to the patient's specific concerns. The accuracy of the information is also paramount. If the therapist does not have the information, he or she should help the patient get it before making a referral to another practitioner. For example, a patient with a recent stroke and complex cardiac history asks whether it is safe to have sex. Although the patient's physician can provide the answer, it is not enough for the therapist to say, "Ask your physician." By bringing up the concern to the therapist, the patient has chosen that person as an advocate. The therapist might respond, "Your physician is best equipped to answer that question. Would you feel comfortable asking her yourself, or would you like me to contact her for you?"

Specific Suggestions

If a patient is experiencing a sexual problem, limited information may not be enough to solve it. The next level of intervention is Specific Suggestions, aimed at solving the specific problem. This type of intervention requires more knowledge, time, and skill from the clinician, but is appropriate for some occupational therapists (Box 18-1). The clinician should meet with the patient (and partner, if appropriate) in a comfortable, private setting and obtain a sexual problem history. This history should include:

Box 18-1

Competencies for Sexuality Interventions at Each PLISSIT Level

PERMISSION

To perform this level of sexuality intervention, the therapist should do the following:

Acknowledge the sexuality of all people
Be comfortable with his or her own sexuality
Believe that interest in sexuality is appropriate for everyone
Be comfortable speaking directly about sexual issues (or be willing to overcome discomfort)
Refrain from projecting personal sexual morals and values onto others.

LIMITED INFORMATION

To provide this level of intervention, the therapist should fulfill the criteria listed for Permission and do the following:

Have a basic understanding of human sexuality and its many variations
Understand the physiology of human sexual response
Be able to analyze the effects of physical disability on various sexual activities
Be willing to seek and provide accurate sexual information
Be aware of the limitations of his or her own knowledge base

SPECIFIC SUGGESTIONS

To perform this level of intervention, the therapist should fulfill the criteria for Permission and Limited Information and do the following:

Be familiar with various sexual activities
Be comfortable discussing specific sexual activities
Be able to conduct a sexual problem history
Be able to adapt various sexual activities to accommodate functional limitations

INTENSIVE THERAPY

To perform this level of sexuality intervention, the therapist should fulfill the criteria for Permission, Limited Information, and Specific Suggestions and do the following:

Have formal training in sex therapy, sexuality counseling, or psychotherapy

---

- The patient's assessment of the problem and its cause, onset and course
- The patient's attempts to solve the problem
- The patient's goals

Just as the occupational therapist would not initiate treatment of other problems without a full evaluation, the clinician must fully understand the sexual problem before making specific suggestions. After the sexual problem history is obtained, treatment goals should be developed in collaboration with the patient. These goals may address learning the effects of stroke on sexual function; adapting to changes in sensory, motor, or cognitive function; adapting to psychosocial and role changes; and improving sexual communication.

One male stroke patient reported sexual problems after a weekend visit home. A sexual problem history revealed that he had always preferred the male-superior position for intercourse. Since his CVA, increased leg extensor *tone* and weakness had prevented adequate pelvic thrusting in this position. With his occupational therapist, the patient discussed various new positions to increase mobility: lying on the affected side with knees bent, and sitting in a chair with his partner seated facing him.

Intensive Therapy

If the patient's problems are beyond the scope of goal-oriented specific suggestions, he or she may require Intensive Therapy. This level of intervention is based on specialized treatment skills and is beyond the scope of most occupational therapists. Finding an appropriate referral for such patients, such as a psychologist, social worker, or sex therapist, is advisable. If the sexual problems predate or are not related to the onset of disability, the patient may require referral.

The PLISSIT model enables the health care professional to adapt a sexuality program to the needs of the setting and the population served. Although permission to express sexual concern is universal, the need for limited information and specific suggestions varies. The best way to assess the need for sexuality intervention is to ask patients about their concerns. Occupational therapist Evelyn Andamo's treatment model uses a written "problem checklist" in which the patient is asked to identify problems in whatever role he or she fills including that of sexual partner.[4] By addressing sexuality in a multiproblem context, this model helps normalize sexual concerns. The checklist includes two items related to sexual problems and concerns about sexual activity.[4] Patients who check either item receive further intervention as needed, including problem clarification, sexual history-taking, and the development of treatment goals and treatment planning. Any evaluation can be adapted to include verbal questions about sexual concerns. This can be repeated before home visits or as discharge approaches because patients' concerns change over time.

Underlying some health care workers' reluctance to address sexuality may be a fear of opening a "Pandora's box" of issues too difficult or intimate for them to handle. This is seldom the case. Most people do not wish to disclose their sexual problems or to include strangers in their intimate relationships. They want and benefit from the least intervention possible to help them solve their sexual problems and deal with their concerns. Other clinicians fear that providing permission to discuss sexual concerns will facilitate inappropriate patient sexual behavior. Recent literature indicates that many health care workers are exposed to inappropriate sexual behavior on the part of patients during their careers, and they often lack training in dealing with these behaviors. Less experienced clinicians and students tend to ignore the behaviors even when they are severe, which may result in high stress and difficult working conditions.[28] Of course, any clinician who is exposed to sexual or other inappropriate behavior by anyone should address the problem immediately. Patient behaviors should be documented in the medical records; other staff members may also be affected. All new therapists and students should be encouraged to report harassment and seek help with difficult situations.

Providing permission to patients to address sexual issues directly actually decreases inappropriate behaviors. Flirting, sexual jokes, and innuendoes are often a patient's way of indirectly expressing doubts and concerns about sexuality after disability. One stroke patient, MG, overheard his occupational therapist inviting some coworkers to her home and asked, "When are you going to invite me over?" The therapist replied, "You know, MG, that I am your therapist and although you're a really nice person, it would be unethical for us to have a social relationship. But tell me, are you interested in developing new social relationships?" This question led to a lively discussion about MG's returning interest in women and sex. The therapist was understanding and supportive. The patient made no further advances to her. By refocusing attention on the patient, the therapist deflected the unwanted attention and responded to the patient's real need for permission to acknowledge his returning sexual feelings.

DEVELOPING COMPETENCY

Competency in sexuality intervention comprises three elements (see Box 18-1): comfort, knowledge, and skill. These elements are interrelated; individuals are more comfortable with things they know well (knowledge) and do well (skill). Suggestions for improving these competencies follow.

Comfort

Reading (See resources and references at end of chapter.)
Films (Be aware that many are related to spinal cord injuries.)
Disability literature
Sexual Attitude Reassessment seminars (These are sponsored regularly by Planned Parenthood.)

Knowledge

Readings (See resources and references at end of chapter.)
Lectures
Inservice education

Skill

Role playing with other staff members

Acquiring skill through practice

Seeking a mentor for private supervision who specializes in sexuality

SPECIFIC SUGGESTIONS FOR TREATMENT

Many performance component deficits that occur after CVA may affect sexual function and sexuality. These deficits include sensorimotor, cognitive, communication, and psychosocial changes. With sexuality, as with other ADL, determining the underlying causes of the performance problem can be challenging. The following section comprises a list of suggestions that may be used during treatment.

Hemiparesis/Sensory Loss

1. Having the hemiplegic partner lie on the affected side frees the uninvolved side for touching; this position also provides support, permits active movement, and focuses attention on the intact side. Early treatment by the rehabilitation team (occupational and physical therapy) should include instructing the patient to lie comfortably on the affected side (Figure 18-2).

2. Impaired motor control (limb and trunk) may require a change in coital positioning because the hemiplegic partner may find it difficult to assume certain positions. Alternatively, the unaffected partner may assume the superior position in bed or on a chair, or lying on his or her side (Figure 18-3).

3. Positioning for comfort with the use of pillows can be incorporated into foreplay.

4. Partners should discuss sensory loss beforehand; in hemiplegia there may be absent or diminished light touch, impaired proprioception, kinesthesia, or loss of stereognosis. Stimulation on areas of intact sensation and incorporation of stimuli to intact senses (e.g., us-

ing scents, keeping lights on for visual stimulation, music, and stimulating language) may help improve sensory abilities.

5. Individuals with severe sensory deficits must consider skin protection during sexual activity to prevent skin breakdown.

6. In the case of impaired hand function, a vibrator can be attached with the use of Velcro to enable stimulation.

7. Treatment of weakened muscles of facial expression to improve body image and facial expression and strengthening of oral-motor muscles may enhance oral sexual activities such as kissing and oral-genital sex.

Cognitive/Perceptual/Neurobehaviorial Impairments

1. Simple positions are recommended. Achieving a routine of sexual activity may be helpful if the person has difficulty moving spontaneously. When the brain becomes used to a routine, it does not have to work as hard to plan movements and the patient does not have to concentrate on how he or she is moving.[33]

2. Hemianopsia or unilateral neglect may cause a person to ignore parts of their hemiplegic partner's body or not respond when approached from the partner's affected side. The unaffected partner must be sensitive to these deficits.

3. Nonverbal communication such as touching and gesturing are encouraged with partners who may have speech or language disorders.[33]

4. Distractions such as loud music should be kept to a minimum.[33]

5. Individuals with memory impairment should keep a log of daily activities, including sexual activities, in an effort to remain oriented.[33]

6. Sexual role changes such as increased sexual initiation by the nondisabled partner can help minimize the effects of cognitive changes on sexual function.

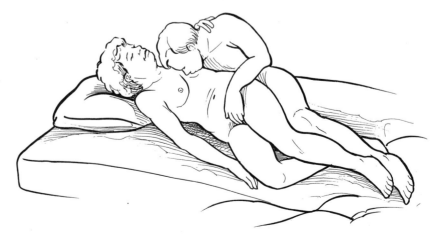

Figure 18-2 This position allows for genital fondling during rear entry vaginal or anal penetration. It is appropriate for opposite or same-sex couples. Either partner can participate fully if lying on the hemiplegic side.

7. Fantasies or intimate thoughts may be shared in writing or by using augmentative communication devices before and after sexual activity.[33]
8. A team approach may be helpful. Speech and language pathologists can help the patient improve or compensate for verbal and nonverbal communication deficits.

Decreased Endurance

1. Sexual activities should be planned ahead. The patient should wait 3 hours after meals before engaging in activities and avoid sex when fatigued. Instead, this may be a good time for intimate cuddling, hugging, or participating in massage.
2. Intercourse can be deemphasized through exploration of other sexual activities such as mutual masturbation and oral-genital sex.
3. Sexual positions that use less energy should be considered.
4. Sexual activities may be easier to do in the morning, when energy may be greater, instead of the evening.

Inadequate Vaginal Lubrication

1. A water-based lubricant should be used.
2. Foreplay should be extended to ensure adequate lubrication of the vagina before intercourse.
3. Lubricated condoms may be helpful.
4. Both partners should keep in mind that impaired vaginal lubrication may also be a normal age-related change.
5. A consultation with a gynecologist may be warranted.

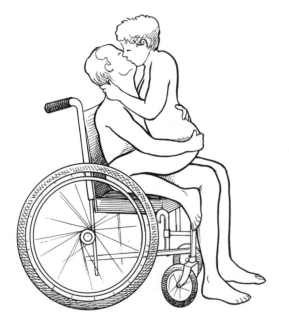

Figure 18-3 This position is appropriate as an alternative to lying on a bed or other surface; it is a nice alternative for wheelchair use and may break the barrier of wheelchair being used only for transport.

Impotence

1. Certain medications may have an effect on erection in addition to the stroke itself. This possibility should be discussed with the patient and his physician.
2. Alternatives to intercourse should be considered.
3. If impotence is related to depression or another psychologic issue, the therapist should suggest that the patient discuss it with the appropriate team member, such as the psychologist or psychiatrist.
4. A ring placed on the base of the penis may help maintain blood flow into the penis and help the patient maintain an erection.
5. For impotence or ejaculatory problems, consultation with a urologist may be warranted. Treatment options include vacuum constrictor devices, injection of vasoactive agents, and penile prosthesis implantation.[21]

Incontinence

1. The patient should avoid fluids before engaging in sexual activity.[33]
2. Men may wear a condom to prevent leakage onto the partner.
3. Patients on a voiding schedule should be encouraged to adhere to the schedule to prevent accidents.
4. Towels should be available in case of accidents, and the patient should discuss his or her situation before engaging in sexual activity to prevent embarrassment.
5. The patient should empty his or her bladder before engaging in sexual activity.

Contraception and Safer Sex

Most stroke patients are past the childbearing years; however, contraception remains an issue for those who are still fertile. Menses may be affected after a stroke, although studies are inconclusive.[27] However, the exploration of contraceptive methods may be needed, depending on the patient's impairments. The functional abilities needed to use condoms, a diaphragm, or a cervical cap include fine motor abilities, motor praxis, and intact cognitive and perceptual function.[33] However, in some cases the nondisabled partner can assist with contraception and work it into the sexual repertoire. For example, if a woman had a stroke and her contraception of choice is the diaphragm but she cannot insert the device because of hemiplegia, her partner might do this for her. If the couple prefers, alternative methods of contraception could be explored. A review of other methods may be warranted, particularly if the patient previously used the pill, which has side effects, some of which affect circulation.[44]

Latex condoms are preferred for safer sexual practices against sexually transmitted diseases; however, an erect penis is required. If the male has difficulty maintaining or achieving an erection, it may not be possible for him to use condoms effectively. Female condoms or alternative sexual practices minimizing contact with body fluids may be explored, and individuals and couples should be educated on options such as mutual masturbation and oral sex with the use of a dental dam, which is a latex sheet placed over the vulva during cunnilingus. The therapist is responsible for staying updated on current guidelines related to safer sex practices if education on safer sex will be included in treatment.

■

CASE STUDY

PR is a 52-year-old married man who previously suffered a hemorrhagic left basal ganglia stroke. He was admitted to a subacute rehabilitation center with right hemiplegia and language and short-term memory deficits. His right upper and lower extremity sensation was absent for tactile stimulation. He demonstrated increased flexor activity and had no active arm movement. PR required maximal assistance with all transfers and ADL, and his activity tolerance was poor. Before admission he had lived with his wife of 1½ years and ran a business requiring frequent travel. PR's wife also worked full time and taught women's exercise classes in her free time.

By his 18-day team conference, PR had made substantial gains. He was independent in stand-pivot transfers and required minimal assistance in dressing. He demonstrated emerging sensation and motor control in his right arm and lower extremities. He was able to walk during physical therapy with a cane and assistance from a therapist. His language function had improved, with only some word-finding deficits remaining. He and his wife attended the team meeting. Her last question to the team was, "When will his sex drive return?" PR said, "Don't worry, honey, it will come back like everything else." The staff recommended discussing this issue with the new neurologist, with whom the couple had an appointment the following day.

On return from his neurologist, PR reported to his speech therapist that he and his wife had "forgotten" to bring up sexuality. He reported achieving only partial erections. The therapist offered him a consultation with a staff member who was knowledgeable about sexuality and disability, and he agreed. The speech therapist had received no training or information about sexuality and had no experience in this area. PR's treating occupational therapist, who was not present at the team meeting, was willing to use part of his scheduled treatment time for the sexuality intervention.

The occupational therapist introduced herself to PR and made an appointment to meet with him the next week in his private room. She asked whether he had any specific questions or concerns so she could prepare information for their meeting. He said the concerns were mostly his wife's and that he was confident his sex drive would "return just like use of my arm and leg are going to return." The occupational therapist suggested including PR's wife in the meeting, but PR said she was unavailable during the daytime so the occupational therapist might as well speak to him alone.

A brief sexual history revealed that PR had been single for 11 years before this second marriage and that he had been sexually active with a variety of women during that time. He and his wife considered sex an extremely important part of their relationship. "People can be very sexy even though they don't look it," he explained. PR volunteered that he and his wife would not need help with sexual positioning for intercourse because they preferred the female-superior position. PR admitted to decreased sexual desire, which he attributed to fatigue, separation, and the nonconducive environment. He reported having erections that he estimated at "three quarters of normal hardness," which was an improvement. He reiterated that he was sure everything would come back.

The intervention included three levels of the PLISSIT model.

Permission

The therapist assured PR that concern about sexuality was common among stroke survivors and their sex partners and that, after a life-threatening event, sexual concerns are a sign of returning health. They discussed the myth that middle-aged people are not attractive and society's insistence in portraying only young, thin, beautiful people as "sexy." The therapist explained that although health care workers are sometimes reluctant to bring up sexuality, PR had the right to be assertive in getting any assistance he needed in this area.

Limited information

PR was provided a verbal summary of the research on stroke and sex. He was informed that some people experience sexual dysfunction after stroke and that desire, libido, erection, ejaculation, and orgasm may be affected. The therapist emphasized the lack of correlation of sexual dysfunction to motor or sensory deficits and the high correlation between prestroke and poststroke sexual function. The therapist and PR discussed the effect of antihypertensive medications on sexual function. PR reported telling his physician that he would not take any medication that had side effects on sexual function. The physician prescribed a medication without sexual side effects.

Specific suggestions

Although PR reported no need for ideas to improve his sexual function, a level of denial was evident in his assurances that "everything would come back." The occupational therapist said, "Just as you're participating in therapy to improve your arm, leg, and speech, your sexual function will improve faster if you don't just sit around waiting for its return." PR agreed that he felt as if he had a new, different body and that he would find it helpful to explore and learn the "new" body's responses. They discussed including his wife in the sexual explorations, but she was uncomfortable with the lack of privacy in the facility.

Because PR would be unlikely to have sexual relations with his wife before discharge in 6 weeks, strategies were discussed for initiating sexual activity in a positive, nonthreatening way because early problems with erectile function are not necessarily predictive of continuing problems. Alternative sexual activities are also considered "real sex."

Because of their prestroke sexual function, motivation, interest, maturity, and willingness to communicate, PR and his wife were likely to make a good sexual adjustment to the effects of stroke. However the therapist did offer information on treatment of erectile or other sexual dysfunction in the future should problems arise because she would not be available to PR after discharge. She also reported the latest medical interventions for erectile dysfunction, which would be familiar to any urologist. Although he felt he wouldn't need it, PR seemed glad to know that treatment was readily available.

At this facility, sexual concerns were not addressed by any rehabilitation discipline. While treating PR, the therapist had provided written information on the sexual effects of CVA and the role of speech and language therapists in sexuality counseling to the speech therapist who referred him and summarized the results of the counseling session. Staff members became aware that other patients might have sexual concerns but lacked the comfort level or assertiveness to initiate the communication. The therapist was asked to provide an inservice on sexuality, which was well attended by members of the OT department and other interested staff.

■

CASE STUDY

WA is a 62-year-old woman who previously suffered a right MCA stroke with resulting left hemiparesis. After her initial and rehabilitation hospitalizations, she was discharged home for continued occupational and physical therapy. She lived in a senior housing development, which had a social room on the premises. WA had been widowed for more than 15 years and reported that her husband had been an alcoholic and a "terrible man." During WA's initial evaluation at home, the occupational therapist asked what her goals for rehabilitation were. WA was quick to reply, "I want to be able to get out of the wheelchair so I can chase a man." Sexuality had not been addressed until this point in the evaluation. The therapist took the opportunity to ask WA whether she had a significant man in her life, to which WA replied "no". The therapist asked WA whether she had any concerns about resuming sexual activities after the stroke; again WA replied no. She explained that she was not looking to marry again and simply wanted to be exposed to people so she could flirt. During this conservation the therapist realized that further exploration of sexual function was geared toward getting WA out into the community again. WA had been limited in this endeavor because of poor mobility and wheelchair dependency.

In this example the therapist used the Permission level of the PLISSIT model. The patient brought up the topic herself, and it was discovered through further questioning that WA was really referring to a need to socialize, not so much as to act on her sexual desires. In subsequent conversations, WA's occupational therapist reassessed this situation, particularly as WA made progress with ADL and functional mobility. After 6 months of treatment, WA was getting back out into the community, attending an adult day care center, and participating in bingo games in her building. She was taught how to transfer on and off the furniture in the social room to allow greater independence and a sense of normalcy. All areas of function, including sexuality, were reevaluated periodically during WA's treatment program, and her goals remained unchanged from her initial evaluation.

In this example the issue of sexuality was less directly related to actual sexual activities than to socialization and flirting. Had the therapist neglected to pursue WA's early statement about wanting to "chase a man," the patient's needs might never have been met.

■

CASE STUDY

LE was a 57-year-old woman with an unknown social history who was admitted to a rehabilitation hospital who previously suffered a right CVA with left hemiplegia and perceptual deficits. At the initial evaluation the occupational therapist asked whether LE had any sexual concerns. "Yes, I want to know whether I'll ever have sex again," she said tearfully. The occupational therapist realized that such a question could not be answered and that the client's concerns needed clarification. Was LE concerned about being able to find a partner? About "performing" sexually? The therapist helped LE clarify her question with some probing, "What are you concerned about specifically? What do you think might get in the way of your having sex again?" LE reported having a male friend with whom she had an active sex life. Her major concerns were whether she would regain enough function to return home and whether sexual activity would provoke further strokes. The occupational therapist reassured LE that most people can safely resume sexual activity after a stroke and offered to help her consult her physician for medical clearance. The therapist provided the limited information LE was looking for through reassurance and by obtaining medical clearance through another team member (that is, the physician). The therapist was able to tie in all the rehabilitation goals with the patient's desire to return to her home and previous lifestyle, which strengthened the collaboration between LE and the rehabilitation staff.

Program development

The therapist should have support, resources, and referrals available when sexual issues are addressed. The therapist should inform supervisors and others on the rehabilitation staff of activities. Resources and referral services should be identified in other departments and outside the facility, if appropriate. The therapist should check the facility's existing policies on sexuality (if any) and strive to be in compliance. The therapist should report experiences and provide education to others. If possible an interdisciplinary committee should be formed to address sexual issues and develop appropriate programs.

Documentation and billing

Sexuality interventions may be billed and documented in various ways, depending on the billing system and the issues discussed. Appropriate categories include ADL training, patient and family education, discharge planning, and psychosocial training.

As in treatment, sexuality is best addressed in a multiproblem context. Patient privacy and confidentiality must be maintained. Examples of goals include the following:

1. Patient will identify proper bed positioning for sleep and sexual activity.
2. Patient's spouse will accurately assess patient's safety to engage in physical and sexual activities.

■

SUMMARY

All people are sexual, and sexual activity is important to most people throughout their lives. Interest in or desire for sexual activity does not necessarily diminish as people grow older. Stroke may interfere with sexual expression by affecting the survivor's desire, libido, erectile or lubrication response, orgasm or ejaculation, and sensorimotor, cognitive, psychosocial, ADL, and role function. Stroke may also affect the partner's response or the patient's ability to find a sexual partner. Research has shown that sexual desire is most often affected; however, prestroke sexual activity is the strongest predictor of poststroke sexual activity. Occupational therapists can use a holistic approach and training in activity analysis and adaptation to assist people who have had strokes in regaining their desired sexual function. A team model is best for sexual rehabilitation, with each team member knowledgeable about sexuality and providing special expertise. The PLISSIT model helps the practitioner identify the type of sexuality intervention required. All occupational therapists should be able to provide patients with permission, limited information, and specific suggestions and should be able to make appropriate referrals for sexual concerns related to stroke. Therapists must be sensitive to the multiple components of sex.

REVIEW QUESTIONS

1. What are the stages of the sexual response cycle and the associated physiologic changes in males and females?
2. What are some of the normal changes in sexual function in aging men and women?
3. Why does sexual activity decline among older people?
4. What are the four levels of sexuality intervention in the PLISSIT model? Which may be performed by occupational therapists?
5. What skills are needed to provide sexuality counseling to patients who have had strokes?
6. What common effects of stroke interfere with sexual function and sexuality? What are the best predictors of poststroke sexual function?

■ COTA Considerations ■

- Sexuality is considered an ADL.
- Strive to feel comfortable discussing sexual issues with a patient; this topic should be addressed during a therapy session.
- If you are uncomfortable, tell the patient, but offer to find a team member who can speak with the patient about these issues.
- Sexual dysfunction may be related to several physical, neurologic, social, and psychologic causes. The solutions vary from individual to individual.

REFERENCES

1. Aloni R, Ring H, Rosenthal N, et al: Sexual function in male patients after stroke a follow up study, *Sexuality Disabil* 11:121, 1993.
2. Aloni R, Schwartz J, Ring J: Sexual function in post-stroke female patients, *Sexuality Disabil* 12:3, 1994.
3. American Occupational Therapy Association: *Uniform terminology for occupational therapy—third edition*, Bethesda, Md, 1994, The Association.
4. Andamo EM: Treatment model: occupational therapy for sexual dysfunction, *Sexuality Disabil* 4:26, 1980.
5. Annon JS: The PLISSIT model: a proposed conceptual scheme for the behavioral treatment of sexual problems, *J Sex Educ Ther* 2:1, 1976.
6. Boldrini P, Basaglia N, Calanca MC: Sexual changes in hemiparetic patients, *Arch Phys Med Rehabil* 72:3, 1991.
7. Bray GP, DeFrank RS, Wolfe TL: Sexual functioning in stroke survivors, *Arch Phys Med Rehabil* 62:286, 1981.
8. Burgener S, Logan G: Sexuality concerns of the post-stroke patient, *Rehabil Nurs* 14:4, 1989.
9. Chipouras S, et al: *Who cares? A handbook on sex education and counseling services for disabled people*, ed 2, Baltimore, Md, 1982, University Park Press.
10. Cole TM, Cole SS: Rehabilitation of problems of sexuality in physical disability. In Kottke FJ, Lehman JF, editors: *Krusen's handbook of physical medicine and rehabilitation*, ed 4, Philadelphia, FA Davis.
11. Coslett HB, Heilman, KM: Male sexual function: impairment after right hemisphere stroke, *Arch Neurol* 43:10, 1986.
12. Cushman LA: Sexual counseling in a rehabilitation program: a patient perspective, *J Rehabil* 54:2, 1988.
13. Evans J: Sexual consequences of disability: activity analysis and performance adaptation, *Occup Ther Health Care* 4:1, 1987.
14. Finger WW: Prevention, assessment and treatment of sexual dysfunction following stroke, *Sexuality Disabil* 11:1, 1993.
15. Fugi-Meyer AR, Jaasko, L: Post-stroke hemiplegia and sexual intercourse, *Scand J Rehabil Med* 7:158, 1980.
16. Garden FH, Smith BS: Sexual function after cerebrovascular accident, *Curr Concepts Rehabil Med* 5:2, 1990.
17. Garden FH: Incidence of sexual dysfunction in neurologic disability, *Sexuality Disabil* 9:1, 1991.
18. Gatens C: Sexuality and disability. In Woods NF, editor: *Human sexuality in health and illness*, ed 3, St Louis, 1984, Mosby.
19. Goddess ED, Wagner NN, Silverman DR: Poststroke sexual activity of CVA patients, *Medical Aspects Hum Sexuality* 13:16, 1979.

20. Goldberg RL: Sexual counseling for the stroke patient, *Medical Aspects Hum Sexuality* June 1987.
21. Hatzichristou DG, Bertero EB, Goldstein I: Decision making in the evaluation of impotence; the patient profile-oriented algorithm, *Sexuality Disabil* 12:29, 1994.
22. Hawton K: Sexual adjustment of men who have had strokes, *J Psychosom Res* 28:243, 1984.
23. Hellerstein HK, Friedman EH: Sexual activity and the postcoronary patient, *Arch Intern Med* 125:987, 1970.
24. Kaplan SA, Brown WC, Blaivas JG: When stroke patients suffer urologic dysfunction, *Contem Urol* January 1990.
25. Laflin M: Sexuality and the elderly. In Lewis CB, editor: *Aging: the health care challenge: an interdisciplinary approach to assessment and rehabilitative management*, ed 2, Philadelphia, 1990, FA Davis.
26. Mackey FG: Sexuality in coronary artery disease, *Postgrad Med* 80:1, 1986.
27. Masters WH, Johnson VE: *Human sexual response*, Boston, 1966, Little, Brown.
28. McComas J et al: Experiences of student and practicing physical therapists with inappropriate patient sexual behavior, *Physical Therapy* 73:762, 1993.
29. McCormick GP, Riffer DJ, Thompson MM: Coital positioning for stroke afflicted couples, *Rehabil Nurs* 11:2, 1986.
30. Monga TN, Lawson JS, Inglis J: Sexual dysfunction in stroke patients, *Arch Phys Med Rehabil* 67:19, 1986.
31. Monga TN, Monga M, Raina MS, et al: Hypersexuality in stroke, *Arch Phys Med Rehabil* 67:415, 1986.
32. Muller FE, Mittleman MA, Maclure M, et al: Triggering myocardial infarction by sexual activity, *JAMA* 275:18, 1996.
33. Neistadt ME, Frieda M: *Choices: a guide to sex counseling with physically disabled adults*, Malabar, Fla, 1987, Robert E Krieger.
34. Neistadt M: Human sexuality and counseling. In Hopkins HL, Smith HD, editors: *Willard and Spackman's occupational therapy*, ed 8, Philadelphia, 1993, Lippincott.
35. Novak PP, Mitchell MM: Professional involvement in sexuality counseling for patients with spinal cord injuries, *Am J Occup Ther* 42:2, 1988.
36. Parke F: Sexuality in later life, *Nursing Times* 87:50, 1991.
37. Payne MS, Greer DL, Corbin DE: Sexual functioning as a topic in occupational therapy training, a survey of programs, *Am J Occup Ther* 42:227, 1988.
38. Purk JK, Richardson RA: Older adult stroke patients and their spousal caregivers, *J Contemp Hum Serv* 75:10, 1994.
39. Romano MD: Sexuality and the disabled female, *Accent Living*, Winter 1973.
40. Sjogren K, Damber JE, Lilequist B: Sexuality after stroke with hemiplegia. I, *Scand J Rehabil Med* 15:2, 1983.
41. Sjogren K: Sexuality after stroke with hemiplegia. II, *Scand J Rehabil Med* 15:63, 1983.
42. Sjogren K, Fugl-Meyer AR: Adjustment to life after stroke with special reference to sexual intercourse and leisure, *J Psychosomatic Res* 26:4, 1982.
43. Strauss D: Biopsychosocial issues in sexuality with the neurologically impaired patient, *Sexuality Disabil* 9:1, 1991.
44. Szasz G, Miller S, Anderson L: Guide to birth control counseling of the physically handicapped, *Can Med Assoc J* 120:1353, 1979.
45. Thienhaus OJ: Practical overview of sexual function and advancing age, *Geriatrics* 43:8, 1988.
46. US Department of Health and Human Services: *Post-stroke rehabilitation*, Clinical Practice Guideline 16, 1995.
47. Wigg EH: Counseling the adult aphasic for sexual readjustment, *Rehab Counseling Bulletin* December, 1973.
48. Zasler ND: Sexuality in neurologic disability: an overview, *Sexuality Disabil* 9:1, 1991.

Suggested Reading

Neistadt ME, Frieda M: *Choices: a guide to sex counseling with physically disabled adults*, 1987, Robert E. Krieger.
Kroll K, Levy Klein E: *Enabling romance*, Bethesda, Md, 1995, Woodbine House.

Sexuality Resources

American Association of Sex Education Counselors and Therapists
435 North Michigan Avenue, Suite 1717
Chicago, IL 60611
312-644-0828

Coalition on Sexuality and Disability (Publishers of journal *Sexuality and Disability*)
132 East 23rd Street
New York, NY 10010
212-242-3900

Planned Parenthood of America (see local Yellow Pages for listing)

SEICUS (Sex Information and Education Counsel of the United States)
32 Washington Place
New York, NY 10003
212-673-3850

Sexuality and Disability Training Center
Boston University Medical Center
88 East Newton Street
Boston, MA 02118
617-638-7358

Stroke Clubs of America
805 Twelfth Street
Galveston, TX 77550
409-762-1022

The Task Force on Sexuality and Disability of the American Congress of Rehabilitation Medicine
5700 Old Orchard Road
Skokie, IL 60077
708-966-0095

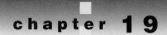

christine m. johann

chapter **19**

Seating and Wheeled Mobility Prescription

key terms

team approach	deformity prevention	functional concerns
seating	mobility	alignment
pressure relief	biomechanics	

chapter objectives

After completing this chapter, the reader will be able to accomplish the following:

1. Understand the evaluation process specific to seating and mobility.
2. List the goals of seating and positioning.
3. Recognize the types of mobility bases and seating systems that are available.
4. Discuss seating and mobility recommendations specific to clients who have sustained a cerebrovascular accident.

Before recommending a wheelchair for a patient with a mobility impairment, the therapist should evaluate the case carefully. Seating and wheeled mobility prescription is an integral part of a patient's functional restoration. Many therapists now recognize the need to learn about rehabilitation technology, which encompasses not only seating and wheeled mobility but also environmental control units, augmentative and alternative communication, and switch access selection for computer, power wheelchair, and augmentative communication use (see Chapter 21).

This chapter focuses on the basic principles of seating and positioning, the evaluation process, and the features and benefits of seating systems and wheelchairs. Although the emphasis is on seating and wheeled mobility

prescription specific to patients with a cerebrovascular accident (CVA), these principles apply to patients of all types and ages who display impaired mobility as a result of a neuromuscular or central nervous system disorder or trauma.

BASIC PRINCIPLES

The therapist's role in evaluating, simulating, and recommending equipment must be viewed differently today than it was 20, 10, or even 5 years ago. Changes in manufacturers of rehabilitation equipment, the style of the equipment, and the health care system have all dramatically influenced this process. Diane E. Ward[7] identifies several paradigms that affect the delivery of prescriptive seating. These are as follows:

Paradigm Shifts in the Focus of Health Care

A paradigm shift has occurred in health care, which now focuses on prevention. Health care professionals now emphasize training and educational models that help people attain and sustain healthy lifestyles rather than waiting until they become ill or develop further problems. Many seating systems and accessories are available that can help decrease the progression of deformities, pain, and problems. Someone who is seated properly feels happier, healthier, and better able to function.

Paradigm Shifts From Disability to Ability

The paradigm shift from disability to ability involves the way people who sustain an injury or disease that causes permanent orthopedic, neuromuscular, or central nervous system damage are described. These people are no longer viewed as disabled; rather, the condition they were born with or have acquired has created a conflict between their capabilities and their desire to interact with the environment and lead a meaningful life. Wheeled mobility and seating systems can enable people with these conditions to move about in their environment and lead active, productive lives. Without these devices, people with disabilities would be unable to function independently.

Paradigm Shifts in the Role of Health Practitioners

The therapist and patient are partners. Therapists must educate and empower their patients to make careful and responsible choices, while respecting each patient's disability, lifestyle, ethics, and cultural background. Health care reimbursement has changed the process whereby patients receive medical care or products. This process is governed by certain rules and regulations that therapists must address to ensure adequate care of patients. Therapists must then prepare patients to integrate this equipment into their daily life. The therapeutic interaction is extremely important, with profound cultural and societal implications. Equipment that enhances patients' abilities should be viewed as a positive experience. Cultural and societal barriers must be changed through therapist and health care practitioner education and involvement.

Paradigm Shifts in Efficacy Measurement

The rehabilitation technology industry has been challenged to prove its effectiveness. Organizations such as the Rehabilitation Engineers Society of North America (RESNA), National Registry of Rehabilitation Technology Suppliers (NRRTS), and many others are developing standards and measuring tools to ensure proper design, fabrication, prescription, and delivery of this equipment. Functional outcomes of a patient's health and ability to function are being studied and measured to determine whether these products are truly effective. Therapists and other health care practitioners must become involved in education, research, and product development to ensure that their patients receive the best possible equipment if and when needed.

FUNCTIONAL ENHANCEMENT OF SEATING AND POSITIONING

Approaching patients to discuss wheelchair use is often difficult. Therapists should present the topic in a positive way, emphasizing the potential for enhanced independence and functioning. They should also address postural discomfort or problems that may occur as a result of muscle imbalance caused by the neuromuscular insult.

Therapists often focus solely on the wheelchair, but the seating system should be the initial concern. Patients must understand that the seating system is the primary unit influencing their body posture and preparing them for proper postural control and function. The wheelchair-mobility frame is an accessory that allows for movement in the environment. Without a proper, customized seating system interfaced with a wheelchair frame at optimum angles for the patient's postural needs, patients do not benefit from mobility. Although they may be able to move about their environment, their posture, energy level, comfort, and health are at risk.

Primary Goals of Seating

The primary goals of seating and positioning are as follows:

1. Provide overall stability and control
2. Promote proximal stability, thereby enhancing distal extremity control
3. Decrease development of muscle contracture and skeletal deformity
4. Enhance comfort and appearance
5. Minimize the development of pressure sores
6. Improve function of autonomic nervous system
7. Increase sitting tolerance and energy level
8. Enhance function of the patient

Provide Overall Postural Stability and Control

Patients with neurologic insults are often influenced by abnormal skeletal muscle activity and pathologic reflexes. Proper seating can help balance muscle activity and decrease abnormal reflexes and posturing. Proper positioning provides an adjunct to therapy and affects goals in all areas of daily living.[1] Improved postural stability allows patients the freedom to interact, move their extremities, and hold their heads in the midline position.

Promote Proximal Muscle Stability, Thereby Enhancing Distal Muscular Control

A stable base of support for the pelvis allows patients to develop control and balance of their trunk musculature. When the pelvis is stable, the patient's center of gravity passes through the base of support, which helps promote stability.[4] This central stability allows for distal extremity control. The patient is able to make better use of arm or leg movement, head control, or oral motor control to perform functional tasks (e.g., hand function for dressing, leg movement for wheelchair propulsion, midline head orientation for improved visual tracking of objects, and oral motor control for speech articulation or swallowing).

Decrease Development of Muscle Contracture and Skeletal Deformity

Decreased pelvic stability, muscle weakness, and muscle imbalance can cause abnormal posture. Abnormal posture results in shortening or tightening of muscle groups, which can lead to a decreased range of motion in joints, muscle contractures, and skeletal deformity. Abnormal posture must be corrected as soon as possible so the patient does not develop fixed abnormal body positions. If soft tissue and skeletal flexibility is preserved, the patient can be successfully encouraged to sit properly through seating and seating system accessories. This proper positioning serves as a guide that can eventually promote the development of proper muscle control in that desired position. If muscle control cannot be improved, proper positioning provides adequate support.

Enhance Comfort and Appearance

With appropriate seating, patients feel and look better. Much like a splint or orthotic, the seating system must sometimes be introduced gradually, leading to full time use. Once patients can tolerate proper seating alignment, the benefits are tenfold. Not only do patients look and feel better; their circulation and skin has improved health and function. People who feel comfortable and good about themselves are much more productive and functional. Increased social interaction and communication are immediately apparent.

Minimize the Development of Pressure Sores

When impaired sensation, motor control, or judgment affects patients' ability to shift their weight as needed, patients may be at risk for development of pressure sores. A seating intervention that increases surface area support and equalizes weight distribution decreases the development of pressure sores.[1]

Improve Function of the Autonomic Nervous System

Abnormal posturing, muscle shortening, and an inability to shift weight can increase pressure on internal organs and other structures. When a patient is leaning forward or to the side because of poor pelvic or spinal muscle control, a strain on circulation, digestion, and cardiopulmonary function can result. Proper positioning encourages appropriate pelvic, spinal, and trunk alignment, which allows for improved physiologic functioning of the autonomic nervous system. Proper head and neck support can decrease the potential for aspiration when swallowing problems exist.[1]

Increase Sitting Tolerance and Energy Level

If patients are comfortable and feel they are functioning better, they will probably be more compliant in using a seating system. This compliance improves sitting tolerance and furthers therapeutic goals. Seated patients who receive proper support experience less fatigue and pain than those who struggle against abnormal muscle activity or reflexes to support their body position. Improved energy levels allow patients to interact with their environment, which enhances their function and quality of life.

Enhance Function of the Patient

Enhanced function of the patient can be seen as the outcome of the seven previous goals. Although stated last, this goal is the ultimate outcome of all aspects of therapeutic intervention. Improved function is specific to each patient. Functional improvements depend on the severity of the patient's neurologic insult and the potential for rehabilitation. The prevention of pressure sores, improvement of attention span, increased interaction with the environment, ability to assist in or perform activities of daily living, and independent mobility may all represent functional improvement. All functional abilities and goals are enhanced by improved seating and positioning in the wheelchair.

BASIC BIOMECHANICS OF SITTING

For proper seating of patients, a basic understanding of biomechanics is necessary so that proper posture can be understood and evaluated. One of the main components of proper seating is the distinction between flexible and fixed abnormal posture or deformity.

If a patient is sitting in an abnormal posture, such as a posterior pelvic tilt, and the examiner can manually correct the position, the posture can be termed a *flexible deformity*. Therefore the seating system selected must have components that correct and enhance this desired position because the patient cannot maintain it independently.

If a patient is sitting in an abnormal posture and the examiner cannot manually correct the position, the posture is termed as a *fixed deformity*. The recommended seating must compensate for this deformity and support the patient in this posture. Proper seating that provides the appropriate surface area of support for unique body contours helps decrease the progression of the deformity and minimize excessive pressures, thereby maintaining skin integrity and preventing decubitis ulcers.[3]

Normal and Abnormal Skeletal Biomechanics

Therapists must recognize the biomechanical features of the pelvis and its relationship with the spine to understand abnormal pelvic positions and their influence on the spine.

The pelvis moves anteriorly and posteriorly in the sagittal plane around a coronal axis, laterally tilting in a frontal plane around an anteroposterior axis and rotationally in a transverse plane around a vertical axis. A stable neutral position of the pelvis must be attained to provide the proper postural alignment of the spine (Figure 19-1). In a neutral pelvic position the anterior superior iliac spine (ASIS) is level with or slightly lower than the posterior superior iliac spine (PSIS). A neutral pelvis is also appropriately positioned when both iscial tuberosities are bearing equal weight (Figure 19-2). Palpating the ASIS and PSIS, then both right and left ASIS, can help determine the normal posture and alignment of the pelvis. Appropriate sitting posture can be observed in Figure 19-3, where a stable neutral pelvic position leads to symmetric positioning of the lower extremities and trunk.

Abnormalities of the pelvic position can be viewed in Figures 19-4, *A*, *B*, and *C*. Lateral tilting of the pelvis, in which one ASIS is higher than the other, is demonstrated in Figure 19-4, *A*. This unequal weight distribution of the ischial tuberosities, or pelvic obliquity, can lead to scoliotic spine curvature, trunk weakness with excessive lean-

ing to one side, and high risk for decubitus ulcer development on the weight-bearing ischial tuberosity. This problem is commonly seen in patients with asymmetric muscular problems, lower extremity muscle imbalance, spasticity, and midline orientation deficits.

Posterior pelvic tilt is demonstrated in Figure 19-4, *B*. A posterior pelvic tilt occurs when the ASIS is higher than

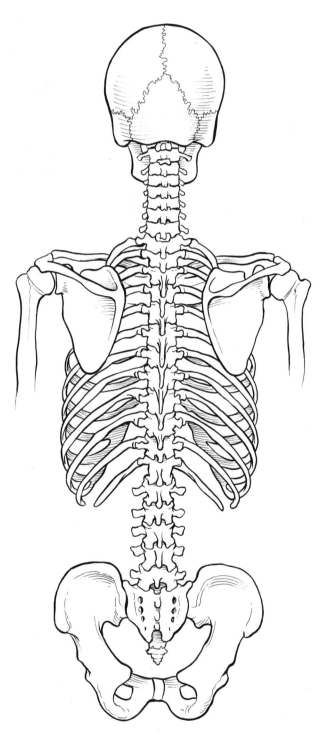

Figure 19-1 Lateral view of the spine and pelvis with appropriate alignment and spinal curvatures.

Figure 19-2 Appropriate spinal and pelvic alignment viewed posteriorly.

the PSIS. This abnormal pelvic position can lead to a kyphotic spinal position. A posterior pelvis with lumbar and thoracic spinal kyphosis can lead to unequal weight distribution, with increased pressures on the sacrum and coccyx structures, and a compensatory cervical hyperextension. This causes neck and back pain and limits the visual field. A posterior pelvic tilt is seen in patients with weakness, muscle imbalance, and limited pelvic mobility or shortened hamstring muscles stressed by forcing a knee angle that cannot be tolerated. Therapists should evaluate the pelvis in conjunction with the hamstring muscle so that patients who are sitting with their knees and feet in the leg rests do not have excessive stress on the hamstring. This problem is commonly seen in patients who are seated in a wheelchair with elevating leg rests. If the patient's hamstring muscle cannot sufficiently elongate to tolerate the open knee angle of an elevating leg rest, the patient will compensate by shifting to a posterior pelvic tilt posture.

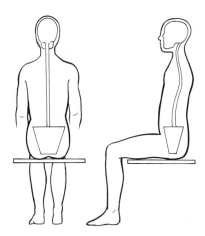

Figure 19-3 Appropriate alignment in seated posture. Note symmetric pelvis and spinal alignment.

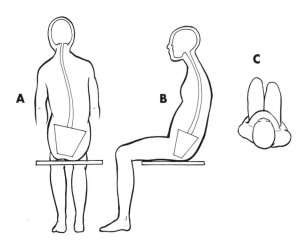

Figure 19-4 Common malalignments after a stroke. **A,** Lateral tilting of the pelvis in a patient with scoliosis. **B,** Posterior pelvic tilt with kyphosis. **C,** Trunk and pelvic rotation.

In anterior pelvic tilt the ASIS is lower than the PSIS. This abnormal pelvic position can cause a lordotic curve in the spine. This is typically seen in patients with decreased muscle recruitment and overall muscle weakness.

In pelvic rotation, one ASIS is farther forward than the other (Figure 19-4, **C**). It can also be observed by abnormal trunk rotation and unequal leg length posturing when the patient is seated. This abnormal pelvic rotation influences the spine to move into a rotated position and predisposes the patient for a scoliotic curvature of the spine. Pelvic rotation can create unequal weight distribution of the ischial tuberosities, which can lead to decubitus ulcers. This posturing is commonly seen in patients with muscular imbalances, asymmetries, and spasticity.

Pelvic positioning is affected by intrinsic factors such as the muscular influences of the hamstrings, abdominals, hip extensors, rectus femoris, trunk extensors, muscle length, muscle tone, and lumbar mobility.[6] Pelvic positioning is also affected by extrinsic factors such as the seating system, seat cushion, back support, seat-to-back angle interface, pelvic positioning belts, and foot placement.[6]

THE EVALUATION PROCESS

The evaluation process for seating and mobility is specific to each patient's needs. It determines the patient's strengths and weaknesses with regard to seating and wheelchair prescription and use. Extensive documentation is required for ordering equipment. The therapist must document not only evaluation results but also medical justification for the equipment so payment can be approved by the reimbursement or funding agencies. The seven strategic steps[5] in the following section help therapists simplify this process.

Step 1: Implement a Team Approach

The team involved in evaluating and recommending seating and mobility includes the patient and family, primary occupational and physical therapists, speech pathologists, physicians, and rehabilitation technology suppliers (RTSs). All team members are crucial and provide information necessary to determine the full spectrum of the patient's physical and functional needs.

Step 2: Conduct a Comprehensive Evaluation

The team members must complete a comprehensive evaluation documenting the patient's physical status, including orthopedic, neuromuscular, cognitive, perceptual, and visual function. Each team member provides unique information that results in the appropriate seating and mobility recommendation.

The occupational and physical therapists share the responsibility of providing evaluation results of the patient's orthopedic and neurologic status, motor control, muscle strength, influences of abnormal reflexes, joint range of motion and muscle contractures, past or future surgical intervention, static and dynamic sitting balance, muscular control in sitting, visual and cognitive-perceptual abilities, and functional abilities. Speech pathologists provide information regarding the client's oral motor control and speech or augmentative communication needs.

The patient, family, and caregivers must be interviewed to obtain vital information on the patient's lifestyle; vocational abilities; work-site requirements; and home, car, or van accessibility. The implementation of seating and mobility recommendations to the patient can have a dramatically positive or negative effect on the entire family. Therefore all evaluation areas must be carefully assessed before recommendations are presented.

The therapists and RTSs should organize and guide the evaluation so it addresses the following topics: reevaluation of used or old equipment; need for modification of present equipment or replacement with new equipment; ability of chosen equipment to provide proper postural support, increase comfort, and decrease pain; follow-through with therapeutic intervention; management of documentation for funding reimbursement or payment.

A physical mat evaluation of the patient assessing physical status and setting current goals is necessary. The evaluation should examine the patient's functional abilities and limitations in prone, supine, and upright sitting positions to determine the type of postural control required. This evaluation is most effectively performed on a therapy mat.

Step 3: Simulate Equipment

Simulating the type of seating design and components a patient requires before they are ordered is extremely important. Before looking at specific manufacturers' products, the team should discuss the components required in a general way, then select designs based on those criteria. The RTS can provide sample equipment from the manufacturers, which allows the patient and family to compare products before making a final decision.

Step 4: Provide Patient Education

The therapists and RTS should thoroughly explain to the patient and family the reasons that certain equipment is being recommended. Instruction on the seating system or mobility base and the way it supports or enhances the patient's posture must also be provided. If a patient has a condition that requires preventive measures, such as a decubitus ulcer, it should be clearly stated to the patient and family so that they understand why certain products have been recommended. The patient's funding sources must be reviewed with regard to approval of products.

Providing this information empowers both the patient and family to be educated consumers, reinforces their confidence in the team's recommendation, and increases their satisfaction with the final product.

Step 5: Document Essential Information

During this process, all information obtained should be documented on evaluation forms. Goals of seating should be formulated based on the patient's physical assessment. Recommendations are determined by the patient's specific goals and should also be documented.

The medical justification letter is based on this information. This letter, along with a physician's prescription, is necessary for funding approval.

Step 6: Perform Follow-Up

After the team has recommended and documented the patient's equipment needs, the job is only half over. On delivery of the equipment, the team must ensure that it is appropriately fitted to the patient. This effort enhances the patient's confidence in the product and allows the therapist to see the end product.

Step 7: Review Functional Outcome

The evaluation and fitting process determines the functional enhancement the seating system and mobility base provides for the patient. The funding agencies sometimes prolong the approval process and question the teams's recommendation. The team must focus on their goals and the importance of clearly communicating them to the funding agency.

After delivery the goals should be reevaluated, and therapists should schedule time to assist patients with their equipment. The team should implement measurable goals that reinforce the functional enhancement the equipment provides. Therapists should evaluate whether the equipment has improved the patient's quality of life, such as by improving an area of function, promoting independent mobility and increasing comfort or sitting tolerance.

MATCHING EQUIPMENT TO PATIENT FUNCTION

Manual Wheelchair Frame Styles

Wheelchair frame styles have been evolving since the 1930s. Two basic types of manual wheelchair frame styles are available: rigid and folding. Because this chapter's focus is on seating and mobility specific to patients with CVA, the manual and power wheelchair frames most commonly recommended for this diagnosis are emphasized.

The patient's medical condition and the availability of funding reimbursement determine the style of wheelchair frame recommended. The most frequently recommended wheelchair frame style is the folding frame. Folding wheelchairs are designed with a crossbrace that allows the chair to be folded for ease of transport and storage. Wheelchair frames are made of different materials designed for various chair weight requirements. The weight of the wheelchair is important if the patient's strength, endurance, and propulsion abilities are in question. A basic wheelchair is constructed of aluminum and is appropriate in weight for a patient with average upper body strength. They are durable enough for everyday use and reasonably priced. Lightweight wheelchair frames are typically constructed with aircraft aluminum or titanium. These chairs are extremely durable but more costly than standard wheelchairs. The basic wheelchair-frame style can be viewed in Figure 19-5. Both frame style and chair accessories are crucial to ensure proper postural support and function in the wheelchair.

The following outline depicts wheelchair-frame accessories and functional concerns that should be considered.

Wheelchair Frame Seat-to-Floor Height (*Figure 19-6*)
- Standard: 19½ inches from seat to floor
- Hemi height: 17½ inches from seat to floor
- Super-low: 14½ inches from seat to floor

Functional Concerns
Based on the patient's lower extremity and knee-to-heel measurement, the seat-to-floor height is crucial for the following reasons: comfort of the lower extremity on the foot rest and propulsion of the wheelchair with one or both lower extremities.

Wheel Style
Two styles of inner wheel support structure are available: mag wheels and spoke wheels.

Functional Concerns
Wheel style is chosen based on the patient's ability to care for and maintain the wheelchair. Mag wheels require no maintenance. Spoke wheels require periodic tightening of the individual spokes. Spoke wheels are lighter in weight than mag wheels.

Tire Style
Three types of tires are available for standard wheelchairs—pneumatic, pneumatic with flat-free inserts, and solid rubber.

Functional Concerns
- Pneumatic tires roll better on varying terrain. They have good shock absorption ability. They require maintenance of air pressure and can be punctured.
- Pneumatic tires with flat-free inserts are pneumatic tires injected with a substance to replace the air. This prevents the need for air pressure maintenance and the possibility of flats. Flat-free inserts decrease the shock absorption qualities and add weight to the tire.
- Solid rubber tires are the most inexpensive but handle varying terrain poorly. The patient needs more energy to propel a wheelchair with solid rubber ties. They are, however, very durable.

Wheel Hand Rims and One-Arm Drive Wheelchairs
Hand rims are placed on the outside of the tire so that the wheel can be stroked or propelled. Hand rims are available in aluminum or plastic-coated styles. One-arm drive wheelchairs have two hand rims on one wheel only (Figure 19-7).

Functional Concerns
- Aluminum hand rims are standard on most wheelchairs. Aluminum hand rims can become slippery or cold in different weather conditions, and most active wheelchair users wear specific gloves for this reason.
- Plastic-coated hand rims are the same as aluminum, with the exception of their plastic covering, which provides a better grip surface for the user. One problem is that without proper maintenance the plastic coating can irritate or cut the user's hand.

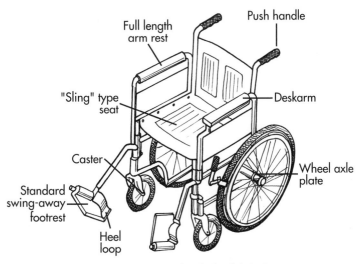

Figure 19-5 Basic style of wheelchair frame.

- One-arm drive wheelchairs: This standard wheelchair has both right- and left-hand rims on the same side. It was designed for patients with only one functional upper extremity (See Figure 19-7). The double hand rim allows one arm to control the wheelchair in all directions. To use this wheelchair properly, the patient must be able to understand its use.

Wheel Axle Plate

The wheel axle plate (see Figure 19-5) allows for wheel alignment up and down and back and forth.

Functional Concerns

Most standard chairs do not allow for axle plate adjustment. Axle plates typically increase the cost of the chair. However, they allow the chair to be fine-tuned by adjustment of the tire to the best position for propulsion. This results in improved control and muscle energy conservation.

Casters

Caster wheels (see Figure 19-5) are in the front of the wheelchair and are available in several diameters.

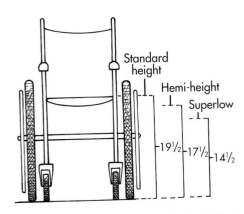

Figure 19-6 Seat-to-floor heights of wheelchair frames.

Functional Concerns

- Large casters handle terrain better but have an increased rolling resistance on smooth surfaces. They also increase the chair's turning radius.
- Narrow-width casters handle smooth surfaces well but can get stuck in bumpy terrain.
- Small casters are typically seen in sporty wheelchairs. They handle smooth terrain well but can get caught in cracks and bumps on rough terrain.
- Caster wheel options should be considered along with the patient's knee-to-heel measurement and the type of legrest or footrest that is being ordered. If this combination is not carefully considered, the caster wheels can bump the legrests or footrests.

Elevating Leg Rests and Footrests

- Elevating leg rests raise or lower the lower extremities if the patient requires this because of a medical condition (Figure 19-8).
- Footrests have a fixed knee angle and support the lower extremity in sitting.

Functional Concerns

Elevating leg rests are typically recommended for patients with limited knee angles, poor circulation in the lower extremities, or edema. These leg rests are typically overprescribed and must be carefully considered. If patients do not have adequate hamstring muscle elongation to tolerate a knee angle change, they will sit with a posterior pelvic tilt to compensate for the lack of muscle flexibility.

Footrests are available in different knee angle degrees—typically 60, 70, and 75. The angle degree recommended should be based on patient need. Proper adjustment of the footrest length is important to ensure lower extremity stability and support in sitting. Swing-away removable footrests should also be ordered so the patient will be safe during transfers.

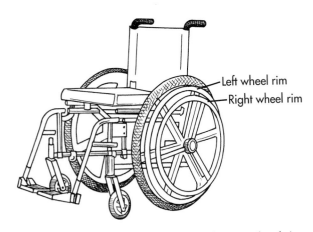

Figure 19-7 One-arm drive wheelchairs have two hand rims on one wheel only.

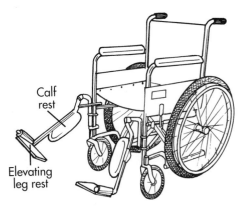

Figure 19-8 Elevating leg rests raise or lower the lower extremities.

Armrests (Fixed or Removable)

Two different armrest lengths are available: full and desk. Armrest heights also come in two varieties: fixed and adjustable (see Figure 19-5).

Functional Concerns

- Full-length arms provide full arm support at rest and upper extremity support during transfers. Because of their front arm cut-out, desk-length arms enable the patient to pull up closer to a table.
- Because they are not removable, fixed arms restrict a patient from transferring sideways.
- Removable arms allow for ease of side transfers. They can also be removed from the wheelchair frame during storage.
- Fixed-height arms are one standard height and cannot be adjusted.
- Adjustable-height arms allow for varying height adjustment to provide upper body support.

Power Mobility Products

Power mobility products are frequently recommended for patients who do not have the upper body strength and co-ordination to propel a wheelchair manually. Power mobility enables patients to move about independently and be productive and active. Safe use of power mobility requires sufficient visual, perceptual, and cognitive functioning. Many different types of power mobility products are available. This chapter focuses on two basic power products that are frequently ordered for patients who have sustained a cerebrovascular accident (see Chapter 21).

Basic Power Wheelchair

The most basic power wheelchair (Figure 19-9) available is a direct-drive, joystick-operated power wheelchair. This type of power wheelchair is available with either a power base frame or a folding frame.

Functional Concerns

A basic power wheelchair can handle varying terrain and is fairly durable. Different sizes of tires are available from the various manufacturers. Joystick operation is the most basic form of power wheelchair control. Different hardware accessories are available to position the joystick in the best location for the patient. Alternative switches are available for patients who do not have the functional control necessary to operate a joystick. Although these switches cannot be discussed at length, it should be noted that many varieties are available and that the power wheelchair must be designed to accommodate these switches.

Power Wheelchair Bases

Power wheelchair bases are much more durable than power folding frames. The power base can handle different terrain and usually has better shock absorption capability,

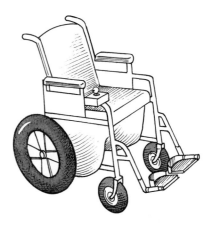

Figure 19-9 The direct-drive, joystick-operated power wheelchair is the most basic power wheelchair available.

which ensures a smoother ride. Power bases can be transported only by an accessible van or bus.

Power Folding Frames

Power folding frames are practical in theory but deceiving in reality. Although the frame can be folded by pulling out the batteries and battery tray, the unit is still quite heavy. Two strong adults could handle lifting the folded power frame in and out of a van or car, but everyday use with one person assisting the patient is extremely difficult. Therefore power mobility must be carefully considered with regard to transportation and accessibility issues.

Because of its folding crossbar and flexible frame, a power folding frame does not handle terrain as well as a power base. However, for basic power mobility, it is an efficient and reasonably priced alternative.

Power Scooters

Power scooters are another option available in power mobility (Figure 19-10). Patients who have good functional control of their upper extremities and appropriate visual, perceptual, and cognitive skills can use power scooters.

Functional Concerns

Although power scooters can be beneficial for some patients, seating is difficult to customize and is usually not appropriate for patients with moderate to severe neurologic impairment. Use of a power scooter requires the ability to transfer by stepping on and off the platform base or maneuvering the rotating feature of the seat.

Power scooters are available in three- and four-wheel frame options. Four-wheeled scooters handle terrain outdoors much better but are heavier and more difficult to transport. Three-wheeled scooters do not handle varying terrain as well. Scooters can be broken down to transport in a car, but as with folding power wheelchairs, they are extremely difficult for one person to handle because the pieces are heavy. Accessible vans and buses are

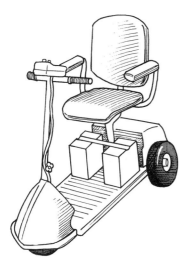

Figure 19-10 Power scooters can be used by patients who have good functional control of their upper extremities and appropriate visual, perceptual, and cognitive skills.

necessary unless two strong adults are available to lift the scooter.

Scooters have a wider turning radius than power wheelchairs and can be difficult to handle in a home. If either a power wheelchair or a scooter is appropriate for a patient, the decision is generally based on the patient's preferences.

Seating Systems

The importance of seating, goals, and assessment of biomechanics and posture were all reviewed earlier in the chapter. This section describes the types of seating systems available and their various features.

Three basic styles of seating exist: linear, contoured, and custom contoured. All three provide the same basic benefits:

- They allow for proper positioning in correct alignment.
- They maintain alignment of the trunk and extremities.
- They decrease or slow the progression of contractures and deformities.
- They are essential for comfort, pressure relief, support, and enhancement of function.

Linear Seating Systems

Linear seating systems are flat, noncontoured planes of support. Linear seat cushions or backs can be custommade or factory-ordered in various sizes, densities, and fabrics.

Functional Concerns

Linear seating provides a firm, rigid seating base that can be beneficial for active patients. Independent transfers are usually easily achieved from a linear cushion. Patients with moderate-to-severe neuromuscular or central nervous system insults tend to benefit more from contoured seat-

ing. Patients with minimal musculoskeletal involvement typically benefit the most from linear seating. Linear seating systems do not provide a great deal of posture support because our bodies are contoured. Patients who require more support because of muscle weakness or imbalance usually benefit more from contoured seating.

Contoured Seating/Custom Seating

Contoured seating is designed to ergonomically support the body. Contoured seat cushions and backs can be custom-built with carved-out or specially molded foam. They are also available in various predetermined shapes.

Functional Concerns

Contoured seating provides an excellent surface area for support that benefits patients by enhancing postural alignment, decreasing abnormal posturing, and increasing pressure relief. Independent transfers can be more difficult from contoured seating if patients do not have the upper extremity strength or control to move away from the cushion or back support. Patients with minimal neuromuscular or central nervous system insults benefit the most from seating that has slight contours. Moderately to severely impaired patients benefit more from highly contoured seating. Manufacturer-determined contoured seating benefits minimally to moderately impaired patients more than severely impaired ones. The patient's degree of deformity and whether it is fixed or flexible must be assessed very carefully. Patients with fixed deformities typically require custom-built carved foam seating or custom-molded seating. Without careful seating assessment the patient is at risk for decubitus ulcers.

The different styles, designs and accessories for seating systems are described in Table 19-1. This table depicts the seating component, its indication for use, the postural control components it provides, and the functional achievement that can occur.

EVALUATING THE PATIENT WITH CVA

Special Considerations with CVA Diagnosis

Therapeutic intervention for patients with brain damage caused by a CVA focuses on physical, cognitive, and visual-perceptual motor treatment. Patients who have a CVA experience functional disturbances as a result of the brain damage. These functional disturbances do not differ fundamentally according to age, but therapeutic intervention and rehabilitation are more difficult for elderly patients who have multiple lesion sites, other medical conditions, spreading vascular disease, a lack of plasticity in the central nervous system, and permanent brain damage.[2]

Patients with hemiplegia resulting from CVA have difficulty controlling posture, balance reactions, and smooth movement patterns that enable the performance of functional tasks. Davies[2] describes the typical patterns of adult hemiplegia (Table 19-2, p. 450).

Table 19-1

Seating Systems

SEATING COMPONENT	INDICATIONS FOR USE	POSTURAL CONTROL PROVIDED	FUNCTIONAL ASSISTANCE
Solid wood insert	Slide it inside the cover, under the cushion; cushion can then be attached with Velcro to sling upholstery of wheelchair	Prevents hammocking of wheelchair upholstery; provides a solid base of support for the cushion; prevents internal hip rotation and posterior pelvic tilt related to stretched-out wheelchair upholstery	Improves pelvic position and spinal alignment; enhances upper body control
Solid seat	Remove wheelchair upholstery; solid seat hooks lock down on seat rails of wheelchair; hooks on solid seat can be adjusted to provide anterior or posterior tilting of solid seat and cushion on wheelchair frame	Prevents hammocking of cushion by providing a stable base of support; easy to remove so wheelchair can be folded; allows anterior/posterior tilting for enhanced sitting alignment; easy adjustment of angle between wheelchair seat and back	Anterior/posterior tilting beneficial for patients with weak pelvic and truncal musculature; adjustable angle beneficial for patients with progressive disorders
Foam cushion	Foam linear cushions provide a stable base of support; foam comes in varying densities and can be layered in different densities to provide increased comfort and some pressure relief	Can enhance sitting posture and increase comfort	Recommended for patients with minimal seating needs, particularly those who have good alignment of pelvis and hips; enhanced ability for side transfers
Contoured foam cushion	Contoured foam cushions provide increased surface area of support and pressure relief; a variety of foam densities are available.	Ergonomically shaped to enhance pelvic and lower extremity alignment in sitting; provides a greater surface area of support, thereby increasing pressure relief and comfort	Recommended for patients with moderately impaired postural control; enhances pelvic alignment and control as well as alignment of hip and lower extremity; benefits patients who have progressive disorders and may require support changes over time
Pressure-relieving cushion (fluid medium)	Contoured cushion with pressure-relieving fluid pad on top allows for a stable base of support for proper seating alignment	Provides pelvic and lower extremity alignment; provides pressure relief without changing seating support; can be attached by Velcro to solid seat or upholstery (with solid wood insert)	Imperative for patients at risk for decubitus ulcers; good for patients who need more stability in the pelvis to enhance trunk control; requires no maintenance
Pressure-relieving cushion (air medium)	The air-bulb shape allows for some contouring that is caused by the seated patient's weight	Various designs to assist with minimal postural control; provides pressure relief through air medium; attaches by Velcro to solid seat or upholstery (with solid wood insert)	Imperative for patients at risk for decubitus ulcers; beneficial for patients who have good trunk control; requires maintenance of air pressure and volume
Lumbar back support	This component provides support for patients who need assistance to sit with natural lumbar curve	A simple, low-cost lumbar back support that attaches by Velcro to back post with straps; lumbar component supported by upholstery on wheelchair back	Comforting for patients needing minimal seating support; evaluation of lumbar spine flexibility very important for this support to enhance posture

Continued

Table 19-1

Seating Systems—cont'd

SEATING COMPONENT	INDICATIONS FOR USE	POSTURAL CONTROL PROVIDED	FUNCTIONAL ASSISTANCE
Solid back support 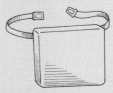	This component provides support that is easily removed	Helps enhance upright sitting; usually made of foam covered by nylon or vinyl fabric; can be easily made to attach and detach with a buckle strap	Beneficial only if patient can maintain upright sitting at 90- to 95-degree seat-to-back angle (depending on degree of back posts on the wheelchair)
Pita back	This component provides back support with little change to wheelchair	Helps enhance upright sitting; placed inside back upholstery of the wheelchair; can be attached with Velcro or straps for wheelchair folding	Beneficial only if patient can maintain upright sitting at 90- to 95-degree seat-to-back angle (depending on degree of back posts on the wheelchair)
Linear back support	This component provides back alignment support but attaches to wheelchair differently than others, through hook hardware; it is usually made of linear foam covered in vinyl or nylon fabric	Helps enhance upright sitting; possible to open up seat-to-back angle to improve sitting posture; removable or permanently mounted hardware, depending on need	Angle-adjustable hook hardware for fine-tuning the seat-to-back angle to improve posterior pelvic support and trunk and upper extremity alignment and control; beneficial for patients with upper body weakness
Adjustable back support 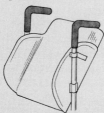	This is an angle-adjustable back shell that can be used for contoured foam, foam in place, or custom-molded foam backs; the shell can be reused if foam insert needs to be changed or removed	Enhances full surface area support for the back and relieves pressure; helps correct abnormal spinal alignment or support a fixed spinal deformity through contoured foam cushions; can be factory shaped by the manufacturer or custom-molded to patient's body	Beneficial for patients with moderate to severe involvement who require a greater surface area of support to improve alignment or decrease progression of a deforming posture; angle adjustment for fine-tuning the support to enhance spinal alignment and upper body control
Pelvic strap or seat belt 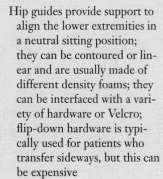	This component is designed to prevent posterior pelvic tilt and sliding out of chair	Pelvic strap or seat belt positioned on wheelchair frame at a 45-degree angle to the patient's hip; pelvic strap positioned so that it is below the patient's anterior superior iliac spine (ASIS)	With proper positioning, enhances pelvic alignment by preventing patient from sliding into a posterior pelvic tilt
Leg adductors 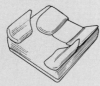	Designed for patients with leg adduction weakness, this component prevents the legs from rolling into external hip rotation	Helps reinforce lower extremity or femur alignment; enhances posture and increases comfort while sitting	Proper alignment of lower extremities or femur leading to better pelvic and spinal alignment; decreased fatigue while sitting
Hip guides 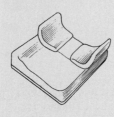	Hip guides provide support to align the lower extremities in a neutral sitting position; they can be contoured or linear and are usually made of different density foams; they can be interfaced with a variety of hardware or Velcro; flip-down hardware is typically used for patients who transfer sideways, but this can be expensive	Prevent the lower extremities from posturing into external hip rotation, which can be caused by a neuromuscular insult that results in hypertonicity or spasticity of the lower extremities or from insult or injury that results in hypotonicity or paralysis	Optimal postural alignment while seated is essential for function; align the lower extremities in a neutral hip position, which enhances pelvic control and position; stability and sitting control derived from pelvis and hips

Table 19-1

Seating Systems—cont'd

SEATING COMPONENT	INDICATIONS FOR USE	POSTURAL CONTROL PROVIDED	FUNCTIONAL ASSISTANCE
Medial knee block (pommel) with flip-down hardware 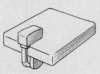	Medial knee blocks, or pommels, prevent internal hip rotation or extreme leg adduction; they can be custom-made in a variety of shapes and sizes; they are typically constructed of a variety of foams and interfaced with different hardware, depending on the severity of the postural muscle overactivity	Align the lower extremities and prevent excessive hip adduction or internal hip rotation, which is typically caused by a neuromuscular insult that results in hypertonicity or spasticity (Hypotonicity or paralysis can also cause this but is not as common)	Optimal postural alignment essential for function; align the lower extremities to help provide a stable base of support for the pelvis and spine
Pelvic obliquity build-up 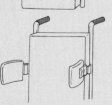	This component enhances proper pelvic alignment; excessive lateral tilting of the pelvis is an indication for use if the patient has the flexibility to benefit from the correction	Possible for malalignment of the pelvis to result in permanent deformity; levels out the ischial tuberosities and encourages symmetric sitting; prevents the occurrence of excessive weight bearing on one ischial tuberosity, which can cause a decubitus ulcer	Stable base of support created by symmetric pelvic alignment, which enhances functional sitting; necessary to perform a thorough evaluation to determine if the patient has enough muscular flexibility (Forcing a pelvic obliquity build-up when a patient cannot be corrected can lead to excessive pressure and a decubitus ulcer)
Lateral trunk supports, straight and curved 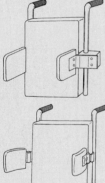	Patients with trunk weakness or excessive leaning to one side benefit from lateral trunk supports	Prevent lateral trunk flexion, which can be caused by muscle weakness or abnormal posturing; can be straight or curved with hardware that is permanently mounted or swing-away, depending on the patient's need for support and transfer ability	Enhance function with lateral trunk supports by helping maintain a midline trunk position, thereby freeing up the upper extremities; midline orientation of the spine and neck/head also physiologically important
Harness/anterior chest support 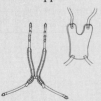	Anterior chest supports are usually required when a patient is unable to maintain an upright trunk while sitting	Decreased head control, upper extremity function, and physiologic function of vital organs caused by excessive forward leaning of the trunk; supports the chest and shoulder girdles to enhance upright sitting caused by trunk weakness and abnormal posturing	Enhances function by promoting upright sitting, improving head and neck alignment, and freeing up the upper extremities for function; can be any shape or size, depending on the patient's needs; easy to remove as necessary
Head/neck support 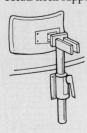	Head/neck supports are recommended for patients with poor head control or weak neck musculature	Maintains a neutral cervical spine and head alignment; available in various shapes and sizes, with different attachment hardware	Imperative to support the head and neck in cases of neck weakness or posturing which can affect breathing, swallowing, and vision; with proper neck alignment, overall oral muscular control enhanced and vision and cognition/socialization stimulated

Continued

Table 19-1

Seating Systems—cont'd

SEATING COMPONENT	INDICATIONS FOR USE	POSTURAL CONTROL PROVIDED	FUNCTIONAL ASSISTANCE
Brake extension	Brake extensions are required when a patient is either too weak to adjust the brakes or unable to reach them	Allows patients to lock and unlock their wheelchairs independently	Promotes independence and sense of safety and responsibility
Upper extremity support, full and half lap trays	Lap trays can be beneficial for patients who require a support surface on which to rest their upper extremities	Can help position patients with weakness in the trunk or lower extremities into an upright sitting alignment	Allows for positioning and weight bearing of the upper extremities, which can correct trunk, spine, and head and neck posture
Arm trough	An arm trough can be either separate or part of a half lap tray; it allows for positioning of an upper extremity	Can further position the extremity into neutral alignment in cases of flaccid or paralyzed upper extremities; typically wedged to decrease edema of the extremity	Benefits patients who are unable independently to move their extremity, which often causes edema; provides proper support contact and alignment; can also help to increase patient's awareness of the extremity, which is important in cases of visual neglect or sensation problems

For patients with limited or absent ambulation, seating and mobility recommendations must address these typical patterns of adult hemiplegia.

Seating and Wheelchair Considerations

The seating goals that must be addressed for patients with hemiplegia are as follows:

- Provide support and stability to the pelvis and lower extremities
- Decrease abnormal postural patterns in the lower extremity
- Improve alignment of the trunk and spine
- Provide upper extremity support and proper shoulder girdle alignment
- Decrease neck posturing
- Provide appropriate foot support

The pelvis should be evaluated first, followed by the lower extremities, trunk, upper extremities, head and neck, and feet. By following this sequence when seating a patient, the therapist addresses all physical areas and provides the most appropriate seating system.

Table 19-2

Typical Patterns of Adult Hemiplegia

BODY PART	COMMON MALALIGNMENT
Head	Flexion toward hemiplegic side, neck rotation toward unaffected side
Upper extremity (flexion pattern)	Scapula retraction, shoulder girdle, depression, adduction, and internal rotation; Elbow flexion, forearm pronation or supination; Wrist flexion and ulnar deviation; Finger and thumb flexion and adduction
Trunk	Trunk rotation backward on hemiplegic side with lateral trunk flexion
Pelvis	Backward rotation, obliquity, and frequent posterior pelvic tilt
Lower extremity	Hip extension, adduction, and internal rotation; Knee extension; Foot plantar flexion and inversion; Toe flexion, adduction

Fitting the Patient Based on Functional Status

The following list describes the seating components that can be prescribed for patients with hemiplegia, based on their functional status and degree of impairment.

- Pelvis: A cushion with a solid base of support (such as a solid seat or wood insert) should be provided. The patient should never sit on a seat upholstery or a cushion placed directly on upholstery. Wheelchair upholstery stretches out over time, causes a hammock effect, and can add to internal hip rotation and pelvic obliquity. Most patients who either are newly injured or have a good deal of muscle flexibility can achieve proper postural alignment from a cushion placed on a stable solid insert. Typically the pelvic rotation and obliquity either decreases greatly or disappears with the stable support.

- Lower extremities: The affected side typically has the postural influence of leg adduction and internal hip rotation. Most patients experience a decrease in this posture when seated on a stable cushion. In more severe cases, hip guides or medial knee blocks must be added to control the posture.

- Trunk: The affected hemiplegic side typically postures in lateral trunk flexion. If the pelvis is positioned adequately, the lateral trunk flexion can decrease or disappear. For patients with severe weakness, lateral trunk supports can be added to support the upper body in proper alignment. Having a slightly contoured back can also help enhance erect spinal posture through lumbar support. This decision must be carefully evaluated to ensure that the patient has the necessary lumbar spine flexibility.

- Upper extremity: The affected upper extremity requires support and stability from a lap tray or arm trough to decrease posturing and stabilize the shoulder.

- Head/neck: Usually if a patient is seated with a stable base of support at the pelvis and lower extremities and has adequate trunk control or support, the neck posturing will decrease or disappear. For patients with moderate to severe involvement who require more support a head or neck rest can be placed on the chair to ensure proper support of the cervical spine and head. This is important to address, especially if the patient has a visual field neglect or perceptual motor damage.

- Feet: Foot support is typically determined by the patient's functional level. Most patients with hemiplegia who propel their wheelchairs prefer to propel with the unaffected arm and leg. Therefore the wheelchair base seat-to-floor height must allow the patient's foot to reach the ground to propel the chair. The depth of the seat cushion must also be assessed and should be slightly short or have a beveled carved front to permit freedom of movement. The affected lower extremity should be supported by a leg rest or footrest. Patients with CVA should not generally use elevating leg rests. Elevating leg rests tend to cause overstretching of hamstring muscles and posterior pelvic tilt posturing when muscle imbalance or spasticity is present.

REVIEW QUESTIONS

1. If patients cannot use their bilateral upper extremities to propel a wheelchair, in what three ways could they become mobile?
2. What muscle can lack flexibility or the capacity for elongation and cause abnormal posturing in a posterior pelvic tilt?
3. What are the three basic styles of seating systems?
4. What functional abilities or skills (other than physical) does a patient need to operate a power mobility product?

■ COTA Considerations ■

- Seating systems should be prescribed to enhance function and prevent postural deformity.
- Consider reimbursement issues before performing a wheeled mobility and seating system evaluation.
- For most patients a thorough evaluation of the discharge environment (e.g., door widths, turning radius) must precede wheeled mobility prescription.
- At the initial evaluation a patient's skin integrity and weight-shifting ability should be evaluated so that a pressure-relieving cushion can be issued if needed.
- Familiarize yourself with the restraint policies of your agency or institution before prescribing seating equipment.

REFERENCES

1. Bergen AF: *Positioning for function*, Valhalla, N.Y., 1990, Valhalla Rehabilitation.
2. Davies PM: *Steps to follow: a guide to the treatment of adult hemiplegia*, Heidelberg Germany, 1985, Springer-Verlag.
3. Hetzel TR: Skin integrity, Proceedings from the 10th International Seating Symposium, Vancouver, British Columbia, 1992.
4. Hetzel TR: Stable pelvis recline, *Jay Medical Wheelchair Seating Update Newsletter*, Fall 1993.
5. Johann CM: Keys to clinical success, *Team Rehab Report*, p 44, June 1995.
6. Kreutz D: Seating and positioning for the newly injured, *Rehab Mgmt*, p 67, Dec/Jan 1993.
7. Ward DE: *Prescriptive seating for wheeled mobility*, vol 1, Kansas City, 1994, Health Wealth International.

SUGGESTED READING

Angelo J: *Assistive technology for rehabilitation therapists*, Philadelphia, 1997, FA Davis.
Carr Ek: Positioning of the stroke patient: a review of the literature, *Intl J Nurs Stud* 29(4):355, 1992.
Ferido T: Spasticity in head trauma and CVA patients: etiology and management, *J Neurosci Nurs* 20(1):17, 1988.
Minkel JL: *Sitting solutions: principles of wheelchair positioning and mobility devices*, New Windsor, N.Y., 1996, Minkel Consulting.
Norkin CC: *Joint structure and function*, ed 2, Philadelphia, 1992, FA Davis.

catherine a. salerno

chapter **20**

Home Evaluation and Modifications

key terms

home environment	mobility	adaptations
architectural barriers	safety	durable medical equipment
accessibility		

chapter objectives

After completing this chapter, the reader will be able to accomplish the following:

1. Apply methods of assessing the home environment for barriers.
2. Understand architectural guidelines as established by the American National Standards Institute.
3. Implement methods for modifying the home environment and increase safety and mobility independence for patients recovering from CVA.

A barrier-free environment in both the home and community is essential to successful independent living for individuals who are elderly or physically disabled and particularly for individuals who have suffered stroke.[2] Throughout the rehabilitation process, therapists work with patients toward the goal of achieving independence in mobility and self-care. However, this process usually occurs in an institutionalized setting that is relatively free of architectural barriers. *Architectural barriers* are defined as architectural features (e.g., stairs, doors) in the home and community that make negotiating at will difficult or impossible for an individual.[3]

Most individuals with disabilities wish to return to their own homes. For many, some type of durable medical equipment and home modifications are necessary to achieve easy access.[5]

Understanding the patient's home environment is an integral part of treatment and discharge planning. A home visit with the patient should occur well before the discharge date to provide recommendations to facilitate safety and independence. Information gained from this home visit is used to modify the existing treatment plan and establish appropriate therapy goals. This chapter focuses on architectural barriers commonly found in the home, ways to eliminate them, basic wheelchair information, and a general overview of methods for assessment appropriate for patients who have had a CVA. This chapter—with its bulleted, quick-reference format—is intended to be used as a resource for practical suggestions that will assist the occupational therapist's clinical reasoning process when evaluating the homes of stroke survivors.

BASIC GUIDELINES AND WHEELCHAIR INFORMATION

The wheelchairs shown in Figures 20-1 through 20-6 are based on a standard adult-size chair. Dimensions vary with the size of the patient using the chair. See Chapter 19 for information regarding specific wheelchair adaptations. The therapist must know the specific size and type of wheelchair being prescribed for the patient before making recommendations for home modifications.

Evaluating the Home

Evaluation for architectural barriers is usually organized by room.[6] In this approach the following information is considered during the home evaluation process.

Exterior

Suggestions include the following:

- Assess type of residence—Note whether dwelling is a house or apartment building; determine whether dwelling has elevator or staircase access; examine steps (their number, height, width, and depth); note walkway railings and width; assess distance and grade between the dwelling entrance and the curb or driveway

- Note protection from the weather—Examine condition of surfaces over which wheelchair must travel (e.g., grass which becomes mud, concrete with cracks, shaded bricks covered with moss, asphalt that softens in the hot summer sun)
- Examine driveway—Note size and ability to accommodate a wheelchair van; assess composition (solid, boulevard style with a strip of dirt in the middle); determine whether surface is paved or gravel
- Survey surrounding area—Look for trees that drop nuts, branches, leaves, and pine cones; note location of mailbox

Entrances

Suggestions include the following:

- Consider all entrances to evaluate accessibility; note any entrances inaccessible to the patient
- Measure steps and landings and note the presence and height of railings
- Measure all doorway widths and heights, including interior doors to closets and between rooms
- Note the direction of each door swing, the presence and height of any sills, and the height of any installed

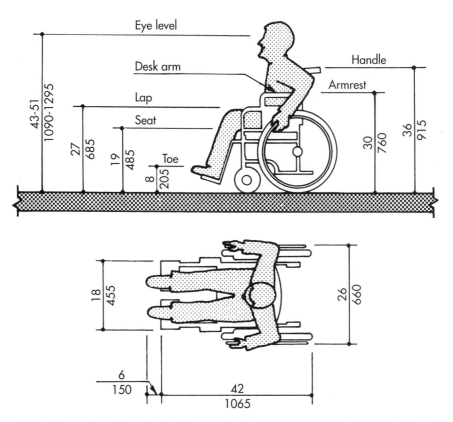

Figure 20-1 Dimensions of standard adult manual wheelchair. Width: 24 to 26 inches from rim to rim. Length: 42 to 43 inches. Height to push handles from floor: 36 inches. Height to seat from floor: 19 to 19.5 inches (excluding cushion). Height to armrest from floor: 29 to 30 inches. Note: Footrests may extend farther for very large people. (From American National Standards Institute: *Accessible and useable buildings and facilities*, New York, 1992, The Institute.)

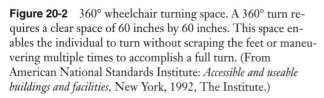

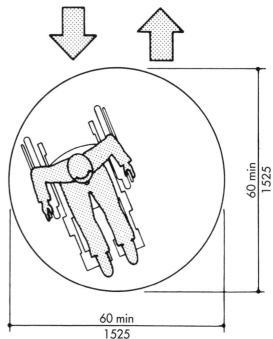

Figure 20-2 360° wheelchair turning space. A 360° turn requires a clear space of 60 inches by 60 inches. This space enables the individual to turn without scraping the feet or maneuvering multiple times to accomplish a full turn. (From American National Standards Institute: *Accessible and useable buildings and facilities*, New York, 1992, The Institute.)

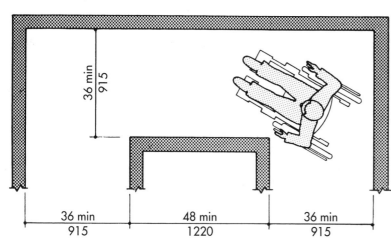

Figure 20-3 90° wheelchair turning space. A 90° turn requires a minimum of 36 inches for the wheelchair user to have clear space for the feet and prevent scraping the hands on the wall. (From American National Standards Institute: *Accessible and useable buildings and facilities*, New York, 1992, The Institute.)

Figure 20-4 Minimum clear width for doorways and halls. A minimum of 32 inches of doorway width is required; the ideal is 36 inches. Hallways should be a minimum of 36 inches wide to provide sufficient clearance for wheelchair passage and allow the user to propel the chair without scraping the hands. (From American National Standards Institute: *Accessible and useable buildings and facilities*, New York, 1992, The Institute.)

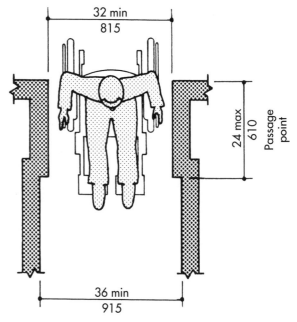

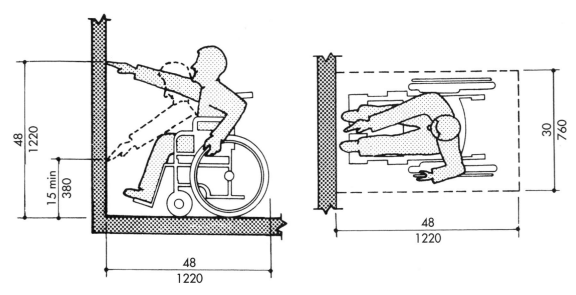

Figure 20-5 Forward reach. The maximal height an individual can reach from a seated position is 48 inches. Height should be at least 15 inches to prevent the wheelchair from tipping forward. (From American National Standards Institute: *Accessible and useable buildings and facilities*, New York, 1992, The Institute.)

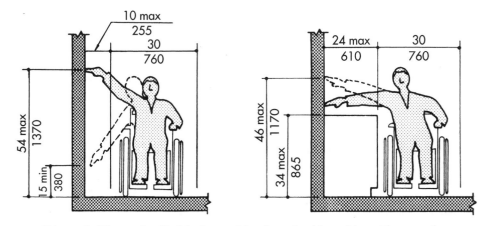

Figure 20-6 Side reach. The maximal height for reaching from the side position without an obstruction is 54 inches. If an obstruction such as a countertop or shelf is present the maximal height for side reach is 46 inches. (From American National Standards Institute: *Accessible and useable buildings and facilities*, New York, 1992, The Institute.)

locks; determine whether screen doors open out and solid doors open in; assess the weight of the doors and whether they can be moved from a wheelchair
• If patients lives in a building with an elevator, note whether the chair can be maneuvered into the elevator; assess whether the elevator stops flush with the landing; consider whether the patient can reach the buttons

Interior
Suggestions include the following:

• Assess the number of levels and whether the bedrooms are located upstairs or down; consider relocating a bedroom downstairs for improved mobility

• Count and measure all steps (their height, width, and landing), and note whether handrails exist on both sides
• Measure the dimensions of the staircase; note the stair height, width, and depth

Living Room and Hallways
Suggestions include the following:

• Consider phone accessibility; height of light switches, thermostats, and electrical sockets; furniture arrangement; floor covering; doorway width and thresholds; note the width of the hallway and number of turns
• Determine whether the patient will be able to open and

close windows; note whether the windows slide up and down or swing out; measure the height of the latches

Bedroom

Suggestions include the following:

- Measure doorway width, threshold height, and mattress height
- Consider space for hospital bed and bedside commode; note floor space and covering (i.e., carpet, wood, tile, linoleum) because these may have an impact on walking and wheelchair mobility
- Note whether the bed is stable for transfer
- Assess the accessibility of dressers and closets
- If a mechanical lift is being prescribed, ensure enough room is available to maneuver it around the bed.

Bathroom

Suggestions include the following:

- Measure the door width and threshold height, and note the direction of the door swing (in or out)
- Measure the entry width and note the type of entry of the shower or bathtub; determine the inside and outside sill height and sill width; measure the length, width (inside top and bottom), and height of the faucet; note the type of shower head
- Note whether the wall is plasterboard, tile, or fiberglass; the type of wall has an impact on installation of grab bars
- Measure the height of the toilet, the available space on the left and right, and the space in front of it; check whether the toilet paper roll is within easy reach; consider the sink height and counter distances to the left and right
- Determine the presence of any nonslip treatment in the tub; note whether the patient has a shower curtain or a glass door

Kitchen

Suggestions include the following:

- Measure the height and depth of the basin of the sink, the distance to the faucet knobs, cabinet and counter heights, and refrigerator door heights
- Consider table height in relation to wheelchair fit
- Note outlet height and location, type of controls and location on the stove and microwave, and height and accessibility of light switches

Laundry

Suggestions include the following:

- Note location and measurements of washer and dryer if relevant

- Determine whether washer and dryer are front loading or top loading
- Assess whether the washer and dryer are permanently installed or must be moved into place and set up each time for use

Basement

Suggestions include the following:

- Examine staircase, railings, windows, furnace controls, fuse box, and lighting

Sketches of each room with notations of problematic areas are useful for the therapist attempting home simulation during treatment sessions. A brief summary of findings with recommendations for modifications and safety should be provided to the family.

HOME EVALUATION FORMS

Evaluation formats differ from simple to complex, depending on the clinician's and patient's needs. Samples of home assessments are provided in the Appendix.

MODIFICATIONS

The therapist's recommendations should meet the patient's need to function with the greatest level of independence and safety. Consideration must be given to the patient's budget and the extent of the structural changes necessary to attain the patient's goals. Building contractors should be consulted and bids obtained for extensive reconstruction needs and to assist with determining the feasibility of structural modifications. Generally modifications should be made in accordance with the guidelines established by the American National Standards Institute (ANSI).[1]

The ANSI publishes the document *American National Standards for Buildings and Facilities*. It provides specifications to make buildings and other facilities accessible and usable for individuals with physical disabilities. The examples provided are reprinted to increase occupational therapists' understanding of specifications needed for patients recovering from a cerebrovascular accident (CVA) who rely on wheelchairs for independent mobility.

Exterior

A parking space with a 4-foot aisle adjacent to it allows an individual to maneuver a wheelchair alongside the car. Pathways and walkways should be a minimum of 48 inches wide and have smooth surfaces to prevent tipping and difficult wheelchair mobility. Motion-sensitive or automatically timed lighting along walkways provides safety.[7] At least one entrance to the home should have easy access. If all entrances are reached by stairs, the number of steps influences the solution to creating a "no-step" entrance. Options include ramps, stair gliders, or porch lifts.[7]

General Comments on Ramps

- Ramps should be a minimum of 36 in wide and have nonskid surfaces
- The ideal ratio of slope to rise is 1:12—for every inch of vertical rise, 12 inches of ramp is required (Figure 20-7)
- Ramps should have level landings at the top and bottom of each run; the landing's width should be at least as wide as the ramp; to allow for unobstructed ability to open the door, a 24-inch area is needed.
- Handrails should be waist high for individuals who can walk (a minimum of 34 to 38 inches) and should extend a minimum of 12 inches beyond the top and bottom runs
- Ramps require either railings or curbs at least 4 inches high to prevent individuals from slipping off the ramp

General Comments on Stairs

- According to ANSI, all steps on a flight of stairs should have uniform riser heights (a maximum of 7 inches) and tread depth (a minimum of 11 inches)
- All stairs should have handrails; the handrail grasping surface should be ½ to 2 inches in diameter and have a non-slip surface; handrails should be mounted approximately 1½ inches away from the wall to allow for adequate grasping space.

General Comments about Doors and Landings

Standard door width should be a minimum of 32 inches. Several solutions to narrow door problems do not require replacing the entire frame and door with a wider doorway. Existing hinges may be replaced with swing-clear hinges. The clear opening of the door may thus be enlarged by 1½ to 2 inches. Doorstops may be removed, adding an additional ¼ inches to the clear opening width of the doorway. If existing doors are removed, an additional 1½ to 2 inches can be provided. By removing doors and doorstops, a total of 2¼ to 2¾ inches in width can be gained.[6]

Small landings on either side of the door present problems for a wheelchair or walker user because pulling a swinging door open is difficult if the assistive device is already occupying the landing area over which the door must swing.[7] A minimum of 18 inches for walkers and 26 inches for wheelchairs is needed outside the door swing area (Figure 20-8). Rather than enlarging a landing by removing walls and partitions, three options are available. The door can be removed, an automatic door opener can be installed, or a door pull loop with Velcro-type attachments can be devised. The latter can assist individuals with closing a swing-in door. It can be constructed from 2-inch wide webbing material and should be at least 30 inches in length. A loop sewn at one end assists patients with weak grasps. The other end can be fastened to the door lever or knob using 1-in wide Velcro-type loops and hooks.

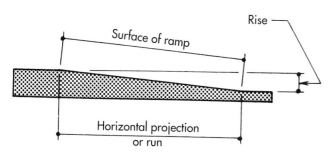

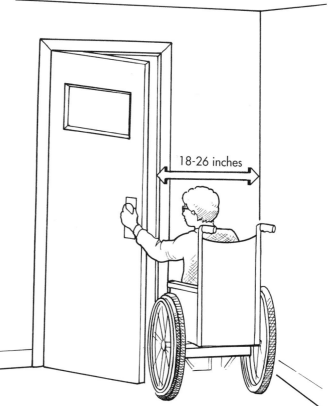

Slope	Maximum rise		Maximum horizontal projection	
	in	mm	ft	m
1:12 to 1:15	30	760	30	9
1:16 to 1:19	30	760	40	12
1:20	30	760	50	15

Figure 20-7 Slope and rise of ramps. This diagram provides the components of a single ramp run and a sample of ramp dimensions. The slope ratio is an important consideration when designing a ramp; slope creates hazardous wheelchair propulsion conditions if it is too steep. (From American National Standards Institute: *Accessible and useable buildings and facilities,* New York, 1992, The Institute.)

Figure 20-8 Door swing area. A minimum of 18 inches for walkers and 26 inches for wheelchairs is needed outside the swing area.

If doors are to be replaced, several options are available. If space is a limiting factor, sliding doors are useful (Figure 20-9). However, their weight and lateral movement can make maneuvering difficult. Moreover, some sliding doors require floor tracks, which are obstacles for wheelchairs and people who have difficulty walking. Pocket doors are effective if only occasional privacy is necessary (Figure 20-10). Folding doors require lateral movement but are lighter in weight (Figure 20-11). Door thresholds higher than ¼ inch should be removed or beveled to prevent tripping hazards and remove barriers for wheelchair users.

Hardware

Lever door handles or doorknob adapters are preferable to round twist doorknobs. Slide bolts, which can be reached from a seated position, may replace dead bolt locks. Kick plates can be installed on doors to prevent gouging and scratches from wheelchairs and walking aids. They should be as thin as possible to allow clear door width opening. They should extend from the bottom of the door to a height of 10 to 16 inches.

Hallways, Living Room, and Dining Area

Hallways should be a minimum of 36 to 48 inches wide. They should be free of protruding objects such as low tables, coat racks, and planters. Thresholds should be eliminated. Nonslip and low-friction surfaces are recommended. Scatter rugs should be removed. Carpeting should be removed or tacked or taped down to eliminate

trip hazards. Furniture should be rearranged to accommodate a wheelchair turning area of 5 square feet. Coffee tables, ottomans, and other trip hazards should be eliminated for patients who walk with assistive devices. A favorite chair can be increased in seat height by adding medium-density foam cushions. Telephone and appliance wires should be taped or tacked down. Easy access to light fixtures and outlets is recommended. Appropriate height for wall switches is 36 to 48 inches. Outlets should be a minimum of 18 inches above the floorboard. Rocker switches and dimmer switches can reduce the fine manipulation required for operating light switches, or automatic timer lights can be installed. Inexpensive environmental control units can aid in independent operation of television sets, radios, and other appliances (see Chapter 21).

Bedroom

The bedroom should be free of clutter and scatter rugs. A minimum of 3 feet should be available on the side of the bed to allow for wheelchair transfers.[3] The height of the bed should be equal to the height of the wheelchair for safe transfers. If the bed is too low, it may be elevated on blocks or a platform. This also increases ease for sit-to-stand transitions if the patient is ambulatory. A firm mattress is recommended to improve bed mobility. A trapeze can assist with mobility in bed if necessary. Side rails provide safety from falls. They also can be used as assistive devices for rolling in bed. Dressers should have toe space

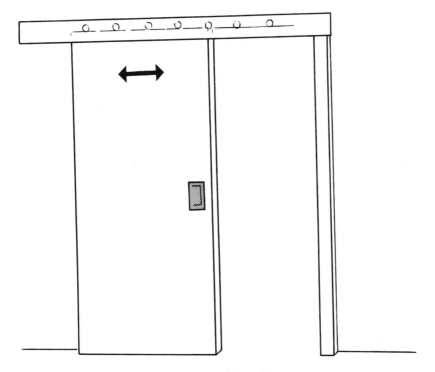

Figure 20-9 Sliding door.

underneath and easy-glide drawers. Stackable baskets may be a substitute for clothing storage. Closet doors should be removed or replaced with folding doors or a curtain. The height of the clothing rod should be a maximum of 48 inches.

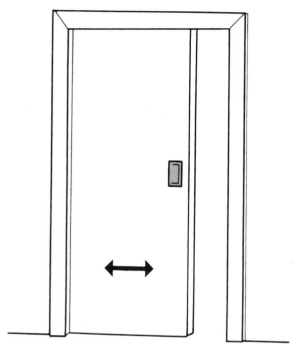

Figure 20-10 Pocket door.

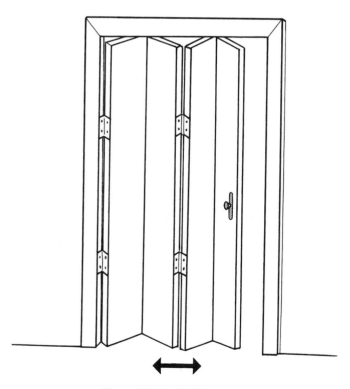

Figure 20-11 Folding door.

Bathroom

Doorway width may preclude bathroom access for the wheelchair user. Removing the door, installing a pocket or sliding door, or using a narrow rolling commode chair are options for entry to the bathroom for nonambulatory individuals. The optimal toilet seat height should be 17-19 inches. This allows for level transfers from a wheelchair and decreases the amount of bending required to get up and down for those who can stand. Options for raising the height of the toilet include a raised toilet seat, an over-toilet commode, or a drop-arm commode. For individuals who have greater weakness in their lower extremities than in their upper extremities, a toilet safety frame may assist with sit-to-stand transitions. Grab bars should be installed throughout the bathroom because surfaces become slippery and falls are more likely. The height of horizontal bars should range from 33 to 36 inches above the floor. The width of the bar should be 1¼ to 1½ inches to accommodate grasp efficiently. When bars are mounted adjacent to the wall, the distance between the wall and the bar should be 1½ inches so that the patient's fingers can reach around the bar but the arm cannot slip through. Walls around the tub or shower stall should be reinforced. Bars should be mounted securely into the wall studs. Towel racks should be removed if they are likely to be used for support.

Glass doors on tub and shower stalls should be removed and replaced with a curtain. Glass doors can detach from tracks and fall on the person. This renovation increases accessibility for transfers and improves safety conditions. Recommended height for tub rims is 17 to 19 inches. Shower stall thresholds should be ½ inch high. A roll-in shower may be recommended for nonambulatory individuals. It should be a minimum of 30 by 60 inches. Some tubs have rounded bottoms. This can present stability problems if a stationary leg of a tub bench is supposed to be positioned inside. A clamp-on tub bench is more suitable for such tubs. Regardless of the type of tub the individual's balance and transfer method and architectural constraints should be carefully evaluated to determine the most appropriate and safe type of seat. A flexible shower spray unit assists with rinsing; the hose should be a minimum of 60 inches long. The handle can be adapted for individuals with limited hand dexterity. Nonskid tub strips or a rubber bath mat should be applied to the floor of the tub or shower stall and outside the tub to prevent falls. See Figure 20-12 for samples of shower stall and shower seat dimensions.

Sink and Lavatories

The height of the sink should be a maximum of 34 inches above the floor. Wheelchair users need a minimum of 29 inches of height underneath the sink to enable them to have close access to the faucets and basin. Access problems may be eliminated by removing cabinets or doors. The mirror above the sink should be angled ¼ to ½ inch for in-

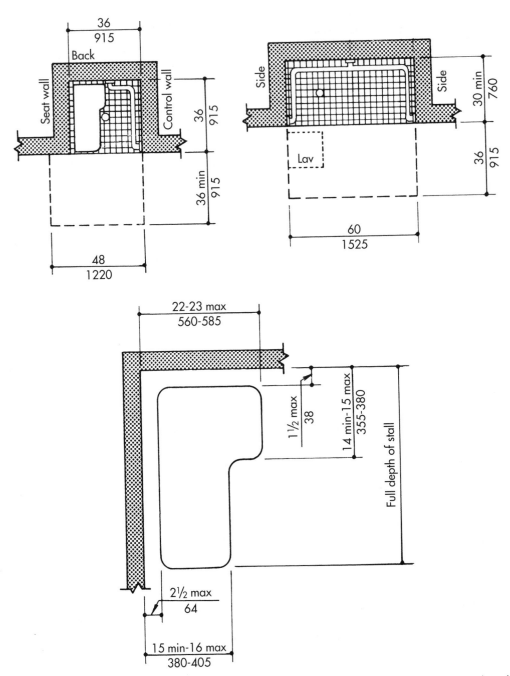

Figure 20-12 Transfer-type shower stall, roll-in shower stall, and shower seat design. (From American National Standards Institute: *Accessible and useable buildings and facilities*, New York, 1992, The Institute.)

dividuals who are seated. Water pipes should be insulated to prevent contact burns. Hot and cold water should mix and empty through a single faucet to mix water of variable temperatures. Water temperature controls should be set no higher than 115° F. Ordinances in some cities mandate a fixed maximum temperature for hot water for safety. Single-lever faucet controls are recommended because they provide visual indication of water temperature and do not require fine motor dexterity to operate.

Kitchens

Three kitchen layouts are most commonly seen: L-shaped, aisle, and U-shaped. The L- or U-shaped configuration can improve efficiency (Figure 20-13).[6] Work surfaces should be free of clutter, and small appliances that are frequently used should be placed within reach.

Counter tops are generally 36 inches high, making accessibility difficult for wheelchair users. Alternate counter or work surfaces can be adapted by adding pull-out cutting

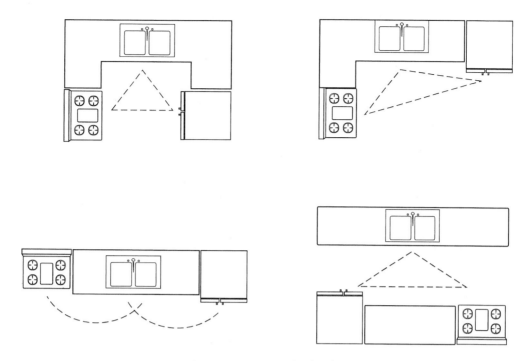

Figure 20-13 Common kitchen layouts.

boards or placing a cutting board on top of a drawer that has been partially opened. Height-adjustable counter tops and cabinets provide easy access for individuals with limited reach; however, this option is expensive. The countertop should have a maximum depth of 24 inches. The corners and edges should be rounded. Base cabinets should have enough toe space at the bottom to accommodate wheelchair footplates. Retractable doors and lazy Susans increase accessibility to stored items. Adapted knobs or D-loop handles assist individuals with decreased coordination and grasp strength. Easy-glide drawers and pull-out shelves may decrease energy expenditure.

Appliances also must be taken into account. A side-by-side refrigerator is recommended for increased access to the refrigerator and freezer. Shelves should be adjustable; lazy Susans may provide easier access to stored food items. A wall-mounted oven and range top with staggered burners are recommended for wheelchair users. A mirror placed above the stove allows seated individuals to see the cooking process. Transparent pots are another alternative. Range controls should be located at the front or side to eliminate the need to reach over hot elements. Controls can be adapted for individuals with limited hand dexterity. Tactile or audible cues can assist individuals with limited vision. For wall-mounted ovens the controls should be no higher than 40 inches above the floor for wheelchair user access.[6] Microwave and toaster ovens may be convenient and safe alternatives for cooking.

Sink basins should be a maximum of 6½ inches deep. A plastic or wooden rack can be used to raise the working level. A retractable hose can increase the ease of rinsing dishes. Single-lever faucet controls are recommended and should be positioned no farther than 21 inches from the edge of the counter.

FALL PREVENTION

The checklist in Figure 20-14 is an adaptation from the fall prevention checklist used at the Rehabilitation Hospital of the Pacific located in Honolulu, Hawaii. This checklist was originally used as a tool to provide education to family members and caregivers after the home evaluation process. The adjustments incorporate options for durable medical equipment.

■

CASE STUDY

JJ is a 72-year-old woman who was admitted to the hospital with a diagnosis of right CVA. Her hospital course was uncomplicated, and she was transferred to the rehabilitation unit 4 days later.

An occupational therapy evaluation was performed and clinical findings were reported. Passive range of motion was within functional limits throughout all joints in the upper extremities bilaterally. Strength was good in the right upper extremity. Minimal active movement was present in the left shoulder, and one-finger subluxation was noted. Sensation was intact for light touch, pain, and temperature. Functional abilities were moderately impaired because of decreased ability to bear weight on the left upper and lower extremities. Sitting balance was fair. Standing balance was poor. She required moderate assistance for bed mobility. Sit-to-stand required maximal assistance of

Exterior

___ Walkways have a smooth surface and are clear of objects.

___ Outdoor lighting is sufficient for safe ambulation and wheelchair maneuvering at night.

___ Step surfaces are nonslip and edges are clearly marked to prevent tripping.

___ Steps are sturdy and handrails are secure.

Living Room

___ Entryway and room are free of clutter to allow safe walking or wheelchair mobility.

___ Stepstools, ottomans, coffee tables, and other low-lying objects are out of the way to prevent trip hazards.

___ Chairs have armrests and are sturdy.

___ Telephone and lighting are accessible; cords are tucked down.

___ Environmental controls are accessible.

Hallway

___ Doors that open into halls are removed.

___ Floor is clear of objects.

___ Carpet borders and runners are secured.

Bathroom

___ Door width is wide enough to permit wheelchair access.

___ No thresholds are trip hazards.

___ Scatter rugs are removed.

___ Grab bars are installed near toilet, tub, and entryway.

___ Toilet is proper height.

___ Nonskid bath mat or strips are installed on floor of tub or shower.

___ Tub or shower seat is available for bathing.

Bedroom

___ Doorway entry is proper width.

___ Bed is proper height and firmness.

___ Night lights are present.

___ Hospital bed is available.

___ Side rails are installed.

___ Bedside commode is available.

Kitchen

___ Table is sturdy.

___ Frequently used items are located at waist level.

___ Use of range top is avoided.

___ Microwave or toaster oven is available.

___ Throw rugs are removed.

___ Electrical cords are tied up or taped down.

Figure 20-14   Fall prevention checklist.

one person, and transfers required moderate to maximal assist depending on the surface. She was unable to walk at the time of evaluation, and wheelchair mobility skills required moderate assist. In self-care a left neglect was noted during all activities. JJ required setup assistance for eating and grooming. Dressing and bathing required moderate to maximal assist.

JJ was treated in both occupational and physical therapy for 6 weeks. During her fourth week of treatment a home evaluation was scheduled. The therapy team felt having the patient present during the visit would be useful because she lived alone and still required the use of a wheelchair. She lived in a two-bedroom rental apartment in a building with a no-step entry and elevator. The apartment had large rooms, but wheelchair accessibility was limited because of excessive furniture and thick carpeting. The hallway was narrow. Her bedroom and bathroom were located off to the right of the hallway, and the second bedroom was located at the end of the hallway. She was unable to negotiate the turn into her bedroom with the wheelchair because of the hall and door width. The therapist suggested that she switch bedrooms and use the second bedroom as her own. The bed was low with a soft mattress and the closet was not accessible because of narrow paths and excessive furnishings. The bathroom was spacious and could easily accommodate a wheelchair; however, the door was only 19 inches wide, preventing wheelchair access. The bathroom had a combination tub and shower with sliding glass

doors. The toilet was located behind the door. The sink had round fixtures that were difficult to turn. The kitchen was wheelchair accessible. The refrigerator door opened to the right and the stove had controls at the back of the range top. The cabinets were high and not accessible from a seated position. The following recommendations were made:

Living room

1. Remove one couch and coffee table.
2. Remove the area carpet and scatter rugs.
3. Relocate the lamps for easier access.

Bedroom

1. Elevate the bed 4 inches on cinder blocks to equal the height of the wheelchair.
2. Place a plywood board beneath the mattress to increase firmness.
3. Remove the closet door and one dresser.
4. Lower the height of the closet rod to 40 inches above the floor.
5. Place a drop-arm commode chair next to the bed.
6. Place a night-light in the wall socket.

Bathroom

1. Remove the sliding glass doors and replace with a shower curtain.

2. Use a tub transfer bench and flexible shower hose for bathing.
3. Place a 24-inch grab bar on the wall of the tub 33 inches from the floor.
4. Park the wheelchair in front of the bathroom door and walk with assistance.
5. Place a chair in the bathroom in front of the sink to perform grooming and dressing tasks.
6. Tilt the mirror ½ inch.

Kitchen

1. Reverse the door swing on the refrigerator.
2. Relocate frequently used items to the counter.
3. Relocate the toaster oven to the kitchen table.

Communication

1. Purchase a portable cordless phone.
2. Consider registration with an emergency call service.

JJ was in agreement with the above recommendations and requested permission from the landlord to install the grab bar. During the rest of her inpatient rehabilitation stay the focus of treatment was placed on achieving independence in bed-to-commode transfers, short distance walking, light meal preparation and kitchen tasks from wheelchair level in a home-simulating environment. At the time of discharge, JJ was independent in all self-care, transfers, and meal preparation. She required contact guard for short distance ambulation with a hemiwalker and was independent with wheelchair mobility. She was recommended for home care services for follow-up therapy and assistance from a home health aide.

■

SUMMARY

In 1991, Cooper and associates published an article in the *American Journal of Occupational Therapy* entitled "Barrier Free Design: A Review and Critique of the Occupational Therapy Perspective."[2] In their review of occupational therapy literature on barrier-free design, they identified both insufficient research on this topic and a lack of a common conceptual base with which to guide the development and use of environmental assessments.

Two themes emerged from the literature: an increased awareness among occupational therapists regarding accessibility standards as developed by the ANSI and a consistent reference to accessibility and mobility concepts. The review makes clear that occupational therapy has declared an interest in barrier-free design.

The educational curriculum of occupational therapy includes the teaching of methods used to conduct home evaluations and modifications for both functional and architectural features. In spite of the emphasis placed by the profession on the importance of barrier-free design, a computer search of the major international occupational therapy journals revealed that few articles of rele-

vance on the topic have been published over the past 20 years.

Among the articles reviewed from 1971 to 1991, the earliest article, a position paper of the American Occupational Therapy Association (AOTA), presented a historical perspective on architectural barriers in relation to people with physical disabilities. In 1984, another historical overview was presented focusing on the needs of the geriatric population. In that overview, four survey studies resulting from occupational therapy class projects were described. A funded study described in the overview addressed public building access. This study revealed that none of a variety of public buildings was completely compliant with ANSI standards. A grocery and convenience store accessibility study yielded descriptive results indicating little difference in the compliance with ANSI standards between urban and rural centers. A subsequent follow-up indicated that 25% of the stores had complied with accessibility standards and recommendations. The authors described the role of occupational therapists as advocates for community accessibility as being key to the resultant changes.

The present review appears to indicate that research on barrier-free design is in an early stage of development. The home-based checklist found in occupational therapy educational programs is evident in the literature but lacks a common conceptual framework. Because the demand for accessible environments is increasing, occupational therapy consultation and input also can be expected to increase. To provide optimal care and improve quality of life for stroke survivors, this area of intervention must continue to be challenged and researched.

REVIEW QUESTIONS

1. What options can an occupational therapist consider if existing doorways are too narrow for a wheelchair?
2. What issues does an occupational therapist need to address for a wheelchair-dependent patient recovering from stroke who is returning home?
3. What modifications should be considered to make bathrooms safe and accessible?
4. What are architectural barriers?

■ COTA Considerations ■

- If a wheelchair does not have an accurate turning axis within an apartment or house, visualize ways to change or modify the environment to allow accessibility.
- Sometimes low-tech solutions such as rearranging contents of cupboards so that high-use items are in easy reach are the best to implement.
- Suggesting the removal of furniture or rugs to improve access within the home is more practical than proposing more assistance to navigate around tight corners or move to another space.

• Survey the home environment for obstacles that can cause injuries and note the way they can be removed or changed to improve safety. Obstacles may include exposed pipes and surfaces that are slippery when wet such as bathtubs.

REFERENCES

1. American National Standards Institute: *Accessible & usable buildings and facilities*, New York, 1992, The Institute.
2. Cooper AB, Cohen U, Hasselkus B: Barrier-free design: a review and critique of the occupational therapy perspective, *Am J Occup Ther* 45:344, 1991.
3. Datona R, Tesster B: Architectural barriers for the handicapped, *Rehab Lit*, February 1967.
4. Farzan DT: Reintegration for stroke survivors, *Nurs Clin North Am* 26:1037, 1991.
5. Law M, Stewart D, Strong S: Achieving access to home, community, and in workplace. In Trombly CA, editor: *Occupational therapy for physical dysfunction*, ed 4, Baltimore, 1995, Williams and Wilkins.
6. Salmen JPS: *AARP the do-able renewable home*, 1991, Washington, DC, AARP.
7. Shamberg S, Shamberg A: Blueprints for independence, *Occup Ther Prac* 1:22, 1996.

beverly k. bain

chapter 21

Assistive Technology

chapter objectives

After completing this chapter, the reader will be able to accomplish the following:

1. Integrate assistive technology interventions into treatment plans focused on increasing the independence of the stroke survivor.
2. Identify commonly used assistive technology for the following performance deficits: communication dysfunction, mobility dysfunction, and decreased ability to access the environment.
3. Understand the use of environmental control units, augmentative communication, powered mobility, and computer access in the stroke population.

George is aphasic and has minimal use of his right upper extremity (RUE) and right lower extremity (RLE) because of a stroke he sustained 2 days ago. When he wants to turn on the hospital television, he can use a portable augmentative alternative communication (AAC) device to call for assistance or use his left hand to press the large buttons on a remote environmental control unit (ECU) that has been attached within easy reach with the use of Velcro.

Marie has been discharged from the hospital to her daughter's home and will undergo outpatient rehabilitation. She will be alone several hours a day. Rather than hurry to answer the tele-

phone, she can use an answering machine. She can prepare a cup of coffee by using a remote ECU to turn on the coffee maker and other electronic appliances.

Harry can move about his apartment with a cane, but when he wants to go shopping or to visit friends he uses a one-arm drive wheelchair or add-on power pack attached to a standard wheelchair or a powered scooter. Rather than travel to the post office, he can use his computer to send e-mail to his granddaughter working in another state or to pay bills or check his bank statement.

These are but a few ways in which assistive technology (AT) can improve the quality of life for persons who have had strokes. A reflective therapist can be creative in evaluating clients in this age of technology. People of all ages and abilities can use AT to increase their function, compensate for loss of bilateral function, conserve energy, ensure safety, develop self-reliance, and enhance independence.

Historically, occupational therapists have used adaptive equipment to enhance the functional abilities of the patients they treat. AT devices (ATDs) are an extension and expansion of adaptive equipment and are wondrous tools in the total rehabilitation process of persons who have had strokes. AT services (ATSs) are the therapeutic processes that therapists use to evaluate, select, train, and reevaluate the AT user, tasks, environments, and devices that are most appropriate. According to the American Occupational Therapy Association (AOTA) Technology Competencies,[22] "low-technology" devices are inexpensive, readily available, and easy to adapt; "high-technology" devices may be expensive, be available only from selective rehabilitation vendors, require special training for both the professional and the AT user, and require modifications or fabrication by a rehabilitation engineer. A computer is considered a high-technology assistive device for written communication, and a communication board is considered a low-technology assistive device; however, a creative therapist might use a low-technology universal cuff to help a patient use a computer.

Occupational therapy practitioners are vital members of the AT rehabilitation team. They are educated to evaluate the patient holistically, analyze tasks, and consider all environments in which the patient must perform these tasks to become independent. In addition, occupational therapy practitioners usually work with interdisciplinary teams—an attribute in the area of rehabilitation technology—which requires the collaboration of physical therapists, therapeutic recreation specialists, nurses, physicians, speech pathologists, social workers, and most important the patient and caregiver.

DEFINITIONS

The 1988 Technology-Related Assistance for Individuals with Disabilities Act[35]—referred to as the *Tech Act*—defined an ATD as "any item, piece of equipment, or product system, whether acquired commercially off the shelf, modified, or customized, that is used to increase, maintain, or improve functional capabilities of individuals with disabilities." Examples range from a $15 device purchased from an electronics store or through a catalog that may be screwed into a lamp for touch activation to a $3000 voice-activated computer purchased from an AT vendor. The Tech Act defines an ATS as any service that directly assists an individual with a disability in the selection, acquisition,

or use of an assistive device.[35] This act also provided grant appropriations for the development of projects to provide states with information and technical assistance. In 1994, after a year of congressional hearings and deliberations, the second Tech Act was passed. It requires states to conduct activities leading to the development of systems change and encourage advocacy services.

ASSISTIVE TECHNOLOGY MODEL

When an occupational therapy practitioner determines that a patient might benefit from adaptive equipment, there are four elements in an effective and efficient treatment model to consider: (1) the patient/user, (2) the tasks the patient must perform, and wants to perform, (3) all the environments in which the tasks will be performed, and (4) the devices required to accomplish the tasks. The four parts are interdependent and must be considered if a device is to be used to its fullest potential by a contented person who wants to enhance functional abilities at home or in the community. In the past 10 years there has been an explosion in the development of technology devices to enhance quality of life. The prudent therapist must have a model to follow when selecting AT devices and rendering AT services as part of the total rehabilitation process (Figure 21-1).

In this interdependent model, the patient's physical, cognitive, and psychologic needs are considered in conjunction with those of the family and caregivers. Not every new device is appropriate for every person. The tasks most people must accomplish are (1) hand manipulations (e.g., to turn on appliances or write), (2) communicating with others verbally with the use of gestures or writing, and (3) transverse mobility—up and down—for short or long distances. Most tasks are performed in various environments (e.g., home, school, workplace, community, clinic). All present and future environments must be considered so the client does not underuse or abandon the device.[12,31] The ATDs most commonly used by people who have had

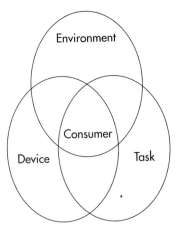

Figure 21-1 Interdependent AT model.

strokes are powered scooters, adapted vehicles, verbal communication aids, ECUs, and computers.

THERAPEUTIC FOUNDATION

The therapeutic foundation for the use of AT as a tool in occupational therapy rehabilitation is based on three frames of reference: (1) biomechanical—specifically energy conservation and work-simplification principles, (2) acquisitional—learning theories, and (3) rehabilitation—adaptation of devices and the environment.

The use of a powered scooter to travel long distances, use of a remote control to activate appliances, and a computer are all in the biomechanical frame of reference. By reducing the energy expended for these activities, patients can increase their endurance for other activities of daily living (ADL) and leisure activities. When patients use AT to increase function, they also conserve the energy of the caregiver.

The acquisitional frame of reference is associated with a person learning new ways of performing desired tasks,[29] perhaps with the use of a computer or AAC device. The appropriate application of ATDs can enhance a person's ability to interact in the environment and accomplish purposeful activities. For example, a patient who could write before a stroke (but not after) could learn to use a computer and again correspond with family and friends. By learning to use an augmentative communication device, the patient could convey needs and hold meaningful two-way conversations.

Compensation and adaptation of equipment and the environment are the elements in the rehabilitation frame of reference that form the theoretical bases for using ATDs. Devices such as "stove minders" that signal a person when a pot is boiling or automatically turn off the burner at a preset time may be considered adaptive or low technology equipment. Such devices also compensate for memory loss as a result of a stroke. Environmental modifications have been enhanced by tool redesign, such as electric door openers, adapted one-hand computer keyboards, special computer wrist supports, and electric lifts for powered scooters and wheelchairs. In addition, the use of ECUs can reduce the number of needed modifications of home, school, and work environments while increasing the patient's quality of life.[23]

ASSESSMENT

No standard AT assessment instrument exists. A systematic nine-step problem-solving approach to evaluating each component of the model is summarized in Table 21-1.[10]

Table 21-1

Problem-Solving Approach to the Assessment of Consumers for Assistive Technology Devices			
STEPS	PART OF SYSTEM	PROBLEM	ACTION
1	Task	Tasks the consumer must accomplish with the ATD: • Communication • Mobility • Environmental controls • Computer adaptation • Switch interface	Review records; interview consumers, caretakers, and family; and observe.
2	Consumer/user	Consumer's abilities in the lying, sitting, and standing positions	Conduct formal testing: motor, manual muscle testing, reflexes, range of motion (ROM), coordination, endurance, sensory, psychosocial, cognitive, social; interview; and observe.
3	ATD	On the basis of information from steps 1 and 2, possible devices that can be used	Characteristics to consider include input, processing, output, display; commercial availability; safety and reliability; practicality; and affordability.
4	Environment	Present and future: Bed/chair Home School/work Community	Interview, observe, and conduct on-site visits.
5	All	Trial period	Try various devices in a variety of environments.
6	ATD	Selection	Order, adapt, or fabricate.
7	Consumer/user	Application	Train in use and maintenance.
8	All	Documentation	Record in all intradepartmental and interdepartmental files.
9	All	Reevaluation	Periodically reevaluate consumer, ATD, environment, and tasks.

The occupational therapy practitioner is familiar with sensorimotor, cognitive, and psychosocial standard and non-standard evaluations of patients. For all ATD assessments the input, throughput, output, and feedback characteristics, as well as the safety and reliability of all devices, should be included. Other references for AT assessment are the AOTA Technology Special Interest Newsletters.[7] Samples of AT assessment instruments are included in the references.[8,11,33,34,38] The key factor in all assessments is the collaboration of the client with the AT rehabilitation team members.

GUIDELINES FOR USING ASSISTIVE TECHNOLOGY EQUIPMENT

Because most ATDs contain electronic components, professionals, users, and caregivers must be aware of and should routinely check the following parts when using AT equipment:

- All appliances, wall outlets, lamps, electric cords, and extension cords should be carefully checked.
- All electric cords should be kept out of pathways.
- Never wrap cords around appliances or bind them tightly, because the extra stress can damage the wires.
- Batteries should be routinely recharged or replaced (especially in powered scooters, AACs, and IR or RF ECUs).
- Batteries have memory and require a full charge the first time they are used. (Read and study the manufacturer's label.)
- Cellular phone batteries must be recharged.
- Telephone answering machine tapes should be checked for readiness.
- Computers should always be connected to surge protectors (especially in old buildings).
- Any ATD selection starts with readily available devices that can be purchased from reliable electronics stores or catalogs.
- A conventional backup for electronic high-technology devices (especially AACs) should always be available. Some manufacturers have devices they will loan to patients to use while equipment is being repaired.
- Written instructions, catalogs, diagrams, telephone numbers, and pictures of ATDs should be given to the user, caregiver, or both.
- The warranty of any equipment should be checked. (The warranty is not valid if modifications are made.)
- All environments should be barrier free. (Small scatter rugs should be removed, hallways and stairs illuminated, and door widths checked.)
- Many people who have had strokes are older and may have decreased vision, hearing, sensation, and cognitive abilities. The patient should be observed daily for changes.
- Many older people are not as familiar with computers and high technology and may be reluctant to try ATDs. Devices should be kept simple to increase the patient's function; too many gadgets may overburden or infringe on the patient's independence.
- A network list of long-time ATD users, professional consultants, reliable manufacturers, and dependable vendors should be kept.
- As a patient's physical, cognitive and psychosocial abilities change, environmental changes occur, or tasks and needs change, there may also be changes in the ATD requirements; therefore reevaluation is an ongoing process. If a patient cannot return to the occupational therapy department, a phone call or a mailed checklist can substitute.

MOBILITY

Most persons who have had a stroke use standard wheelchairs that they learn to propel with the nonaffected arm and leg during the early phase of rehabilitation. Some patients progress to using only a cane, a leg brace, or both; and a few need powered mobility in the home or immediate work environment. However, many mobility technology devices have been developed for the comfort of older patients that may enhance the function of people who have had strokes: powered scooters; add-on–powered systems for standard wheelchairs; electronic lifts; porch lifts; and portable, lightweight ramps.

Powered Scooters

In the past 5 years, major advances have been made in powered scooter design: bucket seats, adjustable telescopic handle or tillers, front- or rear-wheel drive option, and ease in disassembly or folding for transport in cars or vans. (Several electronic trunk lifts are also available.) The new scooter seats provide additional comfort and stability, with armrests that may be flipped up for ease in transfer. Some seats swivel and may be fitted with special seat cushions or custom molded seats, depending on the person's sitting balance (see Chapter 19).

It should be noted that front-wheel drive scooters have small wheels that maneuver well in tight spaces and on hard surfaces but not on thick carpet, grass, or uneven surfaces. Rear-wheel drive scooters have greater traction to maneuver over grass, dirt, gravel, and hills (10° or less). All scooters require a battery charger. Most have built-in battery chargers permanently mounted in the base, meaning the entire scooter must be taken in for service; others have external chargers that must be transported separately if the user plans a trip or the scooter needs an unexpected charge. It is highly recommended that the user's visual ability and all environments be carefully evaluated and that an interdisciplinary team decision be made after the user has practiced with different models. Scooters have many advantages for patients in need of mobility technology because they are lighter, easy to disassemble for transport in a car, easy to maneuver, and cost less than powered wheelchairs.

Add-On Power Units

Another ATD that may increase function for persons who sometimes need power mobility are known as "power pack" or portable power conversion or add-on power units that fit most manual wheelchairs. Some of their advantages are ease of assembly and portability in the overhead storage compartments of airplanes. However, the large rear wheels of a manual wheelchair (which use friction drive) may wear down when a pack is used for a prolonged time, and they are expensive if used infrequently. As with any ATD, careful evaluation of the advantages and disadvantages must be discussed with the user.

VERTICAL MOBILITY

Mobility in some environments may require vertical mobility, which can be accomplished with a chair lift; chair glide; or small, wall-mounted elevator. All can be expensive. When the AT user needs to use stairs only to reach a bedroom, the environment may be modified with a downstairs room (e.g., dining room, study, or den if bathroom facilities are available on the same level) as the bedroom. Many homes, buildings, and workplaces have one flight of stairs outside that may be fitted with a porch lift for a wheelchair; portable ramps may also be used for inside or outside accessibility.

Other ATDs to conserve energy and increase the mobility of users are electric, hydraulic, and battery-operated lifts. An Abledata[1] search is an excellent way to find information on the various available lifts. All caregivers should know all lift operations, and the manufacturer should supply the user with warranties, instructions, and catalogs.

Powered Wheelchairs

If a severely affected person does need a powered wheelchair, the following steps should be taken:

- Proper positioning is essential (see Chapter 19).
- The user should be evaluated for an appropriate control site.
- It should be determined whether an AAC or ECU will be used.
- Add-on equipment should be mounted securely.
- An interdisciplinary team should select all the equipment with collaboration of the user and caregiver.[36]

Public Transportation

With the passage of the Americans with Disabilities Act (ADA),[4] there has been an increase in accessible public transportation for persons with disabilities. Buses, trains, airplanes, and ship companies have made an effort to improve this accessibility. People who have had strokes must carefully plan each trip and consider the following:

- Getting to and from the station
- Getting up and down stairs
- Locations of elevators or escalators
- Getting through turnstiles
- Getting through doors
- Walking distances in the station
- Availability of accessible bathroom facilities
- Available assistance
- Availability of lifts into and out of mode of transportation

Seat belts should always be used in automobiles, and any wheelchair or scooter should be securely tied down or wheel-locked.

ENVIRONMENTAL CONTROL UNITS

An ECU is "a means to purposefully manipulate and interact with the environment by alternately accessing one or more electrical devices via switches, voice activation, remote control, computer interface, and other technologic adaptations. The purpose of an ECU is to maximize functional ability and independence in the home, school, and leisure environment."[10]

Commercially readily available ECUs are the devices of choice for patients who need to turn lights and appliances off and on, use portable telephones and telephone answering machines, and in some cases use devices to summon assistance. ECUs can be practical for use in the hospital or long-term care facility, at home, in bed, in chairs, or any situation in which the patient needs to increase the function of manipulative skills.

Assessment

In the assessment of a patient for an ECU (or any AT or adaptive device), the proper positioning of the client, both in bed and when mobile, should be considered first. Next, an evaluation of the client's abilities in the following areas should be carried out:

- Physical/motor: ROM, reflex coordination, and endurance should be evaluated. Usually the nonaffected extremity can be used to activate the device, but an assessment of the person as a whole is important.
- Sensory, visual, and auditory ability: Assessments of these areas are important in determining the best means of access and feedback.

- Cognitive ability to follow instructions: For example, can the patient remember which device is activated by which button and in what sequence?
- Psychosocial factors: Patient and caregiver expectations and motivation to use an ECU should be determined.

After evaluating the patient's abilities, goals, needs, and all tasks that could be accomplished with an ECU now and in the future should be discussed. A written list of needs is suggested and should also be discussed with the family and all caregivers (Figure 21-2).

The characteristics of the ECU should then be evaluated with emphasis on (1) input method and required distance of the throughput or transmission (e.g., one room, several rooms in a small apartment, inside and outside a house); (2) the output (the number of lights and appliances that must be controlled); (3) portability (because most ECUs are used in bed, in a wheelchair, or in various rooms in a home or office); (4) safety, reliability, and durability; (5) ease of assembly, operation, and maintenance; and (6) current and future affordability.

Environmental Control Unit Remote Transmission

The major means of ECU transmission are infrared; radio frequency; sound, ultrasound, or voice; and AC house current. Most ECUs are remotely controlled with no physical attachment between the input (switch, button), throughput (transmission), and output (lights, appliances) (Figure 21-3).

Guidelines for ECU Transmission Selection

- Infrared transmission travels only in line-of-sight, but the distance can be extended with the use of extending devices such as Powermids or Leap Frogs. An infrared controller can teach a television controller or an X-10 infrared receiver to accept signals (Figure 21-4).
- Sound waves, both voice and ultrasound, travel in only one room. Ultrasound waves can bounce off walls, and voice-activated ECUs may require a microphone or close proximity to the controller. Use of ultrasound devices is easy to learn because it involves color coding of modules and buttons. Ultrasound devices have several methods of input (e.g., large buttons, large pads, joystick).
- Radio frequency transmission travels from room to room. The signal is sent from a portable input device to a radio frequency receiver (plug into house outlet) that sends the signal through an X-10 module and house current to an appliance or light.
- Using AC house current, ECUs transmit inside and outside a house or building. This method uses a controller to send signals to designated modules that have plugged in lights or appliances. Each controller has a "house code," and each module must have the same house code and a "unit code" for each light or appli-

ance. The controller and module must be connected to the same house circuit. However, different controllers can be used in the same house if different house codes are designated. For example, if two patients were sharing the same hospital room, one patient's house code would be set on A and the other patient's code would be set on C. The patients would be able to control their own nurse call button, television, radio, lights, or fan. The patient with house code A could use unit code 1 for the lamp, 2 for the television, 3 for the nurse call button; the patient with house code C could use unit code 1 for the nurse call button, 2 for the fan, and 3 for the television (Figure 21-5). Many ECUs incorporate the X-10 system into their units; therefore it is important that the occupational therapy practitioner understands the basis of this means of transmission. A variety of input controllers are commercially available, so the number of devices that need to be controlled must be carefully evaluated (Figure 21-6). A point to remember about AC house current ECUs is that they can receive stray signals from airplanes, radio-operated garage door openers, and electrical storms. For additional information on ECUs see the references.[10,11,14,15,17,25,28]

TELEPHONES

Telephones are important for the safety of, as well as the convenience and socialization for, people with disabilities. Many technologic telephone advances benefit people with hearing, speech, visual, and motor impairments. For visual impairments, there are telephones with enlarged number pads or enlarged stick-on numbers that may be applied to any telephone. For the person who can function with one hand, speaker phones, shoulder holders, gooseneck holders, and telephone clips are available. For severely impaired people who need assistance dialing an operator, an overlay may be placed over the buttons; it requires only a gross motion to push down the "0" button. Telephones may also be controlled by computers, AACs, and ECUs. Other modifications include the following:

- Portable, lightweight headset telephones
- Telephones with a four-button emergency attachment
- Memory storage of frequently called numbers
- Battery backup
- Redial capacities

For people with poor voice quality, there are telephones that amplify the voice; for those with poor voice volume, there are electronic artificial larynxes. Several voice-activated telephones have been developed and refined in recent years. The great advances in technology have increased the telephone capabilities of older persons with hearing impairments and those who are deaf. The hearing-impaired may attach small amplifiers to any handset or purchase a

Name _____ Date _____ Age _____ Sex _____

Date of Onset _____ Diagnosis _____

Reason for Referral _____

Major Functional Problem Areas: Communication _____ Manipulation _____ Motor _____ Other _____

I. DEVICES TO BE CONTROLLED

Devices	Quantity	Comments
		Location (bed, wheelchair, school, workplace, other); remote transmission: IR, ultrasound, RF
Call Bell		
Emergency Call System		
Telephone		
Intercom		
Lights: Lamps		
Overhead		
Bed Control		
Television		
VCR		
Stereo		
Radio		
Tape Recorder		
Fan		
Temperature		
Computer		
Page Turner		
Door Opener		
Door Lock		
OTHER		

II. POSSIBLE ACCESS METHODS

Direct Selection _____ Scanning _____ Encoding _____ Voice Activation _____

Switch(s) _____ Mounting Hardware _____

Comments:

III. FEEDBACK

Offered by ECU: Auditory _____ Visual _____

Offered by USER: Auditory _____ Visual _____

IV. INTEGRATION WITH OTHER EQUIPMENT (check all that apply)

Equipment	Manufacturer/Model
Wheelchair	
Computer	
Communication Aid	
OTHER:	
Comments:	

V. EXPENDABILITY FOR FUTURE USE

A. What are the user's goals?

Vocationally:

Avocationally:

Educationally:

B. Medical Status (Prognosis/Potential for Improvement)

VI. FUNDING

Additional Comments: _____

Figure 21-2 Environmental control systems needs assessment form (Courtesy American Occupational Therapy Institute; Bain et al, 1991; revised 1995.)

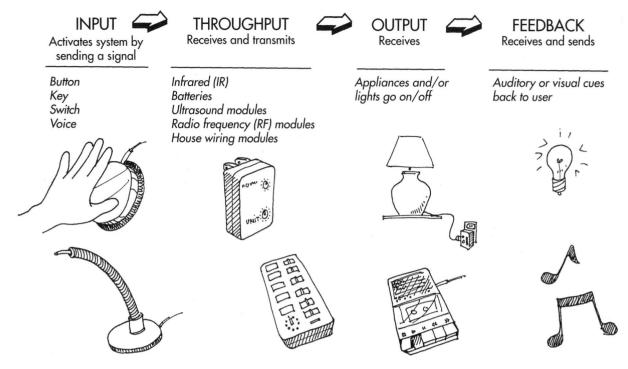

Figure 21-3 ECU control. (Courtesy Cristina Burwell, Boston, Mass.)

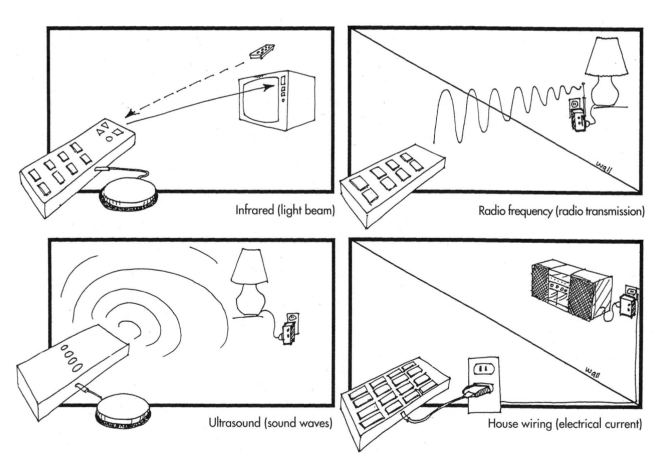

Figure 21-4 ECU transmitters. (Courtesy Cristina Burwell, Boston, Mass.)

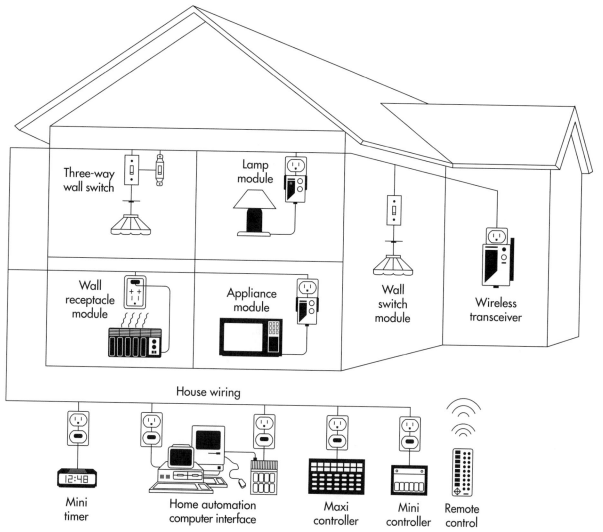

Figure 21-5 Control of lights and appliances throughout house with an ECU. (Courtesy X-10, [USA], Inc., Closter, NJ.)

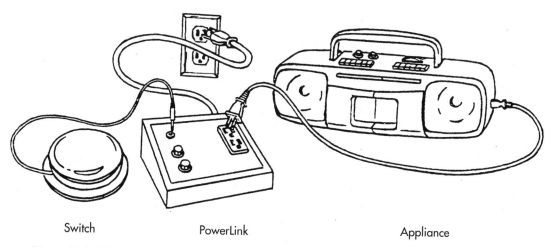

Figure 21-6 Diagram of PowerLink 2. Switch activation of radio. (Courtesy AbleNet, Inc., Minneapolis, Minn.)

handset with adjustable amplification built in. With the passage of the ADA, many more public telephones also have amplification capabilities. Special telephone modifications can be purchased at local telephone stores and electronics stores and through office supply catalogs.

The occupational therapy practitioner must assess the patient's telephone needs, collaborate on the selection, train the patient and caregiver, be sure the installation is satisfactory, and conduct routine follow-ups. In a study of aging by the Rehabilitation Engineering Research Center (RERC), the State University at Buffalo found that when older subjects were satisfied with their phone systems, they actually increased their use by almost 50%. Another important result of this study was the finding that the cost for telephone-solutions equipment averages $70.45, not including labor charges.[27]

Persons who have had strokes rely on the telephone to communicate daily, call for assistance if they fall, report a fire, or call police in an emergency. The AT rehabilitation team must consider phones necessities.

MONITORING SYSTEMS

Personal-response systems are technologic devices worn or carried by people who live alone. These devices are activated with minimal pressure; some have voice activation. The switch sends a signal to a monitoring center that puts the user in touch with a relative, friend, neighbor, or emergency services. Most cardiac users are linked directly to hospital monitoring centers. This device can be cost-effective in reducing nursing home or hospital stays while granting safe independence to the user and comfort to relatives who cannot offer constant care.[24] Several systems exist throughout the United States and in many European countries. Most require a monthly monitoring fee, and some equipment is either rented or must be purchased. The 24-hour monitoring centers have all the patient's vital information. The patient, therapist, and family must evaluate each system according to the patient's and family's needs.

A low-technology solution for monitoring people in the same house is an inexpensive (i.e., less than $50) portable baby monitor, which is sensitive enough to hear breathing anywhere in the house. These monitors are available in department stores and electronics stores.

COMPUTERS

Computers have become part of daily life and can be used to compensate for deficits in written communication; conserve energy; socialize on the Internet or by electronic-mail; and build self-esteem by helping the patient accomplish "tech-age" tasks and play games such as bingo, chess, mah-jong, or bridge. Occupational therapists with basic computer skills can use computers as an effective tool for those with visual, cognitive, or physical impairments.

Assessment

The assessment of the patient (which should begin with proper positioning) includes the following:

- Cognition—especially attention span, short-term memory, following directions, and decision making
- Visual ability—with emphasis on lateral neglect, figure-ground, visual attention, and acuity
- Motor control—noting whether the person can use the affected hand to assist in simultaneous striking or only the nonaffected hand is being used and whether the person has sufficient ROM to reach all the keys on the keyboard

An interview or discussion with the patient is necessary to determine which tasks the patient wants to accomplish with the computer because many people have "computer phobia." (It is often helpful if another patient can demonstrate the ease of word-processing a letter or show a computer-prepared flyer to a computer novice.) A grandparent's task might be to increase social interaction skills; playing computer games with their grandchildren could help the individual meet this goal if the occupational therapy practitioner evaluates the cognitive and visual skill requirements of several games.[30]

All present and future environments in which the computer will be used should also be assessed. Considerations are physical factors (e.g., accessibility of the room, computer table height, light in the room) and psychosocial factors (e.g., determine who will be sharing the computer and who will set up the computer).

When the characteristics of the computer are evaluated, the following factors should be noted:

- Input methods—single- or two-handed, scanning or direct-selection mouse, keyboard
- Throughput or processing—by batteries or AC current, model type (e.g., desktop, notebook)
- Output—print size, color, contrast of letters on the background
- Feedback—size and color on the monitor, auditory sounds of printer and central processing unit

An excellent computer assessment resource is Deterding and Dustman's *Computer Access Checklist*.[16] It comprises two parts: an evaluation of the consumer's performance components (motor, sensory, cognitive) and contextual issues related to the consumer's computer use. Another beneficial resource is the article by Anson, which has flow charts to describe physical access and sensory and performance enhancements.[6]

Computer Adaptations

Computer adaptations might be required for the patient to compensate for deficits in cognitive, visual, and motor skills (Table 21-2). Low-technology solutions should be attempted first, followed by software and hardware solutions.

Table 21-2

Computer Problems and Solutions

PROBLEM AREA (CONSUMER'S DEFICITS)	POSSIBLE SOLUTIONS (LOW-TECHNOLOGY, SOFTWARE, HARDWARE)
Visual • Acuity • Figure-ground • Light sensitivity • Eye control • Lateral neglect	• Large, color, stick-on tabs • Enlarged text size • Large monitor • Magnifier on monitor • Enlarged screen commands • Screen reader • Antiglare screen
Motor • Simultaneous key striking (holding one key, pressing one or more keys at the same time) • Mouse use • Energy conservation	• Key latches/locks • Key guard locking adapters • Holding typing stick in affected hand • Track ball • Mouse-key program • Minikeyboard • Word prediction programs • Macros • One-handed keyboard
Cognitive Mainly software retraining programs • Attention span • Short-term memory • Following directions • Decision-making	• HELP key • Abbreviation expansion • Work prediction • Macros • Synthesized speech • Gradation from one step to multiple steps

Additional considerations when assessing a computer include the following:

• Hardware should be adapted so that the top of the monitor is lined up with the top of the user's head.
• The keyboard and central processing unit should be separate from the monitor to allow positioning flexibility.
• Desk height and width should be adjustable to accommodate wheelchair.
• Proper seating position should never be compromised.
• Users with hearing loss or who work in a noisy environment may require visual prompts.
• Synthesized speech computers can be useful as communication devices or training aids for users with aphasia.

Computer Activities

In the rehabilitation process, computer applications are used to compensate for deficits, conserve energy, and en-

hance psychosocial skills. The therapeutic applications for persons who have had strokes are numerous. Besides the previously mentioned activities, other examples are word-processing a favorite recipe book, preparing and keeping schedules of important names and dates, corresponding through electronic mail, shopping from catalogs by faxing and using databases to research information on specific equipment, learning safety and wellness measures, and socializing on Internet support groups. The list is only limited by the occupational therapy practitioner's experience and the patient's motivation.

For additional information on computers, see the references.[15,20,26,39]

AUGMENTATIVE ALTERNATIVE COMMUNICATION

The basic areas of communication are verbal, conversational, written, and gesture. Usually the occupational therapist screens, evaluates, and trains persons in the area of written communication. Use of computers as writing aids and speech synthesizers is increasing.

The term *augmentative communication* is defined as any form of communication that does not require speech. An aphasic person may communicate through gestures, facial expressions, body or sign language, picture-letter-word boards, communication boards, alternative augmentative communication (AAC) aids, or a combination of these. An effective speech system includes both standard nonelectronic and electronic aids.

Communication aids are defined by the American Speech-Language-Hearing Association (ASHA) as "physical objects or devices used to transmit or receive messages (e.g., a communication book, board, chart, mechanical or electrical device or computer)."[3] AAC systems "attempt to compensate (either temporarily or permanently) for the impairment and disability pattern of individuals with severe expressive communication disorders."[2]

When an AAC aid is used, the speed at which the user can locate and select a key, the number of required selections before the aid offers an output, and the quality of the output must be considered, as well as the user's sex, age, and dialect. The most frequently used nonelectronic communication system requires the user or communication partner to point to choices to convey messages. Pointing may be performed by the patient with the nonaffected hand.

An electronic AAC system uses a form of electronic technology, usually with batteries as throughput. The input must be properly mounted and readily accessible to the user. Output can be conducted by spelling; abbreviation; pictographic; coding of words, phrases, and sentences by synthesized speech; visual display; printed copy; or a combination of these outputs.

Assessment

A communication evaluation should begin with the identification of all the tasks, needs, and goals of the patient and communication partners. The patient's cognitive, motor, and hearing abilities should be assessed because communication is a sender-receiver feedback system. All the environments in which the aid will be used should be assessed, including factors such as mounting of the aid (e.g., in bed, for walking, in a wheelchair), sound level, and light. (Some AAC aids use light-emitting diodes that decrease visibility in bright sunlight.)

The key characteristics of any communication system are the following:

- Speed at which a message can be conveyed
- Portability of the aid
- Accessibility of the aid to the user in various positions
- Dependability of both manual and electronic power sources

- Quality of the output
- Durability of the aid
- Independence of the user
- Vocabulary flexibility (programmable or fixed)
- Time required for repairs and maintenance of the aid[14,19,20,28]

Role of the Occupational Therapy Practitioners

Team cooperation is required to deliver the appropriate augmentative communication services to a client and to integrate the AAC aid with other ATPs. In the service delivery of electronic communication the four substantial contributions of the occupational therapist are (1) a holistic evaluation of the patient that includes evaluation of physical abilities (e.g., seating and positioning, ROM, coordination), cognitive skills (e.g., following directions, memory, sequencing), and sensory abilities (visual and auditory); (2) evaluating and recommending the most effective control interface and selection technique; (3) training the patient to use the aid (especially if switches are used); and (4) collaborating with other team members.[5,14,19,37]

The speech therapist usually determines the patient's communication needs, assesses the patient's language ability, collaborates in the selection of the aid, and trains the patient and major communication partners. Other professional members of the team may include a physician, who is required to sign orders for equipment; a social worker, who may counsel the patient and family; a rehabilitation engineer, who may modify the control interface and mounting system; and the vendor or manufacturer, who designs and produces the electronic aid. To be effective, this professional team must work closely with nonverbal patients and their communication partners.

In addition, the occupational therapy practitioner should be aware of various aids that are available—from simple, small, battery-operated aids that can be used bedside for nonspeaking persons to complex, programmable, wheelchair-mounted systems that integrate with computers and ECUs. Communication is required all day in many different situations; therefore, any AAC device should not interfere with other activities and should use an appropriate power source.

For additional information, speech pathologists, manufacturers, and vendors are available for inservice training, workshops, and training institutes. Three valuable comprehensive resources are the ASHA booklet *Augmentative Communication*[2]; the International Society for Augmentative and Alternative Communication journal, which includes proceedings of its biennial conference; and the *Trace Resource Book*.[13] The occupational therapist must know what equipment is available and the most appropriate control interface. The speech pathologist is responsible for evaluating the patient's language communication abilities and training the patient in communication.

Recently occupational therapists have learned to use AT to extend the abilities of patients of all ages and with varying degrees of function. The occupational therapy practitioner should seek more information, knowledge, skills, and competency by attending conferences and workshops, enrolling in technology courses, visiting electronics stores, reading catalogs, and talking with other professional groups and users.

In 1991, AOTA formed a special-interest group in technology; additional information can be obtained from the AOTA Division on Practice. Another informative interdisciplinary professional group is Rehabilitation Engineering and Assistive Technology Society of North America (RESNA), which publishes a journal, newsletter, proceedings of conferences, special topic booklets, and other excellent resources in their *Assistive Technology Sourcebook*.[18] RESNA holds national, international, and regional meetings each year; in addition, some states have local groups that meet bimonthly.

As with any specialty area, AT builds on the body of professional knowledge. It is advisable to first learn low technology solutions and then to progress to the areas for which the occupational therapy department or clinical site is responsible: positioning, mobility, ECUs, AAC aids, and computers. It often seems impossible to stay informed about the rapid advances in technology, but discussion with occupational therapists, other professionals, and consumers is beneficial. AT is one of many tools of the occupational therapy profession. As Mary Pat Radabough said, "For most people, technology makes things easier. For people with disabilities, however, technology makes things possible."[32]

■
CASE STUDY

MP, a 64-year-old widow, had a stroke 6 months ago. She lives alone on the second floor of her married daughter's house.

MP independently carries out all personal hygiene tasks except bathing. The day MP had her stroke she was found by her daughter on the bathroom floor, unable to speak or to move her right hand and leg. She can lightly clean her one-bedroom apartment, prepare meals, and do laundry by hand. She needs assistance shopping for food. MP attends outpatient therapy once a week, plays cards with friends once a week, and attends church when someone drives her.

MP was referred to the AT rehabilitation team so that she could (1) increase her mobility on stairs and over long distances, and (2) learn to use safety devices in cases of emergency so she can continue to live independently.

While in the hospital, MP used a simple AAC device until her speech became clear. She also used an on/off ECU to control her television, radio, and lights. After discharge, she was transferred to her daughter's home, where she used her grandson's bedroom on the first floor. She attended outpatient

rehabilitation three times a week. MP's occupational therapist taught her work-simplification and safety skills, such as using a microwave oven placed at table height to prepare meals and an automatic electric teapot that turns off after boiling; installing bathroom bars near the toilet and bathtub; using an answering machine for telephone messages; and carrying a simple ECU in her pocket to control her lights, fan, television, and radio. MP's physical therapist continued to work on her gait and stair-climbing ability. She no longer needed speech therapy.

The AT rehabilitation team recommended that (1) MP and her daughter investigate a "life emergency system" to summon assistance (preferably a pendant that MP would wear at all times to summon her daughter and then the hospital), (2) the daughter contact a rehabilitation technology supplier to determine whether a porch or stair lift or a one-floor elevator might be installed to allow her mother to continue to live on the second floor (to avoid disrupting her daughter's family life and to increase MP's independence and quality of life), (3) the occupational therapy practitioner supply MP with literature on the emergency system and suppliers and (4) the social worker discuss funding of the AT equipment with MP and her family.

■
REVIEW QUESTIONS

1. When considering whether a person should use an AT device, which factors must be evaluated according to the technology model presented in this chapter?
2. What are the three frames of reference that form the theoretical basis for using AT with stroke patients? Give an example of each.
3. Which powered mobility devices would you recommend for a stroke patient to use while shopping in a mall? State your rationale.
4. What are the four major transmission methods for ECUs? Give examples of each.
5. What would be the most cost-effective and safe ECU for a consumer whose tasks include turning lights and appliances off and on and who also needs a telephone system?
6. Give two possible solutions for a problem in each of the three problem areas that might limit a stroke patient using a computer (visual, motor, cognitive).
7. What are the major occupational therapy contributions on the AT team in the area of AAC?
8. Briefly discuss the value of RESNA for the occupational therapy practitioner working in the area of AT.
9. Give two examples of AT devices that could enhance the function of stroke patients in (1) mobility, (2) manipulation, and (3) communication tasks. State your rationale.
10. List five ways an occupational therapy practitioner can increase knowledge about and skills in AT.

■ COTA Considerations ■

- Before assistive technology devices are prescribed, a thorough evaluation of the patient's physical, cognitive, and psychosocial needs must be performed.
- When any ATD is recommended, the emphasis of evaluation is on the input method, the output, portability, safety, ease of learning, and affordability.
- Use of assistive technology can mean the difference between returning to a safe home environment or not, as well as decreasing the number of hours that a caregiver is required.
- AT is a rapidly expanding practice area; it is crucial to remain up to date by attending conferences and seminars and reading current literature.[22]

REFERENCES

1. *Abledata*, Silver Spring, Md, 1994, National Rehabilitation Information Center.
2. American Speech-Language-Hearing Association: Report: augmentative and alternative communication, *ASHA* 33(suppl 5):9, 1991.
3. American Speech-Language-Hearing Association: Report: competencies for speech-language pathologists providing services in augmentative communication, *ASHA* 31:107, 1989.
4. *Americans with Disabilities Act*, Public Law 100-366, 42, USC 12101, 1988.
5. Angelo J, Smith RO: The critical role of occupational therapy in augmentative communication services, *American Occupational Therapy Association technology review '89: perspectives on occupational therapy practice*, Rockville, Md, 1989, American Occupational Therapy Association.
6. Anson D: Finding your way in the maze of computer access technology. *Am J Occup Ther* 48:121, 1994.
7. Bain BK: Assessment of assistive technology, *AJOT Technology Special Interest Section Newsletter* 5(1,2), 1995.
8. Bain BK: *Assessment of clients for technological assistive devices: American Occupational Therapy Association technology review '89: perspectives on occupational therapy practice*, Rockville, Md, 1989, American Occupational Therapy Association.
9. Bain BK et al: *Environmental control systems: assessment, selection, and training*. Cincinnati, Ohio, June 1991, AOTA Annual Conference.
10. Bain BK et al: Technology. In Hopkins H, Smith H, editors: *Willard and Spackman's occupational therapy*, ed 8, Philadelphia, 1993, Lippincott.
11. Bain BK, Leger D, editors: *Assistive technology: an interdisciplinary approach*, New York, 1997, Churchill Livingstone.
12. Battvia A, Hammer G: Toward the development of consumer-based criteria for the evaluation of consumer-based criteria for the evaluation of assistive devices, *J Rehabil Res Dev* 27:425, 1990.
13. Borden P, Lubich J, Vanderheiden G: *Trace resource book: 1996-97 edition*, Madison, Wisc, 1996, Trace Research and Development Center.
14. Church C, Glennen S: *The handbook of assistive technology*, San Diego, 1992, Singular Publishing Group.
15. Cook A, Hussey S: *Assistive technologies: principles and practice*, St Louis, 1995, Mosby.
16. Deterding C: Computer access options. In Hammel J, editor: *Technology and occupational therapy: a link to function*, Rockville, Md, 1996, American Occupational Therapy Association.
17. Dickey R, Loeser A, Specht E: Environmental control for persons with disabilities. In Bedford J, Basmajian J, Trautman P, editors: *Orthotics: clinical practice and rehabilitation technology*, New York, 1995, Churchill Livingstone.
18. Enders A, Hall M: *Assistive technology sourcebook*, Washington, DC, 1990, RESNA Press.
19. Fishman I: *Electronic communication aids*, Boston, 1987, College-Hill Press.
20. Flippio K, Inge K, Barcus J: *Assistive technology: a resource for school, work, and community*, Baltimore, 1995, Paul HJ Brookes.
21. Hammel J, editor: *Technology and occupational therapy; a link to function*, Rockville, Md, 1996, American Occupational Therapy Association.
22. Hammel J, Angelo J: Technology competencies for occupational therapy practitioners. *Assistive Technology* 8:34, 1996.
23. Hopkins HL, Smith HD, editors: *Willard and Spackman's occupational therapy*, ed 6. Philadelphia, 1983, Lippincott.
24. Joe BE: International symposium focuses on emergency response devices. *Occupational Therapy Week* 4:4, 1990.
25. Lange M: Selecting environmental controls. *Team-Rehab* 6:43, 1995.
26. Lee K, Thomas D: *Control of computer-based technology for people with physical disabilities*, Toronto, 1990, Toronto Press.
27. Mann WC et al: The use of phones by elders with disabilities: problems, interventions, costs, *Assistive Technology* 8:23, 1996.
28. Mann WC, Lane JP: *Assistive technology for persons with disabilities*, Bethesda, Md, 1995, American Occupational Therapy Association.
29. Mosey AC: *Psychosocial components of occupational therapy*, New York, 1986, Raven.
30. Nunnally MR: Technology as a therapeutic modality for older adults: a continuum of tasks for improved function, safety, and quality of life. In Hammel J, editor: *Technology and occupational therapy: a link to function*, Rockville, Md, 1996, American Occupational Therapy Association.
31. Phillips B: Technology abandonment from the consumer point of view. *NARIC Q* 3:2, 1992.
32. Radabough MP: Keynote address, Washington, DC, June 1990, RESNA Conference.
33. Scherer MJ: Assistive technology device predisposition assessment. In *The Scherer MPT model: matching people with technologies*, Rochester, NY, 1991, Scherer Associates.
34. Smith R: *Administration and scoring manual: OT fact*, Rockville, Md, 1990, American Occupational Therapy Association.
35. *Technology-Related Assistance for Individuals with Disabilities Act*, 29 USC 2202 (2) and (3), 1990.
36. Warren CG: Powered mobility and its implications. In Todd SP, editor: *Choosing a wheelchair system*, Washington, DC, 1990, Veterans Health Services and Research Administration.
37. Webster JG, Cook AM, Tompkins WJ, et al, editors: *Electronic devices for rehabilitation*, New York, 1985, John Wiley & Sons.
38. Williams BW et al: *Lifespace access profile: assistive technology planning for individuals with severe or multiple disabilities*, Sebastopol, Calif, 1993, Authors.
39. Wright C, Nomura M: *From toys to computers: access for the physically disabled child*, ed 2. San Jose, Calif, 1990, Wright.

jennie w. sullivan

patricia a. ryan

chapter 22

Activities of Daily Living Adaptations: Managing the Environment With One-Handed Techniques

key terms

basic activities of daily living

instrumental activities of daily living

adaptive techniques

adaptive devices

environmental modifications

work simplification and energy conservation

chapter objectives

After completing this chapter, the reader will be able to accomplish the following:

1. Explore a variety of adaptive techniques and assistive devices to allow for completion of activities of daily living.
2. Enhance performance of activities of daily living using principles of energy conservation and work simplification.
3. Explore environmental modifications to enhance safety and ease of mobility in the performance of activities of daily living.

Occupational therapy intervention for stroke survivors is geared toward ameliorating deficits resulting from stroke and varies tremendously from one patient to another. For certain individuals, limited return of functional use of the involved extremity makes performance of both self-care and instrumental activities of daily living (IADL) uniquely challenging. According to the study *Compensation in Recovery of Upper Extremity Function After Stroke*,[4] the emphasis of intervention during rehabilitation for patients with extensive upper extremity paralysis should be on teaching one-handed compensatory techniques. The occupational

therapist is called to use creative problem-solving abilities to enhance independence in a wide range of activities, helping the patient achieve meaningful, realistic goals. (See Chapter 15 for a comprehensive overview of instrumental ADL.)

BASIC ENVIRONMENTAL CONSIDERATIONS

Before initiating basic ADL training, considerations regarding the variety of environments in which the patient is required to perform should be addressed. While surveying the patient's environment, the therapist should consider the following criteria:

1. Safety factors
2. Ease of mobility and performance of ADL

Safety

Helping patients negotiate the bedroom environment safely is a priority, because this is an area in which many self-care activities are performed. The height of the bed should allow the patient to sit comfortably with both feet flat on the floor so that a good base of support is provided. If the bed is too high or low, the following adaptations can be considered. Several inches can be sawed off or added to the bed posts of a wooden bed to adjust the bed height. Leg extensions are commercially available from a variety of rehabilitation catalogs. Another alternative is to remove the bed frame entirely and use only the box spring and mattress. Ideally a double mattress should be used to improve ease of mobility and provide an increased sense of security. The mattress should be firm to allow for increased postural stability and improved balance. The bed should be placed within the room to allow access from both sides. Use of a transfer handle positioned on the patient's noninvolved side improves safety and ease of mobility in and out of the bed (Figure 22-1).

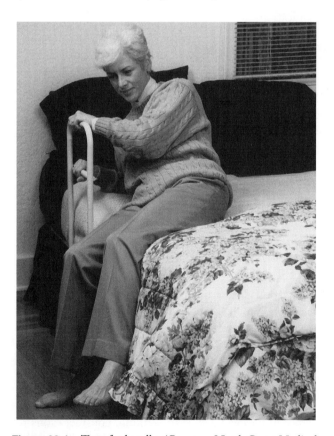

Figure 22-1 Transfer handle. (Courtesy North Coast Medical, San Jose, Calif.)

Bedroom furniture should be rearranged to eliminate obstacles hindering the patient from negotiating a path to the bathroom or room exit. If possible, changes in the floor surface should be avoided. Bare floor surface changing to raised carpeting, for example, may increase the risk of falls.

The sensory environment is another component to be considered. Factors such as sufficient lighting and a comfortable room temperature must be ensured. If inadequate, both conditions present safety obstacles. For example, if the room temperature is too cold, the patient may experience an increase in muscle activity possibly decreasing postural stability and the ability to perform self-care tasks successfully. (See Chapter 20 for a detailed review of home modifications.)

Ease of Mobility and Performance of Activities of Daily Living

In addition to the safety of the environment, the therapist also must consider arrangement of the bedroom to increase ease of mobility and performance of ADL. Energy conservation and work simplification techniques may be used to teach the patient ways to prioritize, organize, and limit work to save time and energy and enhance the successful outcome of task performance. The following techniques should be considered:

1. Eliminate excess space. Enough space must be available for ease of mobility without excess. Excess space forces a patient to travel greater distances, draining personal energy resources. For example, the bathroom should ideally be directly off the bedroom rather than down the hall. If this arrangement is not possible, a bedside commode and sitting table with a mirror that can be set up to allow for performance of toileting and grooming are useful modifications. A living room can be used to replace an out-of-the-way bedroom.
2. Arrange the room so that sequential tasks can be performed with minimal travel time in between.
3. Place appliances and controls where they can be easily accessed. Lamps, alarm clocks, and telephones should be placed where they are most often needed and most convenient for the patient. The use of environmental control units should be considered (see Chapter 21).
4. Eliminate clutter. Thorough cleaning and organization is essential to allow for easy retrieval of commonly needed items.
5. Arrange for easy access of clothing and toileting supplies by eliminating excess reaching and bending. Shelves are easier to access than drawers. If drawers are used, they are easier to open with a central knob rather than handles. Also, closet rods can be lowered to eliminate excess reaching. An alternative solution includes use of a reacher.

Therapists must be aware of the impact of neurobehavioral deficits that impact on both basic activities of daily living (BADL) and instrumental activities of daily living (IADL). These deficits influence equipment choices and training techniques (see Chapter 13).

BASIC ACTIVITIES OF DAILY LIVING

The United States Department of Health and Human Services has published poststroke rehabilitation guidelines in which several BADL instruments are described, including the Barthel index, Functional Independence Measure (FIM), Mini-Mental State Examination (MMSE), and Neurobehavioral Cognitive Status Examination (NCSE). Information regarding validity, reliability, sensitivity, and strengths and weaknesses of each instrument can be gathered by reviewing the guidelines in depth. Guidelines can be obtained by contacting the United States Department of Health and Human Services.[8]

Grooming and Hygiene

When performing hygiene and grooming activities, assistive devices and alternative methods often provide increased independence and safety and decreased energy expenditure.

Toileting

A toilet tissue dispenser should be mounted within easy reach of the unaffected side and allow for easy one-handed retrieval of tissue sheets. Two possibilities include a tissue box dispenser mounted on the bathroom wall or an easy-load toilet paper holder, which eliminates excessive paper roll waste. This alternative gives a more aesthetic appearance, possibly improving acceptance by the patient (Figure 22-2). Moist towelettes can be used in place of toilet paper. This is a viable alternative for patients with urgency or impaired sphincter control. Assistive devices are commercially available for one-handed self-catheterization, as well as one-handed female urinals (see Recommended Resources).

Showering and Bathing

Transferring from a slippery tub, controlling water temperature, and washing adequately in a slippery tub are all safety factors to be considered during bathing.[2] No-slip mats should be placed both inside and outside the tub. All toiletries should be placed where they can be easily reached. Articles should be moved close together if the individual is sitting on a tub bench to ensure safe reaching. To ensure safety of water temperature and ease of bathing, a hand-held shower hose with control of water flow may be used to prevent scalding. This device can be purchased through a variety of catalogues.

Long-handled scrub sponges and bath brushes are excellent assistive devices for washing. A flex sponge is able to bend in any direction to wash all of the body, including the

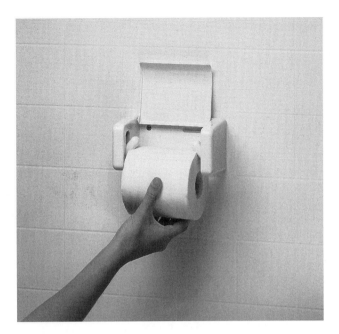

Figure 22-2 Easy-Load toilet paper holder. (Courtesy Sammons Preston, Inc., a BISSELL Company.)

nonaffected arm, axilla, and shoulder, which may be difficult to reach (Figure 22-3). Soap on a rope or a suction soap holder may be used to prevent soap from slipping about or getting lost in the water. The soap on the rope is either hung around the neck or hung within easy reach. Another alternative is to use liquid soap in a pump container. A soaper sponge also may be used to wash without having to hold a slippery bar of soap. If grasp is limited, a terry cloth wash mitt with a pocket to hold the bar of soap can be used. The above devices may be purchased through a variety of rehabilitation catalogues. For those who must rely on another to bathe them, a mechanical lift positions the person in a body sling. This lifting device has a swing arm to allow a person to be suspended in a shower or over a tub.

Shampooing

Shampoo in a pump spray bottle helps avoid waste and reaches a broader area of the scalp. A full spray hand-held shower is convenient for rinsing.

Drying

To decrease energy expenditure while drying, an extra-large towel or terry wraparound robe can be worn to absorb most of the water. The back and nonaffected arm are the most difficult areas to dry. The following procedure can be incorporated:

1. Place the towel over one shoulder.
2. Reach behind and grasp the other end, pulling the towel down across the back.
3. Repeat the same procedure over the opposite shoulder.

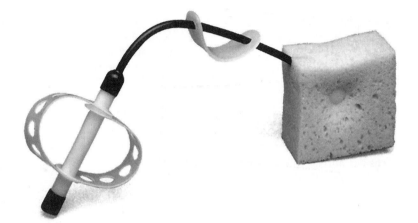

Figure 22-3   Flex sponge. (Courtesy Sammons Preston, Inc., a BISSELL Company.)

An alternative method is to toss the towel over the top of a doorway and shut the door as much as possible to hold the towel in place. The towel can then be pulled across the back and shoulder with the nonaffected extremity.

Washing at the Sink

Some individuals may have difficulty showering or bathing for a variety of reasons. An alternative method is to have body washes at the sink. The easiest position in which to wash the affected arm is to place the arm and axilla in the sink basin. To wash the unaffected arm, the individual steadies the soapy washcloth over the edge of the sink and rubs the arm and hand over it.[1] The rest of the body is then washed with one hand. Again, a flex sponge may be used to wash all of the body, including the nonaffected extremity. A supplement to washing at the sink is the use of a bidet. The Hygenique Plus Bidet/Sitz Bath System is specially designed for personal hygiene needs. This system combines a spray wand for bidet cleansing and a sitz bath (Figure 22-4).

For individuals with very low endurance who are unable to shower or bathe at the sink, a total-body pH-balanced cleanser may be used for shampooing, bathing, and incontinence care. This product is available through a variety of rehabilitation catalogues. Drying techniques are the same as previously described.

Performing Oral Hygiene

Oral hygiene care can easily be done with one hand. A toothpaste dispenser can dispense the correct amount of toothpaste on the brush for individuals with limited hand function (Figure 22-5). The method of brushing (electric or manual) is a personal choice. The use of an electric toothbrush may decrease energy expenditure because the brush vibrates up and down, holding the arm in one position. A Waterpik attachment is excellent for massaging the gums and rinsing between the teeth. Suction toothbrushes may be attached to a suction unit to prevent dysphagia-related aspiration in individuals who cannot tolerate thin liquids.

The simplest method for denture care is to soak them overnight in a commercial denture cleanser. If additional

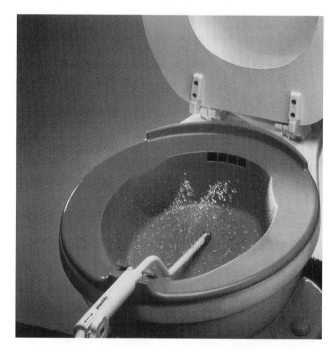

Figure 22-4   Hygenique Plus Bidet/Sitz Bath System. (Courtesy North Coast Medical, San Jose, Calif.)

cleansing is needed, a suction denture brush can be used.

Flossing teeth with one hand can be performed easily and effectively with a dental floss holder (Figure 22-6).

Applying Deodorant

Aerosol sprays are easier to apply to the unaffected arm unless the individual has sufficient function to reach the axilla with a roll-on or stick applicator. The affected axilla must be passively placed away from the body to apply deodorant. This can be accomplished by bending forward at the hips, allowing gravity to assist the arm away from the body.

Caring for Fingernails

Nail care of the affected hand can easily be done with the noninvolved hand. Cleaning, cutting, and filing the nails of the unaffected hand is more difficult.

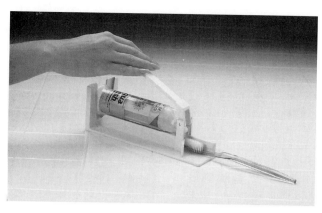

Figure 22-5 Toothpaste dispenser. (Courtesy Sammons Preston, Inc., a BISSELL Company.)

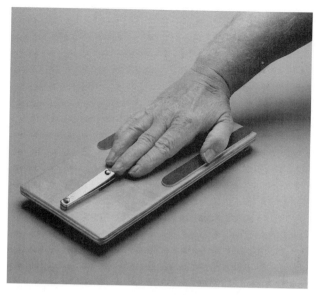

Figure 22-7 One-hand fingernail clipper. (Courtesy Maddak, Pequannock, NJ.)

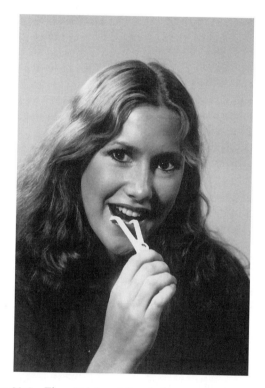

Figure 22-6 Floss Aid dental floss holder. (Courtesy Maddak, Pequannock, NJ.)

The following strategies may be used to ease nail management:

1. To clean the unaffected hand, a nail brush with suction cups can be used for cleaning fingernails.
2. To cut the nails of the unaffected hand, a one-hand fingernail clipper may be used. When the board is pressed down, the jaws of the clipper close (Figure 22-7).
3. Filing the nails of the unaffected hand can be done in a variety of ways. A suction emery board can be used. Other individuals may choose to use a home-made device such as an emery board or sandpaper glued to a piece of wood,[6] a nailfile secured to a table with masking tape,[7] or a file wedged in a drawer.[3]
4. Applying nail polish to the unaffected hand can be done by mounting a clothespin on a piece of wood with a C-clamp to hold the polish brush. The polish is applied when the person moves their nail in relation to the brush.

Caring for Toenails

Cleansing toes can be accomplished with the use of a footbrush or Footmate System (Figure 22-8). Clipping toenails is easier if the feet are soaked in warm water first. A pistol-grip remote toenail clipper is one of several devices designed for one-handed use to clip toenails; it allows the foot to be reached with less bending (Figure 22-9).

Hairstyling

Simple short hairstyles are the easiest to manage with one hand. Combing or styling long hair may be easier if adjustable long-handled grooming accessories, available through various rehabilitation catalogues, are used. Lightweight splinting material also may be used to extend the handles of an individual's favorite grooming tools.

Blow-drying hair can be made easier by using a commercial product called the Hands-Free Hair Dryer Holder, which allows the unaffected hand free operation to style hair (Figure 22-10). An alternative method is a home-devised product such as a position adjustable hair dryer. A lightweight blow-dryer, a desk lamp with spring-balanced arms, a tension control knob at each joint, and a mounting bracket are the only materials needed to fabricate the de-

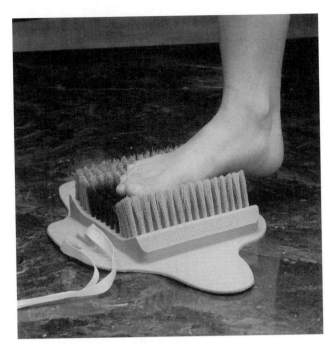

Figure 22-8 Footmate System. (Courtesy North Coast Medical, San Jose, Calif.)

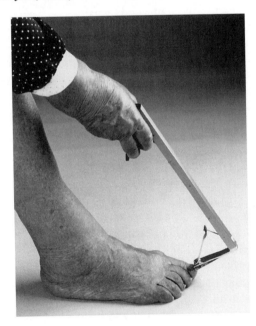

Figure 22-9 Pistol-grip remote toenail clipper. (Courtesy Maddack, Pequannock, NJ.)

vice. The position-adjustable hair dryer requires limited body movement because the dryer can be positioned in any plane desired.[2]

Brush attachments to the hair dryer also can be used for blow-drying styles. A hot brush curling system can be used for setting hair in simple hairstyles.

Shaving

Shaving can be done one handed with any type of razor. If a patient is unsteady with the motor skills, a Silk Ef-

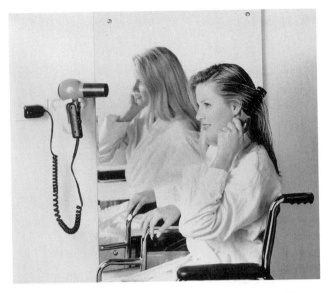

Figure 22-10 Hands-free hair dryer holder. (Courtesy Sammons Preston, Inc., a BISSELL Company.)

fects razor reduces the risks of nicking the skin. An electric razor is easily managed with one hand and is recommended for safety to prevent nicks.

Applying Makeup

Makeup may be applied one handed with practice. Grip and bottle makeup holders are useful to stabilize supplies; suction cups and rubber mats also help stabilize grooming items.

Feeding Techniques

Positioning at the Table

The affected extremity should be supported in a good weight-bearing position on the table. This position promotes appropriate upper extremity alignment, visual awareness of the extremity, and trunk symmetry.

Using Adaptive Devices

To avoid embarrassment while dining with others and reach full independence with feeding, compensatory strategies and adaptive equipment are often used. The following equipment is recommended:

- Nonskid mats should be used to prevent slippage of plates and bowls and to hold them steady during meals.
- Plate guards and scoop dishes are recommended to eliminate food getting pushed off the plate while scooping or when buttering bread.
- A rocker knife or knife with serrated and curved edges is easily used with one hand if safety awareness is intact.
- Combined implements such as knife and fork or knife, fork, and spoon are available for purchase. Safety in using these combined instruments is a con-

cern if loss of sensation or weakness in oral-motor structures is present.[3] Utensils with built-up handles also may be used to assist a weak grasp.

Dressing

Retraining an individual with hemiplegia who is limited to the use of one hand to dress presents challenges to both the patient and the therapist. Specific deficits that must be addressed include the following:

1. Impaired postural stability and balance
2. Decreased dexterity and work speed
3. Impaired ability to stabilize clothing articles and body parts
4. Decreased endurance accompanied by increased energy demands on the body
5. Impaired sensory capabilities
6. Possible cognitive and perceptual limitations

When retraining the patient in dressing techniques, the therapist should incorporate adequate time and allowances for rest breaks into the session. The patient should be able to achieve success without undue effort. Loose-fitting clothes should be selected. Roomy clothes with limited fasteners allow for increased ease of movement and easier donning and doffing.

Dressing and undressing invariably involve awkward movement patterns and a certain amount of sitting down and standing up. Care must be taken to ensure that the danger of falling is minimized. Management of clothes is always difficult at first; the occupational therapist should reinforce to the individual that independence and efficiency are achieved through practice.

Fasteners

Many individuals with hemiplegia can learn to manage fasteners if the following requirements are met:

- Garments fit loosely.
- Buttons and hooks are of a larger size.
- Fasteners are positioned either in front of or on the nonaffected side of the garment and are within sight.

Buttons

If the patient is unable to manage fasteners, the following adaptation can be applied. Remove the buttons from the garment and then sew them back on over the button holes. Using Velcro squares, sew the loop side of the Velcro over the original button side of the garment. Sew the hook side of the Velcro under the buttonholes. The patient then simply uses hand pressure to close the garment.[3]

Zippers

Zippers may be easier to manage if a ring or loop is added to the zipper tab. Open-ended zips should be avoided. Leave the zip fastened at the bottom and don the

garment by pulling it on over the head. A large safety pin left fastened can prevent the zipper from sliding all the way down and detaching during overhead donning.

Adaptive Dressing Techniques

Before initiating dressing training, the therapist should ensure the patient is seated on a stable, supportive surface, preferably a sturdy armchair. Both of the patient's feet should be securely positioned on the floor to establish a solid base of support and increase postural stability. Clothing should be placed within easy reach and in the order in which each item is required. This helps maximize energy preservation.

A wide variety of dressing techniques are described in the literature, depending on the particular treatment theory incorporated by the therapist. Some general principles that facilitate ease of one-handed dressing are described in the following sections.

Upper Extremity Dressing

Donning Garments with Front Fasteners (Figure 22-11)

1. Pull the shirtsleeve onto the affected arm.
2. Pull the shirtsleeve over the affected shoulder.
3. Swing the garment around until the other sleeve hangs down the back or pull the sleeve over the head and around the neck. The patient may even anchor it by biting the sleeve.
4. Reach to the back with the nonaffected arm and place it into the opening of the remaining sleeve.
5. Using a shrugging motion with the nonaffected arm, straighten the sleeve into place.

Shirtsleeves may need to be expanded or loose-fitting to be pulled over the noninvolved hand. This can be achieved by sewing a piece of elastic into the sleeve cuff to allow for easy passage over the hand[3] and to eliminate the difficulty of managing a cuff button.

The top button of a shirt collar is often difficult to fasten. The button is usually small, and the collar fits snugly around the neck. The problem can be eliminated by replacing the button with a Velcro fastener.[3]

Donning Ties

Ties are difficult to manipulate single handedly. The simplest solution is to use a conventional already tied tie. A piece of elastic may be inserted into the back of the tie to replace a small part of the fabric. This allows for easy passage of the tie over the head.[3] Clip-on ties also are convenient to use.

Donning Pullover Shirts

1. Shirt tags or labels should be used to identify the front and back side of the garment.
2. Pull the correct sleeve onto the affected arm, and pull the garment onto the affected shoulder.
3. Bend the head forward through the neck opening.

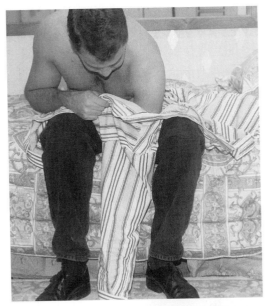
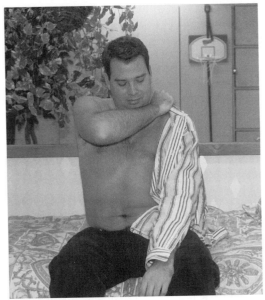

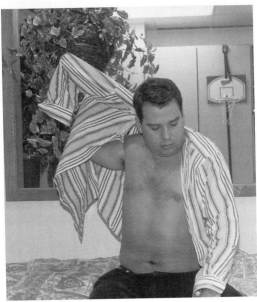

Figure 22-11   Sequence for upper extremity dressing for a patient with left hemiplegia.

4. Put the nonaffected arm into the other sleeve.
5. Straighten the sleeve by rubbing the arm against the leg.
6. Pull the garment over the torso.

Donning Brassieres

Front-fastening bras are easier to manage than bras that fasten in back. The bra should be donned by putting the affected arm in first. Another method is to fasten the bra first and then put the bra on by donning it over the head. Larger hooks can be substituted for smaller hooks, or a Velcro strap and D ring may be sewn in as substitutions for the fastener.[3] A bra extender can be purchased and inter-changed between bras; increasing the girth accommodation can ease donning.

Back-closure bras may be managed in the following way[3]:

1. Align the bra around the waist so that the cups face back. The strap can be held in place by hugging it with the affected arm, by tucking into the elasticized panty waist, or by using a clothespin to hold it onto the pants.
2. Fasten the hooks in front.
3. Swivel the bra around so that the cups are in front.
4. Pull the strap over the affected shoulder.

5. Using the thumb of the nonaffected hand, pull the strap over the nonaffected shoulder.

The easiest solution, although not necessarily the most aesthetic, is a fully elasticized bra such as a sports bra, which can be slipped on over the head. A hook-and-eye bra can be adapted by sewing the back fasteners together.[3]

Lower Extremity Dressing

Donning Pants and Underwear While Lying in Bed
1. Bend the affected leg until the foot is within reach. The unaffected leg may be used to assist with this.
2. Place the pants over the affected foot and allow the leg to straighten into the pant leg.
3. Put the nonaffected leg into the pants and pull the pants up as far as possible.
4. Using the nonaffected leg or if possible both legs, lift the pelvis off the bed. Wriggle the pants up to the waist.
5. Fasten the pants. (Velcro may be used in place of buttons.)

Donning Pants and Underwear While Sitting Up (Figure 22-12)[3]
1. While sitting (preferably on a firm surface), cross the affected leg over the nonaffected leg. Use clasped hands to lift the leg.
2. Put the correct pant leg over the affected foot and pull it onto the leg.
3. Dress the nonaffected leg.
4. Pull the pants up as far as possible while sitting; shift weight over each buttock.
5. Stand up to pull the pants up around the waist. If balance is impaired, lean against a wall or sturdy piece of furniture to provide support and minimize the risk of falling.

Donning Skirts
1. Put the skirt over the head and then pull it down.
2. Make sure to maneuver the fasteners to the front or the nonaffected side for increased ease of fastening.
3. Twist the skirt around to the correct position.

A skirt with an elasticized waist that expands to pass over the head may be simpler.

Donning Socks (Figure 22-13)
1. Cross the affected leg over the other leg, using clasped hands to lift the leg.
2. With the leg in place, open the sock using the thumb and index finger of the nonaffected hand. Roll the sock down to the heel before slipping it on for greater ease in donning.

3. Bend forward at the hips to assist in reaching the foot. Pull the sock over the foot.
4. Don the sock on the nonaffected foot in the same fashion.

Donning Shoes (Figure 22-14)
1. Choose shoes that provide good support. A broad heel can provide better stability if balance is poor. Men's standard dress shoes have a toe spring built into the front. For a patient recovering from stroke, it may assist with toe clearance during the swing phase of gait.
2. Bring the affected foot closer to the body by crossing it over the nonaffected leg or by using a small footstool.
3. With the leg in place, open the shoe as much as possible before attempting to put it on.
4. Bend forward at the hips to reach the foot. Place the shoe over the ball of the foot and pull it on. A helpful technique to aid with getting the shoe over the foot is to mold a small piece of splinting material onto the shoe heel and allow it to harden. This helps to keep the heel rigid, preventing it from buckling under as the foot slides in.
5. Shoes with Velcro closures are quite easily managed with one hand. Shoelaces can be substituted with elastic laces or coilers that do not require tying.

Donning Lower Extremity Orthotics
Lower extremity orthotics can be difficult to manage one handed, and assistance may be required. In general, the donning of orthotics is easier if placed into the shoe first. An adaptation to the pant leg that may be helpful in donning the orthotic is to open the inseam of the pant cuff to the desired length. Stitch the loop side of a Velcro strip underneath the top of the seam and the hook side to the front of the seam. The pant leg can then be opened up, allowing for easier manipulation of the orthotic over the calf.

Adaptive Devices

Adaptive dressing devices should be introduced only if the patient cannot otherwise perform dressing safely or efficiently. Dressing devices that might be considered include the following:

1. A reacher, particularly if a patient has poor trunk control
2. A dressing stick, which can be useful to extend reach if trunk balance is impaired and to push garments off the affected side
3. A long-handled shoehorn, which may assist the patient in slipping on shoes

All of the above devices are available from a variety of rehabilitation catalogues.

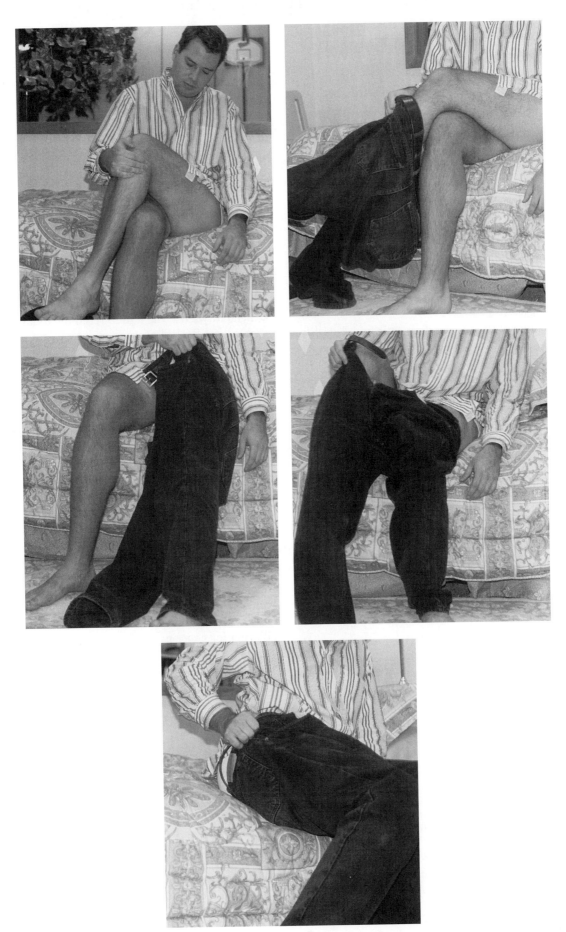

Figure 22-12 Sequence for donning pants and underwear for a patient with left hemiplegia.

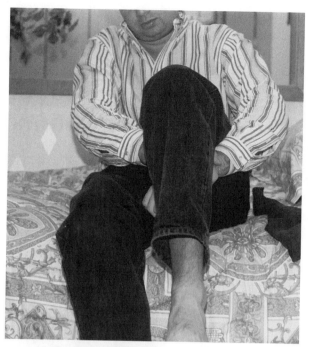

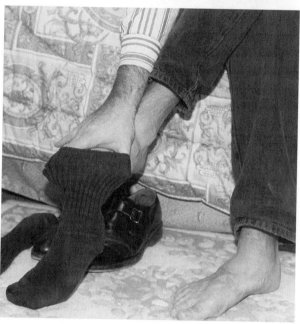
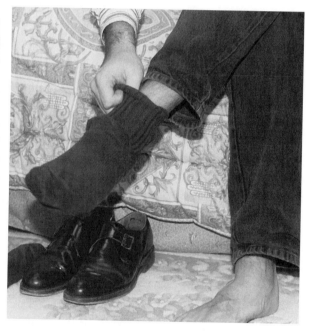

Figure 22-13 Sequence for donning socks for a patient with left hemiplegia.

INSTRUMENTAL ACTIVITIES OF DAILY LIVING

Kitchen Activities

Kitchen tasks can be safely accomplished by an individual with hemiplegia if adequate activity pacing, properly placed secured equipment, and adaptive devices are provided.

Energy Conservation and Work Simplification

A consequence of weakness and impaired upper extremity function is that the individual with hemiplegia tires more quickly and thus needs to work at a slower pace. The following energy conservation guidelines should be included in treatment plans focusing on increasing instrumental activities of daily living (IADL):

- Allow increased time for task completion.
- Take frequent short rest breaks.
- Sit when working, when possible.
- Avoid complicated procedures.
- Use ready-prepared foods when possible.

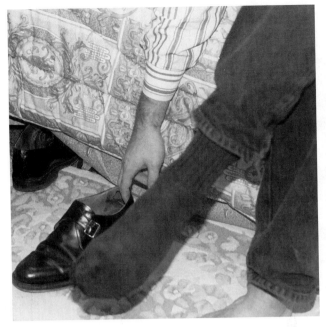

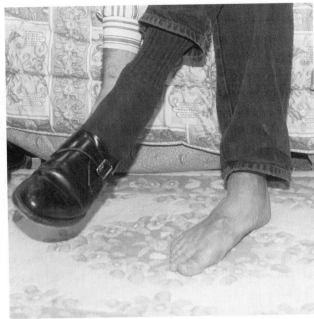

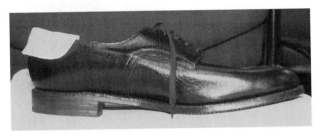

Figure 22-14 **A** and **B,** Sequence for donning shoes for a patient with left hemiplegia. **C,** Heel support fabricated from low-temperature plastic.

- Use labor-saving equipment. (Electrical equipment such as microwaves and food processors with easy-to-control on and off switches and self-cleaning ovens and self-defrosting freezers reduce manual labor requirements.)
- Arrange work surfaces at a height that allows for maximal efficiency.
- Avoid excess reaching and bending.
- Reduce clutter.

To allow for easy access to supplies, items needed most often should be kept on convenient shelves at the front of the most accessible cupboards and drawers or at the back of the work surface.

Storage

A variety of storage devices can be purchased that enhance easy equipment access[3]:

- Plastic-covered racks either slide under or clip to the underside of shelves, increasing visible storage space. They can be purchased at hardware stores.
- Peg-Boards can be hung on the wall and used to hang small pots, strainers, kitchen tongs, and spatulas.
- Magnetic knife racks can be placed over a counter top and can be used to store knives, peelers, and kitchen scissors.

- Lazy Susans, which can be placed in easy-to-reach cupboards or at the back of a counter, are useful for people who have trouble bending or reaching beyond the front of the cabinet; they allow for convenient storage of jars, cans, and bottles.

Transport

Moving supplies safely about the kitchen is another significant challenge for the person with hemiplegia. To avoid lifting and carrying, a rolling cart can be used for transporting items from one side of the kitchen to the other. Ideally, the cart should have a handle at one end to provide support while walking. Dycem can be used to help secure items on the cart shelves. A clip secured to the side of the cart with glue can be used to hold a cane or walking device while the person pushes the cart with the noninvolved hand.[3]

Stabilization

Cooking activities can be successfully accomplished single handedly if adequate stabilization of items is provided. Tasks such as opening packages and containers, peeling, slicing, making sandwiches, stirring, and mixing create problems that can usually be solved by a variety of self-help devices. Commonly used and readily accessible items for self-help are described in the following paragraphs.

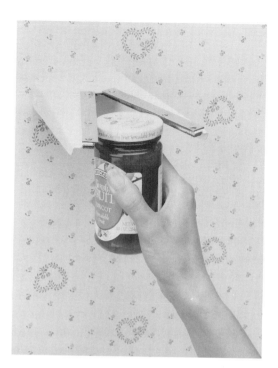

Figure 22-15   Zim jar opener. (Courtesy North Coast Medical, San Jose, Calif.)

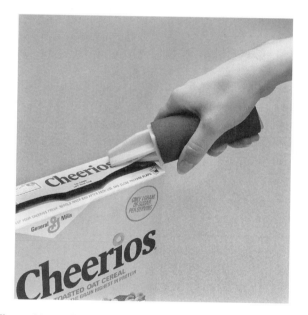

Figure 22-16   Boxtopper. (Courtesy North Coast Medical, San Jose, Calif.)

The Zim jar opener is easily mounted to the wall or underside of a cabinet and allows for one-handed screw cap removal of lids measuring from ½ to 3½ in in diameter (Figure 22-15).

A Sure Shot jar opener combined with a Belliclamp allows for easy opening of jar lids for individuals with weak grasps or use of only one hand. The Belliclamp is used to hold jars and bottles securely during use of the jar opener. Lightweight electric or cordless can openers are easy to

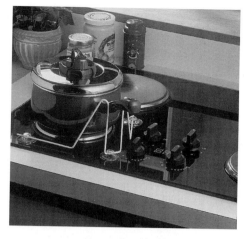

Figure 22-17   Pan holder. (Courtesy Sammons Preston, Inc., a BISSELL Company.)

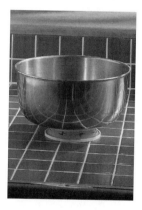

Figure 22-18   Stay Put Suction Disc. (Courtesy Sammons Preston, Inc., a BISSELL Company.)

use with one hand and are available from a variety of product catalogues and appliance stores.

Cardboard boxes containing cereals, rice, and instant potatoes can be opened one handed by stabilizing them firmly in a kitchen drawer and then carefully using scissors or the point of a knife to slit the boxtop open. Boxtoppers are inexpensive devices that easily slide open boxtops and are ideal for one-handed use (Figure 22-16).

Pan holders keep pots and pans stabilized on a range top while the individual stirs or sautés one handed and are important to prevent spillage of hot food (Figure 22-17).

A common device for stabilizing equipment and food items during food preparation is Dycem. It is made from gelatinous material, is nonslip on both sides and is an easy, inexpensive alternative to help secure items such as pans and mixing bowls in place during cooking. The Stay Put Suction Disc provides another means of securing bowls and plates to any smooth surface using vacuum pressure (Figure 22-18). Mixing bowls with suction bases are available from a variety of product catalogues and allow for more vigorous one-handed stirring without sliding or tipping.

Cutting boards designed for one-handed use and designed from wood, formica, or plastic come equipped with rubber suction feet to secure the board in place. Stainless steel nails hold food in place for cutting and chopping. Food guards keep food from sliding while the individual spreads butter or sandwich spreads. Cutting boards can easily be fabricated using 2-in thick wood and nails.

Food Storage

Rigid plastic containers with overlapping lids are usually easily opened and sealed with one hand.[3] Plastic containers with screw top lids are ideal for storing rice, sugar, flour, and other items that pour. Aluminum foil molds easily with one hand and is useful for covering containers and wrapping food that requires refrigeration.

Dish Washing

Nonstick cooking utensils are easy to clean and make the cleanup process go quicker.[3] Oven-to-table cookware cuts down on the number of supplies used. Pots and pans can be stabilized for scrubbing by positioning them on a wet dishcloth positioned in the corner of the sink.[3] For washing cups and glasses, a brush suctioned to the inside of the sink such as a suction bottle brush can be used (Figure 22-19).

Home Maintenance

Work simplification methods should be applied in the performance of household tasks. Housework requires a great deal of mobility and necessitates getting into awkward po-

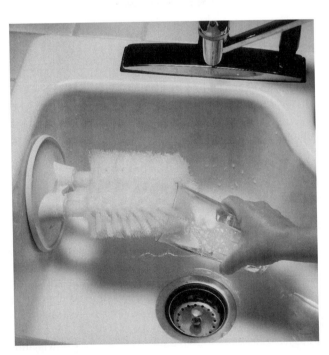

Figure 22-19 Suction bottle brush. (Courtesy North Coast Medical, San Jose, Calif.)

sitions. Housework can be made easier if clutter is removed from the house. Time spent dusting is cut in half without added clutter. To conserve personal energy and ensure ease of performance, adaptive devices such as lightweight, long-handled, and electronic tools may serve as useful supplements.

Caring for the Floor

Long-handled, freestanding dustpans, self-wringing sponge mops, electric floor scrubbers, light upright vacuum cleaners with helping hand attachments, and no-wax floors can ease the maintenance of floor care. While mopping the floor, the individual should use a rectangular bucket.[3] This allows the sponge mop to be fully soaked with water in a half-filled bucket as opposed to a round bucket.[3] The bucket should be filled and emptied on the floor with a plastic jug to avoid heavy lifting.[3]

Cleaning the Bathroom

A long-handled reach sponge mop should be used. This product is available through a variety of rehabilitation catalogues. The risk of falling is great and kneeling or sitting should be considered in the performance of this household task.[3]

Extra cleaning materials should be kept both upstairs and downstairs to avoid unnecessary journeys.[3] Items can be transported in an apron with large pockets, a shoulder bag, or a wheeled cart.

Bed Making

Bed making can be difficult with only one hand. Beds should be positioned so that access to both sides is easy. To conserve energy, bed making can be accomplished by completing each corner of one side from the undersheet to bedspread before moving to the other side to repeat the operation.

Changing Sheets

Sheets can be easily managed if folded or unfolded in position on the bed. Pillows should be kept on the bed during changing of the pillowcases so that the bed takes the weight of the pillow.[3]

Laundry

Machine Washing Clothes

The individual should select fabric and garment designs that are completely machine washable and dryable. Automatic machines should be used.

Hand Washing Clothes

Soaking articles overnight in soap or detergent can minimize the effort to remove dirt with one hand. A washboard can be useful for scrubbing out dirt and stubborn stains.

Wringing Clothes

Small articles can be rolled in a towel and squeezed to remove excess water. Clothes can be wrung out with one hand. Drip-dry clothes should be placed on a hanger before they are removed from the sink.

Ironing

A lightweight iron should be used. Steam irons are efficient at removing creases. Steamers also can remove creases from many materials.

Most ironing boards are height adjustable so that the individual can sit or stand when using them. Ironing boards can be difficult and heavy to manage with one hand. The board may be left permanently standing if space permits. Ironing also can be done on the kitchen table or a counter covered with a folded towel or sheet.

Sewing

Threading Needles

A needle can easily be threaded with one hand if it is held in a pincushion, padded armchair, or bar of soap. Self-threading needles and automatic needle threaders also are available at most major department stores.[3]

Cutting

Material can be cut if it is stabilized by weight to prevent slipping. Although most scissors are for right-handed use, left-handed scissors and shears are available.

Hand Sewing

Hemming and sewing seams can easily be performed by placing material over a curved object such as an armchair and holding it down by weights.

Machine Sewing

Sewing machines can be used with one hand with practice according to safety guidelines.

Communication

Writing

Individuals whose strokes have affected their dominant sides need to consider dominance retraining—learning to write with the noninvolved hand. An important goal for such individuals is to be able to sign their names legibly.

Writing practice begins with exercises consisting of continuous circles and connected up and down strokes. Large strokes are practiced at first, progressing to smaller ones. With increasing proficiency, alphabet letters are practiced. At the initiation of training, a larger-size pencil, crayon, or rubber pencil grip attached to a standard pencil should be used. The paper may be stabilized with Dycem or a clamp or by weighting the paper down.

Except for meeting the requirement of a functional signature, individuals may prefer to use another method of written communication. Equipment such as personal computers, tape recorders, and typewriters all can easily be accessed by the individual with hemiplegia.

Using the Telephone

Providing for easy access to the telephone is not a significant problem. Ease of telephone use can be facilitated by use of a speaker phone. Another product, the commercially available phone holder, frees the noninvolved hand for dialing or taking messages. This device consists of a flexible arm clamped to a table, which holds the telephone receiver in a stationary position; it is available through product catalogues (see Chapter 21).

COMMUNITY-BASED ACTIVITIES

Marketing and Grocery Shopping

Energy conservation should be applied in marketing and grocery shopping. The individual should make a list of necessary items and anticipate weekly expenses to minimize trips to the cash machine. Items should be categorized according to aisles, thus limiting excess walking around the store. A lightweight pushcart can be used to carry items around the store and home if a car is not available. An alternative solution is phone and mail shopping. Individuals using wheelchairs require assistance with shopping trips. Money should be placed in an easily accessed pocket or purse to ensure easy retrieval at the checkout line.

Banking

Banking has become easier during the past decade. Individuals can easily go the bank, access money through automatic teller machines (ATMs), and bank by phone. If a signature has been altered because of loss of function in the dominant hand, the bank must be notified. Banks have varying policies regarding this situation. For the most part, the new signature can easily be placed on file. Some banks, however, require a written and notarized letter from a physician before a new signature can be authorized.

■

CASE STUDY

EB is a 74-year-old male recovering from a left cerebrovascular accident (CVA) with right hemiplegia and a medical history significant for hypertension. EB was employed as an engineer for 50 years but has been retired for the past 2 years. He is currently married, and his wife is employed full time. EB resides in a ground floor apartment with 3 steps up to enter the building.

EB was referred for home care services on discharge from the hospital. Initial occupational therapy evaluation revealed the following: He was alert and oriented to person, place, situation, and time. His cognitive perceptual status was intact. Before his stroke, EB was right-hand dominant. On evaluation, his right upper extremity was flaccid. His left upper extremity had functional range of motion and strength. Sensation was intact throughout. Static and dynamic sitting balance was good. When standing, however, he was unsteady while performing challenging tasks. His endurance for light activity was poor. EB required assistance with the following ADL tasks: bathing, grooming, feeding, dressing, simple meal preparation, writing, and community-based activities.

A number of treatment goals were established with the patient.

Long-term goals

1. EB will be independent in managing BADL using adaptive techniques and assistive devices as required.
2. EB will be independent with simple meal preparation.
3. EB will participate in IADL, such as shopping and banking.

Short-term goals

1. EB will independently bathe himself using assistive devices.
2. EB will independently clean and floss his teeth with use of assistive devices.
3. EB will be able to cut and butter food independently with a rocker knife.
4. EB will independently dress himself using adaptive techniques and devices.
5. EB will independently prepare himself lunch.
6. EB will independently perform home-based financial responsibilities.
7. EB will participate weekly in food shopping outings.

Before initiating basic ADL training, the therapist surveyed the environment to ensure safety and ease of mobility. The following changes were recommended and implemented:

1. Excess clutter was removed from the bedroom, bathroom, kitchen shelves, and drawers to ensure easier access of needed supplies. Closet rods were lowered to allow for easier access of clothing.
2. The bathroom floor rug was replaced with no-slip mats inside and outside the tub. A tub transfer bench with hand-held shower attachment was provided.
3. A board was placed under the mattress to increase firmness, and a bedrail was placed on EB's uninvolved side to increase safe transfers in and out of bed.
4. A lamp was placed on a bedside table next to EB to ensure sufficient lighting.

ADL training was initiated with several implementations made.

Bathing

1. Soap on a rope was used to stabilize the soap.
2. A flex sponge enabled EB to successfully reach all body parts.
3. A pump spray shampoo bottle was used to avoid excess waste and keep shampoo from getting into eyes.
4. One handed-drying techniques were reviewed with EB.

Oral hygiene

1. A toothpaste dispenser allowed for easy one-handed access.
2. The Floss Aid dental floss holder allowed EB to floss his teeth.

Nail management

1. A one-handed home device was fabricated from a nail clipper secured to a piece of plywood with suction feet attached.
2. A pistol-grip toenail clipper enabled EB to cut his toenails with less bending.

Feeding

A rocker knife, nonskid mat, and plate guard allowed EB to cut and butter his food successfully and without spillage.

Dressing

1. Energy conservation techniques were reviewed because of EB's poor endurance.
2. EB was able to don and doff shirts but unable to manipulate fasteners. Velcro was used to substitute for buttons.
3. EB was able to don his pants successfully with the support of a sturdy dresser placed next to the bed, which he leaned against to pull up his pants safely while standing.
4. EB was able to don his shoes after a piece of splinting material was molded into the shoe heel. Elastic laces allowed for easy fastening.

Simple meal preparation

EB was required to make lunch for himself while his wife was at work. His favorite lunch was a ham and cheese sandwich with lettuce and tomato and a glass of apple juice.

The following kitchen adaptations were made:

1. EB used a rolling cart to gather necessary supplies at one time and maneuver them to the kitchen table, where he could sit to complete the task.
2. A cutting board was fabricated using 2-inch thick wood, nails, and a plastic food guard glued to the side of the board. Using the board, EB was able to cut tomato slices successfully, stabilize lettuce, and spread mayonnaise on a slice of bread while stabilizing it against the food guard.
3. Presliced ham and cheese were stored in a plastic zipper bag that EB could easily access and seal using the zipper bag sealer.
4. Using a Zim jar opener, EB was able to open the apple juice bottle top.

Dominance retraining and financial management

EB was initially right-hand dominant. An important goal for him was to be able to sign his name legibly on legal documents. He was put on a program of writing practice exercises.

After a legible signature was obtained, EB contacted the bank and was required to submit a copy of his new signature to be placed on file.

Marketing and grocery shopping

As EB's endurance improved, shopping outings with his wife were encouraged. The following energy conservation guidelines were incorporated:

1. EB made a list of necessary items and grouped them according to aisles in order to limit excess walking.
2. A lightweight pushcart was purchased to carry items around the store and into the home.
3. Before leaving home, EB would place his money in an easily accessible pocket from which it could be quickly retrieved at the checkout line.

■

SUMMARY

This chapter described equipment recommendations and practical and creative solutions that the occupational therapist can incorporate to assist patients in becoming more independent in performing BADL and IADL. For individuals with limited functional return of the involved upper extremity, compensatory techniques are crucial during the rehabilitation process and maximize the potential for reaching meaningful goals. As always, the therapist should concentrate on activities the patient finds most meaningful and curtail activities the individual does not want to perform. For individuals with extensive paralysis resulting from stroke, family members or hired outside help may be required to assist with ADL to ensure safety.

RECOMMENDED RESOURCES

A+ Medical Products
888-843-3334
Available products include:
"ASTA-CATH" female self-catheter guide
"FEMINAL" female urinal for one-handed use in any position

Do it one-handed: a manual of daily living skills for stroke rehabilitation
Lenox House
PO Box 1097
South Orange, NJ 07079

One-handed in a two-handed world
Prince-Gallison Press
PO Box 23
Hanover Station, Mass 02113-0001

REVIEW QUESTIONS

1. When is use of compensatory strategies most advantageous as part of the rehabilitation process?
2. What environmental considerations need to be taken into account before the initiation of activity of daily living training?
3. Where can specific information regarding the reliability and validity of basic activity of daily living evaluation instruments be obtained?
4. What are some compensatory techniques and adaptive devices an individual may use during grooming and hygiene to compensate for loss of one upper extremity?
5. Which specific deficits need to be considered before the initiation of dressing training?
6. What energy conservation and work simplification techniques should be considered during instrumental activity of daily living training?
7. Which compensatory techniques and adaptive devices should be considered to compensate during kitchen-based activities for loss of one upper extremity?
8. What types of adaptive devices should be considered for easier performance of home-maintenance activities?
9. If a signature has been altered as a result of loss of function in the dominant hand, what issues need to be addressed before the patient resumes financial responsibilities?

■ COTA Considerations ■

- Adaptive equipment should be issued to increase the efficiency, effectiveness, and safety of activity of daily living performance.
- Do not overprescribe equipment; for many patients (particularly those with neurobehavioral impairments), less is more.
- Encourage patients to use affected limbs during activities of daily living as much as possible. Issuing equipment too early may lead to learned nonuse of the involved limbs.
- Evaluate safety awareness and cognitive status of the patient before issuing assistive devices that may be potentially harmful (e.g., rocker knives).

REFERENCES

1. Davies P: (1991) *Steps to follow*, Berlin, 1991, Springer-Verlag.
2. Feldmeier DM, Poole JL: The position adjustable hair dryer, *Am J Occup Ther* 41:246, 1987.
3. Jay P: *Help yourselves*, Essex, England, 1979, Ian Henry.
4. Nakayama H et al: Compensation in recovery of upper extremity function after stroke: the Copenhagen stroke study, *Arch Phys Med Rehabil* 75:852, 1994.
5. Ozner M, Materson R, Caplan L: *Management of persons with stroke*, St Louis, 1994, Mosby.
6. Pedretti L, Zoltan B: *Occupational therapy practice skills for physical dysfunction*, St Louis, 1990, Mosby.
7. Trombly C: *Occupational therapy for physical dysfunction*, Baltimore, 1989, Williams and Wilkins.
8. U.S. Department of Health and Human Services: *Clinical practice guideline #16: post stroke rehabilitation*, Rockville, Md, 1995, Author.

nancy c. whyte
denise a. supon

chapter **23**

Leisure: Methods to Improve Skills

key terms

leisure

models of leisure

types of leisure

leisure roles

leisure attitudes

leisure satisfaction

activity analysis

intrinsic barriers

external barriers

communication barriers

Leisure-Ability Model

activities of daily living

adaptive equipment for leisure

chapter objectives

After completing this chapter, the reader will be able to accomplish the following:

1. Define leisure, types of leisure, and functions of leisure activities.
2. Discuss the changes in an individual's ability to engage in leisure tasks after a CVA.
3. Describe problems that may interfere with a patient's participation in leisure tasks. (Evaluation of leisure skills will be analyzed.)
4. Present possible solutions to these problems (treatment techniques).
5. Discuss research addressing leisure participation after stroke.
6. Outline ways occupational therapists can adapt leisure tasks to allow partial or full participation by someone with a disability caused by a CVA.

Occupational therapy includes the consideration of leisure. Although insurance companies may be reluctant to cover this area of intervention, occupational therapists are professionally obligated to address changes in patients' leisure roles, as well as use patients' leisure interests to plan treatment sessions. This area of functioning is critical in the assessment of patients' motivation, quality of life, and self-esteem.

This chapter provides a conceptual framework to help therapists evaluate the leisure skills and improve the leisure participation of patients who have sustained a cerebrovascular accident (CVA). Its focus is to increase the ability of occupational therapists to improve the leisure skills and the quality of life of this population.

DEFINITION OF LEISURE

Many definitions of leisure appear in the literature.* Leisure can be defined according to various theories, including cognitive, sociologic, psychologic, and cultural perspectives. A combination of these theories is necessary to ensure a complete understanding of the complex phenomenon of leisure.

Leisure definitions can be divided into four categories: temporal, activity-based, work-related, and psychologic.

Several authors have defined leisure in temporal terms. Leisure may be defined as planned time off from scheduled, necessary activities such as self-care, sleep, home management, work, and school. Patients who have had strokes may require excessive time to complete their basic self-care routines. Self-care methods may require adaptation to allow time for leisure pursuits. This definition is limited because it addresses only the time spent performing the activity, not the content of the leisure activity. Experiences at work may be similar in quality and fulfill the same purpose as the leisure activity experience.[32]

Leisure can also be defined as an activity, free time, a state of mind or being.[6] Leisure refers not only to a quantity of time but also to a sense of freedom, a decrease in obligations, the chance to gain knowledge, an opportunity for socialization, a symbol of social status, and a physiologic or emotional necessity.[4a] Common definitions of leisure are as follows:

- An attitude or feeling of freedom
- A kind of social activity
- A specific time period

Leisure has also been defined according to activities. Activity-based definitions of leisure are the least common.[27] Leisure can be defined as any activity undertaken by choice. Examples include a specialized group task or lesson, a day trip, and a favorite craft activity. These activities have various functions, including rest, relaxation, stress relief, enjoyment, social networking, and skill development.

Some definitions define leisure according to an individual's work and leisure roles. They focus on the balance of work and play, the perceived needs that are met, and the roles that are performed. A person may develop a professional career based on a leisure interest. For example, someone who enjoys sailing may become a sailing instructor. In this example, work and leisure roles are similar, as opposed to those of a surgeon who also enjoys sailing. The way individuals incorporate leisure into their workday is also relevant. An example of this is eating lunch in an al-

*References 33-35, 38-40.

ternate environment, such as a garden. These work-leisure definitions are difficult to apply to children, persons who do not work because of medical problems, and persons who are retired.

Psychologic definitions focus on the human experience of leisure. Concepts such as state of mind, perceived freedom, and intrinsic motivation are commonly used. These definitions emphasize the person's subjective view of the leisure experience, including the amount of perceived freedom, level of satisfaction, and motivation for the leisure activities. Responses to the same activity vary among individuals. For example, the sailing instructor may experience a low degree of freedom while sailing because it is the primary source of income. The hospital worker, on the other hand, may experience a high degree of freedom while sailing because performance or participation does not affect income.

Many writers have outlined various models of leisure.[10,11,15,17,32] These models draw from various categories in an attempt to fully explain leisure. Box 23-1 summarizes three models of leisure based on the work of Krauss, Murphy, and Neulinger.[31]

The classical view of leisure is best represented by Aristotle, who defined leisure as "a state of being in which activity is performed for its own sake."[31] According to Primeau,[32] "the state of mind definition provides us with the qualities that distinguish leisure from non-leisure activities. Some qualities include freedom of choice, intrinsic motivation, enjoyment, low work-relation, low role constraint, aesthetic appreciation, relaxation, novelty, self-expression, companionship, intimacy, and lack of evaluation."[32]

According to James F. Murphy, the five views of leisure are categorized according to the classical or traditional view, the discretionary-time concept, the idea of leisure as a so-

Box 23-1

Models of Leisure

RICHARD KRAUS

Classic view (state of mind)
Symbol of social class (social status)
Form of activity (nonwork task)
Unobligated time (free time)

JAMES F. MURPHY

Classic view (state of mind)
Discretionary time (free time)
Social instruments (social interactions and networking)
Anti-utilitarian (leisure as an end in itself)
Holistic view (person considered as a whole)

JOHN NEULINGER

Subjective view (meaning of leisure experience to individual)
Objective view (free time)

cial instrument, the anti-utilitarian view, and the holistic model.[31] The American Occupational Therapy Association's Uniform Terminology provides the following definitions: Leisure or Play activities are defined as intrinsically motivating activities for amusement, relaxation, spontaneous enjoyment, or self-expression. There are two divisions of these activities: (1) play or leisure exploration and (2) play or leisure performance. . . . Play or Leisure Exploration is defined as identifying interests, skills, opportunities, and appropriate play or leisure activities. . . . Play or Leisure Performance is defined as planning and participating in play or leisure activities. It includes maintaining a balance of play or leisure activities with work and productive activities and activities of daily living. Also it involves obtaining, utilizing, and maintaining equipment and supplies.[1a]

Kelly determined that individuals participate in leisure tasks for a variety of reasons. Kelly classified four types of leisure performance: unconditional leisure, compensatory and recuperative leisure, relational leisure, and role-determined leisure.[21] Usually a leisure task is chosen based on the individual's needs.

The type of leisure activity chosen for personal pleasure or enjoyment is known as *unconditional leisure*. The individual is free from social influences or limitations.[21] Examples include reading the newspaper and painting.

Rest and relaxation are the purpose of compensatory or recuperative leisure activities.[21] For example, someone may require rest and relaxation to cope with job-related stress. These leisure activities promote relaxation. Examples include knitting, going to a movie theater, and watching television. All individuals have unique stress-reduction strategies; consequently, each individual responds differently to a given activity.

Building and maintaining personal relationships are the goals of relational leisure activities.[21] Examples of this type of leisure include dining with friends, playing with children, and going on outings with a significant other or family. This type of leisure task enables an individual to build supportive social systems, develop social skills, and maintain relationships.

Obtaining the approval of others is the purpose of role-determined leisure activities. The expectations of family members, friends, and coworkers affect the individual's choice of activity and perceived performance or skill level.[21] These leisure activities are an inherent part of the individual's identity. Participation in this type of leisure task varies according to cultural role expectations (Box 23-2).

Box 23-2

Types of Leisure

Unconditional leisure
Compensatory or recuperative leisure
Relational leisure
Role-determined leisure

Many factors affect an individuals's participation in leisure tasks. The next section reviews and discusses these factors and the role of occupational therapists in evaluating and enhancing the leisure skills of patients who have sustained a CVA.

FACTORS AFFECTING LEISURE PERFORMANCE

Many factors affect leisure participation, including the following:

- Skills, physical and intellectual
- Types of leisure tasks available
- Stage of life
- Social and cultural environments
- Leisure attitudes, roles, and satisfaction
- Use of time
- Barriers to leisure participation

A strong, well coordinated person may prefer physical leisure activities such as baseball, soccer, and basketball. Persons with less developed physical skills may be interested in more intellectual leisure tasks such as reading, playing chess, and working puzzles. They may also be interested in creative leisure pursuits, such as painting, photography, and quilting.

Geographic location may also affect participation in leisure activities. If a person lives in a rural environment, leisure activities may include hiking, horseback riding, swimming, and fishing. Someone in an urban environment may go shopping or to theaters, lectures, and museums.

Leisure assumes various forms throughout life. The amount and type of leisure activities depend on the person's developmental stage.[16]

During childhood, gross motor development is enhanced by running, climbing, and playing. The development of creativity is expressed in play activities such as making art and craft projects. Physical and social development in middle childhood is manifested in various games and group play activities. During adulthood, leisure pursuits are important for establishing and maintaining social networks. A balance between work and play is important. Brightbill makes the following observation: "Sustaining leisure interests during middle age and later adulthood is important for constructive use of time, happiness, and quality of life."[4a]

Factors that influence participation in active leisure activities include financial constraints, decreases in functional skills, and decreases in social supports. Many elderly individuals replace active leisure tasks with more passive ones after experiencing decreases in physical and cognitive abilities.

The family structure often reveals the influence of social and cultural factors. Leisure attitudes, roles, and satisfaction are shaped by the family system, which provides the child with a forum to explore play activities and learn appropriate behaviors. Parents value leisure activities to varying degrees. The occupational therapist must appreciate the significance of both the family and the culture on activity participation. Godbey and Parker describe the importance of culture as follows:

"Many people in Western societies view solitary activities as a poor use of time and as nonproductive. On the contrary, many Eastern societies place emphasis on time spent engaging in solitary, reflective activities."[12]

Leisure attitude is defined as the expressed amount of affect toward a given leisure-related object. According to Feibel and Springer, "this attitude is a multiplicative function of a person's beliefs that an object has certain characteristics and a personal evaluation of these characteristics."[9] Many factors affect an individual's leisure attitudes. These factors include social influences, personality, past experiences, and motivation. Leisure attitudes play an important role in the choice and pursuit of leisure activities. A positive experience during an activity usually results in the person continuing to engage in this pursuit.

A leisure role is defined as a perceived identity associated with a leisure task. Changes in a person's roles throughout life are accompanied by shifts in leisure participation. Role changes resulting from disability may cause role strain and role conflict: "*Role strain* refers to the difficulty an individual experiences when attempting to meet role obligations. Role conflict occurs when the occupant of a position perceives that he or she is unable to meet role expectations."[20]

Leisure satisfaction is defined as the pleasure and fulfillment a person derives from leisure tasks.

Use of time is an important factor in leisure participation. If a person spends most of the day at work and returns home with additional work, participation in leisure may be limited. Although the person may derive satisfaction from this schedule, participation in leisure is low. The therapist should analyze the person's schedule to determine whether intervention is necessary. Assistance with time-management skills or strategies to combat stress may be necessary. An individual's leisure participation is also influenced by internal, environmental, and communication-related barriers[23] (Box 23-3).

ROLE OF THE OCCUPATIONAL THERAPIST

Occupational therapists working with patients who have had CVAs are concerned with the way these individuals spend their time. Occupational therapists often forget about leisure and play because they are so focused on self-care and instrumental activities of daily living. However, leisure activities can be equally meaningful to patients as they redefine their life roles.

Occupational therapists should explore patients' leisure needs from the beginning of therapy. As they focus on improving their patients' independence in many activities of daily living, they must also include leisure activities adapted to meet individual needs. For example, therapists may adapt the steps of the leisure task, the environment in which the activity is performed, the positions or movements required, and the tools of the activity (Box 23-4). (These adaptations are further explained in the treatment section.)

Leisure tasks may also be used to improve patients' performance components and thereby increase their functional independence. Valued leisure activities may be incorporated into the treatment plan to improve other functional areas. For example, the patient may be achieving postural and motor goals in a standing position while engaging in a game of air hockey (Box 23-4).

Evaluation of Leisure Skills

Occupational therapists are trained to perform activity analysis to determine the skills needed to perform certain activities. There are many ways to assess an individual's leisure interests, including a leisure interest checklist (Figure 23-1), a structured interview form, and a time log (Figure 23-2) that requires the patient to record previous and current use of time.

It is too easy for occupational therapists to neglect the importance of the leisure roles because of reimbursement issues. By using their skills in activity analysis, occupational therapists can modify leisure tasks to fit patients' needs.

Activity analysis is important when evaluating patients' leisure participation. After a CVA, patients may lose key performance component skills that affect their ability to engage in leisure activities.

Activity analysis is used to determine the performance component skills required for a specific activity. The therapist's knowledge includes identifying the human and

---

Box 23-3

Factors Affecting Leisure Performance

- Skills
- Types of leisure tasks
- Stage of life cycle
- Social and cultural environments
- Leisure attitudes, roles and satisfaction
- Use of time
- Barriers to leisure participation

Box 23-4

Role of the Occupational Therapist

Evaluate patient's physical, cognitive, and perceptual skills and environmental factors (social and cultural) that affect leisure participation.

Provide treatment to improve patient's limitations.

Provide adaptive equipment and adapt techniques to improve leisure participation.

Provide education about various community resources and alternative transportation methods to increase participation.

Date _____

Name _____

Age _____

Cultural background _____

Favorite leisure task _____

Occupation _____

Marital status _____

Onset of stroke _____

Children's ages _____

Male _____ Female _____

Please answer the following questions to enable your therapist to assist you in resuming/persuing your leisure interests:

1. When do you perform leisure activities?

____ Morning ____ Afternoon ____ Evening ____ Weekdays

____ Weekends ____ Holidays ____ Vacations

2. What type of leisure activities do you enjoy?

____ Physical ____ Intellectual ____ Arts ____ Social

____ Solitary ____ Structured ____ Unstructured

3. Place a check mark next to the people who are involved in your leisure activities.

____ Significant other ____ Spouse ____ Children ____ Parent

____ Sibling ____ Friend ____ Co-worker ____ Pets

____ Relatives ____ Grandparents ____ Grandchildren

4. Do you want to resume your past leisure activities?

____ Yes ____ No ____ Do not know

5. If you do not want to resume past leisure activities, please place a check mark next to the reasons.

____ Loss of skills ____ No time ____ Depressed ____ Resources not available

____ Afraid ____ No transportation ____ Decreased leisure performance

____ Decreased communciation skills ____ No interest

____ Other—Please state the reason. _____

_____

6. Are you satisfied with your present leisure activities?

____ Yes ____ No—why? _____ ____ Do not know

Figure 23-1 Leisure interest checklist.

Please check the types of leisure activities you enjoy:

Music

____ Attending concerts

____ Singing

____ Playing instruments

____ Conducting

____ Watching concerts on television

____ Listening to the radio

Dance

____ Tap

____ Ballet

____ Folk

____ Jazz

____ Ballroom

____ Modern

____ Other

Arts and Crafts

____ Carpentry

____ Sewing

____ Knitting

____ Needlepoint

____ Painting

____ Quilting

____ Ceramics

____ Model making

____ Drawing

____ Sculpture

____ Photography

____ Other

Community

____ Volunteering

____ Travel

____ Church

____ Temple

____ Other

Sports

____ Skiing

____ Softball

____ Baseball

____ Football

____ Running

____ Jogging

____ Biking

____ Hockey

____ Basketball

____ Skating

____ Sailing

____ Other

Table Games

____ Table tennis

____ Cards

____ Scrabble

____ Dominoes

____ Puzzles

____ Chinese checkers

____ Checkers

____ Othello

____ Chess

____ Monopoly

____ Backgammon

____ Trivial Pursuit

____ Other

Relaxation

____ Meditation

____ Yoga

____ T'ai chi

____ Horticulture

____ Pet care

Figure 23-1, cont'd   For legend, see opposite page.

Time	Activity	Environment	Physical assistance	Cognitive skills required	Feelings
6:30 AM					
7:00					
7:30					
8:00					
8:30					
9:00					
9:30					
10:00					
10:30					
11:00					
11:30					
12:00 PM					
12:30					
1:00					
1:30					
2:00					
2:30					
3:00					
3:30					
4:00					
4:30					
5:00					
5:30					
6:00					
6:30					
7:00					
7:30					
8:00					
8:30					
9:00					
9:30					
10:00					
10:30					
11:00					

Figure 23-2   A time log is used by patients to record their previous and current use of time.

nonhuman environments and the interaction among all of the factors. This knowledge enables the occupational therapist to break down the activity into a detailed series of steps. The therapist is able to decrease or increase the difficulty of the activity by changing one or more of its components.

When evaluating the leisure roles of patients, therapists must consider seven factors that can affect leisure performance:

- Evaluation findings related to performance components and occupational performance
- Types of leisure activities that interest the patient
- Patient's stage in the life cycle
- Physical, social, and cultural environments
- Patient's previous leisure attitudes, roles, and satisfaction
- Patient's past and present use of time
- Premorbid barriers.

These factors can guide therapists in identifying leisure activities that must be modified and assisting patients with leisure exploration. A checklist (see Figure 23-1) can assist therapists in determining the type of leisure tasks patients enjoyed before their stroke.[14,28]

When evaluating the patient's ability to perform leisure activities, the occupational therapist uses the results from the evaluation of performance components and occupational performance areas. The evaluation uses uniform terminology developed by the American Occupational Therapy Association in 1994. Results of the evaluation should provide the necessary information regarding the patient's strengths and limitations in the performance component areas.

For example, a complete neuromuscular and sensory assessment is necessary to provide information regarding range of motion, skeletal muscle activity, strength, endurance, postural control and alignment, motor control, praxis, fine motor coordination, and visual-motor integration. The complete cognitive and perceptual assessment provides necessary information regarding level of arousal, orientation, recognition, attention span, initiation and termination of activities, memory, sequencing, categorization, concept formation, spatial operations, problem-solving, learning, and generalization.

The type of leisure activities the patient performed before the CVA is important to review. For instance, someone who participated in unconditional leisure tasks most of the time may have been content with little social contact. If the person enjoyed relational leisure tasks, social interactions may assume a greater importance.

The patient's stage in the life cycle must be considered because participation in leisure changes during the aging process. During adulthood, an individual's participation in leisure activities decreases because of demands such as work, household maintenance, and child care. The importance and meaning of leisure also change as a person matures.

The physical, social, and cultural environments are critical in the development of leisure practices and the pursuit of leisure activities during adulthood. Information on the patient's social and cultural networks helps the therapist focus the treatment plan.

The patient's leisure attitudes, roles, and satisfaction before the stroke are important factors to consider after the stroke. The therapist should identify the importance of the selected leisure tasks and the patient's level of satisfaction with them. Identifying the specific aspects of the activity the patient finds enjoyable is helpful. The therapist should also document the patient's leisure roles by discussing topics such as family expectations.

Past and present use of time can be addressed by asking patients to describe the way they spent their time before the stroke, whether they achieved a balance between work and play, and whether they now require additional time for nonleisure activities.

Premorbid barriers to leisure participation must be addressed. These are obstacles that kept patients from participating in the full scope of leisure activities before their stroke. These barriers include intrinsic, environmental, and communication barriers (Box 23-5).

Treatment of Problem Areas to Improve Leisure Skills

The intervention process begins with obtaining the patient's leisure history. The therapist then reviews the results of the evaluation and determines the patient's strengths and limitations in relation to the performance components. Leisure tasks may be used to achieve the goals of occupational therapy treatment. Leisure activities may be used during treatment sessions to remediate component skills, enhance the skill itself, or adapt the leisure activity itself. Therapists must identify the skills necessary to perform the tasks and modify them according to each patient's ability. The occupational therapist may provide treatment for neuromuscular and cognitive deficits that will enable the patient to engage in the leisure activity.

The National Therapeutic Recreation Society (NTRS) proposes a continuum model of leisure service delivery. According to one description, "the 'Leisure Ability Model' serves as a guide for community recreation professionals to facilitate the movement of individuals with disabilities from more intrusive, specialized recreation services into integrated leisure environments."[36] This model consists of a continuum with four levels:

- Noninvolvement
- Segregated
- Integrated
- Accessible

Box 23-5

Factors Affecting Leisure Performance After CVA

PERFORMANCE AREAS AND PERFORMANCE COMPONENTS (EVALUATION FINDINGS)

- Strengths
- Limitations

TYPE OF LEISURE TASKS

- Unconditional
- Compensatory or recuperative
- Relational
- Role-determined

STAGE IN THE LIFE CYCLE

- Childhood
- Young adult
- Middle age
- Later life

SOCIAL AND CULTURAL ENVIRONMENTS

- Support system (i.e., family and friends)
- Nationality
- Religion

LEISURE ATTITUDES, ROLES AND SATISFACTION

- Attitudes
- Roles
- Satisfaction

USE OF TIME

- Present
- Past

BARRIERS TO LEISURE PARTICIPATION

- Internal barriers
- Lack of knowledge
- Decreased skills
- Decreased opportunities
- Environmental barriers
  - Attitudes
  - Architectural
  - Transportation
  - Rules and regulations
  - Barriers of omission
  - Economic
- Communication barriers
  - Social skills
  - Ability to speak
  - Ability to listen

At the first level—noninvolvement—the person who has the disability does not participate in any leisure tasks. At the second level—segregated—the patient participates in structured activities developed for group members with the same disability group. Examples include but are not limited to community activities through local stroke organizations, stroke support groups, and specialized sports programs (aquatics).

The third level—integrated—"provides persons with disabilities the opportunity to be mainstreamed into regular community recreation programs and to participate alongside nondisabled participants. It appears that this approach goes a long way toward helping to change the negative attitudes, stereotypes, stigma and myths associated with persons with disabilities and the systems that serve them."[36] The occupational therapist can instruct patients in the use of adaptive equipment and methods to successfully pursue leisure activities in the community.

The fourth level—accessible—occurs when the individual with a disability "is able to select and access preferred recreation programs with no more effort than his or her counterpart who is non disabled."[36] "The participant is able to realize his or her ultimate goal of achieving a satisfying leisure lifestyle, free of any significant individual and external constraints."[36]

These levels can be used to gradually improve an individual's level of involvement. For instance, if a patient enjoys bowling and wants to return to this activity, the therapist may locate or form a specialized bowling program. When the patients develop skills, they may join an integrated bowling program and eventually an accessible bowling program.

This model can serve as a guide for occupational therapists when introducing resources for leisure services. Occupational therapists can assist patients in exploring alternative types of leisure tasks that fulfill their needs. This may include expanding their leisure activity repertoires to improve the quality of their lives. Occupational therapists educate patients on available services.

Treatment can also focus on helping patients and family members overcome barriers to leisure participation. Common barriers are intrinsic, environmental, and communication-related.

Intrinsic barriers are the results of the disability. These barriers may include but are not limited to lack of knowledge about leisure activities and programs, decreased educational activities, health problems related to the disability, psychological and physical dependence, and decreased skills.[23]

Occupational therapists can address intrinsic barriers in a variety of ways. Remaining informed about current community resources, support groups in the area, and professional leisure organizations designed to serve individuals who have a physical disability is essential.[5] These organizations include stroke support groups, wheelchair sport leagues, and the American Heart Association.

Environmental barriers include attitudes, architectural and ecological obstacles, transportation, rules and regulations, and barriers of omission.[23]

The attitudes of others are a serious problem for persons who have disabilities. Attitudinal barriers result in negative behaviors, stigmas, and decreased acceptance and participation in leisure tasks. Occupational therapists can suggest strategies patients can use to address social prejudices.

Architectural barriers prevent individuals who have physical disabilities from participating in leisure activities. The main problem is accessibility. Many buildings and sport facilities are not wheelchair accessible. Occupational therapists can consult with architects, builders, and contractors to determine necessary modifications, such as installing a lift for a swimming pool.

Transportation barriers are another issue. Many persons who have disabilities cannot drive or take public transportation independently. Public transportation is not always wheelchair accessible. When it is accessible, it does not always foster independence because it may require a driver to operate the lift to enter or a brake-locking mechanism, for example. The Americans with Disabilities Act (ADA) is gradually correcting this problem by requiring wheelchair-accessible transportation. Occupational therapists can educate patients about the ADA and alternate methods of transportation.

Economic barriers also play a role in preventing individuals with disabilities from performing leisure activities. For example, gym memberships are too costly even for many able-bodied persons. Disabled individuals often live on a fixed income and have many medical and living expenses. Occupational therapists can educate their patients about available resources and community groups and encourage participation.

Barriers of omission occur when leisure programs are developed without consideration of all members of society.[23] For instance, a barrier of omission exists when a new leisure program is being developed and the site is in a building inaccessible to persons in wheelchairs. Occupational therapists should instruct their patients to become advocates for themselves and make the public aware of their needs.

The final barrier involves communication. Disabilities that affect the ability to speak, listen, or respond lead to poor social interaction during the leisure task. By training patients in the use of assistive technology to improve communication skills, occupational therapists can play an active role in correcting this environmental barrier (see Chapter 21).

RESEARCH ON LEISURE ACTIVITIES AFTER STROKE

A number of research studies address the issue of leisure activities after stroke. These articles can provide occupational therapists with valuable information on assessment and adaptation of leisure skills for stroke patients.[7,24,26,30]

A review of the literature suggests that occupational therapists can play a major part in helping patients resume or begin leisure activities after CVAs.

Many research articles state that many individuals who sustained a stroke do not resume many of their favorite social and leisure activities.[19,29] Factors that affect leisure participation after stroke include the following:

- Time
- Meaningfulness of activities
- Personal standards
- Internal/external control
- Range of interests
- Performance
- Transportation
- Social relations

Studies have shown that many individuals who sustained strokes do not resume leisure tasks because they do not have time. Their days are usually filled with exercises and self-care tasks. Other individuals who participated in the study reported that time passed slowly and they were bored.[19,29]

The meaningfulness of the leisure task helps determine whether the person will resume the activity. Patients who are retired when they have strokes, tend to have developed more meaningful leisure activities and are able to derive satisfaction from these tasks. However, young patients who received a great deal of satisfaction from work find leisure activities less meaningful.

Personal standards also affect leisure resumption. Many individuals will not participate in a leisure activity unless they can perform it fully or well. Others may not care whether the task requires adaptation, as long as they can perform the task. Another consideration is whether the person performed the task for enjoyment or self-identity.

Whether patients perceive the activity as externally or internally controlled also affects their participation. Many patients do not want to participate in activities they believe are selected and controlled by others. Conversely, patients tend to engage more frequently in activities they control themselves. Depending on the way they are handled, leisure tasks may promote either dependence or independence.

The range of interests patients possess before the stroke appears to be an important factor in the resumption of leisure activities. If they participated in a wide variety of leisure tasks, they usually are able to resume some of them. If these activities required a high degree of physical strength and coordination, participation may be limited. If these leisure activities required skills that were not affected by the stroke, participation is more likely.

Another crucial factor, role balance, relates to the number and types of role changes that occur after a CVA. If patients focus mainly on work-related roles, the resumption of leisure activities may not be important to them.

Performance or skill level may also affect the level of leisure activity. If the stroke resulted in major deficits in cognitive and perceptual skills, the patient will probably not resume leisure tasks.

Environmental factors such as transportation can affect leisure participation. If the leisure activity involved driving a car, patients may be unable to participate after a stroke.

Relationships with friends and family were found to be most influential factors determining involvement in social and leisure activities after stroke. These relationships help patients resume leisure tasks by providing them with the necessary support and resources.

The results of an ethnographic research study by Jongbloed and associates[20] demonstrate that disabilities resulting from stroke can lead to changes in family roles and social relationships, which may result in role strain, or role conflict. This study provides valuable information on ways occupational therapists can help patients and family members adapt to these changes. During the initial interview, occupational therapists can ask patients about their family roles before and after the stroke and the effect of these changes on the family. Occupational therapists may focus the treatment plan on improving or reestablishing these roles. For example, treatment of a woman whose primary role was homemaker may focus on improvement of home management skills. If the patient's primary roles were social, the occupational therapist can explore leisure interests and focus treatment on improving the component areas needed to perform these tasks. Overall, the goal of treatment should be increased motivation and self-esteem.

A research article by Feibel and Springer[9] indicates that depression after stroke is strongly related to a decrease in social activities. The study provides solutions to the problem of deceased participation in social activities. Therapists should address this issue at the beginning of the rehabilitation process. For example, depression should be assessed and treated during the initial stages of therapy to facilitate participation in social activities.

A research study by Labi and associates[25] indicated that many patients do not resume normal social activities after stroke. Factors include social and environmental issues, emotional difficulties, and organic brain dysfunction. Activities outside the home appear more difficult to resume than activities in the home.

Astrom and associates[2] examined the functional, mental, and social factors that affected life satisfaction after stroke. These factors include depression, poor ADL performance, and decreased social activity outside the home.

These studies provide valuable information for occupational therapists and the rehabilitation team to use when evaluating and treating patients after stroke. Other studies[8,41] have examined instruments to measure leisure activities in subjects after they have sustained a stroke. These instruments are a good beginning, but further research is necessary to improve the validity and reliability of these tools. Continued research will further assist occupational therapists in evaluating, treating, and adapting the leisure skills of individuals who have sustained a CVA.

ADAPTING THE LEISURE TASK

Reintroducing leisure activities to patients who have sustained a stroke is extremely important. If the patient does not regain the skills needed to perform these leisure tasks,

many adaptive devices are on the market to enable full participation in these tasks. To select the most effective adaptive aide, the occupational therapist analyzes the skill components necessary to perform the chosen activity. After identifying the components that limit performance, the therapist selects and introduces an appropriate adaptive device. Occupational therapists provide patients with information on various organizations, adaptive methods, and adaptive equipment that enhance and promote participation in leisure activities. Use of these resources enables patients to lead meaningful and productive lives.

Many types of adaptive equipment enable patients who have use of one hand to participate in leisure tasks (e.g., card holders, knitting-needle holders, fishing-pole holders, and needlepoint holders). These products are available from the Internet, catalogs, occupational therapists, and specialized organizations and stores.

SUMMARY

Leisure is a complex phenomenon. A review of the literature reveals that leisure may be defined in various ways. Many factors influence an individual's participation in leisure activities, such as roles, attitudes, satisfaction, stage in the life cycle, and intrinsic and extrinsic barriers. The role of the occupational therapist is multifaceted, including assessment, intervention through techniques and adaptive equipment, and patient and family education, with an emphasis on community resources. Leisure activities may be used to improve a patient's motivation, quality of life, and self-esteem.

■

CASE STUDY

RS is a 74-year-old woman who sustained a right-sided CVA 4 months ago. After completion of the central nervous system assessment, interest checklist, time log, and activity analysis form, the occupational therapist established goals with RS.

Briefly, the results of the central nervous system assessment were as follows: Right upper extremity function was within normal limits. Left upper extremity function revealed poor motor control with synergistic patterns present and impaired sensation throughout. Ability to shift weight anteriorly and laterally while in a seated position was fair. Sustained attention skills were limited. She had a minimal left-sided inattention to self and environment and minimal impairments with spatial relations.

RS has been widowed for 5 years and reports feeling lonely, depressed, and fearful of falling. Her three adult children live out of state, and her social network consists of supportive neighbors, church members, and her dog.

Currently a home health aide assists RS with self-care and home management tasks. RS requires activity set-up for grooming and upper body hygiene, minimal assistance with upper body dressing and bathing, moderate assistance with lower body dressing and bathing, moderate assistance for stand-pivot transfers, minimal assistance for bed mobility, and moderate assistance with meal preparation from a seated level. She is not performing her favorite leisure task of knitting. How can an occupational therapist assist RS?

■
REVIEW QUESTIONS

1. Describe leisure according to the temporal definition.
2. List and define the types and purposes of leisure tasks.
3. What are the seven factors that must be addressed when evaluating an individual's leisure participation and performance after sustaining a CVA? Describe how these factors affect leisure participation and performance.
4. What are leisure attitudes, roles, and satisfaction?
5. List and describe the environmental barriers that affect leisure participation.
6. What is the role of the occupational therapist in assessing and improving a patient's leisure participation after a CVA?
7. How would the occupational therapist assist a patient and family members in resuming leisure activities in their community?

■ COTA Considerations ■

- Use leisure interest checklists to identify relevant treatment activities and areas of intervention.
- Integrating leisure tasks into treatment plans may improve specific performance components as well as the performance area of leisure participation.
- The use of a time log is helpful to understand patients' activity patterns.
- Consider adaptive equipment and technology to increase the level of participation in leisure activities.
- A leisure history interview is required for effective treatment planning.

REFERENCES

1. Angeleri F et al: The influence of depression, social activity and family stress on functional outcome after stroke, *Stroke* 24:10, 1993.
1a. American Occupational Therapy Association: *Uniform terminology for occupational therapy*, ed 3, *Am J Occup Ther* 48:1047, 1994.
2. Astrom M, Asplund K, Astrom T: Psychosocial function and life satisfaction after stroke, *Stroke* 23:4, 1992.
3. Atler K, Gliner J: Poststroke activity and psychosocial factors, *Phys Occup Ther Geriatr* 7:4, 1989.
4a. Brightbill C: *Man and leisure: a philosophy of recreation*, Englewood Cliffs, NJ, 1961, Prentice-Hall.
4b. Brocklehurst J et al: Social effects of stroke, *Soc Sci Med* 15:35, 1981.
5. Dattilo J: *Inclusive leisure services: responding to the rights of people with disabilities*, State College, Pa, 1994, Venture Publishing.
6. DeGrazia S: *Of time, work and leisure*, New York, 1962, Twentieth Century Fund.
7. Drummond A: Leisure after stroke, *Int Disability Study* 12:4, 1990.
8. Drummond A, Walker M: The Nottingham leisure questionnaire for stroke patients, *Br J Occup Ther* 57:11, 1994.
9. Feibel J, Springer C: Depression and failure to resume social activities after stroke, *Arch Phys Med Rehabil* 63:276, 1982.
10. Godbey G: *Leisure in your life: an exploration*, State College, Pa, 1994, Venture Publishing.
11. Godbey G, Goodale T: *The evolution of leisure*, State College, Pa, 1988, Venture Publishing.
12. Godbey G, Parker S: *Leisure studies and services: an overview*, Philadelphia, 1976, WB Saunders.
13. Goodale T, Witt P: *Recreation and leisure: issues in an era of change*, State College, Pa, 1985, Venture Publishing.
14. Holbrook M, Skilbeck CE: An activities index for use with stroke patients, *Age Ageing* 12:166, 1983.
15. Iso-Ahola S: *Social psychological perspectives on leisure and recreation*, Springfield, Ill, 1980, Charles C Thomas.
16. Iso-Ahola S, Jackson E, Dunn E: Starting, ceasing and replacing leisure activities over the life span, *J Leisure Res* 26:3, 1994.
17. Iso-Ahola S: *The social psychology of leisure and recreation*, Springfield, Ill, 1980, Charles C Thomas.
18. Jackson E: Special issue introduction: leisure constraints/constrained leisure, *Leisure Sci* 13:273, 1991.
19. Jongbloed L, Morgan D: An investigation of involvement in leisure activities after a stroke, *Am J Occup Ther* 45:420, 1991.
20. Jongbloed L, Stanton S, Fousek B: Family adaptation to altered roles following a stroke, *CJOT* 60:70, 1993.
21. Kelly J: Leisure styles and choices in three environments, *Pacific Sociological Review* 21:187, 1978.
22. Kelly J, Godbey G: *The sociology of leisure*, State College, Pa, 1991, Venture Publishing.
23. Kennedy D, Austin D, Smith R: *Special recreation opportunities for persons with disabilities*, Dubuque, Iowa, 1987, WC Brown.
24. Krefting L, Krefting D: Leisure activities after a stroke: an ethnographic approach, *Am J Occup Ther* 45:429, 1991.
25. Labi M, Philips T, Gresham G: Psychosocial disability in physically restored long-term stroke survivors, *Arch Phys Med Rehab* 61:561, 1980.
26. Lawrence L, Christie D: Quality of life after stroke: a three year follow-up, *Age Ageing* 8:167, 1979.
27. Loesch L, Wheeler P: *Principles of leisure counseling*, Minneapolis, 1982, Educational Media.
28. Matsutsuyu J: The interest check list, *Am J Occup Ther* 23:323, 1969.
29. Morgan D, Jongbloed L: Factors influencing leisure activities following a stroke: an exploratory study, *CJOT* 57:223, 1990.
30. Niemi M, et al: Quality of life 4 years after stroke, *Stroke* 19:1101, 1988.
31. Neulinger J: *To leisure: an introduction*, Boston, 1981, Allyn & Bacon.
32. Primeau L: Work and leisure: Transcending the dichotomy, *Am J Occup Ther* 50:569, 1996.
33. Roberts K: *Leisure*, New York, 1970, Longman Group.
34. Rojek C: *Leisure for leisure*, New York, 1989, Routledge Chapman & Hall.
35. Rosenfeld M: *Wellness and lifestyle renewal*, Rockville, Md, 1993, The American Occupational Therapy Association.
36. Schlelen S, Ray M: *Community recreation and persons with disabilities: strategies for integration*, Baltimore, 1988, Paul B Brookes.
37. Stein T, Sessoms H: *Recreation and special populations*, Boston, 1973, Holbrook Press.
38. Torkilkdsen G: *Leisure and recreation management*, London, 1992, Thompson Science.
39. Veblen T: *The theory of the leisure class*, New York, 1899, Economic Classics.
40. Yukic T: *Fundamentals of recreation*, New York, 1970, Harper & Row.
41. Wade DT et al: Social activities after stroke: measurement and natural history using frenchay activities index, *Int Rehab Med* 7:176, 1985.

A Survivor's Perspective

THE EVENT

It happened during breakfast, on a bright December morning, unannounced, almost gently, and absolutely painlessly. I was wearing a thick terry cloth robe, which buffered my slumping to the floor and gave it (at least in my visual memory) a slow-motion appearance.

I ended up on my left side on the parquet floor, rejecting my father-in-law's offers of help, thrashing my right leg, holding onto the seat of my chair with my right hand, a little embarrassed and miffed that I did not seem able to stand up. I also remember distinctly my irritation at my mother-in-law's plaintive demands that her husband remove a piece of bread I was chewing on when the stroke hit. She, a keen observer with an artist's eye for detail, had noticed that chewing motions had ceased on the left side of my mouth and food was stuck under the cheek.

Because I was recuperating from open-heart surgery—a mitral valve repair that had been performed 2 weeks earlier—little diagnostic acumen, especially for a neurologist, was required to conclude that I had suffered a stroke. Lying on my dining room floor waiting for the ambulance, I ruminated about the inappropriateness of the word *stroke*

to describe what had happened to me, which had been more like the gentle snuffing of a candle than a violent hit. Nevertheless, the term *stroke* (from the Latin *ictus*, which is still widely used in medical jargon) is universally accepted and has equivalent words in most Western languages. I concluded one of two things: either stroke referred to the suddenness of the event rather than to its outward manifestations or I had had an unusual stroke. Now I know both things are probably true.

The fact that I was musing about words minutes after my stroke illustrates the most important "lucky" feature of this unfortunate event: it had spared mentation and speech. Although at times I suspect that my friends and relatives may have welcomed a little aphasia on my part, talking, reading, and soon enough, working have been a vital part of my recovery, and I am certainly grateful for whatever forces, natural or supernatural, pushed the blood clot into the right rather than into the left carotid artery.

Finding myself totally incapacitated in a hospital bed was not as traumatic an experience as it would be now, maybe because it occurred so shortly after a similar postoperative intensive care experience. Or else, unbeknown to me, I was in a slightly stuporous state that blessedly quenched the emotional reactions to what was happening. Although I seemed to remember every detail of those first days after the stroke, later I discovered some curious gaps.

Acknowledgment: This chapter is dedicated to Maria Laura, Beppe, Giorgio, and Alessandra. My recovery would have been a lot slower without their loving assistance and support.

For example, I have no memory of having received a Doppler scan. Months later, when a repeat scan was performed and I was shown the results of the first examination, I had to admit to myself that I must have been in that same laboratory, which I did not remember, subjected to the same procedure, which seemed new to me, by the same technician, who greeted me cordially but whom I did not recognize.

The question most often asked, especially by other neurologists, is "what does it feel like to be hemiplegic?" I had asked myself the same question when seeing patients who had lost various degrees of motor control. The answer, again, at least in my case, is disappointingly simple: it really felt like nothing, like I had never been able to use my left limbs; no exasperating feeling of formulating a mental command and getting no action occurred. Nor do I think that this was because of loss or diminution of left-body awareness (asomatoagnosia) or sensation, because I had neither to any detectable extent. Peculiarly, the frustration and anger with the sluggish and clumsy left limbs, especially in the hand, came later as I was gradually regaining function and continue to this day. I do not remember how many times I have cursed and actually punched my left hand for not performing adequately, knocking things over, being in the way, or simply being ridiculously (and embarrassingly) tremulous in reaching for objects.

However, at the time of admission to neurology, my only frustration was related to being totally dependent on others for everything, from turning in bed to performing bodily functions. As an intensely (maybe a bit neurotically) private person as I had been all of my life, the loss of privacy that comes with major illness was initially a big problem for me. The "silver lining" has been, in fact, the acceptance of my physical frailty as a matter of fact.

How does a neurologist live with a neurologic disease? I cannot answer this question appropriately because I lived my stroke as a patient, not as a neuroscientist. I asked few neurologic questions and never wanted to see my magnetic resonance imaging (MRI) films. As I had done at the time of my heart operation, I had full trust in the skill of my physicians and colleagues first and my physical and occupational therapists later and took a passive though cooperative attitude throughout the healing process. I think this consciously ignorant and trusting position may have done me more good than a critical, controlling approach.

Of course, seeing my own left toe go up in a classical Babinski sign, witnessing my own excessive knee jerk, feeling odd paresthesias in the left side of my body and "pins and needles" in my left hand were strangely interesting experiences. Some peculiar phenomena may have escaped an untrained observer: for example, I noticed at some point (perhaps 2 months after the stroke) that a spontaneous Babinski sign occurred whenever I initiated urination. This happened without exception and consisted of two or three jerky dorsiflexions of the left toe that promptly subsided as the stream of urine became steady. This "urinary Babinski" persisted throughout the first year after the stroke and continues to occur sporadically to this day. My colleagues in the stroke unit swear they have never heard of a similar phenomenon, but physicians and therapists may find inquiring about this systematically with patients recovering from stroke a worthwhile task. Who knows, perhaps the "urinary Babinski" (DiMauro's sign?) will be added to the spontaneous Babinski sign observed by H. Houston Merritt on removing a patient's slippers.

As every patient does, I worried about the extent of recovery I could expect. I was encouraged by the fact that I could bend my leg from the very beginning. I would show this proudly to visitors and colleagues with the expectation of rosy prognostic pronouncements. I was concerned by the total lack of movement in my left arm, but I learned later from a good friend, a pediatric neurologist, that he had felt optimistic about my future recovery because from the first day I could flex my fingers. Wisely, however, he kept his own council about his positive prognosis until much later, when my arm had in fact regained a good deal of function.

Another weird aspect of my stroke (and as it turned out a positive one) has been the complete lack of spasticity, which has greatly facilitated the rehabilitation process. The only hint of spasticity appeared during automatic reactions such as stretching and yawning, when both left limbs would spontaneously and uncontrollably go into extreme flexion.

THERAPY

When one of the editors of this book, who had been my occupational therapist, asked me to write about my experiences as a patient recovering from stroke and suggested the title "Notes of a Survivor," I asked him whether he meant survivor of the stroke or survivor of physical and occupational therapy. Lest my later comments sound too enthusiastic or be considered self-serving on the part of the editor, let me start with a few negatives.

Both physical and occupational therapy are boring, consisting as they must of highly repetitive exercises and activities: the patient soon learns to count "reps," longing to reach the magic number (usually 10—do therapists have a functional rationale for this quota?) requested by the therapist. And no cheating is tolerated: therapists have mastered a secret way of keeping track of reps automatically and privately even as they keep up a conversation with you, and they will not be defrauded of even a few reps.

Another thing: therapists have a bit of a sadistic trait that may be innate and predisposing to the job or else part of their professional training. As soon as you feel comfortable doing the required number of reps for any given exercise, the number of reps usually goes up by five. The idea, I think, is to keep you challenged, and you are. Furthermore, consider pain: did you know that therapists distinguish between "good" pain and "bad" pain? Good pain is the muscle soreness that comes from those five cycles of ten reps, a guarantee for the therapist that you are doing your exercises and using the proper muscles. Bad pain is classified in imaginative ways: my occupational therapist, a man, used a scale of severity that ranged from "paper cut pain" to "labor pain," at which point the secretary on the occupational therapy floor, a woman, invariably reminded us that we men did not know what we were talking about.

One other piece of good news and bad news: exercise works, but only as long as you keep exercising. The moment you stop, you start losing ground, so that you are in fact condemned to exercising for life, which to a Mediterranean soul such as I is a pretty harsh sentence. My way of surviving this torture is to make exercise part of a highly routinized wakeup ritual, something I do almost automatically, like brushing my teeth. This way you feel slightly guilty when you skip the routine and, conversely, when you do exercise, you enjoy that little heady virtuous feeling I remember from my jogging days.

So much for the negatives. The positive side of the ledger is much larger. As a neurologist and a student of neuromuscular diseases, I am ashamed to confess that I had virtually ignored physical therapy and occupational therapy—a never-never land where patients usually ended up after the physicians concluded their brilliant diagnostic workups—and I had a vague notion of physical and occupational therapists as robot-like technicians. A few sessions of occupational therapy and physical therapy sufficed to change my views drastically. The first thing that impressed me was their knowledge of muscle anatomy and physiology; I thought I knew muscles! Throughout the rehabilitation process, I was amazed at their understanding of movement and lack thereof, muscle coordination, and compensatory mechanisms. Thus I had at all times the comforting notion that all exercises and activities were rationally planned on the basis of my specific deficits and needs and were not part of a "canned" program. Another encouraging sign was the therapists' obvious satisfaction at every sign of improvement; far from being automata, these people clearly loved their profession and took pleasure in a job well done. In fact, I came to admire both the dedication and the professionalism of my therapists so much that I developed the conviction—which I expressed to the chairman of our Department of Neurology—that all neurology residents ought to spend at least a few weeks observing occupational and physical therapists at work. All too often we neurologists are content with our diagnostic workup of stroke patients and our intervention in the acute phase, only to lose sight of patients' progress.

I developed a pain syndrome in my left shoulder that not only gave me sleepless nights (partly because of pain, partly because of an exaggerated fear of dislocating my arm by sleeping on the left side) but also resulted in a "frozen shoulder," a very painful condition that interfered with my occupational therapy. Again, I was impressed by the variety of approaches used by my therapists not just to alleviate the pain but also to resolve the problem, including slinging, supporting my arm on an over-the-shoulder bag, and taping my shoulder in conjunction with passive mobilization and massage. On that occasion, I found myself in another situation I usually experience from the other side: I volunteered to be the subject of a teaching conference for occupational therapy trainees. Although I derived some satisfaction from being materially useful to the medical profession (something akin to but fortunately short of donating your body to the Department of Anatomy), at our clinical conferences I am now much more aware of the discomfort caused to the patient by being an object of study.

GOING HOME

Falling is, of course, the big fear. I had fallen once in my hospital room, and I fell once again a few days after my return home. Finding myself on both occasions next to a wall, I went through the steps my therapists had so carefully rehearsed with me in the hospital gym, and on both occasions I got up on my own. However, after my relatives left, I had nightmares about falling in the middle of a room and not being able to get up and reach the phone or the intercom. The problem was solved by the acquisition of a portable phone, which I slipped into my pocket every night as soon as I entered my house. I never had to use it, but it served its purpose as a "security blanket."

Showering and getting dressed in the morning also took some adjusting, but I soon learned that what had appeared in the hospital as slightly ridiculous procedures (left sleeve and pants leg first; hook the sock on your big toe first, then slip in the other toes) were in fact precious clues to a highly routinized and reasonably rapid process. I took several months to remaster the tie knot, but I remember with joy the pride of my occupational therapist when I appeared at a clinic appointment wearing shirt and tie instead of the usual turtleneck.

Lest all this appear an exceedingly smooth return to normal life, let me dwell for a moment on the frustrations to which I alluded in my opening paragraphs. Even a mild residual hemiparesis is an endless source of frustration in just about every aspect of daily life. I find dropping objects especially irritating and often remember with new empathy my son's frequent outbursts as a clumsy adolescent—"I hate gravity!" Buttoning shirts, especially cuffs, can be a trying experience, and I have more than a few shirts with ripped-off buttons to prove it. Frustration at times turns to rage, and I have occasionally punched my sluggish left hand with my agile right one; even worse, I have punched a table, with the only result of having still a sluggish left hand and a painful right one. One less disruptive way to deal with frustrating experiences is to curse: I have invented a peculiar English/Italian hybrid curse (unprintable in either language) that I use as a mantra many times a day. Naturally, the level of frustration and the threshold for the "tantrums" vary considerably from day to day and are influenced by mood: on some "bad days," I notice that I am almost looking for a frustrating experience so I have an excuse to explode, thus using the stroke as a scapegoat for my bad mood.

Although I have never been a sportsman (library mouse would be a more fitting definition), as my rehabilitation progressed I have repeatedly had vivid dreams in which I ran, I just ran for the sake of running, and it felt both exhilarating and as easy as it had been before the stroke. I actually tried the motions of running while holding onto a shopping cart in the hallway of my apartment building, but somehow the exhilaration of the dream wasn't there.

CONCLUDING REMARKS

Although I cannot run, I can walk without a cane, I am independent in my daily activities, I have been able to resume my (fortunately sedentary) job, and I travel around the world. To be sure, this is not the typical outcome of stroke. Every patient is different, and I have been unusually lucky in that I was spared speech impediments and spasticity. This in turn has made my rehabilitation easier and more effective.

However, my left side was totally paralyzed only 2½ years ago (at age 54) and I am now enjoying a nearly normal life. Much of my progress has been because of the patient, steady, intelligent, and compassionate work of my physical and occupational therapists. The punchline of these "Notes of a Survivor" has to be that not only can one survive a stroke, but brain plasticity does exist, and good physical and occupational therapy do improve the condition of every patient recovering from stroke to a remarkable degree. Some improvement continues to occur (if you exercise, that is!) for a long time, although at a reduced pace. So, who knows, maybe I will be able to run again before I turn 60.

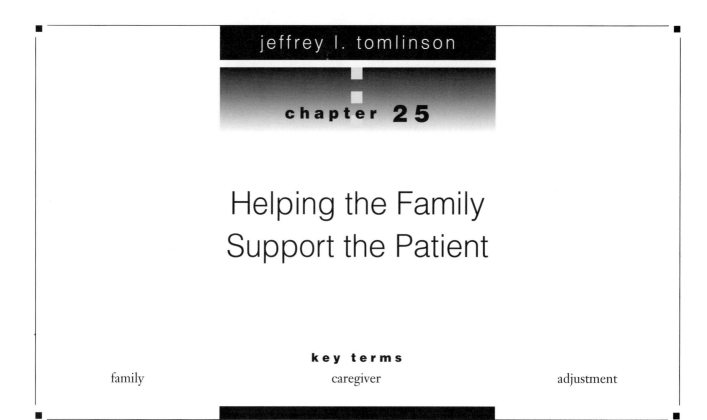

jeffrey l. tomlinson

chapter 25

Helping the Family Support the Patient

key terms

family   caregiver   adjustment

chapter objectives

After completing this chapter, the reader will be able to accomplish the following:

1. Develop treatment plans that integrate families and caregivers.
2. Recognize the family's impact on the recovery of the stroke survivor.
3. Develop strategies to deal with difficult families.

FAMILY'S ROLE

The patient who sustains a stroke is quickly thrown into crisis, both physically and emotionally. It will take all the patient's resources to survive and recover. The patient's family is one of the most important resources. The stroke patient may need extensive support in many facets of life: emotional support, financial aid, physical assistance, and long-term care. As Caplan states, "During the frustration and confusion of struggling with an at-present insurmountable problem, most individuals feel weak and impotent and tend to forget their continuing strengths. At such times, their family reminds them of their past achievements and validates their precrisis self-image of competence and ability to stand firm."[4]

The family serves many functions in our society. One of the first, most important, and most natural roles is caring for those in need of physical and cognitive assistance in the family. Initially, a family usually focuses on the care and nurturing of children. However, in later years the same

function often applies to the care of an individual who is ill. The family provides assistance and resources, such as food, shelter, money, clothing, and transportation. Families also interpret the meaning of events in the outside world and their meaning to the affected family member. This function may affect how the patient responds to health care providers and their services. The family functions as a source of ideology, values, and codes of behavior that guide its members in how to respond to life's events. This effect on the family member of course also affects how the patient responds to the stroke and subsequent care by health professionals. Finally, people in need of a haven for rest and recuperation often turn to their family.[4]

Because the family's impact on recovery from a stroke is not completely clear,[17] several investigators have attempted to determine the contributing factors involved. In one study of 60 families of stroke patients, the patients and families were assessed 5 months after the patient's discharge from the hospital. The authors examined the relationship between family functions and adherence to treatment. Family function was assessed with the McMaster Family Assessment Device, a 60-item evaluation of seven family dimensions. The authors found a strong correlation between compliance with treatment regimens and families that had effective involvement, functional communication, and problem-solving skills.[7] Evans et al state, "If rehabilitation services can affect family behavior early in the course of recovery, there is often a positive influence on other outcomes."[8] For example, education of the family about the stroke has been shown to improve communications between the family and the patient.[8] Another investigator noted that patients with positive, constructive attitudes toward the challenge of a stroke were more likely to eventually achieve their fullest potential.[3]

The family's role as an important resource for fostering these positive attitudes may be one of its most important contributions to recovery. The shared positive outlook of the family and the patient provides a sense of support and hope and focuses collective energies toward recovery. Finally, as a patient begins to recover, families who have taken over some of the roles and tasks of the patient must once again have the flexibility to allow and even encourage the patient to resume some productive occupational role in the family. Dysfunctional families may have great difficulty shifting roles in the home. Such changes in roles can also be difficult for family members who have benefited from their present roles.

Patients who do not fully recover from a stroke may depend on others for extensive assistance and care. This care is often provided at least partially by the family. Of the home care recipients in the United States, 80% receive part of their care from a relative.[20] Of those relatives providing care, 72% are women. Adult daughters represent 29%, and wives represent 23%. The demands on family will most likely continue to grow as our population ages. Those older than 65 years represented 31.2 million in the 1990 census. By 2020 this part of our population will have grown to approximately 52 million. Population projections suggest that the number of potential family caregivers will keep pace with this aging population because the caregivers will comprise baby-boomer generation. However, the availability of these relatives will depend on many other factors, including the continued increase in the number of women in the workforce and divorce rates.[13]

In addition to the aging population, the growing emphasis in our economy on control of health care costs—including long-term care—will put greater pressures on families to provide even more care for their aging and disabled members. Efforts to control costs may include abbreviated rehabilitation contacts and more use of family members to perform rehabilitation activities. Rehabilitation of a stroke patient must include the active involvement of the family as a team member.

FAMILY RESPONSE TO ILLNESS AND DISABILITY

In collaboration with a family, it is important to consider the possible responses of the family. Often therapists and other health care providers feel burdened or exasperated when families act angry, demanding, controlling, or unrealistic. Such behavior may affect the therapist's ability to work with the family, the rehabilitation outcome and finally, the success of the discharge plan.

The initial onset of a stroke is generally sudden and not anticipated. The family may experience a sense of loss of control or helplessness. Seemingly little can be done by the family initially to speed recovery. The family may have a deep sense of loss and disruption, especially when the patient and the family had expected a vital, productive future for the patient. Disruption of the family may be especially severe when the patient's disability affects the other family members' activities and hopes for the future.

Retired couples often speak of the plans they once had to travel or pursue other interests that they had delayed until retirement. Adult children of stroke victims who become caregivers may complain of loss of freedom to leave the home, the problem of social isolation, or the loss of time for personal interests. Families may also be fearful for the patient's safety.[10] Concerns about avoiding any stimulus that might cause another stroke are not uncommon. The embolic or hemorrhagic process of stroke is often understood at a rudimentary level, and the patient's condition is generally perceived as delicate. Information from physicians indicating that future strokes may occur often add weight to this concern. The family may be fearful of physically moving the patient because they worry it may affect vascular stability. The family may avoid exciting or upsetting the patient because they are concerned it will increase the patient's blood pressure and cause another stroke. These concerns lead families to change their behavior around the patient and transmit a message of fear to the patient that may be detrimental.

The response of the family to the stroke changes over time. It is interesting to note that during recovery the patients and their health care providers—who have only known the patients since the stroke—generally compare gains in function with the patient's disabled state after the stroke, whereas the family is much more likely to compare recovery gains with the patient's previous level of function.[3] The authors of one study examined families 7 to 9 months after a member had a stroke and found a substantially higher prevalence of depressive symptoms among both the primary caregivers and the patient.[19] The responsibilities of caring for a family member who has sustained a stroke may lead to greater social isolation for both the patient and the caregiver. Aphasia can cause even greater changes in social function, often resulting in social withdrawal by both the patient and the family.[12] The caregivers of patients with aphasia are more likely to identify their relationship as worse than before the stroke.[3] The family's complaints may include changes in the patient's behavior, mood lability, confusion, constant demands, and changes in sleep patterns.

The need to appreciate the responses of families to the sustained, long-term care of a family member is a growing concern in health care; indeed, some consider family caregivers unidentified patients. Families that functioned well before the onset of illness generally have the capability to adapt to the challenges posed by the illness. Families that have been disrupted naturally strive for a new balance. Roles and responsibilities in the family are gradually reapportioned in an unconscious adjustment process that protects the function of the family.[1] For example, a husband, who previously paid the bills and handled insurance forms, is hospitalized with a stroke. His tasks are considered the father's role of family financial manager. The wife lacks confidence in assuming the responsibility for this task and part of her husband's role. Indeed, a time of such great stress is a difficult time to assume any new responsibility. These responsibilities may be transferred to an adult child—if possible, a man. Likewise, when a wife becomes disabled, her husband may have difficulty assuming many of the traditional roles that the wife had assumed.

When a person with a disability from a stroke plans to return home, the assignment and assumption of caregiver roles may be very stressful for the family. Assisting with activities of daily living (ADL), home management, and cooking can be time-consuming and physically demanding. Many ADL tasks such as bathing, grooming, and toileting are intimate, and some family members may be uncomfortable assisting the patient with them at first. Although home care services are available in many regions, the extent of care may be limited. In addition, increased effort by the health care industry to control the costs of health care (e.g., managed care, utilization review) decrease the availability and increase the cost of home care supports for the family.

The assumption of new roles in the family, especially the caregiver role, may lead to the abandonment of previous roles. This shifting of roles may affect more than one household and may affect others indirectly. Other roles family members may assume include source of emotional support, energy source, spiritual guide, organizer, comedian, cleaner, and initiator of events.

Dysfunctional families and families who were in conflict before the stroke have greater difficulty adjusting to the challenges imposed on them. Marital relationships that were strained before the stroke may be further strained by this crisis.[5] Families with maladaptive patterns of function provide less constructive support and may at times hinder rehabilitation efforts.[7] Families with idiosyncratic, paranoid, or negative ways of interpreting events in the outside world may have a negative impact on the patient.

Families characterized as centripetal in their function are focused inward: family activities, emotional investments, values, interests, and expectations are directed toward the family. The members of such a family have been socialized to fulfill their needs with only family assistance and have difficulty using outside resources.[22] Therapists working with this type of family may sense that they are not openly and completely accepted and that the suggestions made about management of the illness and adaptations of the home are met with skepticism or hesitation. To enhance a more collaborative relationship with a centripetal family and increase the chances that the family follows through with the treatment and management plans suggested, the therapists may have to make a greater effort to gain trust and acceptance. Without such an effort, other therapy interventions offered to the patient may be rendered ineffective by an unsupportive family.

Therapists who must work with angry, demanding families may try to reduce the extent of their contact with them. Contact may make therapists uncomfortable and defensive. Such a reaction diminishes the opportunity for effective communication of the information necessary for continued treatment. Families' emotional responses to a stroke must be considered objectively by therapists. Families often become anxious or angry because they are frightened by the trauma and loss created by the illness. Families often vent to or focus their anger on individuals unrelated to the events that have caused the anger. Indeed, experiences in hospitals often do little to comfort families and sometimes add to their distress. When responding to a family's anger or complaints, the therapist's must remain calm and be an empathic listener. The family's complaints and concerns should be addressed. Attention to complaints is not only a basic responsibility of a therapist as a member of the health care team but an initial opportunity to demonstrate respect for and responsiveness to the family, which in turn helps the family feel more in control at a time when they feel out of control. The family's emotional reaction to the traumatic event should be validated by the therapist. Validation is not indiscriminate agreement with everything the family says—it is emphatically listening to the family's reactions, helping them clarify their thoughts and feelings, and sharing similar experiences of other families and individuals. Consider the following scenario, and note the therapist's responses.

Deborah, a 76-year-old, was returning home from the hospital after 10 weeks of rehabilitation. The occupational therapist from the home care agency immediately received complaints from Deborah's family abut the hospital care. The therapist focused on Deborah's physical needs, ordering durable medical equipment and initiating treatment. However, the family then complained about the equipment. The home care agency addressed these complaints quickly by providing satisfactory replacements. Rather than becoming defensive, the therapist listened to the husband's multiple complaints. At the beginning of the third session, the husband, feeling more comfortable and becoming more trusting, started to express his concerns about his wife's condition. He was worried about how frail his wife had become, that she could have died as a result of the stroke, and that she was still at risk for another stroke. The therapist recognized these concerns as the core issues driving the husband's anxiety. The therapist listened carefully and validated the husband's concerns. This allowed the husband to disclose his fear that he would lose his wife and be alone. The therapist was able to offer some reassurance that Deborah was in stable condition. The therapist then shared this information with the social worker, who was able to counsel the husband and help him come to terms with Deborah's stroke and her health status.

Therapists must also have the support of the administrators of their facilities to intervene with families who may display extreme dissatisfaction. Administrators must understand the family's reactions and be willing to empower their staff to handle family complaints.

COLLABORATING WITH THE FAMILY

Because the family has such an impact on the patient's ability to respond to health care services and may actively deliver some of the care and services during later phases of rehabilitation, engaging of the family in the functions of the treatment team is essential. The initial stages should include an assessment of the family's understanding of the patient's status and the intent of the services being offered. The therapist should simply listen to the type of questions asked by the patient and pose a few evaluative questions in return. Families should then be educated about the illness so that they may effectively use the information to respond appropriately to the patient and health care providers. Each member of the treatment team collaborates with the family in a different context. The physician will most likely educate the family about the cause and anatomy of a stroke, as well as the course of medical treatment during onset and throughout the course of illness. The social worker may be the person who will make initial and continuing formal contact with the family, first to assess the family and home environment, then to help the family develop a long-term care plan and discuss financial needs. The nurse may educate the family about daily management and the new needs of the patient: how to handle and position the patient safely, comfortably, and therapeutically to prevent the development of a decubitus ulcer and how to administer medications and other treatments.

The occupational therapist must educate the family about many aspects of managing the care of a stroke patient.[9] The family must learn about paralysis, ineffective movement, and protection of the impaired extremity: how to manage and adapt to perceptual deficits, hemianopsias and unilateral neglect; how to apply positioning devices and orthotics, keep schedules of orthotic wear, care for the skin, and clean the orthosis; and how to position the patient in bed. Learning safe transfers of the patient to a variety of surfaces may require many practice sessions with the family. The therapist may think every transfer situation has been taught to the family until an accident occurs, such as the patient injuring an ankle falling off a street curb while entering the family car. Transfer training should include transfers to automobiles, beds, toilets, regular chairs, and bathtubs. Education about the handling and care of wheelchairs and the proper use of adaptive equipment helps ensure proper use and increased patient safety. Sharing a supplier's durable medical equipment catalog with the family may help give the family a better idea of available products and generate some questions or ideas about other home adaptations that may be needed. Home visits by the occupational therapist before the patient's discharge may help the family predict adaptations that will be needed in the home and reduce the number of obstacles encountered and frustrations experienced in the first few days at home. The therapist's suggestions for changing the home environment should be tempered by sensitivity to personal property and financial limits (see Chapter 20).

The occupational therapist should share detailed information with the family about the patient's ability to perform various ADLs because the family may overestimate or underestimate the patient's abilities. Instructions on setting up tasks and providing proper assistance helps the family feel they are contributing to the patient's recovery and may relieve the family's worry that all tasks will have to be done for the patient. At the same time the therapist must be sensitive to the family's need for ADL to be completed in a reasonable time to maintain a home routine. (Allowing 15 minutes for the patient to don a shirt may seem reasonable in a hospital, but it may not be practical in a busy home.) The therapist should instruct the family or primary caregiver on helping the patient perform safe, passive range of motion and active exercises and perhaps practice these exercises with the family. When designing an exercise or therapeutic program for the family to perform with the patient, the therapist must consider the availability and needs of the family and caregiver. Tasks that are time consuming, very detailed, or cause discomfort or pain for the patient may discourage the family from following through with the program. Tasks that fit into the family's routine and perhaps incorporate activities the family enjoys may meet with greater compliance.[2]

The therapist should encourage the family to maintain their previous relationship with the family member as much as possible and not assume the role of therapist or home health aide. Although assuming this role may seem to be a constructive way for family members to respond to the negative effects the stroke, it alters the existing patient/family relationship and may be considered an additional problem for the patient.

Both the patient and family should be involved in the goal-setting process. Evaluations such as the Canadian Occupational Performance Measure are helpful in this process (see Chapter 15). If the family is to support the patient and the rehabilitation effort, it is important that they understand and are invested in the goals. This involvement begins with the therapist asking the patient about goals for rehabilitation and then making the patient aware of what is realistic and which goals are priorities. The therapist then asks the family what they consider to be important goals, and this information is then given to the patient. This process can be cumbersome, especially when the family and patient disagree or unrealistic goals have been set. However cumbersome, the goal-setting process is an opportunity to clarify perceptions about the patient's status; the prognosis and course of the illness; the expected efficacy of the rehabilitation; the restorative and compensatory approaches; and short-term, step-by-step incremental goal-setting.

The treatment-planning process is an opportunity to make certain that expectations and demands on all parties are reasonable and consensual. When the family, patient, and therapist have different goals, help them compromise. Usually the similarities in goals can be identified and a common goal reached. When a compromise cannot be reached, the therapist should help the patient and the family prioritize or sequence goals. The patient's wishes should be given some extra consideration. If the patient and the family have been actively involved in treatment planning and the measure of outcomes, the eventual end of rehabilitation services will be better understood and accepted. The patient and family members will more likely agree with the therapist's observation that the patient has reached the optimal level of recovery for the present setting and is therefore ready to move to a different level of care or be discharged from treatment.

A common assumption of families is that the more therapy the patient receives, the better the patient's recovery. The therapist must explain how much therapy is appropriate and why. Families should be taught that rest, socialization, and recreation are essential aspects of recovery (see Chapter 23). Too many hours of intensive therapy may be overwhelming to someone trying to recover.

The therapist and other health care providers can more subtly educate the family by modeling appropriate behaviors. The therapist's comfortable and positive interactions with the patient can help put the family at ease and encourage more natural interactions. Humor can play an important role in this process. The therapist's comfort with touching, holding, and handling the patient, especially the paralyzed extremities, may help the family begin to do the same. An illness and subsequent physical disability may cause the patient or the patient's partner to avoid intimacy and sex (see Chapter 18). In addition, many hospitals and residential health care facilities deter physical intimacy. The authors of one study found that only 17% of couples

continued sexual contact.[6] Touching and embracing may be the first way a couple begins to become intimate again. Physical intimacy can be comforting and affirming for the patient. Accepting and discreetly handling situations in which the patent is incontinent can also set a good example for the family. If the therapist is to help the family address these issues, therapy sessions should occasionally be open for family members to observe or participate. This may seem an additional burden on the therapist and meet with some objections by administrators; however, the benefits of engaging the family in this way can be immeasurable, especially because treatment periods are becoming shorter and greater reliance is being placed on families to become caregivers and extend therapy.

Some hospitals and outpatient clinics have developed structured educational series for families. Hinckley, Packard, and Bardach describe a successful family education program focused on patients with aphasia and their families. The program's topics included communication, intimacy and sexuality, vocations, driving, and volunteering. This type of program can be labor intensive, which should be considered when developing similar programs. The authors were unable to identify outcomes related to more effective management of the patient by family members; however, attendance by families and positive results on satisfaction surveys suggested that the families benefited from this program.[14]

HELPING THE FAMILY ADJUST

Professional assistance in helping the family adjust to the stroke and its impact can have positive long-term results by strengthening the natural family support system that will be helping the patient. The education approach discussed previously is one step toward that adjustment. Professionals can help the family in several other ways. The therapist should acknowledge the efforts the family is making to be with, assist, and care for the affected family member.[15] Often families and caregivers who devote significant effort to caring for their family member feel their devotion is not being reciprocated. Reciprocity is a natural element of social relations. When an object or service is offered to one individual, that individual usually reciprocates in some manner.[16] In a relationship in which someone is ill and dependent, reciprocation is altered. For health care providers, reciprocation can be indirect—remuneration by a third party, an altruistic sense of social reward, or a focus on the further development of professional skills. Some patients and families with limited socioeconomic resources whose services are paid for by government or other programs may feel an absence of social reciprocation and try to reciprocate with a gift or friendly gesture. For family caregivers the absence of reciprocation from the affected family member may leave them feeling angry, empty, or unrewarded. However, the findings of one study suggest that many caregivers experience reciprocity in a dependent relationship. In one study, mothers who received care from their daughters were able to reciprocate through expressions of love. Of the daughters in a caregiving relationship, 87% were able to identify some form of reciprocation that they valued, such as sharing information and advice.[21]

The professional can support the family by acknowledging their efforts and appealing to the family's sense of altruism. Professionals can also help family caregivers identify small, everyday forms of reciprocation. Often this reciprocation occurs in the context of an activity: a smile of appreciation after assistance with care or the reintroduction of music, old recipes, or a craft from a previous era or culture of origin. The identification, spoken or unspoken, of these rewards may help the caregiver sustain their efforts and care for the family member with an increased sense of the value of their assistance.

Professionals may also support family caregivers by monitoring their health promotion activities. Asking caregivers periodically about their own health and feelings can remind them that their health and stress levels are important also and allow them an opportunity to share their experiences and feelings. The therapist should observe caregivers for signs of fatigue or excessive stress and encourage them to schedule and pursue social and leisure interests.[15] The occupational therapist can help caregivers identify these interests and determine how they fit into the routine of caring for the affected family member. The family and the caregivers should be encouraged to use respite periods for travel or leisure.[15]

Respite can be achieved in several ways, including temporarily placing the patient in a residential program, hiring a 24-hour attendant, or relying on other family members to provide temporary care. The therapist should not be discouraged if the family and the caregivers do not respond immediately to these suggestions. The therapist should encourage the family to increase use of home care and day care programs to help reduce stress. Health care providers should help the family identify when the extent of care needed by the patient exceeds the family's resources, capabilities, and home care supports. It may be necessary to consider long-term residential care. The family and the patient may have some emotional difficulty discussing this issue. Professional support, clear information about nursing homes, and assistance in finding the best home for the patient can help make this transition smoother and more successful.

DYSFUNCTIONAL CARE

The demands of caring for a family member who has sustained a stroke may not only exceed the family's resources but may also exacerbate dysfunctional aspects of the family or the individual caregiver. Previously strained relationships may be placed under greater stress and can lead to a breakdown of the family.

It is estimated that 3.2% of older Americans are victims of abuse or neglect[18]; chronic disability is believed to be one of the risk factors.[11] It is also estimated that only one out of six cases of elder abuse is brought to the attention of authorities.[11] Therapists working with patients disabled by a stroke should be sensitive to the signs of abuse and neglect and be prepared to contact authorities. There is often more disagreement among professionals about what constitutes neglect than what constitutes inadequate care. Fulmer and O'Malley[11] suggest that defining neglect and abuse cases as situations of inadequate care helps reduce resistance when attempting to constructively deal with the issue—the welfare of the patient.

DOCUMENTING FAMILY CONTACTS

Many therapists who have traditionally focused on physical rehabilitation express concerns abut documenting their work with the family. Often therapists believe they must document the only physical and functional restoration for reimbursement purposes. This leads therapists to avoid intervening in family-related problems or to avoid reporting these interventions to others. This decision is unfortunate because it eventually harms the patient and the family and does not promote the idea that family interventions need to be provided and reimbursed.

Many interventions with family members can be directly tied to improving the patient's level of function or increased safety in the home. Interventions can help the family to assist the patient safely and effectively with transfers, dressing, and bathing. Other goals that may be documented include the following:

- The family will encourage the patient to perform the self exercise program daily.
- The family will demonstrate a more accurate understanding of the patient's safety needs by maintaining a hazard-free home environment.
- The family will engage the patient in an active leisure pursuit at least twice a week.

REVIEW QUESTIONS

1. Which natural functions does the family provide for its members?
2. How should a therapist respond to an angry, complaining family?
3. What are some of the family attributes that may lead to difficulty helping a member who has sustained a stroke?
4. How should the therapist educate the family?

5. What can a therapist do for family caregivers to improve compliance with treatment?
6. How should the family and the patient be engaged in treatment planning?
7. How can the therapist help the family adjust to the stroke and chronic disability?

■ COTA Considerations ■

- Include family and significant others in the treatment-planning process.
- Consistent family training is a prerequisite for providing a patient with a safe home environment.
- Consider your patient's occupational roles before and after stroke and the impact of this change on the family unit.
- Consider and address the level of stress and anxiety the family is experiencing during the rehabilitation process.

REFERENCES

1. Ackerman NW: *The psychodynamics of family life*, New York, 1958, Basic Books.
2. Anderson J, Hinijosa J: Parents and therapists in a professional partnership, *Am J Occup Ther* 38:452, 1984.
3. Anderson R: *The aftermath of stroke: the experience of patients and their families*, New York, 1992, Cambridge University.
4. Caplan G: The family as a support system. In Caplan G, Killilea M, editors: *Support systems and mutual help: multidisciplinary explorations*, New York, 1976, Grune & Stratton.
5. Diller L: Hemiplegia. In Garrett J, Levin E, editors: *Rehabilitation practice with the physically disabled*, New York: 1973, Columbia University.
6. Drummond AE: Stroke: the impact on the family, *Br J Occup Ther* 51:193, 1988.
7. Evans RL et al: Family interaction and treatment adherence after stroke, *Arch Phys Med Rehabil* 68:513, 1987.
8. Evans RL et al: Stroke: a family dilemma, *Disabil Rehabil* 16:110, 1994.
9. Evans RL, Held S: Evaluation of family stroke education, *Int J Rehabil Res* 7:47, 1984.
10. Figley CR: Catastrophes: an overview of family reactions. In Figley CR, McCubbin HI, editors: *Stress and the family: Volume II. coping with catastrophe*, New York, 1983, Brunner-Mazel.
11. Fulmer TT, O'Malley TA: *Inadequate care of the elderly: a health care perspective on abuse and neglect*, New York, 1987, Springer.
12. Herrmann M et al: The impact of aphasia on the patient and family in the first year poststroke, *Top Stroke Rehabil* 2:5, 1995.
13. Himes CL: Future caregivers: projected family structures of older persons, *J Gerontol* 47 (suppl):17, 1992.
14. Hinckley JJ, Packard MEW, Bardach LG: Alternative family education programming for adults with chronic aphasia, *Top Stroke Rehabil* 2:53, 1995.
15. Kahana E: *Family caregiving across the lifespan*, Thousand Oaks, Calif, 1994, Sage.
16. Levi-Strauss C: The principle of reciprocity. In Coser L, Rosenberg B, editors: *Sociological theory*, New York, 1957, MacMillan.
17. Norris VK, Stephens MAP, Kinney JM: The impact of family interactions on recovery from stroke: help or hindrance? *Gerontologist* 30:535, 1990.
18. Pillemer K, Finkelhor D: Causes of elder abuse: Caregiver stress versus problem relatives, *Am J Orthopsychiatr* 59:179, 1989.
19. Schulz R, Rau MT, Tompkins CA: A longitudinal study of the psychosocial impact of stroke on primary support persons, *Psychol Aging* 3:131, 1988.
20. Silliman RA et al: Families of elderly stroke patients: effects of homecare, *J Am Geriatr Soc* 34:643, 1986.
21. Walker AJ, Pratt CC, Oppy NC: Perceived reciprocity in family caregiving, *Family Relations* 41:82, 1992.
22. Walsh F: *Normal family processes*, New York, 1993, Guilford.

SUGGESTED READING FOR CHILDREN

de Paola T: *Now one foot, now the other*, New York, 1980, GP Putnam's Sons.

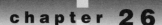

ann burkhardt

chapter **26**

Total Quality Management
of the Adult Stroke Population

key terms

total quality management	quality assurance	quality improvement
risk management	process improvement	

chapter objectives

After completing this chapter, the reader will be able to accomplish the following:

1. Understand the concept of total quality management.
2. Articulate the difference between quality improvement and the process of improvement.
3. Conceptualize how incident reporting relates to risk management.
4. Describe several clinical monitors for the care of individuals surviving stroke.
5. Share tools available in a clinical setting that address the concerns of case management of individuals surviving stroke.

One of the criticisms often made concerning the cost effectiveness of rehabilitation services is the general lack of sufficient outcomes research. This assertion in particular has been used as a basis by some health maintenance organizations (HMOs) and managed care organizations (MCOs) as a reason to deny coverage of occupational therapy services. The occupational therapy profession needs to focus on how its benefits can be measured so that others can appreciate its value. One of the ways clinical research can be generated is through preliminary investigation by clinically based continual quality improvement (CQI) monitors.

Total quality management (TQM) comprises two levels: CQI and risk management (RM).[10] The aim of each CQI monitor is to define an aspect of care that is the essence or crux of professional interventions. The goals of intervention are quantified in measurable terms, which allows data to be gathered that will predict a reproducible and verifiable outcome. Through the provision of a reporting structure the TQM process assists the clinician with formulating outcome measures and setting the standards for provision of patient care according to the process of performance improvement (PI) standards (benchmarking).

CQI monitors direct outcomes of prevention of disease complications or success in treatment. These data should be readily retrievable from charts or through surveys of patients and health care workers (e.g., nurses). Their follow through with occupational therapy's recommendations impacts the success of the treatment intervention. The process that is now called *process improvement* (PI) was once called "quality assurance." The terminology and underlying management philosophy changed, resulting in a model that is progressive and less based on monitoring the status quo. The term *improvement* clearly suggests that quality patient care or treatment must continually increase and also implies that change is an inherent aspect of the monitoring process.

In contrast, risk management defines morbidity, or aspects of patient care that could put the individual or a caregiver at risk for personal injury. Occupational therapists may work with individuals who have survived a stroke in an inpatient hospital, clinic, home, or work setting. One of the more common risk management issues concerns the risk of falling because of changes in balance and equilibrium.[1] Therapists are often consulted to recommend the parameters for safely participating in activities. Physical or chemical restraints may be needed for patients with cognitive changes impairing judgment, attention, or short-term memory to reduce the risk of injury. Federal law limits the conditions under which restraints may be used. Therapy staff and other members of the interdisciplinary team must be aware of the law and adhere to compliance measures yet continue to act in the best interest of the patient. Misuse of exercise equipment may result injuries. For example, if a person who has had a stroke and has glenohumeral joint malalignment uses an upper body exerciser (UBE), it could lead to tendonitis and development of a pain syndrome. When limbs have decreased sensation, particularly when the patient's protective sensation is impaired, participation in activities places the patient at risk for a cut or burn. Certain physical agent modalities also carry a risk when protective sensation is impaired because patients could get burned (e.g., by superficial or deep heat modalities) or shocked (by electrical modalities) if precautions are not followed and equipment consistently checked for safe operation (Figure 26-1).

TQM is an essential part of any occupational therapy setting today. Not only do credentialing agencies such as the Joint Commission on the Accreditation of Hospitals Organization (JCAHO) or the Committee on the Accreditation of Rehabilitation Facilities (CARF) require TQM activities but so do individual contracts for private practices with managed care companies. The managed care industry promotes the idea that cost effectiveness does not imply reduced quality. All practitioners must see practice from this perspective if they are to continue practicing within the changing health care system.

One way in which implementation of treatment and rapid discharge are combined is through the use of critical pathway models.[14] Critical pathways are standardized multidisciplinary care plans through which care is introduced on a timed continuum. Critical pathways efficiently coordinate inpatient care so that the patient receives intervention from all critical care services and is discharged to the community as rapidly as feasible. The rapid discharge reduces the inpatient length of stay (LOS) and is financially desirable for the system providing primary care. Occupational therapists must seek out opportunities to participate in the critical pathway planning committees that coordinate the design and implementation the pathway. Therapists must define the parameters of their staff's involvement, an optimum treatment time frame, and the content of evaluation and treatment to ensure the patient has the skills needed to survive at home following discharge. The level of anticipated function at the time of the discharge should be defined as well. Discharge planning is still the method for recommending the appropriate level of home care or outpatient service for each individual case.

Most of the resources concerning TQM arise out of the medical and nursing literature. Early articles on the topic describe the necessity for defining functional outcome in reference to quality of life.[2] When studies are physician generated the outcomes tend to be measured in terms of the development of medical complications following inpatient discharge or an inpatient's LOS.[12] These factors are related to issues of delaying discharge from the hospital or readmitting to an inpatient setting because of a medical complication. These issues are directly related to reimbursement for care[15] and funding to the provider calculated using the diagnostic related groups (DRGs). The facility receives a flat rate to treat the patient for the primary medical diagnosis regardless of complications. The rate is regionally controlled and is derived by averaging the actual length of hospital stay for persons with a particular diagnosis. The system promotes treating the disease quickly and discharging the patient early. Theoretically this lessens the possibility of complications such as nosocomial infections.[4,16] The problem with the system is that it fails to account for the differences in the recovery

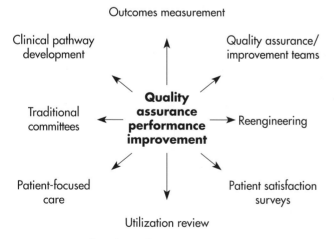

Figure 26-1 The relationship of quality assurance performance improvement to hospital-based care.

times of the healing organ systems and the impact delayed healing has on the ability to participate in basic activities of daily living (BADL) or instrumental activities of daily living (IADL).

For example, joint replacements following fracture will usually heal more rapidly than brain tissue that is damaged because of a stroke. The predicted complications associated with bone healing are more readily quantifiable by nature than those of the central nervous system. For example, learning to dress the lower extremities is less cumbersome if the two upper extremities are functionally intact and visual perception is intact. This concept is simple but may not necessarily be accounted for in physician- or nursing-generated morbidity reviews. There is an inherent dichotomy in nursing-generated CQI because a physician's ability to control a patient's medical status is not necessarily positively correlated with the patient's functional recovery, or ability to participate in the activities that define the patient's life goals.[11] Conflict for therapists working within these models occurs when a philosophical difference in opinion results from team members using inconsistent professional terms because understanding those terms in different ways impedes discharge planning.

Other models attempt to evaluate the severity of impact of disease sequelae on LOS. Several measurement methods were described in 1990 by Thomas and Longo.[13] Individual case review is a method by which charts are retrospectively peer reviewed in an attempt to determine factors that may be prolonging care (and thus increasing cost) beyond the point at which functional ability improves. Difficulties arise when the person reviewing the charts is a member of another profession or not a specialist. A reviewer who is a member of the profession but not a specialist may not understand the nuances or standards of the subspecialty area of practice. Despite these concerns, less than 5% discrepancy exists between accurate charts and the peer reviewers' findings.[13]

Thomas and Longo[13] also describe measuring the impact of disease sequelae on function using several scales including the Acute Physiology and Chronic Health Evaluation II (APACHE II). Although generally used to measure functional impairment severity in intensive care units compared to general acute care, factors used in this scale include the impact of acute illness, age, and chronic disease. The shortcoming of the scale from an occupational therapist's perspective is that it fails to consider the fact that occupational therapy can restore functional control of both the human and nonhuman environments—with or without the use of adapted technology and regardless of the severity of disease.

In comparison, scales have evolved that are used in an attempt to measure categories of function in relation to physical demand. One such scale is the Sickness Impact Profile (SIP).[9] It has 12 categories, including ambulation, mobility, body care, and movement. Another similar scale

in wide use is the Functional Independence Measure (FIM).[5] Although these scales are quantifiable in nature, they fail to account for individual idiosyncrasies or foibles that can enhance or impede functional recovery. In addition, little if any consideration is given to the functional influence of cognition on an individual's ability to successfully participate in and achieve practical or actual desired outcomes in daily life. To an occupational therapist, this fact is incredulous because learning is based on cognition and the ability to utilize problem-solving to successfully plan and complete tasks.

It could be argued that the relationship of cognition to survival from stroke varies so much that using treatment methods in which the influence of this relationship is disregarded may be the only means of achieving any function at all with any degree of consistency.[6] If the goal of treatment for a person with impaired cognition is subcortical execution of daily tasks with habits used before the stroke, then perhaps measurement scales originating from occupational therapy sources are best to consider; the Árnadóttir Occupational Therapy Neurobehavioral Evaluation (A-ONE) (see Chapter 13) and the Assessment of Motor and Process Skills (AMPS) (see Chapter 15) are two such scales. The A-ONE is used to demonstrate the influence cognitive impairment has on an individual's ability to complete BADL, and the AMPS is used as a valid indicator of IADL activity. The use of a similar index, the Activities Index (AI), was used to determine whether the speed of intervention initiation following stroke had an influence on recovery. This possible relationship has implications for occupational therapists working in inpatient settings with interdisciplinary team case management plans. Abbreviated scales with universal application have great value in inpatient and subacute settings in which an interdisciplinary approach is used.

Gross mobility is also an important risk management factor especially in patients with demonstrated motor or sensory impairments, because they are at greater risk for falls.[1,3] Falls increase the risk of developing comorbidities factors such as fractures and soft tissue injuries. A person with a known central nervous system disorder diagnosis should be considered at risk. The patient and caregivers must be educated about the implications imbedded in community mobility. Patients must be taught the least harmful way to fall and the way to get up from the ground if they do fall. If they get up from a fall alone, a system must be in place for them to gain assistance. Supervision is one solution but may be intrusive to an adult patient who is otherwise cognitively intact and able to live alone. For higher functioning individuals a medical alert system, such as a beeper-activated device worn around the neck, may allow independence in the home environment. A fracture superimposed on a neurologically weakened limb will have decreased circulation and delayed healing time. The presence of a fracture will necessitate rehospitalization and a second course of rehabilitation intervention. This clearly is a measurable CQI indicator—both in the inpatient setting as well as on community questionnaire follow-up activities.

CRITICAL PATHWAYS

As managed care has become more prominent in health care systems, provider groups have formed multidisciplinary teams to address cost containment.[7] Two heavily weighted factors affecting cost containment in inpatient settings are (1) LOS and (2) the development of comorbidities. Therefore strategies are being developed to decrease the LOS and provide essential services more quickly and efficiently.

Critical pathways are interdisciplinary team case management plans.[14] The team decides on the ideal inpatient LOS and then tailors an in-depth care map, or treatment plan, that describes the timing and extent of multidisciplinary services. The underlying issues for any health care provider are (1) determining whether it is beneficial to participate in the planning committee for a critical pathway; (2) streamlining intervention plans without sacrificing what MCOs deem quality or cost effectiveness, resulting in realistic staffing that will support a positive outcome; (3) providing the best quality care at the least cost to aid the institution's competitiveness in the managed care marketplace; (4) being proactive in support of the marketability of services; and (5) continuing to guide practice using ethics.

During the planning process for a critical pathway, there is often an aura of open-bidding for the time or opportunity to intervene with the patient. Understanding the timing of making referrals for services and the mechanism used to make referrals is important. If a physician will have to write a prescription for a therapist to initiate an intervention plan, it is often beneficial for the pathway to indicate that the referral be written the day before the planned intervention. One way to simplify this process is to use a general check-off referral form. The physician checks off or initials the request for therapy services; the request indicates the usual time frame for initiation of services (e.g., the first day after a stroke). If blanket referrals are not acceptable, the process of making and receiving referrals increases the multidisciplinary team's labor and decreases available time. For example, there is increased reliance on utilization reviewers to locate the documentation of the physician referral, and the process of relaying the referral to the ancillary services takes the caregiver more time to locate the referral in the written chart.

Once it has been established that each service will deliver care according to the care map, a mechanism must be established to monitor whether the plan is carried out. A care map can be put into the main frame system of the hospital computer. As caregivers intervene, they can initial the computer care map grid. A note is also usually needed to specify the details and outcome of the caregiver sessions (e.g., whether the patient was willing to participate and the patient's tolerance for activity).

The acute inpatient LOS for a stroke patient is currently 4 days. At the end of 4 days the patient either returns home with or without home care (depending on the recovery and resources available for treatment), goes to an inpatient rehabilitation setting for a short LOS (e.g., 2 to 4 weeks), or goes to a long-term care facility for rehabilitation followed by maintenance care. Many long-term care facilities now accept acute care patients and are being reclassified as subacute care facilities. This trend has changed the common perception of a nursing home stay—that it is a terminal care facility and a last resort—because more and more individuals are being discharged to their homes and the community after a short-term nursing home stay.

The role of acute care therapists has become more consultative. Therapists are now members of the primary care team in many acute hospital settings. Because of knowledge of function and safety, they often lead the team when determining discharge planning projections.

As consultants, primary care therapists rapidly evaluate sequelae of stroke and recommend proper positioning and needed equipment for immediate intervention. Because of the limited LOS and therefore of time, patient-centered caregiver education and training must be emphasized.

Handling and alignment during activity participation are duties that are often assumed by home care or subacute care therapists. Handling and alignment must always be a part of functional tasks because outcome is measured by function alone. Therapists can no longer use hands-on treatment methods for months or years on the same patient. Although neurodevelopmental treatment techniques are commonly used with the stroke population, professional survival in the current economic environment is ultimately defined by functional success of patients. Function is the only reimbursable commodity according to third-party payers. Documentation of treatment intervention efficacy is necessary to continue to provide occupational and physical therapy care in the future.

CONTINUOUS QUALITY IMPROVEMENT

The development of CQI monitors should be tied to the context and content of treatment provided to a given population. Therefore the CQI monitors of a stroke population should track the outcome of the care according to the underlying clinical intervention philosophy. For example, if clinical evaluations are used to measure function, one CQI monitor should focus on the outcome of treatment as measured by functional improvement according to the particular measurement tool. Two of the tools used in rehabilitation units are the A-ONE and the AMPS. The A-ONE measures basic self-care functioning in relation to cognitive impairment and recovery after a stroke. Baseline functioning is observed and documented. The person is reevaluated weekly and on discharge. The test is in the form of prefabricated progress note formats and discharge evaluations. Use of prefabricated notes helps therapists adhere to documentation parameters while reporting functional improvements applicable to the deficits identified at the initiation of therapy. Improvement of function continues to be documented throughout the LOS. Although it is true that a patient's neurologic status can be improved without therapy, many cases reveal clinical trends. If CQI monitoring demonstrates an inability to reach projected benchmarks, the need to change the focus of therapy could be demonstrated.

Another CQI monitor that could be used on a stroke service is tracking the development of secondary conditions, such as painful shoulder. Therapists using shoulder protection or positioning programs for their patients, the clinical standards for positioning the shoulder, training the caregivers, and providing education to the patients and caregivers could be routinely monitored. Patient compliance could also be documented. The outcome (i.e., percentage of patients who develop shoulder pain) could be compared to current data on the national norms. The effectiveness of the program could be demonstrated if the outcome is above the national average.

Interdisciplinary CQI monitors are intrinsically valuable to credentialing agencies such as the JCAHO and CARF. An area of stroke patient care that naturally lends itself to interdisciplinary monitoring is dysphagia assessment and treatment outcome. Individuals who develop dysphagia are at greater risk for increased in-hospital LOS or repeatedly being admitted to the hospital because of resulting aspiration pneumonia. The interdisciplinary team treating dysphagia often consists of representatives from occupational therapy, speech pathology, nutrition, radiology, nursing, and otolaryngology. Information could be collected about whether a swallowing assessment was done, the incidence of aspiration pneumonia, the appropriateness of the alternative methods recommended to the patients, and findings when the patient is reassessed.

Another emerging issue is the use of conscious (physical or chemical) restraints. The Omnibus Budget Reconciliation Act (OBRA) of 1981 mandates that restraints of any kind will not be used without proper justification and/or agreement from the patient or the appointed proxy. This decision must be documented in the medical chart and communicated to the interdisciplinary team. Many facilities have formed restraint committees to set facility standards that comply with federal and state laws.

Patient satisfaction may be difficult to assess in the stroke population because of the potential sequelae of stroke and patients' overall dissatisfaction with quality of life—issues over which the therapist has no control. These are inherent problems associated with studying CQI po-

tential in this specific population. Satisfaction must be specifically defined in quantifiable terms and directly relate to functional improvements in basic self-care activities and IADL.[17,18]

Safety is a key area of concern in the stroke population. CQI monitors could track risk management issues such as reducing the incidence of falls in the inpatient or the home setting. Compliance with therapists' recommendations for removing potential safety hazards (e.g., throw rugs) could be monitored. Documenting safety education is often a good way to contain risk management liability.

Theoretically, a CQI monitor could be a pilot for a clinically based outcomes research project. The data could be saved over extended periods of time and retrospectively studied. If therapists could not carry out this degree of analysis independently, graduate students or academic peers could assist with analyzing and documenting the outcomes. Pairing clinical practice with academic preparation for practice may help future generations of therapists develop the skills to routinely collect and analyze their practices, which could improve the efficacy of our professional involvement in health care.

RISK MANAGEMENT

Liability—one of the key underlying concepts of risk management—is always a concern when an industry provides a service to the public. Responsibility for injury must be contained to protect the public as well as the industry providing the services. In a patient care setting, numerous risk factors exist, the most common of which are (1) physical environment that is unsafe, (2) management of injury under conditions that are not ideal, (3) mishandling by a trained care provider or professional resulting in injury or harm, (4) mishandling by nonprofessional personnel resulting in injury or harm, and (5) equipment malfunctions.

A key to risk management is documentation of incidents. When anyone is involved in an incident, whether it initially appears to have resulted in injury, the incident should be documented within the time frame required by the credentialing agency or institutional policy. In many settings, this window of time is 24 to 48 hours. The forms usually require a description of the incident, a list of witnesses, the location of the incident, findings of a medical review, and a plan for action to change the contributing factors and decrease the chance of an incidence occurrence again in the future. Institutional policy may require that these incidents be reported to the state and become part of the morbidity and mortality review standards by which the institution is judged.

DOCUMENTATION OF THE TQM PROGRAM

The TQM (CQI and RM) policies and procedures should be kept in the departmental policy and procedure manual.

If the practitioner is in sole practice or private practice, the practice should also have a policy and procedure manual. In addition to having general policies and procedures, the practice should have a mission statement that agrees with the TQM documents. The staff should participate in risk management and quality improvement initiative training that is documented on a yearly basis. If CQI monitors indicate a need to revise the departmental policies and procedures, the plans for the revision can be documented in the CQI plan. For consistency and context validity, changes should be monitored for efficacy to ensure that they result in improved care and management.

REVIEW QUESTIONS

1. What types of administrative activities should be included in any occupational therapy department's program to ensure quality? (i.e., TQM=RM + PI/QA)
2. Describe a method that can be used to measure and monitor risk in any practice setting.
3. Name three clinically based performance improvement initiatives that could be developed for a setting in which persons who have survived a stroke are treated.
4. What benefit is there for therapists to use the A-ONE, COPM, and AMPS scales to measure function in comparison to other researched and popular tests or scales?
5. From a rehabilitative manager's perspective, what benefits or hindrances are inherent in the use of critical pathways?

■ COTA Considerations ■

- Assist with collecting and reporting data for the process improvement monitor.
- Ask the supervisor about the current process improvement issues.
- Clinical indicators should measure outcome of interventions provided that they have inherent risk. If something should be evaluated that is not being evaluated, communicate the idea or a process of measuring it to the supervisor.

REFERENCES

1. DeVincenzo DK, Watkins S: Accidental falls in a rehabilitation setting: *Rehabil Nurs* 12:248, 1987.
2. Deyo RA, Inui TS: Toward clinical applications of health status measures: sensitivity of scales to clinically important changes, *Health Serv Res* 19:275, 1984.
3. Hamrin E: Early activation in stroke: does it make a difference? *Scand J Rehabil Med* 14:101, 1989.
4. Holloway JJ, Thomas JW: Factors influencing readmission risk: implications for quality monitoring, *Health Care Financ Rev* 1:19, 1989.
5. Kaira L, Dale P, Crome P: Improving stroke rehabilitation: a controlled study, *Stroke* 24:1462, 1994.
6. Kaira L: The influence of stroke unit rehabilitation on functional recovery from stroke, *Stroke* 25:821, 1994.
7. Kaira L, Fowle AJ: An integrated system for multidisciplinary assessments in stroke rehabilitation, *Stroke* 25:2210, 1994.
8. Longo DR, Daugird AJ: Measuring the quality of care: reforming the health care system, *Am Coll Med Qual* 9:104, 1994.
9. Nelson E et al: Functional health status of primary care patients, *JAMA* 249:3331, 1983.
10. Shartell SM et al: Assessing the impact of continuous quality improvement/total quality management: concept versus implementation, *Health Serv Res* 30:377, 1995.
11. Stewart AL et al: Functional status and well-being of patients with chronic conditions: results from the medical outcomes study, *JAMA* 262:907, 1989.
12. Tarlov AR et al: The medical outcomes study: an application of the methods for monitoring the results of medical care, *JAMA* 262:925, 1989.
13. Thomas JW, Longo DR: Application of severity measurement systems for hospital quality management, *Hosp Health Serv Admin* 35(2):221, 1990.
14. Underwood R: Developing critical pathways: management strategies, *AOTA Admin Manag SIS Newsletter* 12(2):1, 1996.
15. Ware JE et al: Comparison of health outcomes at a health maintenance organization with those of fee-for-service care, *Lancet* pp 1017-1022, 1986.
16. Weinberg J: Which rate is right? *New Eng J Med* 314:317, 1986.
17. Wells KB et al: Agreement between face-to-face and telephone-administered versions of the depression section of the NIMH diagnostic interview schedule, *J Psychiatr Res* 22:207, 1988.
18. Wells KB et al: The functioning and well-being of depressed patients, *JAMA* 262:914, 1989.

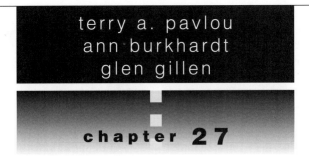

terry a. pavlou
ann burkhardt
glen gillen

chapter 27

COTA/OTR Partnerships:
Teamwork to Enhance Living Skills

key terms

certified occupational therapy
assistant

occupational therapy practitioner
supervision

teamwork

chapter objectives

After completing this chapter, the reader will be able to accomplish the following:

1. Develop strategies to integrate COTA/OTR teams in the rehabilitation of stroke patients.
2. Recognize evaluation and treatment philosophies for occupational therapy practitioners providing services to stroke patients.
3. Understand supervision guidelines for COTAs working with stroke patients.

The management of patients who have had strokes is a challenging and often frustrating process. Positive functional outcomes rely on team communication, organized treatment planning that supports the goals of each discipline, patient-centered interventions, and interventions focused on the patient's acquisition of life skills for enhanced quality of life.

Multiple settings, from intensive care units to community-based programs, provide interventions for stroke survivors through teams consisting of certified occupational therapy assistants (COTAs) and registered occupational therapists (OTRs). This partnership can greatly benefit patients who are receiving services. The focus of this chapter

is to provide these teams with guidelines for intervention. Areas to be addressed include treatment philosophy, evaluations, intervention strategies via case studies, communication, role delineation, and supervision guidelines.

CONSIDERATIONS WHEN WORKING WITH PATIENTS WHO HAVE HAD STROKES

The complexity of stroke rehabilitation stems from the variety of functional deficits observed after a cerebral vascular accident (CVA). The resultant functional limitations depend on the location of the CVA (e.g., cortical, subcortical), the size of the damaged area, the number of CVAs, the age of the patient, comorbidities, and other factors. Therefore communication between the COTA and OTR is essential for optimal care. An occupational therapy practitioner may have a full caseload of patients who have survived a stroke, all of whom are different in terms of functional level.

A CVA can affect the following areas:

- Performance areas: activities of daily living, work and productive activities, and play or leisure[2]
- Performance components: the elements of performance (sensorimotor, cognitive, psychosocial, and psychologic aspects) that are assessed and, when needed, intervened for the goal of improved performance[2]
- Performance contexts: situations or factors that influence an individual's engagement in desired or required performance areas; performance contexts include temporal aspects (e.g., age, life stage) and environmental aspects (physical, social, and cultural aspects)[2]

More specific examples of performance areas and performance components that may be affected by a CVA are outlined in Boxes 27-1 and 27-2.

Several questions must be considered when planning interventions for stroke patients:

- What were the patient's life roles (e.g., parent, homemaker, volunteer, retiree) before the CVA?
- What activities were important to the patient before the stroke? What activities are important to the patient now? This information is critical for goal setting, treatment planning, and assuring that intervention activities are purposeful, meaningful, and relevant.
- What are the goals of the patient, the patient's significant others, and the primary caretakers?
- Is the patient able to learn? What limits the patient's learning capacities (e.g., education, cognitive impairment, language disturbance, depression)?
- What are realistic occupational therapy goals given time constraints, reimbursement, and patient carryover?
- What are the intervention priorities (e.g., pain control, safety, adaptive equipment, transfer training)?
- In what environments (e.g., home, community, work) will the patient be functioning?
- What level of assistance will be available to the patient after discharge? Does the patient need physical or verbal assistance?
- What other disciplines are involved in the patient's care? This information is critical to prevent duplication of services and integrate the goals of other disciplines into the treatment plan.
- What community resources (e.g., stroke support groups, return-to-work programs, prevention programs, social groups) are available to the patient?

Box 27-1

Performance Area Dysfunction After CVA

Dressing	Clothing care
Feeding	Meal preparation
Grooming	Cleaning
Oral hygiene	Shopping
Medication routine	Money management
Community mobility	Household maintenance
Sexual expression	Care of others
Functional mobility	Educational activities
Emergency response	Work/job performance
Bathing/showering	Volunteerism
Toileting	Play/leisure exploration and performance

Modified from American Occupational Therapy Association: Uniform terminology for occupational therapy—third edition, *Am J Occup Ther* 48(11):1047, 1994.

THE ASSESSMENT PROCESS

During the assessment of the CVA patient, interaction between the COTA and OTR varies depending on the level of patient functioning, the experience level of the COTA, and the factors interfering with successful intervention (e.g., pain, unsupportive families, poor response to treatment). Regular communication between the COTA and OTR ensures correct interpretation of assessment information and development of appropriate goals and treatment interventions. Periodic reevaluation by the OTR or the COTA/OTR team is mandatory to upgrade goals and modify the treatment plan as needed.

Patient/Client-Centered Assessment

Assessment by all occupational therapy practitioners, including COTAs, should be patient/client centered. Occupational therapists in Canada have been the most effective in promoting this approach to assessment.

[Patient]/client-centered practice is an approach to providing occupational therapy which embraces a philosophy of respect for, and partnership with, people receiving services. Client-centered practice recognizes the autonomy of individuals, the need for client choice in making decisions about occupational needs, the strengths clients bring to a therapy encounter, the benefits of client-therapist partnership, and the need to ensure that services are accessible and fit the context in which a client lives.[7]

Law, Baptiste, and Mills[8] summarize several concepts that form the basis of a patient-centered approach:

- Autonomy/choice: This concept recognizes that all patients are uniquely qualified to make decisions about their occupational functioning. Only patients can understand the experiences of their daily lives and make choices about their treatment.

Box 27-2

Performance Component Dysfunction After CVA

SENSORY

Tactile
Proprioceptive
Vestibular
Visual

PERCEPTUAL PROCESSING

Stereognosis
Kinesthesia
Pain response
Body scheme
Position in space
Figure-ground
Depth perception
Spatial relations
Topographic orientation

NEUROMUSCULOSKELETAL

Reflexes
Range of motion
Strength
Endurance
Postural control
Postural alignment
Soft tissue integrity

MOTOR

Motor control
Gross coordination

Praxis
Dexterity
Oral-motor control
Visual-motor integration

COGNITIVE INTEGRATION

Arousal level
Orientation
Recognition
Attention span
Initiation of activity
Termination of activity
Memory
Sequencing
Problem-solving
Learning
Generalization

PSYCHOSOCIAL SKILLS

Values
Interests
Self-concept
Role performance
Social conduct
Self-expression
Interpersonal skills
Coping skills
Self-control
Time management

Modified from American Occupational Therapy Association: Uniform terminology for occupational therapy—third edition, *Am J Occup Ther* 48(11):1047, 1994.

- Partnership and responsibility: An ideal patient-therapist relationship is an "interdependent partnership to enable the solution of occupational performance issues and the achievement of patient goals."[8] This approach offers patients a more active role in defining their goals and desired outcomes. The occupational therapy practitioner serves as a resource to help patients meet these goals and achieve desired functional outcomes.
- Enablement: This concept implies a shift from the remediation of deficits to a model in which therapists work with patients to enable them to meet their own goals. "Achievement of these goals is facilitated through a variety of means, including changes in individual skills, changes in environments, and changes in occupations."[8]
- Contextual congruence: This concept places primary importance on individualizing the assessment and intervention process for each patient. The use of diagnosis-specific protocols is discouraged. The contexts in which patients live, their roles and interests, and their culture are of primary importance.

- Accessibility and flexibility: All services should be provided in a timely and accessible manner. Interventions are developed to meet the needs of patients rather than to fit patients into a particular service model.
- Respect for diversity: This concept focuses on respecting the diversity of patients' values and visions. Therapists must avoid imposing their personal values on their patients.

Pollock[9] states the following:

The use of rater judgment in scoring assessments may only reinforce the passivity of clients and the sense of the professional as the answer to the problem. If the person is no longer the problem definer, it is unlikely that he or she will be the problem solver either. This disparity can reduce the client's self-determination and sense of control over health, often leading to what may appear as noncompliance. If the therapy goals are set by the client through a process of client-centered assessment, the potential for active participation is enhanced.

Top-Down Approach to Assessment

Trombly[13] has discussed the distinctions between a "top-down" approach to assessment versus a "bottom-up" approach. According to Trombly, "a bottom-up approach to assessment and treatment focuses on the deficits of components of function, such as strength, range of motion, balance, and so on, which are believed to be prerequisites to successful occupational performance or functioning."[13] An example of this approach to assessment is evaluating and treating the performance components of an upper extremity dressing task (e.g., spatial relations, postural control, upper extremity range of motion and sensation) with the expectation of improving the original task (i.e., dressing). Trombly notes that the occupational therapy practitioner may not clarify the relationship of these components to the task, which leads to the patient becoming dissatisfied with treatment. This lack of clarification may also prevent the patient from understanding the true goals of occupational therapy services (i.e., the acquisition of life skills). Bottom-up approaches to assessment focus on the evaluation of performance components. Many of these assessments are borrowed from other disciplines (e.g., neurology, neuropsychiatry) and are not effective in the evaluation of life skills. Because these assessments do not have a clear link to function and do not include the use of functional tasks, the use of a strictly bottom-up approach makes it difficult to develop goals and treatment plans focused on the acquisition of functional skills. Examples of bottom-up assessments that are commonly used for CVA patients include the Motor-Free Visual Perception Test, Lowenstein Occupational Therapy Cognitive Assessment, Benton Block Construction Evaluation, Purdue Pegboard, Minnesota Rate of Manipulation Test, Allen Cognitive Level, Stroop Test, Draw a person/clock, and Letter Cancellation Task. The usefulness of this evaluation strategy in occupational therapy must be seriously reconsidered if the profession is to retain its unique perspective on function.

Trombly explains the contrasting approach, a top-down assessment, as follows:

One that starts with inquiry into role competency and meaningfulness would clarify the purpose of occupational therapy for the client. . . . A top-down assessment further determines which particular tasks define each of these roles for that person, whether he or she can now do those tasks, and probable reasons for an inability to do so.[13]

Because the top-down approach focuses on the evaluation of performance areas, the functional perspective is clearly evident to patients as well as third-party payers. This type of assessment clarifies the goals of treatment for the patient and allows the therapist to identify barriers to independent living. This approach is useful to both COTAs and OTRs. Examples of top-down approaches to assessment follow.

Recommended Assessments

According to the Clinical Practice Guidelines for Poststroke Rehabilitation,[1] assessments are evaluated in terms of their practicality (ease of use and reasonableness), validity (the instrument measures what it is intended to measure), reliability (consistency of results and the ability of two different individuals to achieve similar results), and sensitivity to change (the ability to detect clinically important changes). In addition, the evaluations chosen should reflect a function-based approach to assessment. The following are examples of currently available assessment tools that may be useful to COTA/OTR teams treating CVA patients.

- Árnadóttir Occupational Therapy Neurobehavioral Evaluation (A-ONE)[4]: This evaluation is based on the structured observation of several performance areas including transfers and mobility, grooming and hygiene, feeding, and dressing. The goal of this evaluation is to determine which neurobehavioral deficits commonly seen after stroke are interfering with independent functioning in the above-stated performance areas. The neurobehavioral deficits assessed in a strictly function-based approach include ideational apraxia, motor apraxia, spatial neglect, body neglect, spatial relations, topographical disorientation, and organization and sequencing.

  This evaluation is standardized and reliable. A training seminar is required for standardized administration and interpretation. The evaluation bridges the usual gap between performance components and performance areas (see Chapter 13).

- Assessment of Motor and Process Skills (AMPS): Developed by Anne G. Fisher, the AMPS is an "observational assessment that permits simultaneous evaluation of motor and process skills and their effect on the ability of an individual to perform complex or instrumental activities of daily living."[5] In the context of this evaluation, the term *motor skills* refers to observable actions that subjects may use to move their bodies or objects in the context of daily living tasks. Examples of observable motor skills include reaching, bending, walking, lifting, moving, and transporting. *Process skills* refers to a series of observable actions used to organize and adapt a person's behavior for completion of a chosen task. Examples of process skills include organizing, gathering, handling, attending, and initiating.

  Overall, the AMPS evaluates 16 motor skills and 20 process skills. Patients may choose to be evaluated on 50 instrumental activities of daily living (IADL) tasks. The evaluation has been standardized using over 7000 subjects internationally and crossculturally. Valid administration and interpretation require training (see Chapter 15).

- Kohlman Evaluation of Living Skills (KELS): Developed by Linda Kohlman Thomson,[11] the KELS is used to determine a person's ability to perform basic living skills. The evaluation combines interview questions and tasks and takes approximately 30 minutes to complete. Seventeen living skills are tested under the five general areas of self-care, safety and health, money management, transportation and telephone, and work and leisure. The stated goal of the KELS is the successful integration of patients into their environments. The KELS can be used to identify tasks that can be completed independently and tasks that require assistance. Six research studies have established the reliability and validity of the KELS.

- Canadian Occupational Performance Measure (COPM):[7] This patient-centered assessment tool and outcome measure is administered through a semistructured interview based on the patient's perception of functioning in self-care, productivity, and leisure. The tool is used to encourage patients to identify the performance areas in which they are having difficulty. After identifying problem areas, patients score their current performance and their level of satisfaction with their performance. Use of the tool ensures that occupational therapy intervention is based on activities that are important to the patient. Because it is an outcome measure, it should be administered early in the provision of services and followed by periodic reevaluations. This tool allows patients to become immediately involved in their treatment and encourages them to be responsible for their own well-being. Because the COPM is not diagnosis specific and crosses multiple developmental stages, it is clearly a useful tool for patients who have had strokes. Therapists who incorporate this tool into their practices will find that writing functional and meaningful goals and establishing function-based treatment plans are easily placed into perspective. (See Chapter 15 for an example of the use of the COPM in planning treatment interventions for a CVA patient who is having difficulty performing IADL tasks.)

- Functional Independence Measure[6] (FIM) and the Barthel Index:[14] Both of these assessment tools have been recommended in the Post-Stroke Rehabilitation Clinical Practice Guidelines for evaluating basic activities of daily living (BADL). Both are widely used in clinical practice and stroke research. Research supports the validity, reliability, and sensitivity of both tools. The Barthel Index includes ten items (bowel management, bladder management, feeding, grooming, dressing, transfers, toilet use, mobility, stairs, and bathing) scored on an ordinal scale from 0 to 20.

The FIM features 18 items, including motor function, cognition, self-care, sphincter control, mobility, locomotion, communication, and social interaction. The FIM is scored on a 1 to 7 ordinal scale.

SUGGESTED TREATMENT APPROACHES

When planning treatment interventions for patients who have had strokes, COTAs should consider the following general principles. Treatment plans should be reevaluated and upgraded as needed with the input of the OTR.

1. Treatment interventions should be based on previously practiced activities that are meaningful and culturally relevant to the patient. When possible, they should be chosen by the patient. Given these criteria, contrived activities, such as inserting pegs in pegboards and placing clothespins on vertical sticks, are highly discouraged. Activities such as completing body puzzles, stacking cones, and transferring beanbags from one bowl to the next not only lack meaning and purpose but infantilize patients. Practitioners should be wary of purchasing and using catalog-order activities; although many are advertised as cognitive-perceptual and sensorimotor activities, they may incorporate objects that patients have never used as adults. These novel activities are not only unnecessarily difficult but usually irrelevant to the patient's daily life. Interest checklists, interviews such as the Canadian Occupational Performance Measure, and conversations with the patient's family are better ways to choose appropriate activities.

2. The use of a "hands-on" approach should not be the major focus of a treatment session. The overuse of physical handling makes patients passive recipients of treatment. In contrast, the use of functional activities allows patients to be active problem-solvers with the goal of successful task completion.

   The majority of movement patterns achieved through therapeutic handling can be just as effectively achieved through functional activities that are relevant to daily life. For example, patients can be made to shift their weight in the standing position by means of the therapist's hands, but this is more effective when patients reach into kitchen cabinets, wash a wall mirror, set a table, make a bed, play a variation of soccer, or perform similar activities (see Chapters 4, 5, 6, 10, and 11).

   If using a hands-on approach, the therapist must clearly explain the rationale to the patient (e.g., "I'm going to stretch your trunk so that you can move with greater ease; now I want you to move with my hands and feel how your body responds.") After any hands-on treatment, the movement pattern must be repeated immediately in the form of a task. This approach provides the opportunity for practice and carryover into daily life (see Chapter 2).

3. During all treatment interventions the patient should be positioned in proper alignment to promote greater ease of motion and enhance effective and efficient movement patterns (see Chapter 19).

4. Treatment interventions should be based on principles of learning. The Clinical Practice Guidelines for Stroke Rehabilitation[1] states the following:

> Rehabilitation is predominantly a learning process. Adherence to basic principles of learning require that:
> - Careful assessment is done to determine tasks that a patient can perform.
> - The skills or knowledge being taught are meaningful to the patient.
> - Training is graded by level of difficulty, and less complex or demanding tasks are addressed first, so that the patients can experience success.
> - Instructions are phrased as concretely as possible and are short, direct, and simple.
> - Instructions are understood.
> - Tasks to be mastered or information to be learned is tailored in order to avoid 'overload.'
> - Steps are taken to slow patient responses if impulsivity causes a person to perform too rapidly or unsafely.
> - Feedback on performance is provided by the therapist . . . .
> - Steps are taken to stimulate responses . . . in order to overcome periods of hypoarousal or lethargy.
> - Repetition and practice are used between training sessions. . . .[1]

(See Chapter 2 for more information on learning strategies.)

5. Patient and family education should be initiated as early in the intervention process as possible.

> Patients, families, and involved others should be given information and provided with ample opportunity to learn about the causes and consequences of stroke and the goals, process, and prognosis of rehabilitation. Family members and other potential caregivers should receive thorough training in techniques and problem-solving approaches required to provide effective support.[1] (See Chapter 25.)

6. "Occupation-as-end": Trombly coined this term to describe interventions that focus on occupation as the goal to be learned. According to Trombly, "Occupation-as-end is not only purposeful but also meaningful because it is the performance of activities or tasks that a person sees as important."[12] Trombly[12] explains that occupation-as-end is brought about by directly teaching the activity or task to be learned. In this model, patients use whatever abilities are available to them, including the use of adaptive techniques or equipment. This model is similar to the Rehabilitative Approach and the Skills Training Approach. Steps of intervention include the following:
   - Occupations are analyzed to ensure that they are within the capabilities of the patient. The task is not used to bring about changes in the capabilities of the patient.

- The therapist assumes the role of teacher and adaptor to facilitate learning.
- The demands and contexts of the task are adapted as necessary.
- The therapist organizes the subtasks so that the patient will succeed.
- The therapist provides feedback to ensure a successful outcome.
- The therapist structures practice to promote improved performance and learning.[12]

Trombly states that the therapeutic principles for this approach derive from cognitive information processing and learning theories. Using the "occupation-as-end" model ensures that the task is apparent and meaningful to the patient.[12]

7. Occupation-as-means: "Occupation-as-means refers to occupation acting as the therapeutic change agent to remediate impaired abilities or capacities."[12] Trombly created this term and provides examples such as arts, crafts, games, sports, exercise routines, and daily activities that are selected according to the patient's needs. According to Trombly, this model assumes an intrinsic healing property in the activity that will change organic or behavioral impairments. Use of this model during treatment interventions includes the following steps:
   - The therapist analyzes the occupation to determine that it demands particular responses from the patient. These responses must be slightly more challenging than those the patient can easily produce.
   - The therapist provides the opportunity to engage in the therapeutic occupation.
   - As the patient attempts the activity and succeeds, the impairment for which the occupation was chosen is remediated.

   The chosen occupation must be challenging but have some potential for success, and the activity must be purposeful and meaningful.[12]

   The preceding principles of intervention should guide occupational therapy practitioners, including COTAs, in the treatment planning process. Therapists should remember that one activity, such as putting on a shirt, not only promotes independence in the task itself (occupation-as-end) but also addresses a multitude of underlying impairments (Figure 27-1).

SUPERVISION OF THE CERTIFIED OCCUPATIONAL THERAPY ASSISTANT

The Roles Document adopted by the American Occupational Therapy Association[3] (AOTA) in 1994 provides guidance for the amount and frequency of supervision all occupational therapy practitioners should seek according to their levels of education, training, and work experience. All professionals have an ethical obligation to seek super-

Possible behavioral deficits interfering with function:

Premotor perseveration: pulling up sleeve

Spatial-relation difficulties: differentiating front from back on shirt

Spatial-relation difficulties: getting an arm into the right armhole

Unilateral spatial neglect: not seeing shirt located on neglected side (or a part of the shirt)

Unilateral body neglect: not dressing the neglected side or not completing the dressing on that side

Comprehension problem: not understanding verbal information related to performance

Ideational apraxia: not knowing what to do to get shirt on or not knowing what the shirt is for

Ideomotor apraxia: having problems with the planning of finger movements in order to perform

Tactile agnosia (asterognosis): having trouble buttoning shirt without watching the performance

Organization and sequencing: dressing the unaffected arm first and having problems with dressing the affected arm; inability to continue the activity without being reminded

Lack of motivation to perform

Distraction: becoming interrupted by other things

Attention deficit: difficulty attending to task and quality of performance

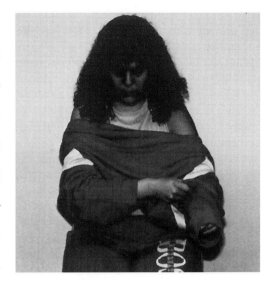

Irritation or frustration when having trouble performing or when not getting the desired assistance

Aggressiveness when being touched and assisted by therapist (tactile defensiveness)

Difficulties recognizing foreground from background or a sleeve of a unicolor shirt from the rest of the shirt

Figure 27-1   A single functional task can be used to evaluate multiple deficits and treat a variety of blocks to functional independence. (From Árnadóttir G: *The brain and behavior: assessing cortical dysfunction through ADL*, St Louis, 1990, Mosby.)

vision as it is needed. This concept has historically been difficult for many occupational therapy practitioners because the profession does not address the need for supervision outside of the workplace. However, occupational therapy practitioners should recognize this obligation, even if their employers deny them adequate supervision.

Occupational therapy practitioners at all levels are often confused by the ways in which the official standards of practice (SOPs) of a professional association, such as the AOTA, differ from state law. For example, most states in the United States currently have practice acts governing occupational therapy. These acts are usually licensing or trademark laws (for use of the name *occupational therapy*). Not every state that regulates the practice of occupational therapy defines the level of supervision the OTR must provide for the assistant practitioner (COTA). Most practice acts defining licensed professions are general, allowing for some legal interpretation and not overrestricting practice. When a state has regulations in reference to the assistant level of practitioner, the laws governing practice in that state supersede the official documents of the professional association. State regulations and official AOTA documents may conflict. AOTA official documents are often consulted even when

they are not law. States that do not have provisions for the occupational therapy practitioner at the COTA level of practice are referred to as *unregulated states.* In an unregulated state, practice models are generally influenced by insurance law and the inclusion of occupational therapy as a mandated, reimbursable, or eminent service. State regulations may also carry mandates for level of practitioner in provision of care, especially under the health care finance administration (HCFA), which is the reimbursing agency for Medicare. Medicare is federally mandated. Block grants are given to the states to fund services provided under Medicare. Individual states regulate the reimbursement of care within the laws of practice and are guided by HCFA guidelines in that state. Therefore the role and function of a COTA in a regulated state may differ from those of a COTA in an unregulated state because of reimbursement guidelines for the provision of care.

COTAs practice in numerous settings (clinical, academic, and research). The ability to assume any of these roles depends on their experience in the practice of occupational therapy, additional training from an experienced practitioner, continuing education, and experiential learning through on-the-job training. The Roles

Document defines several levels of experience: COTAs at all levels of experience who practice in clinical settings as occupational therapists must work under the supervision of a registered therapist (OTR). Several official documents of the Association that discuss occupational therapy specialty settings or areas of practice further define the role of the COTA in each context. For example, for a COTA to work as a case manager the AOTA states that the COTA should have 5 years of experience, 3 of which are in the specific practice area. It further indicates that a COTA who practices as a case manager should have attained additional skills in areas such as management, communications, and systems theory. Under all circumstances, COTAs cannot accept cases according to their own discretion. COTAs must work collaboratively with an OTR and under the supervision of an OTR. Notes may or may not require an OTR's signature. Often, such procedures are mandated by the institution where the practitioner works or third-party payers.

Therefore in specific reference to the care of stroke patients in an inpatient acute-care setting, the OTR and COTA generally work as a team. A COTA trained in standardized tests may administer these tests during evaluations. For example, a COTA may measure range of motion, muscle strength, and hand strength with a dynamometer or pinch meter and use the Canadian Occupational Performance Measure (COPM) and the Assessment of Motor and Process Skills (AMPS). If the COTA is not trained or has insufficient proficiency in portions of the evaluation, the COTA and supervising OTR should collaborate to complete that evaluation and set goals for occupational therapy intervention.

In long-term care settings, COTAs often work without the daily supervision of an OTR, but they must have direct supervision at defined intervals, depending on state regulations, reimbursement requirements, and the policies and procedures of their facilities. Similarly, in home-care and community settings, COTAs often work with a greater degree of independence, seeking out the OTR when this expertise is needed or when collaborative treatment planning is the rule.

The professional ideal is that both levels of occupational therapy practitioner, the OTR and the COTA, work as a team to provide superior patient care within the ethical guidelines of practice. It should go without saying (but probably never will) that misuses or abuse of the trust implied in this relationship constitutes unethical practice. Both levels of practitioner should clearly understand and accept their professional limitations. Foolish pride has no place in occupational therapy.

Cost containment through the judicious use of professional services is consistent with current standards of practice in the insurance industry. Insurance companies provide reimbursement for some services that occupational therapists provide. OTRs must be aware of these reimbursement policies and function as consultants rather than direct care providers when the situation demands. To provide affordable, high-quality care to patients, OTRs must work in conjunction with COTAs.

■

CASE STUDY

ML is a 66-year-old man who was brought to the emergency room after being found on the bathroom floor with left-sided facial drooping and an inability to stand. After a complete workup, he was diagnosed with a right middle cerebral artery (MCA) CVA.

ML received occupational therapy and physical therapy on the acute service. ML was unable to look toward the left side and was tearful during sessions. He drooled (because of the facial droop) and inconsistently followed one- and two-step commands. He was oriented only to name at that time. Further assessment revealed severe deficits in spatial relations and depth perception, an inability to maintain static sitting, and a need for maximal assistance to perform BADL tasks.

On the acute service the treatment plan set up by the OTR and carried out by the COTA focused on the following:

- Bed positioning
- Shoulder protection
- Promotion of awareness of the left upper extremity during activities of daily living (ADL) and mobility functions.
- Education of staff in the handling of extremities during ADL tasks and transitional movements
- Initial BADL training focusing on hygiene and grooming tasks

During the ADL training, items were placed on both sides of the work space to promote scanning and spatial awareness. ML required several verbal cues to initiate the tasks, scan to the left, and sequence the steps of the activity. He was unable to open the toothpaste, mouthwash, and shaving cream. In addition, ML required physical assistance from the therapist to place the toothpaste on the brush. Overall, he required moderate assistance and verbal cues for grooming.

Dressing activities were attempted on the acute service, but ML required assistance because of his neurobehavioral deficits and an increasingly obvious impairment in postural control (i.e., an inability to shift weight and an impaired perception of midline posture).

Treatment during this stage focused on daily repetition of grooming tasks (without changing the activity sequence), seated balance activities using graded reaching tasks, and transfer activities that required two therapists to complete a safe sit-pivot transfer.

ML was transferred to the inpatient rehabilitation unit after 8 days. His initial evaluation by the OTR included the following results:

- Is alert and oriented × 2 (i.e., required two verbal cues to state correct date)
- Follows one-step commands consistently; follows two- and three-step commands 50% of the time

- Has a nonfunctional flaccid left upper extremity with a one-finger inferior subluxation
- Complains of shoulder pain during rolling and repositioning of affected upper extremity
- Requires verbal cues (two or three) to attend to upper extremity during ADL and mobility functions
- Has decreased ADL status secondary to the following neurobehavioral deficits: spatial relations dysfunction, spatial neglect, body neglect, difficulties sequencing tasks
- Requires maximum assistance in IADL functions
- Requires maximal assistance × 1 for transfers and bed mobility
- Requires moderate assistance to maintain static sitting
- Experiences episodes of lability
- Experiences fear that he is at imminent risk of another stroke

The OTR and COTA discussed the initial treatment plan and implemented the following treatment procedures:

- Scapula mobilization and passive range-of-motion exercises
- Staff education regarding shoulder protection
- Daily self-care training for feeding and grooming
- Fabrication of splints to maintain alignment of the wrist and hand and prevent injury during mobility
- Bed mobility activities
- Wheelchair propulsion in open halls
- Family training and observation of treatment sessions
- Participation in a unit group focusing on the physical, psychosocial, and educational needs of stroke survivors

ML responded well to the initial treatment plan. The COTA periodically scheduled cotreatments with the supervising OTR to review procedure and reevaluate and upgrade the treatment plan as necessary. Initial improvements in status included increased awareness of the upper extremity, decreased shoulder pain, increased trunk control as evidenced by an improved ability to reach, improved bed mobility (requiring contact guarding and verbal cues), and improved BADL status in terms of feeding and grooming independently (the former performed with the aid of a rocker knife).

Because the discharge plan was for ML to return home with assistance from his wife and a home health attendant, family training was a critical component of the treatment plan. ML's wife received training and written information on bed positioning, range of motion, promotion of independent performance of self-care, and transfer techniques. By the third week of his inpatient stay, ML was ambulating short distances with a wide-based quad cane. Several sessions focused specifically on safety and guarding during ambulatory bathroom transfers. Both ML and his wife stressed their concern about his inability to toilet independently. They both felt that increasing ML's independence during this activity would ease the transition to home and help them retain their roles as husband and wife.

Because ML was ambulating only short distances (approximately 10 feet), wheelchair propulsion and management were important goals. Colored tabs were placed on the wheelchair mechanisms (e.g., red on brakes, green on leg-rest releases) and one-arm, one-leg propulsion was taught daily. ML's family and friends also learned this technique so they could encourage him to practice when he was not in therapy.

At this point in the treatment program, ML demonstrated independence in grooming, although the combination of oral care, hair care, and upper body washing required at least 45 minutes. The OTR and COTA administered the Árnadóttir Occupational Therapy Neurobehavioral Evaluation (A-ONE—see Chapter 13) to identify the neurobehavioral deficits that were preventing independent performance of self-care. In terms of upper extremity dressing, spatial relations dysfunction was the major deficit influencing his performance. ML could not orient the shirt correctly to his body; he confused right and left as well as front and back. ML required verbal cues to correctly orient the shirt in his lap before donning it. Once the shirt was properly oriented, ML could complete the task. Based on this evaluation finding, ML was trained to use the tag of the shirt as a cue for proper positioning. With this technique, ML achieved independence in upper extremity dressing.

In terms of lower extremity dressing, spatial relations dysfunction was again evident, although ML was able to correct this problem himself. The greatest limiting factor involved organization and sequencing of the task. ML required physical assistance to place the affected leg in his pants first. Treatment focused on training the home health attendant and ML's wife to provide verbal cues during the task rather than physical assistance. The cues were written for consistency.

The Assessment of Motor and Process skills (see Chapter 15) was administered. Two of the three tasks used for the evaluation were retrieving a beverage from the refrigerator and making a lunch-meat sandwich. Motor and process skills that interfered with independent task performance included transporting items, heeding instructions, continuing the task, gathering items, navigating in the environment, and pacing the task. These skills were addressed in therapy by repetition, practice, and performance of similar tasks that challenged the same skills. In addition, ML was provided with a wheelchair bag to transport items, and his wife was encouraged to modify the kitchen setup to allow greater access to needed items.

A home visit was made 1½ weeks before discharge. ML's wife and daughter were present for the evaluation. The following suggestions were implemented by the family:

- Remove throw rugs to increase ease of wheelchair navigation
- Place commode over existing toilet
- Remove reclining chair from living room and move coffee table away from center of room to allow turning radius for wheelchair
- Place foam cushion in ML's favorite chair to increase ease of sit-to-stand transitions

- Install grab bars and tub transfer bench to increase independence and safety in transfer to tub

Before discharge, ML and the home health attendant were provided with a list of tasks that ML should be encouraged to perform at home. ML had worked on these tasks in occupational and physical therapy sessions.

ML received the following home care services: occupational therapy, physical therapy, and assistance from a home health attendant. The home care OTR's initial evaluation revealed that ML was not ambulating at all (the commode had been moved to the bedside); the home health attendant was performing 90% of ML's BADL functions; and ML was increasingly tearful, refusing to leave the apartment. The OTR developed a treatment plan that included increased participation and decreased reliance on the home health attendant, participation in weekly outdoor therapy sessions focusing on community reintegration, and independent ambulation to the bathroom for toileting.

To document his progress toward increased participation in ADL tasks, ML began a self-care log with the assistance of his wife. The log revealed that ML was not attempting to walk to the bathroom because he was afraid of falling. At the next cotreatment session the OTR and COTA concentrated on getting ML on the floor and reviewing techniques for floor-to-chair (or floor-to-couch) transitions. Although ML required moderate assistance ($\times$1) to perform this task, he expressed relief that it could be done by one person.

Before ending home occupational therapy, ML was ambulating to the bathroom independently, toileting independently 100% of the time, performing BADL tasks independently 90% of the time, and participating in simple IADL tasks such as getting a snack for himself independently. ML felt comfortable when his wife took him out in the wheelchair to perform community tasks and leisure activities (e.g., visiting friends, going out to dinner, participating in a stroke support group).

■
CASE STUDY

AM is a 72-year-old woman who was admitted to the hospital with complaints of a "clumsy" and numb right hand and right lower extremity weakness. Her workup revealed that she had suffered a CVA. AM lives alone in a first floor apartment.

Acute care occupational therapy was initiated the day after admission to the hospital. The initial evaluation revealed the following requirements:

- Minimal assistance with bed mobility
- Minimal assistance with dressing (specifically with closures and fasteners)
- Moderate assistance with IADL functions secondary to impaired coordination of her right hand; memory, organization, and sequencing deficits; and decreased vision (secondary to a field cut).

Specific tasks on which AM wanted to focus were handwriting, dressing, and preparing meals.

Initial treatment interventions on the acute service involved participation in tasks that challenged AM's fine motor coordination and functional cognitive skills (e.g., sorting change, playing cards, chopping vegetables). She was provided with elastic laces and a button aid to help with dressing.

On admission to the inpatient rehabilitation unit 6 days later, the treatment plan was continued with additional interventions recommended by the OTR. These included phone use, review of emergency procedures, handwriting exercises, and higher-level meal preparation (with stove use).

At this point in her recovery, AM could independently perform self-care functions using adaptive devices. These activities took longer, but she could do them safely. Her cognitive dysfunction affected her ability to remember phone numbers, manage her money, and recall therapy sessions and unit events.

Treatment intervention included keeping a daily journal of treatment sessions and events both to improve handwriting and compensate for memory deficits. She also practiced counting money, making change, and writing checks during simulated purchases.

As her coordination and limb function improved, AM was weaned off the adaptive equipment she was using to dress herself. AM was proud of this accomplishment and verbalized her relief that she was improving.

At this point in the program, AM informed her occupational therapist that she was unable to comb her wig the way she had in the past. During an evaluation of this task, the therapist observed that AM could not locate items in the right lower visual field. When grooming items (e.g., bobby pins, combs) were placed in this field, AM had difficulty finding them. The therapist reviewed this finding with AM and encouraged her to turn her head to the right and place her hand on the right edge of the work surface, using it as an anchor for scanning. These two strategies were effective in helping AM locate objects in the environment.

IADL tasks were evaluated after an interview focusing on commonly performed activities. Tasks that AM stated she performed and would like to attempt in therapy included sweeping the floor, making the bed, and preparing scrambled eggs. These tasks were evaluated during an OTR/COTA cotreatment session, and the following deficits were found to interfere with task performance:

- Sweeping the floor: Although AM was able to sweep debris into piles without difficulty, she had problems using the dustpan and broom simultaneously. The dustpan slipped from her hand several times, and she was unable to sweep the debris into the pan. She moved slowly and appeared unsure of herself during task performance.
- Bed-making: AM stumbled several times after catching her foot on the bedposts. She was able to complete the task, although the sheets frequently slipped from her hands and she had difficulty tucking in the corners of the sheets.

- Preparing scrambled eggs: This task was the most problematic. AM demonstrated difficulty in locating spices in the cabinets while preparing her work space. She required assistance to select the correct knob on the stove to control the burner. After lighting the stove and placing butter in the pan, she appropriately began cracking the eggs in a bowl. Unfortunately, this task took an extremely long time to perform, and because AM never rechecked the stove, the butter burned. AM did not stabilize the pan while scrambling the eggs, and it began to shift on the burner.

The therapist deemed this task unsafe and recommended that AM not use the stove unsupervised. This recommendation was relayed to AM's best friend, who lived down the hall. AM was discharged to home independent in BADL tasks and able to perform simple homemaking tasks with supervision. She required maximal assistance to perform shopping, stove-top cooking, and heavy housecleaning. In addition, she was able to make simple change and print her name legibly, although her signature remained illegible.

Three days after AM returned home (with 4 hours of assistance from a home health attendant), home occupational therapy was initiated. The initial treatment plan set up by the OTR focused on preparing cold meals independently. This task was broken down, and the components were practiced. Components included scanning and locating items in the refrigerator and cabinets, opening cans, chopping, mixing, and cutting.

The task was graded by the number of steps and objects required to prepare the meal. Tasks included sectioning an orange, preparing tuna fish, and making a cold salad. AM learned to leave commonly used objects on the countertops and in the dish rack to decrease the time she spent locating items.

Another treatment focus was on AM's decreased handwriting skills. Several interventions were implemented, including use of built-up pens, graded handwriting exercises, and simple writing activities, such as signing thank-you cards to friends who helped her while she was in the hospital. As her writing progressed, the COTA engaged AM in activities that would continue to challenge her writing skills, such as updating her personal address book and writing a shopping list for her home health assistant.

Because she was concerned that AM was forgetting to take her medications when unsupervised, the visiting nurse contacted the OTR assigned to the case. The therapist and nurse devised a system for AM to track self-medication using a pillbox and calendar check-off system. The nurse filled the pillbox weekly and wrote the daily medications on a large calendar. AM crossed off the medication after she took it. The COTA on the case posted reminders to check the calendar in several key areas, such as the bathroom mirror, refrigerator, and alarm clock.

AM was discharged from home occupational therapy independent in BADL tasks; independent in home management, including preparation of cold meals (the only hot meal she was able to make was coffee from an electric coffee maker); and able to perform light shopping at the corner store and participate in her church group, where she was responsible for light bookkeeping.

■

REVIEW QUESTIONS

1. Explain the differences between a "top-down" and "bottom-up" approach to the evaluation of a stroke patient.
2. Give two examples of occupational therapy assessments that use a "top-down" approach.
3. Give three examples of using "occupation-as-means" and "occupation-as-end" intervention strategies.

REFERENCES

1. Agency for Health Care Policy and Research: *Clinical practice guidelines: post-stroke rehabilitation*, number 16, Waltham, Mass, 1995, Center for Health Economics.
2. American Occupational Therapy Association: Uniform terminology for occupational therapy, third edition, *Am J Occup Ther* 48:1047, 1994.
3. American Occupational Therapy Association: Occupational Therapy Roles TASK Force: *Am J Occup Ther* 47:1087, 1993.
4. Árnadóttir G: *The brain and behavior: assessing cortical dysfunction through activities of daily living*, St Louis, 1990, Mosby.
5. Fisher AG: *Assessment of motor and process skills*, Fort Collins, Colo, Three Star Press, 1995.
6. Keith RA et al: The functional independence measure: a new tool for rehabilitation. In Eisenberg MG, Grzesiak RC, editors, *Advances in clinical rehabilitation*, vol 1, New York, 1987, Springer-Verlag.
7. Law M et al: *The Canadian occupational performance measure*, ed 2, Ottawa, 1994, CAOT Publications ACE.
8. Law M, Baptiste S, Mills J: Client-centered practice: what does it mean and does it make a difference? *Can J Occup Ther* 62:250, 1995.
9. Pollock N: Client-centered assessment, *Am J Occup Ther* 47:298, 1993.
10. Schell BAB: Use Document TASK Force: career exploration and development: a guide to the occupational therapy roles document, *Am J Occup Ther* 48:844, 1994.
11. Thomson LK: *The Kohlman evaluation of living skills*, ed 3 Bethesda, Md, AOTA, 1992.
12. Trombly CA: Occupation: purposefulness and meaningfulness as therapeutic mechanisms, *Am J Occup Ther* 49:960, 1995.
13. Trombly CA: Anticipating the future: assessment of occupational function, *Am J Occup Ther* 47:253, 1993.
14. Wade DT, Collin C: The Barthel index: a standard measure of physical disability? *Int Disabil Stud* 10:64, 1988.

Glossary

acalculia An acquired inability to solve basic mathematical problems

accessible environment An environment that is usable by an individual, including those with mobility impairments

accommodation The adjustment of the eye to variations in distance

activity analysis A process by which properties inherent in an activity or task are gauged for their ability to elicit individual motivation and fullfill patient needs in occupational performance and performance components

activities of daily living (ADL) The activities usually performed in the course of a normal day, such as eating, toileting, dressing, washing, and grooming

acuity The clarity or sharpness of perception (e.g., visual acuity)

adaptation Coping with the changing characteristics of a task, the environment, or the method of carrying out a task so that an activity can be completed

adhesive capsulitis Thickening and contracture of a joint capsule (specifically the glenohumeral joint) in which the capsule adheres to the humeral head; also known as a *frozen shoulder*

adjustment to disability The point at which an individual with a disability demonstrates self-acceptance and capability of adjustment to disability by using productive strategies for dealing with the handicapping effects of the disability

Affolter approach A treatment approach that emphasizes habit formation and relies heavily on the use of nonverbal stimuli (specifically tactile-kinesthetic input) to guide movement during functional activities

aging The process of becoming older during which cells replace themselves more slowly and are lost through infections and disease

agoraphobia An anxiety syndrome manifested by an abnormal fear of being in open or public places

agraphia An acquired writing disturbance

alexia An acquired inability to read or comprehend written language as a result of brain damage

alignment The placment or maintenance of body structures in their proper anatomic positions

anatomy of the eye The structure of the eye, which is a spherical body contained in a bony orbit and is composed of the iris and pupil, lens, retina, vitreous humor, and eyelids

angioplasty The surgical repair of a narrowed blood vessel (e.g., unclogging a vessel by inserting a balloon-tipped catheter and blocking a weakened area of the vessel wall [aneurysm] or by replacing or remodeling a part of the vessel)

ankle strategy An automatic postural response that occurs when movement is centered about the ankles to maintain the center of mass over the base of support; utilized to control small, slow, upright sway

anomia Loss of the ability to name objects or remember names of people

anosognosia Denial of ownership of a paretic extremity accompanied by a lack of insight about the paralysis

anteroposterior splint An orthotic device that has points of contact on both the front (anterior or volar) and back (posterior or dorsal) surfaces of a limb or the trunk

antihypertensives Drugs used to lower blood pressure in individuals with abnormally high blood pressure

anxiety A disorder characterized by a sense that something bad will occur; tension, fear, or worry out of proportion to the situation, racing thoughts, physiologic symptoms (such as a dry mouth, heart palpitations, cold hands and feet, stomach and bowel upset, and bladder frequency or incontinence)

aphasia The loss of the ability to speak or understand spoken or written language

apraxia The inability to plan or execute a movement to function or participate in activity

aprosody Difficulty expressing or recognizing emotions; often associated with nondominant parietal lobe lesions

architectural barriers Obstacles inherent in the structure or design of buildings that hinder individuals with impaired mobility

arousal The general state of readiness in which an individual is prepared to process sensory information and organize a response

aspiration Penetration of food or liquids into the airway below the level of the vocal folds before, during, or after swallowing

assistive devices Tools that allow an impaired individual to function

assistive technology device Any item, piece of equipment, or product system that is used to increase, maintain, or improve functional capabilities of individuals with disabilities

astereognosis Failure to recognize objects, sizes, and shapes of objects by touch alone; also called *tactile agnosia*

attention The ability to focus on an interaction or activity long enough to grasp its meaning and prepare an appropriate response

auscultation Listening for sounds in the body for evaluation purposes either directly or with a stethoscope; used during dysphagia evaluations to detect signs of swallowing dysfunction

balance The ability to control the center of mass over the base of support within the limits of stability, resulting in the maintenance of stability and equilibrium

benchmarking Setting goals for process improvement; formerly known as "threshold"

biofeedback A process that provides a person with visual or auditory information about physiologic aspects of the body (such as muscle tension)

biomechanical approach An approach that is applicable to the ability and capacity levels of physical function; deals with increasing strength, range of motion, endurance, and alignment in patients with physical dysfunction

bivalve cast A cast that has contact with both surfaces of the limb it surrounds and has been cut in half lengthwise to allow it to be removed and replaced

blocked practice Practice that consists of drills and requires many repetitions of the same task in the same way

bottom-up assessment An evaluation that focuses on the deficits or components of function (e.g., strength, range of motion) that are believed to be prerequisites to function

Broca's aphasia Expressive aphasia characterized by a loss of speech ability

caring Compassion for others and concern for their well-being

carotid plaque A hardened, abnormal deposit on the wall of an artery believed to be related to elevated serum cholesterol blood levels

casting Use of casting tape and plaster or fiberglass (which forms a solid when placed in water) to immobilize a limb in a position of function; when used with neurologically impaired individuals, is usually applied to provide slow, prolonged stretch to a limb with excessive skeletal muscle tightening and/or shortening

cataracts An abnormal progressive condition of the lens of the eye characterized by loss of transparency and a gray-white opacity that can be seen in the lens behind the pupil

center of mass The midpoint or center of body weight

cerebellar strokes Strokes or cerebrovascular accidents involving the cerebellar lobes or blood vessels of the cerebellum of the brain

cerebrovascular accident A stroke; can be caused by numerous factors including cardiac factors, hemorrhagic factors, abnormally increased platelet levels, carotid plaques, infection, and neoplasm

circumduction The circular motion of a limb or the eye

client-centered practice An approach to providing occupational therapy services that embraces a philosophy of respect and partnership with the persons receiving services

closed tasks Activities that take place in a stable and predictable environment; consistent methods of performance over time

cognition The thought process combining sensory function, learning, and the ability to choose an effective response; knowing, thinking, learning, and judging

coital frequency The incidence of periods of coitus; may diminish with aging or disability

color agnosia A deficit in ability to recognize colors as a result of a brain lesion; characterized by an inability to name or recognize colors

concrete thinking Interpreting thought strictly, without processing implied meaning; inflexible thinking

cone A photoreceptor cell in the retina of the eye that enables a person to visualize colors

confabulation An unconscious fabrication of stories or excuses to fill in memory gaps

confrontation Movement of an object through the visual field toward the observer

context Circumstances associated with a particular environment or setting

contextual interference Factors in the learning environment that increase the difficulty of initial learning

contracture An abnormal and usually permanent condition of a joint; characterized by flexion and fixation and caused by atrophy and shortening of muscle fibers or by loss of the normal elasticity of the skin

convergence Coordinated turning of the eyes inward to focus on a certain point

coping Psychologically adjusting to change

cortical blindness Blindness that results from a lesion in the visual center of the cerebral cortex of the brain

cranioaxial tomography (CT) scan A serial X ray that can create an image using multiple attenuation readings

deconditioning Decreased body tolerance to fluctuations in vital function (e.g., blood pressure, heart rate, respiratory rate) in response to exercise or activity

decubitus Skin breakdown (usually adjacent to a bony prominence or weight-bearing surface) that is observed in individuals who continuously remain in a static position; caused by a loss of oxygen in the skin surface that causes tissue necrosis (death), resulting in an ulceration

deep venous thrombosis (DVT) A blood clot positioned statically in a deep vein of a limb

degrees of freedom Elements or variables that are free to vary; a term used to classify the number of planes in which joint segments move or the number of primary axes they possess (e.g., joints that move in one plane such as the elbow joint—1 degree of freedom)

denial Lack of acceptance or disavowal that a circumstance or condition exists

depression A state of being characterized by sadness, feelings of helplessness and hopelessness, low self-esteem, sleep and appetite disturbances, and psychomotor agitation or retardation; in stroke survivors, may be reactive or organic in origin

diabetes A disease resulting from decreased functioning of the islets of Langerhans (which produce insulin to utilize sugars in the blood stream) in the pancreas resulting in organ damage caused by the free circulating sugars; also causes small blood vessel disease, which contributes to the organ tissue death (including target organs such as the heart, kidneys, peripheral nerves, retina of the eyes, and blood vessels)

diabetic retinopathy A disorder of retinal blood vessels characterized by capillary microaneurysms, hemorrhage, exudates, and the formation of new vessels and connective tissue; most often occurs in patients with longstanding, poorly controlled diabetes

disability The inability to perform daily life tasks

disorientation The inability to give personal information regarding self, disability, hospital stay, and time without language disturbance

dissociation The separation of body parts during movement patterns (e.g., dissociation of the scapula from the thorax while reaching)

distractibility Diversion of attention

divergence A separation or movement of objects away from each other (e.g., a simultaneous turning of the eyes outward)

drop-out cast An immobilization cast that has a portion cut out in the direction of desired movement so that the person can volitionally move the limb after initial muscle relaxation is gained (or gravity can assist stretch)

dual obliquity Refers to the anatomy of the hand and has two anatomic ramifications: (1) the progressive decrease of length of the metacarpals from the radial to the ulnar aspect of the hand and (2) the immobility of the second and third metacarpals in relation to the first, fourth, and fifth metacarpals

durable medical equipment Devices primarily manufactured to assist persons with impaired mobility; includes wheelchairs, bathtub equipment, bedside commodes, and ambulatory devices

dynamic splinting Employing traction devices in a splint to alter the range of passive motion of a joint

dysarthria Weakness or altered neuronal control of the muscles responsible for speech production or defective sensory feedback regarding their movement

dysphagia Impairment of the ability to swallow

ejaculatory dysfunction An interruption in the ability to ejaculate or reach sexual plateau; may be caused by a lack of available seminal fluid for the ejaculate and premature loss of the ejaculate

embolism A blood clot that is moving; may travel to an organ and enter a vessel smaller than itself, blocking circulation and contributing to organ dysfunction; can be life threatening

empathy The ability of a person to have compassion for others who are dealing with issues and feelings the person has never experienced

endarterectomy Surgical removal of the lamina of an artery to eliminate plaque and restore blood flow

enteral feeding Provision of nutrients through the intestinal tract

environment The external and internal surroundings that influence a person's development (including the person's own psyche)

environmental control unit A device such as a switch, voice activator, remote control, computer interface, or other technological adaptation used to purposefully manipulate and interact with the environment

epiglottis The cartilaginous structure that hangs over the larynx like a lid and prevents food from entering the airway

erectile dysfunction Difficulty achieving or maintaining an erection during sexual relations until plateau is reached; inability to ejaculate and resolve an erection

executive functions The skills utilized in problem solving, recognition, goal formulation, planning and organization, initiation, and self-regulation and monitoring

extracranial-intracranial bypass A surgery originating outside the cranium in which the cranium is entered, and circulation is rerouted around an obstruction

far transfer Introduction of an activity that is conceptually the same but physically different from the initial task initially performed

feedback Information about a person's environment and the person's relationship to it; can provide knowledge of performance as well as knowledge of results

fiberglass casting tape Soft, rolled synthetic tape that is combined with water and hardens as it cools; used to immobilize a limb

fiberoptic endoscopic evaluation of swallowing (FEES) A functional, diagnostic test of deglutition in which a contrast dye, a flexible endoscopic catheter (inserted nasogastrically), a light source, and an air source (which is used to test sensation of the cricopharyngeal region) connected to a videocamera to test and document the oropharyngeal phase of a swallow reflex

figure-ground discrimination Discrimination of the foreground from the background (e.g., locating a particular object in a cluttered drawer)

fixation patterns A natural strategy used to maintain select body parts in certain positions when in posturally threatening situations

force control strategy A movement strategy characterized by frequent stops and step-like movements requiring more effort or force for progression

fovea The center of the retina where cone cells (color receptors) are concentrated and rod cells (low-light adapting cells) are absent

functional optometry Analyzes active ocular ability and perception

gait analysis Observation and qualification of rhythm, pattern, cadence, and speed while walking

gait training patterns Combinations of intact aspects of gait (rhythm, cadence, and speed) that are used to train persons in an attempt to restore functional ambulation

glaucoma An abnormal, usually progressive condition in which elevated eye pressure caused by obstruction of the outflow of aqueous humor results in decreased visual acuity and vividness of perception and generally involves the entire visual field; progression controlled by treatments such as use of medicated eye drops

handicap Social dysfunction resulting from outward signs of disease or impairment; a limitation in social role performance

handling The manner in which therapists use their hands to provide input to a patient to enhance the quality of motor output and prevent abnormal movement; is associated with NDT/Bobath

hemianopsia Defective vision or blindness often in one half of the visual field; may involve a portion of the field of each eye and tends to follow predictable patterns associated with the decussation (crossing over) of ocular nerve fibers

hemiplegic gaits Ambulation patterns used as a response to unilateral weakness involving a lower extremity

hemorrhage External or internal loss of a large amount of blood in a short time

heterotopic ossification A benign overgrowth or deposition of bone in soft tissues that is usually associated with an increase in the blood level of alkaline phosphatase; may be increased by forced, resisted movement of the affected body part; active (rather than active assistive or passive) movement emphasized in rehabilitation

hip strategy An automatic postural response involving movement about the hips that maintains or restores equilibrium

hydrocephalus A pathologic condition characterized by an abnormal accumulation of cerebrospinal fluid that is usually under increased pressure in the cranial vault

hyperopia Farsightedness; a condition resulting from an error of refraction in which rays of light entering the eye are brought into focus behind the retina

hypertension A common disorder characterized by elevated blood pressure persistently exceeding 140/90 mm Hg; may be caused by a number of factors including failure of the organs regulating homeostasis such as the cardiovascular and renal systems; tends to be a strong hereditary component; can usually be well controlled by a variety of oral medications including diuretics and β-blockers, but poor control can increase risk of stroke, renal failure, and cardiopulmonary disease

hypertonia Abnormally increased muscle tone or strength

ideational apraxia A breakdown in the ability to perform a task because of a loss of neuronal model or mental representation of the procedure required for performance

impaired initiative The inability to initiate performance of an activity when the need to perform is present

impairment Organ dysfunction; the motor and cognitive residuals of pathology

impingement Restriction of movement of a body part, usually involving soft tissues, because of anatomic limitation; tends to increase as the degrees of freedom of a given joint increase because tendons, muscles, and ligaments act as pulley systems or ceilings to a joint, which structurally protects the joint but causes pain and motion limitation when structures overlap abnormally (e.g., fluctuations in tension of soft tissue during repetitive motion or abnormal posturing)

inhibitory casting A casting technique utilized to decrease spasticity and increase functional movement through slow, prolonged stretch of an involved limb

insight The ability to foresee and comprehend implications of actions on circumstances

instrumental activities of daily living (IADL) Complex activities of daily living performed to maintain independence in the home or community

integrated functional approach An approach in which functional activities are used to directly treat sequelae of a stroke

intermediate transfer Changing a moderate number of task parameters while keeping some similarities to the initial task performed

ipsilateral pushing A syndrome associated with stroke in which the individual physically pushes the body toward one side because of a misperception of the actual center of gravity

ischemia A decreased supply of oxygenated blood to a body or organ part

jargon aphasia A language disorder characterized by speech that cannot be understood by others

knowledge of performance Information about the processes used during task performance

knowledge of results Terminal feedback about the outcome of an action in terms of accomplishing a goal

larynx The voice organ; a part of the air passage connecting the pharynx with the trachea that is protected at its proximal end by the vocal folds (cords)

learned nonuse Lack of use of a body part in normal daily activities or spontaneous movement resulting from weakness, diminished perception, or neglect of the impaired body part that leads to a change in its normal, functional use

learning The acquisition of information or skills that is personalized through experience

lens The anatomic crystal of the eye that functions by refracting (i.e., directing the path of) light onto the retina

limbic system A group of structures in the rhinencephalon of the brain that are associated with various emotions and feelings such as anger, fear, sexual arousal, pleasure, and sadness

limits of stability The boundaries of an area of space in which the body can maintain its position without changing the base of support

long-term memory Consolidated and retained information that has passed through the short-term memory

low-load prolonged stretch A stretch obtained by holding a tissue in a moderately lengthened position for a significant amount of time

macula degeneration Progressive degeneration of the maculae (a central spot) of the retina and choroid of the eye that leads to central visual blindness; is commonly managed by ultraviolet-blocking lenses (because sun exposure is considered a contributing factor) or high doses of niacin (vitamin B)

mania (stroke related) A state of being characterized by euphoria, pressured speech, unfocused and prolific thoughts, grandiose thoughts and delusions, insomnia, hallucinations, poor judgment, paranoia, or hypersexuality

memory The mental faculty or power that enables a person to retain and recall (through unconscious associative processes) previously experienced sensations, impressions, ideas, concepts, and information that has been consciously learned

mental imagery A concept or sensation produced in the mind through memory or imagination

metacognition The knowledge and regulation of one's own cognitive processes and capacities

modeling The utilization of drawings, photographs, videotapes, therapists, or patients as models to enhance motor performance

motor adaptation The ability to adapt postural responses to changing tasks and environmental demands

motor apraxia Loss of access to kinesthetic memory patterns that leads to an inability to perform purposeful movement because of defective planning and sequencing of movements (even though the idea and the purpose of the task is understood)

motor control Control of movement and posture

motor learning The study of the acquisition and/or modification of movement; a set of processes associated with practice or experience leading to relatively permanent changes in the ability to produce skilled movement

mourning A reaction to loss of function, a change in appearance, and a loss of potential or exising life roles; commonly associated with hostility and anger

multicontextual approach An approach in which a combination of remedial and functional learning is used to regain functional participation of persons recovering from stroke

myopia Nearsightedness caused by the elongation of the eyeball or an error in refraction causing parallel rays to be focused in front of the retina

near transfer Performance of an alternate form of the initial task performed

negative symptoms A disturbance in normal behavior or a performance deficit

neoplasm An abnormal growth of new tissue (benign or malignant); also called a *tumor*

neurobehavior Any behavioral response resulting from CNS processing that forms the basis for task performance in activities of daily living

neurobehavioral deficit A functional impairment characterized by defective skill performance resulting from neurologic processing dysfunction that affects performance components

neurophysiologic approach A theoretical framework in which external stimuli are used to influence the functional systems of the body

NPO Abbreviation for "nothing by mouth"

occupation The engagement in daily life activities that are meaningful and purposeful, including self-care, instrumental, vocational, educational, play and leisure, and rest and relaxation activities of daily living

occupation as end Teaching an activity or task by using participation in the particular activity or task

occupation as means Using occupation as the therapeutic change agent to remediate impaired abilities or capacities

occupational functioning The ability to perform the tasks that have a role in their natural context

occupational performance The ability to accomplish the tasks required by a certain role

open tasks Tasks requiring adaptation to unpredictable events because objects in the environment are in random motion during task performance

optical flow Movement of an image on the retina

organization The ability to organize thoughts so that a task can be performed in an organized way with properly sequenced and timed steps

orthokinetics A therapy for spasticity in which an orthotic device is used to enable contraction of one muscle while inhibiting its antagonist

orthotic device An external appliance that supports a paralyzed muscle, promotes a certain motion, or corrects a deformity

parenteral Through a route other than the digestive system

pathology The direct anatomic and physiologic effects (e.g., of a stroke)

penetration Entrance of food or liquid into the larynx above the level of the vocal folds

perception The ability to meaningfully interpret sensory information

performance areas Broad categories of human activity that are typically part of daily life

performance components Fundamental human abilities that are required for successful engagement in performance areas

performance contexts Situations or factors that influence engagement in desired and required performance areas

peripheral vision A capacity to see objects that reflect light waves falling on areas of the retina distant from the macula

perseveration Repeated movements or acts during functional performance resulting from difficulty in shifting from one pattern of response to another; refers to initiation and termination of performance and inertia

pharynx The throat; serves as a passage for the respiratory and digestive tracts

plaster A composition of liquid and powder that becomes chemically active on contact with water and hardens when it dries; used to shape a cast

PLISSIT model of sexual counseling Permission, limited information, specific suggestions, and intensive therapy

positive symptoms Spontaneous, exaggerated disturbances of normal function; symptoms that are reactive to specific external stimuli

postural adjustment Automatic, anticipatory, and ongoing muscle activation to maintain balance against gravity; maintain alignment; and orient the head, trunk, and limbs to the environment

postural control The ability to control the body's position in space for stability and orientation

postural stability The ability to maintain the position of the body in space

praxis Ideation; the programming and planning necessary for the execution of skilled, purposeful movement

problem solving The ability to manipulate a fund of knowledge and apply it to new or unfamiliar situations

procedural memory Recall and/or motor implementation of the steps of a task; situational use of learned sequential behaviors

process improvement Use of an assessment tool or mechanism to monitor problem resolution in a care delivery system; part of quality assurance

prosopagnosia The inability to recognize previously familiar faces

quality assurance Any evaluation that compares services provided and results achieved with accepted standards

quality of life The ability to carry out activities of daily living in patterns and configurations that are acceptable to the individual, have personal meaning, and fit into the context of life

random practice Practice of tasks that vary in the same session

recurvatum Backward thrust of the knee by weakness or a joint disorder that results in hyperextension of the joint

reflexes The involuntary functioning or movement of any organ or part of the body in response to a particular stimuli

refraction The deflection of light from a straight path through the eye by various ocular tissues including the lens and its muscles

refractory Resistant to treatment

remedial approach Using splinter skills to transfer skills to functional applications

reticular activating system (RAS) A functional system in the brain essential for wakefulness, attention, concentration, and introspection; closely related to the limbic system

risk management An administrative function directed toward identification, evaluation, and correction of potential risks that could lead to injury and legal liability

rod One of the eye structures that is perpendicular to the retina and detects low intensity light

saccadic eye movements Fast, voluntary, coordinated movements of the eye that allow the eyes to accurately fix on a still object in the visual field as the person moves or the head turns

selective attention The ability to select or focus on one type of information and exclude others

sequencing Efficiently ordering and timing events

serial casting The process of applying casts of increasingly greater degrees of joint motion to stretch a limb away from a contracted position

sexual dysfunction A change in sexual function that is viewed as unsatisfactory, unrewarding, or inadequate

sexuality The quality of being sexual; the sum of a person's sexual attributes, attractiveness, and sexual impulses

sexual phases Excitement, plateau, orgasm, and resolution

short-term memory Information that is consciously retained and manipulated for brief periods; the registration and temporary storing of information received by the different sensory memory modalities; refers to working memory

shoulder-hand syndrome Classified under the general term *reflex sympathetic dystrophy*; characterized by severe pain, stiffness, swelling, and marked reduction in function of the upper extremity

silent aspiration Penetration of saliva, food, or liquid below the level of the true vocal folds without a cough or outward sign of difficulty

somatoagnosia A body scheme disorder; diminished awareness of body structure and the failure to recognize own body parts and their relationship to each other

somesthetic Pertaining to tactile and proprioceptive sensation

spasticity One type of hypertonus that increases with the velocity of joint movement; attributed to hyperactive stretch reflexes mediated by muscle spindle stretch receptors

spatial relations dysfunction Difficulty in relating objects to each other or self

static splinting Splinting that does not allow movement of the body parts; used to provide support, alignment, stretch, and immobilization

stepping strategy A postural strategy used to widen the base of support in which a step is taken when the base of support is expanded in the direction of the center of mass movement

stereopsis The quality of visual fusion

strabismus An abnormal condition in which the eyes are unable to have their axes cross because of an imbalance of the extrinsic eye muscles, resulting in an inability to accurately focus an object in the visual field that is usually accompanied by impaired saccades

tonic arousal A change in muscle tone and response that occurs as a person wakens from sleep

top-down assessment An assessment that focuses on the evaluation of performance areas

topographic disorientation Difficulty finding way in space as a result of amnesic or agnostic problems

Trendelenberg's sign Occurs when a person stands on the affected limb and the opposite gluteal fold falls rather than rises

unilateral body neglect Failure to report, respond, or orient to a stimulus presented to the body contralateral to the cerebral lesion; refers to personal space

unilateral spatial neglect Inattention to or neglect of stimuli presented in the extrapersonal space contralateral to the cerebral lesion

urinary tract dysfunction Dysfunction of the organs and ducts involved in the secretion and elimination of urine from the body

vergence Movements of the two eyes in opposite directions

videofluoroscopy A technique in radiology for visually examining a part of the body or function of an organ using a fluoroscope; used for dynamic evalution of swallowing

visual pathways Anatomic, physical conduits through which visual information is transmitted from the retina to the brain

visual perception The receipt and interpretation of visual sensation that provides information about the environment

Wallenberg's sign Horner's syndrome; cerebellar ataxia and contralateral loss of pain and temperature

Home Assessments and
Safety Modifications

OCCUPATIONAL THERAPY
HOME ASSESSMENT WORKSHEET*

Address visited _____

Date of assessment _____

Exterior:

Type of residence: Type of terrain:

☐ House   ☐ Own   ☐ Rent   ☐ Incline   ☐ Concrete/asphalt

☐ Apartment   ☐ Smooth   ☐ Rough

☐ Care home

Distance from parked car to home: _____   Walkway width: _____ inches wide

Distance from home to curb: _____

Ramping space: 1 foot of ramp to 1 inch of elevation

Maximum length: 30 ft

Level platform: 5 square ft

Platform at door: 5 square ft

Railings

AREA	IDEAL	ACTUAL	COMMENTS/DIAGRAM
Entrance:			
Most accessible entry:			
Front Rear Side		Front Rear Side	
Steps (ground to porch)	7 inches high with nonskid stripes	Number _____ Height _____ Width _____ Depth _____	
		Carpet Nonskid strip Artificial turf _____	
Landing		Number _____ Width _____ Depth _____	
Railings (ascending steps)	32 inches high— extends 1½ ft beyond top and bottom step	Left _____ Right _____ Height _____	
Porch size	4 or 5 square ft	Width _____ Depth _____	
Height of step from porch to house level	7 inches high		
Doorway width	36 inches wide		
Swing of door		In _____ Out _____	
Screen door swing		In _____ Out _____	
Threshold	Level with floor		

Staff _____   Date _____   Time _____

*Courtesy K. Hatae, V. Tully, N. Wade; Honolulu, Hawaii.

AREA	IDEAL	ACTUAL	COMMENTS/DIAGRAM
Interior:			
Number of levels within the house			
Number of steps			
Steps	7 inches high	Number _____	
		Height _____	
		Width _____	
		Depth_____	
		Left ____ Right ____	
Railings (ascending steps)		Left ____ Right ____	
Landing		Height_____	
		Number _____	
		Width _____	
		Depth _____	
Living room:			
Threshold	Level with floor		
Doorway width	36 inches wide		
Floor covering	Wood/tile		
Furniture arrangement	5 square feet turning space		
Favorite chair	Wheelchair height	Height _____	
Density	Firm		
Armrest	Both sides		
Phone accessibility	No long wire Cordless		
Television accessibility	Remote control		
Outlets	18 inches from floor		
Light switches	36 inches from floor		
Hallways:			
Width	36-48 inches wide	Turns_____ Straight	
Turns	Straight		
Floor covering	Wood/tile		
Bedroom:			
Doorway width	36 inches wide		
Door swing		In _____ Out _____	
Threshold height	Level with floor		
Floor covering	Wood/tile		
Telephone accessibility	Next to bed		
Bed size	Single, double, queen, king		
Mattress height	Wheelchair height		
Mattress density	Firm		
Space for hospital bed	36 inches $\times$ 88 inches		
Space for bedside commode	24 inches $\times$ 24 inches		
Night light	Next to bed		

Staff   Date   Time

AREA	IDEAL	ACTUAL	COMMENTS/DIAGRAM
Bell	Next to bed		
Outlets	18 inches from floor		
Light switches	36 inches from floor		
Wheelchair turning space	5 square ft × 5 square ft		
Dresser accessibility	Toe space below		
Closets:			
Accessibility	Bifold, curtain		
Rod height	No higher than 48 inches		
Bathroom:			
Threshold	Level with floor		
Door width			
Door width (with door)	36 inches wide		
Door swing		In _____ Out _____	
Shower/tub:			
Entry width		Entry width _____	
Type of entry	Curtain	Curtain, glass door	
Sill height (outside)			
Sill height (inside)			
Sill width			
Sill width—wall			
Width (inside top)			
Width (inside bottom)			
Length (inside top)			
Length (inside bottom)			
Faucet height			
Shower head (type)	Removable for hose		
Wall type (e.g., tile, fiberglass)		Tile, fiberglass	
Toilet			
Height			
Distance on left (sitting on toilet)	3-9 inches minimum		
Distance on right	3-9 inches minimum		
Distance in front	30 inches		
Lavatory			
Height	26-30 inches		
Distance on left			
Distance on right			
Distance in front			
Accessibility below			

Staff   Date   Time

AREA	IDEAL	ACTUAL	COMMENTS/DIAGRAM
Electric outlets	Open for knee space	Yes _____ No _____	
Wall surface	Wood		
Floor covering	No scatter rugs Tile/linoleum		
Wheelchair turning space	5 square ft		
Kitchen:			
Door width			
Sink			
Height			
Knee space			
Basin depth	6½ inches deep		
Type		Double/single	
Faucet control		Double/single	
Distance to faucet			
Cabinets			
Stove		Gas/electric	
Height			
Controls	Front	Front/back/top	
Oven-handle height			
Type		Wall/integral	
Refrigerator			
Door height			
Door hinge		Left/right	
Freezer			
Door height			
Door hinge		Left/right/side	
Outlets			
Light switches	36 inches from floor		
Table height			
Chair height			
Counter height	30 inches high		
Telephone accessibility			
Appliances:			

_____ Staff   Date   Time

AREA	IDEAL	ACTUAL	COMMENTS/DIAGRAM
Laundry:			
Location			
Doorway width	36 inches		
Number of steps		Number _____	
		Height _____	
		Width _____	
		Depth _____	
Railings (ascending steps)		Left ____ Right ____	
		Height	
Washer door	Front opening		
Controls	Front panel	Front/back	
Dryer door	Front opening		
Controls	Front panel	Front/back	
Clothes line location		Height _____	
Patio:			
Doorway width	36 inches		
Type of door		Sliding/hinged	
Threshold	Level with floor		
Steps		Number _____	
		Height _____	
		Width _____	
		Depth _____	
Railings (ascending steps)		Left ____ Right ____	
		Height _____	

Staff   Date   Time

HOME VISIT EVALUATION*

Name of patient: _____ M/F   Age: _____
Address: _____ Phone number: _____

Diagnosis and disability: _____
_____
_____

Status of patient on discharge:
Ambulatory Status
Is patient ambulating independently?   Yes _____ No _____
Does patient use assistive device? If yes, what type? _____
Wheelchair?   If yes: Standard _____ Motorized _____

Cognitive Status
Is patient alert and oriented?   Yes _____ No _____
Does patient have memory deficits?   Yes _____ No _____
Judgement and safety awareness: Intact _____ Impaired _____

Vision: _____
Hearing: _____

- -

Who will be home to assist patient?
   Family member _____ Home attendant _____ hours per day
In what capacity?
   Self-care _____ Domestic _____ Total _____
For whom will patient be responsible?
   Self _____ Spouse _____ Children (number) _____
For which activities of home management was patient formerly responsible?
   Cooking _____ Laundry _____ Cleaning _____
   Shopping _____ Child care _____
For which activities of home management will patient now be responsible?
   Cooking _____ Laundry _____ Cleaning _____
   Shopping _____ Child care _____

Actual home visit

Type of residence patient lives in:
   House _____ Apartment _____
                          What floor? _____
                          Is there an elevator?   Yes _____ No _____
                          Width of elevator (for w/c) _____
Are there stairs to enter house/apartment?   Yes _____ No _____
   How many? _____
Are structural alterations allowed in residence?   Yes _____ No _____
How many rooms in house/apartment? _____
Can patient get to all rooms?
   Bedroom _____ Kitchen _____ Bathroom _____ Living room _____
   (If patient is in a w/c, width of doorway must be at least 30 inches.)
If private house:
   Can patient sleep on ground floor?   Yes _____ No _____
   Are there bathrooms on every floor?   Yes _____ No _____

*Courtesy K. Hatae, V. Tully, N. Wade; Honolulu, Hawaii.

Bedroom

Width of doorway: _____

Height of bed: _____

Is there room for bedside commode?   Yes _____   No _____

Kitchen

Width of doorway: _____

Height of: Sink _____   Stove _____   Cabinets _____   Table _____   Chair _____

Where are meals eaten?   Kitchen _____   Dining room _____

How far is table from cooking area? _____   From refrigerator? _____

Living room

Width of doorway: _____

Height of: Sofa _____   Chair _____

Do chairs have armrests?   Yes _____   No _____

Bathroom

Width of doorway: _____

Toilet

Height: _____

Width of space to nearest surface (e.g., wall, sink):   Right _____   Left _____

Are walls sturdy enough for grab bars?   Yes _____   No _____

Is there a shower stall? _____   Bathtub? _____   Bathtub with shower? _____

Does patient shower? _____   Bathe? _____   Shower in tub? _____

Shower stall

Glass doors _____   Shower curtain _____

Is there a step up or down? _____   Height _____

Are there grab bars?   Yes _____   No _____

Height of faucets: _____

Width of shower stall: _____

Length of shower stall: _____

Bathtub

Glass doors _____   Shower curtain _____

Facing tub—where are faucets?   Right _____   Left _____   Straight ahead _____

Height of faucets: _____

Height of bathtub: _____

Width of bathtub: _____

Length of bathtub: _____

Miscellaneous

Carpeting? _____   Area rugs? _____

How many telephones does patient have? _____   Wall phones _____   Desk phones _____

Does patient currently own any adaptive equipment? What type? _____

_____

Equipment recommendations

Home adaptation recommendations

Follow up

Equipment ordered from _____, _____
                                                        (Vendor)   (Phone number)

on _____.
            (Date)

Equipment to be delivered to _____ on _____.
                                                                                                                                          (Date)

Date of home visit: _____

Did patient go? _____

_____   _____
                    (Name of occupational therapist)   (Phone number)

To: _____

Address: _____

From: _____

Date: _____

Purpose:

**RECOMMENDATIONS FOR PREVENTING FALLS
AND/OR INCREASING ACCESSIBILITY WITHIN THE HOME***

Exterior

- ☐ Entrance: Use ☐ Front ☐ Back ☐ Side ☐ Other ☐ Entrance
- ☐ Stairs: ☐ Use nonskid stripes on step edges.
  - ☐ Reinforce stairs.   ☐ Remove: _____
- ☐ Handrails: ☐ Install: Right/left   ☐ Secure handrails.
- ☐ Walkway: ☐ Cover with nonslip material. ☐ Remove: _____
  - ☐ Repair broken walkway.
- ☐ Door: ☐ Assist with door.
  - ☐ Install door-closing mechanism.
  - ☐ Add hook to door and _____

Notes:

Living Room

- ☐ Entrance: ☐ Locate lamp close to entry of room.
- ☐ Floor: ☐ Remove throw rugs.   ☐ Tape or tack down carpet.
  - ☐ Clear walking path of electrical/phone cords.
- ☐ Space: ☐ Clear room of furniture and other obstacles.
- ☐ Furniture: ☐ Ensure that tables and chairs can provide support if leaned on.
  - ☐ Remove furniture with wheels or unsteady bases.
  - ☐ Remove low-lying objects (e.g., coffee tables).

Notes:

Hallway/Stairwell

- ☐ Lighting: ☐ Install light.   ☐ Change light bulb.
- ☐ Handrails: ☐ Install: Right/left   ☐ Secure for sturdiness.
- ☐ Other: ☐ Remove obstacles: _____

Notes:

Bedroom

- ☐ Lighting: ☐ Install nightlight and/or bedside lamp.
- ☐ Path from bed
  - to bathroom: ☐ Remove obstacles: _____
- ☐ Bed: ☐ Rearrange: _____
  - ☐ Lower/elevate bed: _____
- ☐ Clothes: ☐ Arrange closet: _____
- ☐ Other: ☐ Install bell/intercom.

Notes:

*Courtesy K. Hatae, V. Tully, N. Wade; Honolulu, Hawaii.

OCCUPATIONAL THERAPY
RECOMMENDATIONS FOR HOME MODIFICATIONS FOR SAFETY AND ACCESSIBILITY*

Patient name:_____

AREA OF CONCERN	PROBLEM	RECOMMENDATIONS	RESPONSIBLE PERSON
Bathroom entrance	☐ Doorway is too narrow. ☐ Tub/shower entrance is too narrow: _____ inches wide. ☐ Towel rack is unsteady as support. ☐ Throw rugs pose a trip hazard.	☐ Remove /widen door. ☐ Remove tub/shower door and replace with curtain. ☐ Remove and replace with grab bars. ☐ Remove rugs.	
Bathing	☐ Balance is unsteady. ☐ Rinsing is difficult. ☐ Tub/shower floor is slippery when wet.	☐ Sit to bathe. ☐ Use a bath bench. ☐ Use grab bars. ☐ Use a flexible shower hose. ☐ Use a nonskid bath mat.	
Dressing	☐ Balance is unsteady.	☐ Dress on _____.	
Using toilet	☐ Difficulty getting on/off toilet is difficult. ☐ Toilet is too low.	☐ Keep toilet seat raised. ☐ Use right/left toilet guard rails. ☐ Use grab bars on _____.	

Kitchen

_____

Laundry

_____

Comments

_____   _____
Occupational Therapist   Date

*Courtesy K. Hatae, V. Tully, N. Wade; Honolulu, Hawaii.

Incident Report

INCIDENT REPORT

SECTION I—PLEASE PRINT CLEARLY

Inpatient ☐   Outpatient ☐   Private duty nurse or attendant ☐   Visitor ☐

Date of incident: _____   Pt. unit #: _____

Time _____ : _____ AM PM   Exact location of incident: _____ Pt. floor: _____

Name: _____
                          Last   First

Home address: _____

Age: _____ Sex: _____ Admitting diagnosis: _____

Description of incident (Use the facts concerning the incident only.):

_____

_____

_____

_____

                                                                                                                       AM
Name of physician notified: _____ Time notified ____ : ____ PM

Employee(s) who first discovered incident:

Activity order: _____ Restraints (if any): _____

Did patient or family contribute to incident? (If so, how?) _____

Mental status (e.g., alert, confused, uncooperative): _____

Condition of floor: Smooth and dry ☐   Wet ☐   Substance _____

Position of bedside rails: _____ Location of call bell: _____

Is equipment involved? _____ Equipment description: _____

Model number: _____ Serial number: _____

Note: If equipment is involved in a patient-related incident, the equipment should be sequestered and Risk Management should be notified.

Signatures: Reporter _____ Supervisor _____

                          Date _____ Date _____

Witnesses (if any): _____

SECTION II—TO BE COMPLETED BY PHYSICIAN: PLEASE PRINT CLEARLY

                                                               AM
Date of exam: _____ Time ____ : ____ PM   Your beeper #/extension: _____

Findings on physical examination: _____

_____

Type of X-rays: _____ Findings: _____

Clinical impression: _____ No injury ☐

Plan: _____

Discussion with Dr. _____ Attending ☐   Resident ☐

Your name (print) _____ Signature _____

CONFIDENTIAL—PREPARED FOR HOSPITAL LEGAL FILE
THIS IS NOT PART OF THE MEDICAL RECORD.
RETURN TO RISK MANAGEMENT WITHIN 24 HOURS.

Prefabricated Note

Name		Age
Unit No.		
Location		
Phone No.		

Referred by

DIAGNOSIS

PRESCRIBING
PHYSICIAN

DATE:

PRESCRIPTION, TREATMENT, AND PROGRESS NOTES

INITIAL EVALUATION

Subjective Complaints:

General Observations:

Mental Status:

Upper Extremity Status: Dominance: _____

• Subluxation: _____ finger breadth at G-H joint

      Type: anterior, inferior, superior, intact

• Scapula position:

• Edema:

• Skeletal muscle activity:

• Upper extremity function:

Right		Left
	Top of head	
	Reach to ceiling	
	Tuck in back of shirt	
	Comb back of head	
	Fold a sheet	
	Hand to mouth	
	Turn doorknob	

PRESCRIPTION, TREATMENT, AND PROGRESS NOTES—CONT'D

• Upper extremity function—cont'd

Right	Left
	Wring out cloth
	Pick up can
	Hold phone
	Hold key
	Hold pencil
	Pick up a pill

A/PROM Limitations   (Goniometrics):

Manual Muscle Test   (5/5):

	Scapula/shoulder
	Elbow to digits

Fine Motor Coordination:

	Manipulate buttons
	Manipulate zippers
	Turn pages
	Open packages/containers
	Tie laces
	Objective testing

Gross Motor Coordination   (Rapid Alternating Movements [If Applicable]):

Hand Strength:

	Gross grasp
	Lateral pinch
	Three-jaw chuck
	Two-point pinch

Sensation:

	Hot/cold
	Light touch
	Sharp/dull
	Proprioception
	Kinesthesia

	Name	Age
	Unit No.	
	Location	
	Phone No.	

Referred by

DIAGNOSIS   PRESCRIBING
                                    PHYSICIAN

(Evaluation Continued)

DATE: **PRESCRIPTION, TREATMENT, AND PROGRESS NOTES—CONT'D**

Quality of Movement:

Comments on Upper Extremity Function:

Postural Control:

- Sitting posture:

- Anterior/posterior weight shift:

- Lateral weight shift:

Cognitive/Perceptual Status (Assessed During Self-Care Activities):

- Vision:

- Ideational apraxia:

- Motor apraxia:

- Body neglect:

- Spatial neglect:

- Organization/sequencing:

- Spatial relations:

- Topographical disorientation:

- Short-term memory:

- Long-term memory:

Comments:

DATE:	PRESCRIPTION, TREATMENT, AND PROGRESS NOTES—CONT'D	
Activities of Daily Living:		
General Status: W/C Amb.	Feeding:	Utensils
Rolling: Right		Cutting
Left		Swallowing eval?
Supine to Sit:	Dressing:	Pullover
Sit to Supine:		Buttondown
Bridging:		Pants/underwear
Sit to Stand:		Bra
Transfer to Bed:		Socks
Transfer to Commode:		Shoes
Transfer to Tub Bench:	Grooming:	Oral care
Sitting Balance: Static		Hair care
Short		Shaving
Long	Bathing:	
Standing Activity Tolerance:	Toileting:	
Standing Balance: Static	Catheterization:	
Short	Meal Prep:	
Long	Bed Making:	
Handwriting:	Housekeeping:	
Phone Use:	Other IADL:	
Emergency Procedure:	Sexuality Concerns:	
Vital Signs:	Family Involved?	
Comments:		
A/P (Problem List/Frequency of TX):		

The following goals have been discussed with patient who agrees/disagrees:

Long-Term Goals:	1-Week Goals:

_____
Signature

CQI Monitor for Stroke: Swallowing

Dysphagia team evaluations and recommendations will be monitored by multidisciplinary staff as follows:

SPEECH LANGUAGE PATHOLOGY

1. Arrange and perform swallowing evaluations with Dysphagia Team (ST/OT) within 1 business day of receipt of referral.
2. Arrange and perform reassessment of swallow function within 14 days of initial assessment.

OCCUPATIONAL THERAPY

1. Ensure appropriate signs (about precautions) are placed at patient's bedside.
2. Ensure diet recommendations are posted at nursing station.
3. Document appropriate diet recommendations in weekly progress notes.
4. Perform swallowing evaluation with ST.

PHYSICAL THERAPY

1. Physical therapist, assigned by supervisor, will monitor weekly postings of diet recommendations and relay information to physical therapy staff.

THERAPEUTIC RECREATION

1. All staff will indicate patient's swallowing status on assessment sheets.
2. Dysphagia postings will be checked before start of group activities and documented on QA monitoring form.
3. Appropriate adaptations will be made to ensure safe participation.

BENCHMARK: 100%

SAMPLE SIZE: All identified dysphagia patients

DATA SOURCE: Medical record, ST/OT/PT/TR policy and procedure

QUALITY ASSURANCE REPORT

Department: _____

Dates covered: _____ to _____

Submitted by: _____

Date submitted: _____

DATE	EVALUATION OF ISSUE	ACTION TAKEN/FINDINGS	RESOLUTION	FOLLOW UP
	Management of Dysphagia was chosen as a QA/QI indicator for the inpatient Rehabilitation Unit because of its high-risk nature. Inconsistent communication and follow-up of dysphagia evaluation findings and recommendations between disciplines were identified via chart review.	A multidisciplinary QA/QI indicator was established to improve continuity and quality of management of the dysphagic patient across all continuums.	This indicator was monitored over a 14-month period. Improvements include the following: • *Enhanced communication* between disciplines • Increased number of opportunities to facilitate *patient, family,* and *staff education:* –Initiated a dysphagia cooking group –Developed new education material *Continuum of care* • Current diet documented on weekly notes by all therapy departments • Required 2-week reassessment	This indicator will be monitored semiannually because of its high-risk nature and impact on patient care.

Policy and Procedure Manual

TITLE: Dysphagia Team Protocol

POLICY: After physician referral a dysphagia evaluation will be conducted by the
                       dysphagia team on an individual basis for patients who (by observation or
                       medical chart review) indicate they may develop swallowing dysfunction.
                       Evaluation may include bedside clinical evaluation and/or modified barium
                       swallow followed by appropriate treatment intervention, which may include diet
                       change.

PURPOSE: To ensure that individuals who appear to be functioning with a possible
                       swallowing dysfunction will be identified and appropriate intervention provided

APPLICABILITY: Dysphagia team members: speech therapy, occupational therapy, and
                       rehabilitation nursing

PROCEDURE: 1. Physician will generate a referral to dysphagia team (i.e., "Dysphagia
                          evaluation by dysphagia team") for any patient presenting with a possible
                          dysphagia.
                       2. Speech therapy will contact dysphagia team members to schedule a bedside
                          evaluation within 24 hours.
                       3. Further required evaluations will be scheduled (e.g., modified barium swallow
                          PRN).
                       4. Outstanding findings including diet recommendations will be communicated
                          to the physician and nursing staff immediately after evaluation.
                       5. Bedside reminders will be posted for patients at risk for aspirations (e.g., "No
                          thin liquids").
                       6. Results and recommendation will be documented in the medical record by a
                          dysphagia team member within 24 hours of evaluation.
                       7. Dysphagia rounds will be held once per month to discuss difficult cases,
                          review treatment plans, etc.

RESPONSIBILITY: Director of Speech Language Pathology and Occupational Therapy

REVIEW MONTH: April

Policy and Procedure Manual

TITLE: Dysphagia Evaluation Protocol

POLICY: A dysphagia (swallowing) evaluation will be conducted by the dysphagia team
                    after physician referral for patients who are at risk for swallowing dysfunction.
                    Patients will be identified by observation and/or chart review indicating the
                    potential for such dysfunction.

PURPOSE: To ensure that patients who appear to be functioning with a possible dysphagia
                    will be identified and provided with appropriate intervention

APPLICABILITY: Dysphagia team members: speech therapy, occupational therapy, and
                    rehabilitation nursing

PROCEDURE: 1. Bedside evaluation will be completed by dysphagia team after physician
                       referral.
                    2. Swallowing function will be assessed by clinical evaluation in the following
                       manner:
                       A. Patient is NPO: oral peripheral examination and observation of vegetative
                          functions
                       B. Patient is PO: evaluation to include oral peripheral examination and
                          administration of various boluses (preferably at mealtime)
                    3. For further evaluations necessary for difficult cases:
                       A. A modified barium swallow videofluoroscopy of the oral cavity, pharynx,
                          and cervical esophagus will be ordered by the physician. MBS will be
                          scheduled by a speech-language pathologist and will be attended by the
                          swallowing team. The physician is required to complete a radiology
                          requisition. The requisition must accompany the patient's chart to the
                          study.
                       B. An ENT evaluation may be recommended to assess swallow function via
                          endoscopy.
                    4. Radiographic assessment: modified barium swallow
                       A. Purpose of the evaluation
                          (1) To measure the speed of the swallow
                          (2) To measure the efficiency of the swallow
                          (3) To define movement patterns of structures in oral cavity, pharynx,
                              and larynx
                          (4) To determine whether aspiration occurs and when, why, and how
                              often it occurs
                          (5) To evaluate the effectiveness of rehabilitation strategies (e.g., postures,
                              diet modifications, therapy strategies)

B. Required materials
    (1) Food consistencies
        a. Thin barium
        b. Thick barium
        c. Applesauce
        d. Cookie
        e. Other foods as warranted (present diet)
    (2) Equipment
        a. Spoon
        b. Measured cup
        c. Special implements (e.g., laryngeal mirror)
        d. Syringe to measure bolus amounts
C. Procedure
    (1) Patient seated upright: viewed laterally then A/P
    (2) Bolus presented—thin/thick barium depends on patient toleration: 1 ml, 3 ml, 5 ml, 10 ml, straw drinking, cup drinking, applesauce, cookie, other consistencies as tolerated
    (3) If patient aspirates after baseline study or appears to be functioning with an inefficient swallow, consider the following:
        a. Termination of study by the radiologist or team
        b. Selection of appropriate positioning
        c. Selection of appropriate compensatory strategies and evaluation effectiveness with video

5. After the study the dysphagia team may make mealtime management recommendations and monitor the patient's swallowing rehabilitation.

RESPONSIBILITY: Director of Speech Language Pathology and Occupational Therapy

REVIEW MONTH: April

Policy and Procedure Manual

TITLE: Dysphagia Diet Evaluation

POLICY: 1. A modified consistency diet for patients with oral-pharyngeal dysphagia will
                       be provided.
                    2. Before the initiation of the diet, a swallowing evaluation will be conducted by
                       the dysphagia therapist (i.e., occupational therapist) after physician referral.
                    3. Diet progresses from pureed to semisolid to solid.

PURPOSE: To provide foods and fluids modified in texture and consistency to reduce the
                    risk of aspiration

APPLICABILITY: Patients with swallowing disorders

PROCEDURE: 1. The clinical nutritionist will complete a nutritional assessment as identified in
                       the standard of nutrition care.
                    2. The clinical nutritionist will recommend (to the physician) the need for a
                       swallowing evaluation when indicated.
                    3. After physician referral the dysphagia therapist (i.e., occupational therapist)
                       will identify and assist in the therapeutic management of the patient and
                       assign an appropriate diet level.
                    4. The dysphagia therapist (i.e., occupational therapist) will also provide proper
                       instructions for eating and feeding techniques to the patient, family members,
                       and the nursing staff.
                    5. The clinical nutritionist will provide nutrition education to the patient and
                       family members.

RESPONSIBILITY: Clinical Nutrition Coordinator of the Departments of Food and Nutrition Services
                    Assistant Director of Occupational Therapy

REVIEW MONTH: March

REVIEWED BY: Patient Care Committee

MRN

NAME

D.O.B.   SEX

CONTINUATION SHEET

DYSPHAGIA TEAM SWALLOWING EVALUATION

Dx.
Reason for referral: _____

_____

Feeding History

Normal preexisting function?   No/Yes   Comments: _____
Has type of food changed?   No/Yes   Comments: _____
Has volume of food changed?   No/Yes   Comments: _____
Weight loss or gain?   No/Yes _____ lbs Comments: _____
  Comments: _____

Current Nutritional Status

Nutritional route: NPO   PO   NGT   PEG   TPN
Diet type: _____
Special dietary requirements: NCS   Low salt   Kosher   Other

Respiratory Status

Auscultation: Pooling?   No/Yes
Suctioning required?   No/Yes   Frequency: _____   Route: _____
Receiving chest physical therapy?   No/Yes
Tracheotomy?   No/Yes   Type: _____
Position of cuff: Inflated   Partially inflated   Deflated
Ventilator?   No/Yes   Cannnot be taken off   Weaning parameters
Previous history of aspiration pneumonia?   No/Yes
Adequate for feeding trial?   No/Yes

General Observations

Alertness: No deficit   Partial deficit   Mod-Sev deficit
Follows directions: Verbal/gestural   0 Step   1 Step   2 Steps   3 Steps
Recognizes swallowing problems: Good insight   Partial insight   No insight
Perceptual/cognitive deficits: None   Partial   Severe
Adequately expresses basic wants/needs: No deficit   Partial deficit   Severe deficit
Hearing deficits? No/Yes
  Comments: _____

Physical Status

Testing position: Bed   Chair
Assist needed to position: Independent   Min-Mod assist   Max assist
Head/neck control: WFL   Impaired
UE control for eating: WFL   Impaired   Nonfunctional

CLINICAL EVALUATION OF SWALLOWING

Observations

Drooling   Excessive oral secretions   Dry mouth
Poor oral hygiene   Residual food in oral cavity:
Food remnants on lips   Dentate   Tongue thrust
Oral-motor apraxia   Excessive coughing (>2×)   Hoarse/wet voice
Increased clearing of throat   Halitosis   Bites tongue/lips   Ropy secretions
Time since last oral feeding:

Oral Control (ROM, strength, sensation)

_____
_____
_____
_____

Primitive Reflexes

Present: Jaw jerk   Rooting/suck   Bite   Absent: _____

Pharyngeal Control

	Intact	Impaired	Absent	Comments
Soft palate function				
Vocal quality				
Gag reflex				
Volitional cough				
Spontaneous swallow				
Volitional swallow				
Laryngeal elevation				

ENT Evaluation   Done   Not Done   If done, results

Boluses used: _____
_____
_____
_____
_____
_____
_____
_____

Stages of Swallow

I. ORAL PREPARATORY STAGE

	Intact	Impaired	Absent	Comments
Orientation to bolus				
Mouth opening				
Bolus containment/lip closure				
Oral sensation for bolus				

II. ORAL STAGE

	Intact	Impaired	Absent	Comments
Bolus formation				
Mastication				
Bolus propulsion				
Buccal tension (pocketing)				
Oral transit time				

Pocketing?   No/Yes   Right/Left

III. PHARYNGEAL STAGE

	Intact	Impaired	Absent	Comments
Swallow reflex				
Laryngeal elevation				
Vocal quality after swallow				

Pooling with ausculation: No/Yes

General Observations

Complaint of food sticking in throat   No/Yes
Complaint of pain on swallow (odynophagia)   No/Yes
Multiple swallows   No/Yes (number _____)
Cough Reflex   No/Yes   If yes,   Before   During   After swallow
    Comments: _____
_____
_____
_____
_____
_____

IV. ESOPHAGEAL STAGE

Complaint of regurgitation   No/Yes
Complaint of pain on swallow (odynophagia)   No/Yes

Impressions _____
_____
_____
_____
_____
_____

Recommendations

Referrals: ENT   Videofluoroscopy/modifed barium swallow
              GI   Dental   Nutrition
Comments: _____

Nutritional Route

PO   Consider: NPO with alternative nutritional support if clinically indicated

Diet Type

Dysphagia diet stage I   Dysphagia diet stage II   Dysphagia diet stage III
Puree   Mechanical soft   Regular   Kosher   Other: _____

Prefeeding Program (Before commencing PO): _____
_____
_____
_____

Mealtime Management
Upright during and 45 minutes after meal
Compensatory strategies: Chin tuck
                                  Alternate solids/liquids
                                  Small bites/small sips
                                  Chin tuck swallow
                                  Turn head to _____ side
                                  Other: _____
Adaptive equipment: _____
Supervision: Constant   Intermittent   Set-up
  Dr. _____ contacted and nursing informed (re: swallowing evaluation findings
  and recomendations on _____).

_____ _____
                    Therapist's Signature   Date

DYSPHAGIA TEAM MODIFIED BARIUM SWALLOW: VIDEOFLUOROSCOPIC TEST RESULTS

Patient was seen on _____ for a modified barium swallow.
Dr. _____ present.
Patient was viewed in   lateral   anterior/posterior position.
Patient was presented with the following boluses: _____
_____
_____
_____

ORAL STAGE

	Intact	Impaired	Absent	Comments
Bolus formation				
Mastication				
Bolus propulsion				
Buccal tension (pocketing)				
Oral transit time				

Pocketing?   No/Yes   Right/Left

PHARYNGEAL STAGE

	Intact	Impaired	Absent	Comments
Swallow reflex				
Laryngeal elevation				

Pooling noted: None   Valleculae   Pyriform sinus
Patient cleared/did not clear residue with the following compensatory strategy:

The radiologist reported that aspiration did/did not occur.
Comments on anatomical structure: _____

Impressions
This patient appears to present with: _____

This patient does/does not appear to be at risk for aspiration with the following boluses: _____

Recommendation

1. Referrals
   a. ENT
   b GI
   c. Nutrition
2. Diet
   a. Consistency
   b. PO/NPO: consider alternative nutritional support
3. Dysphagia team goals
   a. Continued monitoring of status
   b. No further intervention
   c. Swallowing therapy/prefeeding program
   d. Diet modification
   e. Compensatory strategies
      (1) Chin tuck
      (2) Head tilt (left/right)
      (3) Head turn (left/right)
      (4) Multiple swallows
      (5) Alternate solid/liquid
      (6) Other: _____
4. Mealtime management
   a. Upright during and 45 minutes after meals
   b. No meds given with thin liquids
   c. Alternate solid/liquid
   d. Mouth cleaned of residue
   e. Small bites/small sips
   f. Reduced distractions
   g. Supervision during meals
   h. Other:_____
5. Reevaluation for possible upgraded consistency in _____ weeks.

Signature

MRN

NAME

D.O.B.   SEX

CONTINUATION SHEET

Patient name: _____

Date: _____

The following information is for patients and families/caregivers. If you have any questions or concerns, please contact _____.
(name, phone number)

1. Recommended diet consistency:
   A. Solids: Puree   Souflee   Soft   Regular
   B. Liquids: No thins   Thickened only   Honey   Nectar
   Comments: _____
   _____
   _____
   _____
   _____

2. Recommended mealtime management techniques: _____
   _____
   _____
   _____
   _____
   _____
   _____
   _____

3. The following may be symptoms of a swallowing problem and require attention:
   • Coughing/choking during or following eating/drinking
   • Pain in throat while eating
   • Wet, gurgly voice
   • c/o food stuck in throat
   • Refusal/hesitancy to eat certain food types previously enjoyed
   • Weight loss
   • Wet pillow or head on rising from bed
   • Food remaining in mouth
   • Frequent colds
   Additional comments: _____
   _____
   _____
   _____
   _____
   _____
   _____
   _____
   _____
   _____
   _____

CQI Monitor for Stroke: Shoulder Positioning

DEPARTMENT OF OCCUPATIONAL THERAPY
INPATIENT REHABILITATION CQI

TITLE: Shoulder Supports

DATE: To be initiated the week of _____

AREA: Applicable to patients with shoulder pain and those at risk for/presenting with shoulder subluxation

THERAPISTS: Supervisor and Assistant Supervisor of Inpatient Rehabilitation are responsible for this monitor.

ISSUE: Patients with an inferior subluxation will be provided with a support system to protect the shoulder from injury 24 hours per day deemphasing a sling position. The occupational therapist will attempt follow through with other team members to ensure consistency of this system.

RATIONALE: Patients with an inferior subluxation are at risk for injury to the unstable shoulder; therefore a system must be provided to protect the shoulder 24 hours per day without maintaining the upper extremity in a sling position (i.e., adduction, internal rotation, and elbow flexion) for prolonged periods. The position may lead to pain secondary to immobilization, increased edema, functional disuse, neglect, and shoulder-hand syndrome.

METHODS:
1. Four charts of patients who fit into above criteria will be reviewed by the Supervisor or Assistant Supervisor of Inpatient Rehabilitation on a monthly basis, utilizing the appropriate form.
2. Initial evaluation of upper extremity will be used to identify patients to be included.
3. The occupational therapist will document subluxation status, prescribed shoulder support (e.g., lapboard, saddle-sling, hemisling, bed positioning), and use of the support (i.e., wearing schedules).
4. The occupational therapist will schedule co-treatment with team members to ensure consistent use of support as well as provide written instructions as needed.
5. The occupational therapist will instruct the family about use of shoulder supports and document the meeting.
6. All data will be reported to the Director of Occupational Therapy on a monthly basis.

INDICATOR: Patients who have or are at risk for an inferior subluxation (i.e., have a weakened upper extremity and/or malaligned scapula) will be assessed for (and provided with if needed) a system to support the affected shoulder 24 hours per day. After prescription of supports, the occupational therapist will consult with involved departments (physical therapy and nursing) about use and wearing schedule of supports.

THRESHOLD: 100%

REVIEW OF OCCUPATIONAL THERAPY DOCUMENTATION

	YES	NO	N/A
(Initial Evaluation)			
1. Patient's subluxation status is documented in the initial evaluation by OT.			
2. OT will provide and document shoulder support for w/c (e.g., half lapboard, lap table, trough).			
3. OT will provide and document shoulder support for bed (e.g., pillows supporting scapula into protraction and elbow).			
4. Shoulder support is provided and documented by OT for transfers (e.g., hemisling, saddle-sling, or patient support with unaffected extremity).			
5. Shoulder support is provided and documented by OT (when applicable) for use during ambulation.			
6. OT will schedule and document co-treatments with Nursing to review wearing schedule and application of supports.			
7. OT will schedule and document co-treatment with PT to review support of shoulder during transfers and when applicable, during ambulation.			
8. OT will document that written instructions about wearing schedule of supports have been posted bedside.			
9. OT will train family members in the application, use, and wearing schedule of shoulder supports; this will be documented before D/C.			

SHOULDER PROTECTION

Patient Name:

In Bed:
1. Please remove sling.
2. Please place pillow under _____ shoulder blade and elbow while lying supine or on affected side.

Transfers/Ambulation/Toileting:
- Pouch sling to be worn   ☐
- Saddle sling to be worn   ☐

In Wheelchair:
1. Please remove sling (unless it is a saddle sling).
2. Support _____ arm on lapboard or pillow.

Questions?
Call _____
Ext. _____

CQI Monitor for Stroke:
Neurobehavioral/ADL Assessment

DEPARTMENT OF OCCUPATIONAL THERAPY
CQI

TITLE: Cognitive/Perceptual (Neurobehavioral) Evaluation via ADL

DATE: Review interval to be determined after first quarter

THERAPISTS: Supervisor/Seniors

ISSUE: Cognitive/perceptual (neurobehavioral) deficits have a direct impact on self-care and mobility tasks. Traditionally, cognitive/perceptual dysfunction has been evaluated separately from functional tasks. In addition, evaluation tools used by occupational therapists are poorly related to the principals of occupational therapy (i.e., based on functional performance). Literature does not support the correlation between pen-and-paper tasks and functional activities. The A-ONE was developed in an effort to combine the neurobehavioral literature with principles of occupational therapy to develop a theory that relates factors from these two sources.*

RATIONALE: Patients with vascular disorders, metabolic disorders, TBI, infections, toxins, brain tumors, and degeneration of the nervous system may have neurobehavioral deficits that interfere with self-care/mobility. It is crucial that OTs use an evaluation that will identify deficits and their effect on performance.

INDICATOR: Patients who have above diagnoses will be evaluated using the A-ONE for neurobehavioral deficits while performing self-care/mobility tasks. The therapist will document the relationship (or lack thereof) between neurobehavioral deficits and self-care and mobility tasks.

THRESHOLD: 80%

METHOD: Four charts that fit into the aforementioned categories will be screened monthly. Documentation will reflect that cognitive/perceptual deficits were evaluated via the A-ONE protocol. These deficits include motor/ideational apraxia, unilateral body neglect, spatial relations, unilateral spatial neglect, perseveration, and organization/sequencing.

*Árnadóttir G: *The brain and behavior: assessing cortical dysfunction through ADL,* St Louis, 1990, Mosby.

COGNITIVE/PERCEPTUAL EVALUATION VIA ADL

Patient Name _____   Reviewer _____

Dx. _____   Date of Eval. _____

Therapist _____   Review Date _____

Documentation included	Yes	No	N/A
Task(s) evaluated			
Neurobehavioral deficits noted/ not noted during task performed			
Amount and type of assist required to improve task performed			

Score: _____

Comments: _____
_____
_____
_____
_____
_____
_____
_____
_____
_____
_____
_____
_____
_____
_____
_____
_____
_____
_____
_____
_____
_____

Policies and Procedures for Reporting Incidents

Policy and Procedure Manual

TITLE:
Incident Reporting

POLICY:
All patient and visitor related incidents will be reported to risk management department in writing.

PURPOSE:
To provide a means to evaluate (and prevent) patient and visitor incidents and to ensure compliance with state laws and regulatory bodies

PROCEDURE:
1. All patient and visitor related incidents should be reported in writing using Incident Report form.
2. Before completing form, employee should discuss incident with supervisor or director.
3. An objective description of incident should be recorded in medical record. Before documentation, discuss with supervisor or director and risk management if indicated.
4. After completing form, original portion should be detached and forwarded to the risk management department within 24 hours.
5. Copy of report should be forwarded to Director of Occupational Therapy within 24 hours.

RESPONSIBILITY:
Director of Occupational Therapy

REVIEW MONTH:
February

Index

f indicates illustrations; *t* indicates tables; *b* indicates boxes.

Drug	Use	Dosage	Route	Side effects	Other medical issues
Neurourologics					
Baclofen (Lioresal)	Skeletal muscle relaxant, treatment for detrusor dyssynergia	5-20 mg tid-qid	PO	Drowsiness, confusion, headache, nausea and vomiting, constipation	Has observable effects only in very high doses
Bethanechol (Urecholine)	Cholinomimetic, treatment for enhancing detrusor contractions	10-50 mg tid-qid	PO	Nausea and vomiting, dry mouth, lethargy, constipation, urinary retention	—
Dantrolene (Dantrium)	Skeletal muscle relaxant, treatment for better bladder emptying in detrusor external sphincter dyssynergia	25 mg qd-100 mg qid	PO, IV	Drowsiness, dizziness, headache, diarrhea, hepatitis, seizure	—
Dicyclomine (Bentyl)	Anticholinergic, treatment for detrusor external sphincter dyssynergia	20-40 mg qid	PO, IV	Nausea and vomiting, dry mouth, lethargy, constipation, dyspnea	—
Ephedrine	Treatment for stress incontinence in female patients	—	PO	Nausea and vomiting, dry mouth, lethargy, constipation	—
Hyoscyamine (Levsin)	Anticholinergic, detrusor antispasmodic	0.125-0.25 mg qid	PO, IV, SL, IM	Nausea and vomiting, dry mouth, lethargy, constipation, urinary retention	May be better tolerated than oxybutynin
Imipramine (Tofranil)	Treatment for increasing outlet resistance and decreasing detrusor strength	75-150 mg qd	PO	Orthostasis, heart block, nausea and vomiting, anxiety, confusion, ataxia, dry mouth	—
Oxybutynin (Ditropan)	Detrusor antispasmodic, treatment for detrusor external sphincter dyssynergia	5 mg bid-tid	PO	Nausea and vomiting, dry mouth, lethargy, constipation	—
Phenoxybenzamine (Dibenzyline)	α-Blocker, treatment for decreasing outlet resistance	10 mg bid	PO	Orthostasis, tachycardia, drowsiness, fatigue	—
Prazosin (Minipress)	α-Blocker, treatment for decreasing outlet resistance and detrusor external sphincter dyssynergia	1 mg bid-tid	PO	Syncope, sedation, headache, urinary retention	—
Anticoagulants					
Acetylsalicylic acid, i.e., aspirin	Treatment for permanently acetylating platelets to stop thrombosis	50-325 mg qd	PO	Gastric ulcer, bleeding	—
Heparin	DVT prophylactic, treatment for stroke prevention and PVD	5000 U subcutaneously q12h or titrated IV dose	Subcutaneous, IV	Increased bleeding, hematomas, GI bleeding	—
Ticlopidine (Ticlid)	Treatment for stroke prevention	250 mg bid	PO	Diarrhea, nausea and vomiting, neutropenia, thrombocytopenia, bleeding	—
Warfarin (Coumadin)	DVT prophylaxis, treatment for stroke prevention and PVD	Titrate to prothrombin time	PO	Increased bleeding, hematomas, GI bleeding	—